ANNALS OF THE NEW YORK ACADEMY OF SCIENCES
Volume 621

PHYSIOLOGICAL SENESCENCE AND ITS POSTPONEMENT: THEORETICAL APPROACHES AND RATIONAL INTERVENTIONS

Second Stromboli Conference on Aging and Cancer

Edited by Walter Pierpaoli and Nicola Fabris

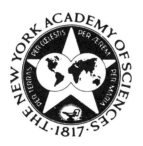

The New York Academy of Sciences
New York, New York
1991

Cover (paper edition): *Snail and turtle emblem of the conference by Paolo Carosone. The snail (Greek, strongylos) refers to the ancient names both of the still active Stromboli volcano and of the spiral of the amnion, two symbols of regeneration. The long-lived turtle with a man-made mechanism connects the prolongation of life with research through introspection, analysis, and technology.*

Library of Congress Cataloging-in-Publication Data

Stromboli Conference on Aging and Cancer (2nd : 1990)
    Physiological senescence and its postponement : theoretical
approaches and rational interventions / Second Stromboli Conference
on Aging and Cancer ; edited by Walter Pierpaoli and Nicola Fabris.
    p. cm. -- (Annals of the New York Academy of Sciences, ISSN
0077-8923 ; v. 621)
    Conference held in Stromboli, Sicily, Italy on May 28–June 1,
1990.
    Includes bibliographical references.
    Includes index.
    ISBN 0-89766-651-8 (cloth : alk. paper). -- ISBN 0-89766-652-6
(paper : alk. paper)
    1. Longevity—Congresses. 2. Aging—Molecular aspects—
Congresses. I. Pierpaoli, Walter. II. Fabris, N. III. Title.
IV. Series.
    [DNLM: 1. Aging—physiology—congresses. 2. Diet—congresses.
3. Endocrine Glands—physiology—congresses. 4. Immunity—in old
age—congresses. 5. Neoplasms—immunology—congresses. W1 AN626YL
v. 621 / WT 104 S921p 1990]
Q11.N5 vol. 621
[QP85]
500 s—dc20
[612.6'8]
DNLM/DLC
for Library of Congress   90-13765
                                                               CIP

                              BiC/PCP
               Printed in the United States of America
                  ISBN 0-89766-651-8 (cloth)
                  ISBN 0-89766-652-6 (paper)
                     ISSN 0077-8923

ANNALS OF THE NEW YORK ACADEMY OF SCIENCES

Volume 621
July 1, 1991

PHYSIOLOGICAL SENESCENCE AND ITS POSTPONEMENT: THEORETICAL APPROACHES AND RATIONAL INTERVENTIONS

Second Stromboli Conference on Aging and Cancer[a]

Editors and Conference Organizers
WALTER PIERPAOLI AND NICOLA FABRIS

CONTENTS

[a] The papers in this volume were presented at a conference entitled Physiological Senescence and Its Postponement: Theoretical Approaches and Rational Interventions; Second Stromboli Conference on Aging and Cancer, which was held in Stromboli, Sicily, Italy on May 28–June 1, 1990.

Part II. Nervous System Plasticity

Part III. Neuroendocrine-Immune Interactions

Part IV. Neuroendocrine-Immune Interactions: Metabolic Aspects

Major funding for this conference was provided by:
  • SIGMA-TAU, INSTITUTE OF RESEARCH ON SENESCENCE

Other financial assistance was received from:
  • THE GLENN FOUNDATION FOR MEDICAL RESEARCH
  • INSTITUT MERIEUX
  • ITALIAN NATIONAL RESEARCH CENTERS ON AGING (INRCA)
  • THE NEW YORK ACADEMY OF SCIENCES

Welcoming Remarks

Dear friends and colleagues,

It has now been three years since we met here to attend the First Stromboli Conference on Aging and Cancer. That conference was really a dive into the mouth of the Volcano, a jump into the unknown, a daring enterprise. Fortunately, all predictable and unpredictable factors contributed to its success: we were supported by the NATO contribution and INRCA's generous help *via* Nicola Fabris; the weather and the sea were sympathetic; "spirits" were high; science and scientists were superb; and even the moon participated in the gala evening by showing its full face. What more? We owe much of the conference's success to the silent, exquisite, and liberal hospitality of the Russo family at the Sirenetta, which is impossible to appreciate fully without realizing the difficulty of maintaining a hotel of the standard of the Sirenetta in a small southern-Italian island like Stromboli, where small problems often become insurmountable hurdles. Everybody was cooperative and immediately felt the strong positive influence of Aeolian Nature, an all-pervasive feeling.

We believe in the power of a harmonic combination of ideas and "hard facts." Natural truth does not allow a dissociation of this combination. In our case, the scientific facts combined perfectly with the ideas, and creative science emerged. This was clearly visible in the welcome given to the proceedings (*Annals* Vol. 521) and in the immediate and later reactions to them of all the participants.

I must admit that we did not harbor any exaggerated expectations; and as a result everybody was relaxed, not feeling nervously obliged to impress the small audience. Epictetus was our teacher and the presence of the Volcano made us shy and respectful.

With the enthusiastic approval of Novera Spector, I dedicated the First Stromboli Conference to Ashley Montagu, who is a living example of the validity of the concept of neoteny. This great anthropologist and humanist has so wonderfully developed the concept of neoteny of man. In his masterpiece *Growing Young,* he succeeded in destroying those devilish, gerontomorphic, necrophilic, and self-punishing theories of life, growth, and aging, which, for centuries, have deceived billions of men and deprived them of the joy of living, hope, faith, and the expectation of the natural maintenance of a youthful mind till very old age.

We invited Ashley Montagu to this meeting. He is well at 85 and, in his own words, "still dancing." He could not come owing to previous commitments, but sent us a message. We expect to see him at the '93 conference and later on. His splendid message is a real "gem" and could not be more appropriate for our present conference.

> Some day after
> Mastering the wind,
> The waves, the tides
> And gravity,
> We shall harness
> The energies of love.
> And then, for
> The second time
> In the history
> Of the world—
> We will have
> Discovered *fire.*

What is *fire?* I think fire is the creative force of Nature, the living fire of the Volcano, the primeval element on this planet, which may inspire us and light a fire in our soul and mind, while we are here and after we depart for home.

There are now so many distinguished guests and experts on aging here, including a key figure missing from our first conference, Vladimir Dilman, for whom I should compose another special speech. He does not need it. . . .

I would like to dedicate this Second Stromboli Conference to a person who also represents a living denial of senescence in his body and spirit, namely, Novera Herbert Spector. My only hesitation in doing this is based on the consideration that it may still be too early to dedicate to him a conference on aging. However, I originally thought of Novera Spector, because he and another living representative of neoteny, Branislav Janković, represent a rare breed of person with inexaustible inner fire. Novera Spector being a master of life, time, and love, I find it appropriate to mention here an aphorism which I wish to dedicate to him:

Life is the art of dosage of time and distribution of love.

I shall conclude by thanking our main sponsor, Dr. Claudio Cavazza, president of the Italian company SIGMA-TAU, Rome, for their financial contribution and their interest in research on aging, which made this conference possible. Also let us thank the New York Academy of Sciences for their generous contribution and for their editorial expertise in preparing the proceedings of this meeting for publication.

Finally, I wish that we could acquire here the ability to interpret the natural processes of aging to the extent that the progressive deterioration of the "aging clock" could really be postponed, if not avoided. This will certainly soon become a reality, because what is good for a mouse may also be good for a man. Death may not be awful if we can adjust the "clock" to its maximum expectancy and thus live long enough to accept death as a well-deserved rest after a joyful and intense life deprived of some of its presently inevitable sorrows, pains, and toils.

Therefore, good luck, and let us grow young together. . . .

Walter Pierpaoli

Human Longevity and Aging: Possible Role of Reactive Oxygen Species

RICHARD G. CUTLER

Gerontology Research Center
National Institute on Aging
4940 Eastern Avenue
Baltimore, Maryland 21224

INTRODUCTION

The number of elderly people in the developed nations of the world is growing at an ever increasing rate. This is evident both in absolute number as well as percentage with reference to total population. The major concern, however, appears to be the negative economic impact such a change in population composition would have on a country. This is because of the steadily increasing cost of medical care of an aging population, particularly for those individuals over 80 years of age, which is the most rapidly growing fraction. There is consequently much interest in gerontology and in exploring a wide range of strategies that might be effective in reducing the cost of a growing aged population.[1,2]

Although the economic burden of the elderly population is clearly evident and is usually most emphasized when discussing the subject of aging and geriatric medicine, I would like to point out that an often overlooked and perhaps even greater cost to society of human aging is the steady decline in many physiological and mental processes that appear to occur shortly after the age of 30 years in the apparent absence of major disease or expensive medical care needs. In this regard, a decrease of productivity and creativity may occur in most people over the some 30 to 40 years of steadily declining health over the normal human life span. We often forget that aging occurs in most individuals without the necessary accompaniment of serious disease, which usually comes much later in life. Thus, the economic as well as the humanist benefits in reducing aging rate may go far beyond the predicted savings in medical cost of just the elderly population.[3]

In this light, a long-term goal in biogerontology should not only be to reduce the medical costs of the growing elderly population but also to increase the healthy and productive years at all ages of our life span.[3] In this regard, we frequently hear from medically-oriented gerontologists that they seek to add "more life to our years and not more years to our life." I would only partially agree with this statement and believe our goal should be more ambitious. That is, to not only add more life to our years but also more years to our life. Indeed, it is probably impossible to simply add more life to our years without also adding more years to our life. It is likely to become more evident in the near future that the only long-term satisfactory method of reducing the medical costs of the elderly will be through a direct intervention of the aging process itself. That is, the development of intervention methods aimed more directly towards treatment of the causes of aging and not simply the effects of aging, as has been the traditional medical approach in the past.

This goal of reducing the overall aging rate in humans runs immediately into the problem of the vast complexity of normal human biology and what little

1

knowledge we presently have in this area of science. In fact, it is usually argued that the mechanisms, whatever they might be, that cause aging are likely to be so complex that we can only hope to begin to understand how to control aging rate after much more is learned of normal biology. Another negative argument is that aging is likely to have many complex and multiple causes and so it is foolish to believe that relatively few genetic or biochemical means of intervention would be effective or could have any significant impact on decreasing human aging rate.

This all may be true, but the arguments given are not too convincing. The fact is that the problem of the complexity of the aging process and of the possibility of developing intervention strategies to increase the healthy years of life span and productivity by reducing human aging rate has simply not received serious scientific attention or evaluation. My objective in this paper is to briefly present an alternative argument indicating that, in spite of the vast complexity of aging, the processes governing aging rate or life span may be much less complex and therefore more subject to intervention in the near future.

The basis of this prediction comes largely from evolutionary and comparative studies of mammalian species closely related to one another biologically and evolutionarily but having substantial differences in their life span and aging rate. These studies led to the formulation of the 'longevity determinant gene hypothesis'[4-7] which predicts that aging is a result of normal biological processes necessary for life but also having long-term negative or aging effects on the organism. These normal biological processes have been divided into two major categories: (a) developmentally-linked biosenescent processes and (b) the continually-acting biosenescent processes. According to this hypothesis, longevity of a species is related to how efficiently the aging effects of these common developmental and metabolic processes they all share have been reduced.

I shall not deal with the processes in the first category but shall note that they include many of the hormones associated with development. For example, most pituitary, thyroid, adrenocorticoid, ovarian and testicular hormones have been found to have long-term aging effects.[8,8a] An important exception may be growth hormone, which does appear to have many rejuvenative effects when administered to old experimental animals.[8] However, long-term studies of growth hormone administration have not yet been conducted to determine possible side effects or degree of life span extension, if any.[9]

Our research has focused on the second category, the continuously-acting biosenescent processes, in testing the longevity determinant gene hypothesis. Here, we have examined the possible aging effects of oxygen metabolism, which is essential for life but is also known to produce what are called 'reactive oxygen species' during normal energy production. Such reactive oxygen species can interact with the cell's genetic apparatus and alter its proper state of differentiation. These changes in differentiation, as they have been predicted to occur during normal aging, have been called dysdifferentiation and could explain many aspects of the normal aging process.

The unique feature of the longevity determinant gene hypothesis is that it suggests that all animal species share common aging causes and common mechanisms of regulating aging rate. Although the processes causing aging may be very complex, it is predicted that less complex key antiaging processes exist that govern aging rate or life span.[4,5,10] For example, human and chimpanzee are closely related to one another, both evolutionarily (about 3–5 million years from a common ancestor) and biologically (DNA sequences are about 98% common).[10a] Because of the remarkable biological similarities between human and chimpanzee, we would expect the aging processes to be also similar qualitatively and, as far as we know, they are. Yet, in spite of these remarkable biological similarities, the chimpanzee has a life span about one half that of human (50 yrs vs 100 yrs) and accordingly appears to age about twice as fast in all biological aspects and exhibits the same age-dependent diseases but occurring in half the time.

So the central question we ask is what is so unique about human biology as compared to the chimpanzee or other shorter-lived animals that allows human to be so long-lived? Because of the strikingly similar biology between human and chimpanzee as well as their close evolutionary relation to one another, it is reasonable to predict that the genetic and biochemical differences governing their life span differences are also not likely to be very great. Thus, we ask, how complex biologically speaking are the processes governing human aging rate? And is it possible from a comparative biological study of animal species closely related to human, but having different life spans, to learn of new mechanisms of how to further enhance human health, vigor and productivity for longer periods of time? According to this approach, we should place equal effort on understanding the mechanisms governing aging rate and health maintenance as well as on understanding the mechanisms causing aging and disease.

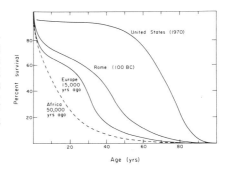

FIGURE 1. Percent survival curve for humans under different environmental hazard conditions. Note different 50% mean values but constant maximum life span potential (MLSP) values of about 100 yrs. Data taken in part from Comfort,[11] Acsádi and Nemereskéri,[12] and Strehler.[13] (From Cutler.[7] Reprinted by permission from Plenum Press.)

Biological Nature of Human Aging and Longevity

Human life expectancy (average survival time) for most of the time *Homo sapiens* has been on this earth ($\approx 100,000$ yrs) is generally believed to have been about 20 to 30 years[11,12,13] (FIG. 1). Only recently over the last 400 years or so in developed nations has life span expectancy increased, and this increase has been rather dramatic (about 40 to 50 years).[12] The reasons causing this increase certainly include reducing infant mortality and environmental hazards, accompanied by better nutrition and healthcare, but these traditional explanations may not be the complete answer.[14] The important point to be made here, however, is that in primitive cultures where life expectancy was about 30 years, few people lived long enough to suffer appreciably from the processes of senescence or aging. Death was almost entirely due to environmental hazards and infectious diseases not aging. Today in developed countries, although people have life expectancies in the range of 70 to 80 years, they are not living younger longer but are instead actually living older longer. Now most people die of problems largely related to the processes of aging and not to environmental hazards. This is because the increased life expectancy occurred with aging rate remaining essentially unchanged. Thus, the increase of life expectancy did not occur as a result of slowing down normal aging processes but instead by reducing the major external environmental hazards to life. This means that the present day problem of an older population in developed nations is actually an artifact of our civilization and not a natural state of human populations.

Some theoretical models of aging predict that normal human aging would result in a steady decline in functional capacity of essentially every physiological and mental process, beginning shortly after the age of sexual maturation[11,15,16,17] (FIG. 2). If this is true, then the slope of the decrease in maximum capacity to function with age could be taken to generally reflect an average or overall aging rate of the body. A fundamental question of biological research in gerontology today is to understand the molecular and biochemical mechanisms leading to this age-dependent decrease in function. What is unique in our laboratory research program is that we have also asked what determines the slope or rate of loss of these physiological functions.

With increasing age there also occurs an increased incidence of disease, which finally results in the death of the individual. An example of such a disease is cancer, which is shown in FIG. 3, indicating the well-known age-dependent increased incidence of cancer.[15] Since we do not yet understand even one mechanism causing aging, it is of course difficult to clearly define what aging actually is, and as a result there is some confusion in separating decline in physiological function as being due to a primary aging process or due to disease both related to and not related to primary aging processes. That is, many diseases could be a result of aging or even a direct manifestation of aging or not related to aging at all but simply related to chronological age. To illustrate this, there is some evidence indicating that the causes of aging and cancer are similar, being based on genetic instability mechanisms. On the other hand, there is much evidence indicating that causes of cardiovascular disease are related to nutrition, which may have little effect in accelerating aging rate. There is also likely to be a positive feedback interaction between aging and diseases of aging, and so both phenomena are likely

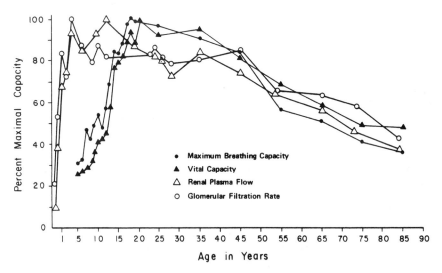

FIGURE 2. Change in organ function with age. (From Bafitis & Sargent.[17] Reprinted by permission from the *Journal of Gerontology.*)

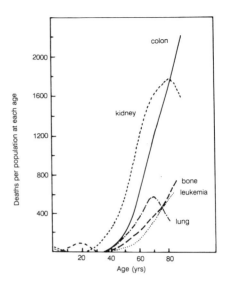

FIGURE 3. Age-specific death rates from several neoplasms: colon, lung, and leukemia per 10^6 people and for bone and kidney per 10^7 people. (Taken in part from Kohn.[15])

to play an important role in determining the overall health status of individuals as they grow older.

It is also expected theoretically that there should be great uniformity in both the qualitative and quantitative nature of aging between different individuals and in the biological functions that are affected. With increasing age, essentially all body functions in every person are found to decline uniformly with increasing chronological age. Persons that are unusually long lived and are able to live past 100 years do so not apparently because they age more slowly but instead because they age more uniformly. That is, they appear not to suffer from any particular weak link in their body functions such as from heart disease or diabetes.[15,15a] In addition, the well-known rectangularization of the human survival curve over the past 400 years or so in developed countries is the result of reducing the random components of survival, leaving largely the nonrandom factor. These nonrandom factors are thought to consist essentially of aging processes.

If found to be correct, such information could be important in the development of effective means to increase the healthy years of life span, as is illustrated in TABLE 1. In this table, the theoretical point is made that, even if the major diseases causing death today could somehow be completely eliminated, the impact on increased life expectancy over the entire country is not nearly so great as one might believe. For example, elimination of all cancer results in an increase of only about 2 years of life expectancy. The reason for this result may be that most people suffering from the major killer diseases today are 65 years of age or older. Thus, the removal of a major disease causing death of the elderly would simply result in uncovering a new disease or health problem since essentially every aspect of body function is being reduced through the aging process.

Such studies indicate that significant increase in the healthy years of life span of the general population of a nation is only likely to be achieved by actually reducing uniformly the rate of aging of the entire body, not by a piecemeal approach of reducing or eliminating specific disease processes.[15b] Thus, efforts being made in the field of cancer or even Alzheimer's disease may not achieve dramatic reduction in medical costs if effective therapy simply uncovers new disease processes characteristic of all people as they grow older.

TABLE 1. Gain in Expectancy of Life at Birth and at Age 65 Due to Elimination of Various Causes of Death[a]

Cause of Death	Gain in Expectancy of Life (Yrs) if Cause Was Eliminated	
	at Birth	at Age 65
Major cardiovascular-renal	10.9	10.0
Heart disease	5.9	4.9
Vascular diseases affecting central nervous system	1.3	1.2
Malignant neoplasms	2.3	1.2
Accidents other than by motor vehicle	0.6	0.1
Motor vehicle accidents	0.6	0.1
Influenza and pneumonia	0.5	0.2
Infectious diseases (excluding tuberculosis)	0.2	0.1
Diabetes mellitus	0.2	0.2
Tuberculosis	0.1	0.0

[a] From life tables published by the National Center of Health Statistics.[18]

The Longevity Determinant Gene Hypothesis

If significant gain to reduce the high costs of human aging to society does indeed require a uniform reduction in human aging rate, then how might this objective be achieved? To begin with, it is first necessary to estimate how complex the problem is that needs to be solved. That is, in-depth studies are seriously needed, for example, to determine the processes governing aging rate and how many genes might be involved. There is unfortunately very little data in this area but a few studies based on an evolutionary comparison of species closely related to one another but having differences in aging rate have suggested that key longevity determinant processes may exist.[5]

The basis of such studies is the fact that different mammalian species do indeed have different aging rates and that they age qualitatively in a similar way (TABLE 2). In addition, estimates have been made as to how fast life span has

TABLE 2. Most Confident Relative Maximum Life Span Potential and Life Span Energy Potential Estimates for Primates[a]

Species (Common Name)	MLSP (Yrs)	LEP (kcal/g)
Human	100	850
Great apes: chimp, orangutan, gorilla	50	450
Macaca, baboon	40	500
Capuchin	40	800
Marmoset, tamarin, squirrel monkey	20	600
Tree shrew	15	500

[a] Rounded-off estimates of MLSP and LEP, showing relative MLSP and LEP values for species where this data is most reliable. There appears to be a 5-fold difference in MLSP and a 2-fold difference in LEP among the primate species.

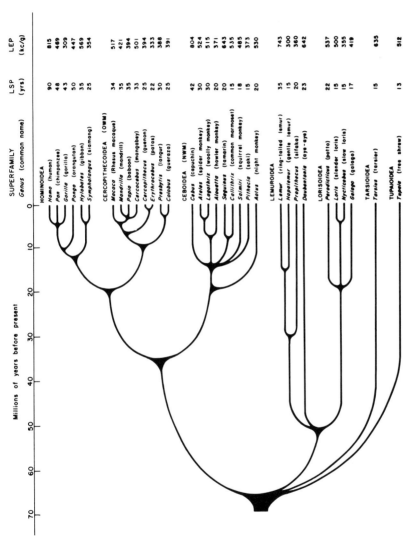

FIGURE 4. Phylogenetic relationship of MLSP and life span energy potential (LEP) estimates for the primate species. Data represent estimates taken from literature values for MLSP and specific metabolic rate (SMR). (From Cutler.[19] Reprinted by permission from the American Physiological Society.)

evolved along the hominid ancestral-descendant sequence leading to the *Homo sapiens* species.[19a,5] In these studies life span was found to increase at a maximum rate of about 14 years per 100,000 years about 100,000 years ago[5] (FIGS. 4–6). Such a high rate suggests that alterations in gene sequence are not likely to be involved in this rapid evolution of life span. Instead, these data are more consistent with the concept that changes in gene regulatory processes occurred during hominid evolution, resulting in a uniform decrease in aging rate.[5,10]

These evolutionary comparative studies have led to the proposal that key longevity determinant genes of a regulatory nature might exist that are capable of governing the aging rate of the entire organism. This concept is in contrast to what has been generally believed,[19b] where aging is thought to be a result of biological

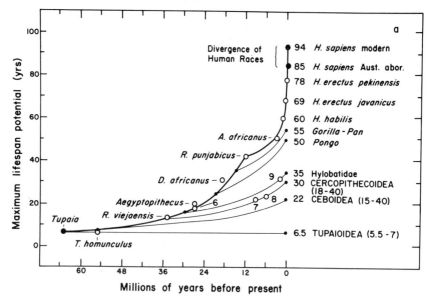

FIGURE 5. Evolution of maximum life span potential for the Anthropoidea. ○, fossil data; ●, living species. (From Cutler.[5] Reprinted by permission from the *Journal of Human Evolution*.)

functions at least as equally complex as the organism itself and that life span or aging rate is determined not by key longevity determinant genes but by thousands of genes operating by highly complex mechanisms unique for each cell and/or tissue of the organism.

Another deduction of the longevity determinant gene hypothesis is that aging is not genetically programmed for some evolutionary survival benefit but instead is the result of normal biological processes essential for life to exist.[19c] TABLE 3 shows the major classes of normal metabolic processes thought to be important as primary causes of aging. Since all mammalian species have remarkably similar biological processes (particularly chimpanzee and human), the question then arises of what normal biological processes are most responsible for causing aging

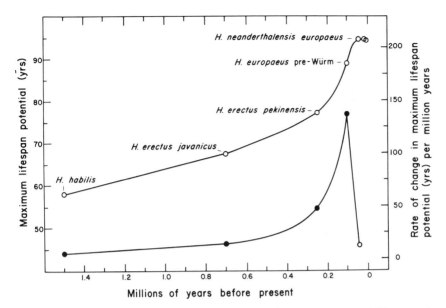

FIGURE 6. Rate of increase in maximum life span potential along the hominid ancestral-descendant sequence leading to modern man. ○, MLSP; ●, rate of change in MLSP per million years. (From Cutler.[5] Reprinted by permission from the *Journal of Human Evolution*.)

and what key mechanisms evolved to control the rate of their expression and consequently the longevity of the organism?

To answer this question, we began a comparison of human biology with that of other closely related species as a function of their life span with the hope of discovering small differences that could help explain why humans are so long-lived. One such comparative study is shown in FIG. 7, showing a plot of life span vs specific metabolic rate. These data suggest that aging rate of different species may be related to their metabolic rate.[20] Thus, it appears that by-products of oxygen metabolism may have a role in causing aging.[20a] This figure also indicates that most animals consume a constant amount of energy over their life span but that humans are exceptional in consuming about four times the energy over their life span. Thus, we humans are already exceptional in not only having more years of life but also in getting more life out of our years as compared to other mammalian species.

TABLE 3. Possible Sources of Products Contributing to the Age-Dependent Destabilization of the Proper Differentiated State of Cells

Basic concept: Aging is a result of normal developmental and metabolic processes:
1. By-products of development (growth and sexual hormones)
2. By-products of stress (adrenocorticoids)
3. By-products of metabolism (oxygen metabolism)

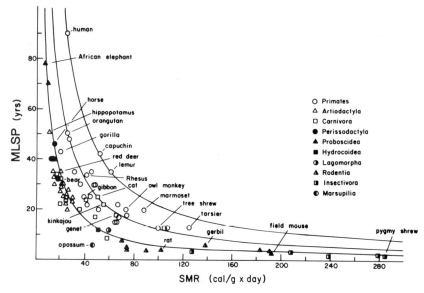

FIGURE 7. Life span energy potential of mammalian species. Data are based on specific metabolic rate (cal/g/day) and life span (yrs) where 90% mortality occurs (LS-90) taken from previously published data. Plots indicate three major classes of life span energy potentials (LEP). (From Cutler.[20] Reprinted by permission from *Gerontology.*)

Oxidative Stress as a Primary Aging Process

It is well known now that utilization of oxygen represents an efficient mechanism for aerobic organisms to generate energy but, during this process, by-products called reactive oxygen species are also created that could damage a cell.[20b] Indeed, all aerobic organisms require a vast complex network of defense mecha-

TABLE 4. Some Endogenous Biological Systems That Generate the Superoxide Radical O_2^-

1. Enzymes:
      Tryptophan dioxygenase
      Intoleamine dioxygenase
      Xanthine oxidase
      Cytochrome P-450
      Peroxidase (*e.g.,* during NADP oxidation)
      Aldehyde oxidase
2. Small molecules:
      Reduced riboflavin, $FMNH_2$, $FADH_2$
      Diphenols (*e.g.,* adrenalin)
      Melanin
      Thiols
3. Cellular organelles:
      Mitochondrial electron transport chain
      Microsomal electron transport chain
         (*e.g.,* P-450 detoxification system)

TABLE 5. Some Antioxidant Defense Mechanisms That May Be Longevity Determinants

1. Nonenzymatic:
   Alpha-tocopherol (membrane-bound)
   Ascorbate (water-soluble)
   Beta-carotene (singlet oxygen quencher)
   Urate (singlet oxygen quencher)
   Ceruloplasmin (plasma protein)
   Ubiquinol-10 (membrane-bound)
   Bilirubin (albumin-bound fatty acids)
   Ergothioneine (muscle tissue)
2. Enzymatic:
   Superoxide dismutase (Cu/Zn and Mn types)
   Glutathione peroxidase (Se and non-Se types)
   Catalase (peroxisomal matrix)
3. Auxillary enzymes:
   NADPH-quinone oxidoreductase (two-electron reduction)
   Epoxide hydrolase (two-electron reduction)
   UDP-glucoronyltransferase (conjugation enzyme)
   Sulfotransferase (conjugation enzyme)
   GSH S-transferase (conjugation enzyme)
   GSSG reductase
   Glucose-6-phosphate dehydrogenase (NADPH supply)
   GSSG export enzymes

nisms to reduce the toxic effects of these by-products of oxidative energy metabolism.[20b] There are many other sources of reactive oxygen species in addition to energy metabolism (TABLE 4), and already a number of defense mechanisms have been identified (TABLE 5). Some strategies that could be used to reduce the oxidative stress state of a cell and/or organism to increase life span are shown in TABLE 6.

Many different diseases, some related to aging, appear to be reduced by dietary antioxidant levels, indicating the biological significance of antioxidants in governing the rate of disease incidence (TABLE 7). There are also data not widely known indicating that the onset frequency of cancer incidence leading to death appears to be related to the aging rate of a species.[20c,20d,21] These data imply that not only does cancer incidence increase exponentially with chronological age but

TABLE 6. Different Strategies to Lower the Toxic Effects of Active Oxygen Species

1. Lower average rate of total body oxygen utilization. Increase body size, lower body temperature, torpor, sleep, hibernation.
2. Increase tissue concentration of antioxidants (superoxide dismutase, alpha tocopherol, carotenoids, urate, ceruloplasmin).
3. Decrease tissue concentration of some antioxidants that may have prooxidant properties (ascorbate, glutathione, catalase (Fe^{++}).
4. Decrease in the intensity of metabolic reactions that produce active oxygen species (cytochrome P-450/NADPH detoxification reaction).
5. Increase intrinsic resistance of cellular constituents to damage and peroxidation by active oxygen species (lowering the peroxidative potential of membranes by possible decrease in percent unsaturated fatty acids).

TABLE 7. Chronic Diseases Found to be Related to Deficiencies in Dietary Antioxidants[30a]

1. Cardiovascular disease
2. Myocardial ischemia/reperfusion injury
3. Cataracts
4. Rheumatoid arthritis
5. Exercise-induced hypoxia reperfusion injury of joints
6. Parkinson's disease
7. Alzheimer's disease
8. Cancer (lung, esophagus, gastric/colon, cervical dysplasia)

that the rate of increased incidence is also related to the aging rate of the species[19] (FIG. 8). This important result suggests that whatever mechanism protects human from cancer so efficiently as compared to other species may also be the same one responsible for the slow human aging rate.[21]

Much evidence indicates that cancer is caused by genetic alterations, resulting in an improper differentiated cell. Such genetic alterations could be caused by

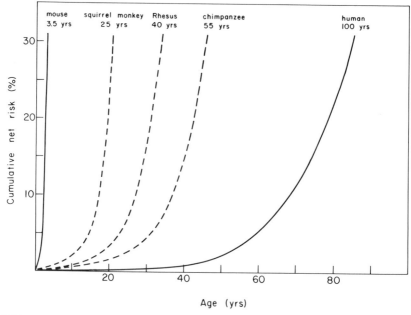

FIGURE 8. Cumulative net risk of death from cancer as a function of age and maximum life span potential. This family of curves represents typical data describing the onset frequency of all types of cancer with age in different mammalian species. The data are plotted as probability being proportional to age.[4] Curves for mouse and human are most reliable (*solid curves*) based on the species' life span and data indicating relative rank order of longer-lived mammals having less cancer incidence with age. (From Cutler and Semsei.[21] Reprinted by permission from the *Journal of Gerontology.*)

TABLE 8. Evidence for the Importance of Oxygen Radicals in Genetic Damage, Disease, and Cancer

---

1. Dietary carcinogens and anticarcinogens, oxyradicals, and degenerative diseases
   Many mutagens and carcinogens act through generation of oxygen radicals.
   Oxygen radicals also play a major role as endogenous initiators of degenerative diseases (cancer, heart disease) through DNA damage, mutation, and promotion effects.
   B. N. Ames, Science **221:** 1256, 1983.[22]
2. Prooxidant state and tumor promotion
   There is convincing evidence that active oxygen, peroxides and radicals can promote or initiate cells to neoplastic growth.
   Prooxidant state can be caused by xenobiotics, metabolites, inhibitors of antioxidant state, and membrane-active agents.
   P. A. Cerutti, Science **227:** 375, 1985.[23]

---

reactive oxygen species[22,23] (TABLE 8). Thus, a common mechanism which could cause both cancer and aging is reactive oxygen species causing a genetic instability. Such an idea is consistent with the dysdifferentiation hypothesis of aging, where aging is predicted to be a result of cells drifting slowly away from their proper state of differentiation.[24] There is considerable evidence supporting dysdifferentiation as a primary cause of aging[25] (TABLE 9) and of reactive oxygen species to be a primary cause of aging (TABLE 10). Taking these data together provides more support that aging may be a result of genetic instability leading to dysdifferentiated cells, which finally causes a decline in physiological function and an increase in disease frequency.

An important aspect of this hypothesis is that it predicts that life span is a result of factors acting to stabilize the proper differentiated state of cells. That is, with human being the longest-lived mammalian species, this hypothesis would predict that human cells should be the most stable in maintaining their proper state of differentiation. If this is true, then it would be important to know what mechanism acts to stabilize states of differentiation. Essentially nothing is known of such mechanisms acting to stabilize the proper differentiated state of cells once the genetic program of development has been completed. Thus, in light of the longevity determinant hypothesis, this area of research should certainly receive increased attention. If reactive oxygen species do play a role in destabilizing the genetic apparatus of cells, then antioxidants and other defense mechanisms acting to lower cellular oxidative stress may be an important component determining genetic stability.

TABLE 9. Some Evidence Supporting Dysdifferentiation as a Possible Causative Factor in Aging

---

1. Cells in tissue culture from longer-lived species appear more stable in terms of spontaneous mutation, greater cell-doubling number to reach a crisis state (Röhm[25]) and lower sensitivity to transformation by chemical mutagens.
2. Rate of accumulation of chromosomal aberrations is related to aging rate of the species.
3. Age-dependent accumulation of abnormal cell types (metaplasias).
4. Qualitative and quantitative age-dependent changes in gene expression, structural proteins, and enzyme levels have been found.
5. Basic housekeeping functions of a cell appear to be adequate in older organisms.

TABLE 10. Evidence Supporting Active Oxygen Species as a Possible Causative Factor in Dysdifferentiation

1. Low concentration of mutagenic/carcinogenic agents induce improper gene regulation, some by induction of transposable elements involved in control of gene expression.
2. Active oxygen species react with chromatin, oxidize specific DNA bases, and cause single-strand DNA breaks.
3. Active oxygen species induce chromosomal aberrations, and longer-lived species have a slower rate of accumulation of chromosomal aberrations.
4. Longer-lived species show a slower rate in accumulation of lipofuscin age pigments.
5. Aging rate is proportional to metabolic rate (cal/g/day) for many different mammalian species.

There is some evidence supporting the prediction that cells from longer-lived species are more stable in maintaining their proper state of differentiation. As shown in FIG. 9, cells from longer-lived species divide more times before reaching a crisis period in cell culture.[25] These and other data suggest the simple hypothesis shown in FIGURE 10 of how oxygen radicals may cause aging. This model can, however, be expanded into what we have called the multistep model of cancer and aging, as shown in FIGURE 11. The important feature of this model is the possibility of taking advantage of much of what has already been learned in cancer research (such as the multistep model of carcinogenesis) and applying it towards an advancement of an integrated model for research in aging and cancer mechanisms. For example, factors governing aging rate could act at the initiation stage (mutagens) or the progressive stage (epigenetic). Thus, dietary factors known to

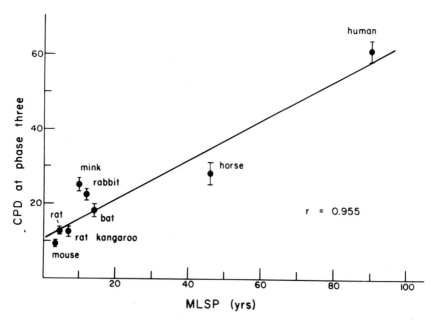

FIGURE 9. Population doubling of cells in culture before a crisis state is reached. (Adapted from Röhme.[25])

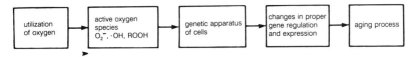

FIGURE 10. Model of how oxygen radicals may cause aging.

be possible causes of cancer (initiators or promotors) may also be acting to accelerate aging rate, and in turn those agents found to protect against cancer (dietary antioxidants) may also be of some benefit in protecting against abnormally high aging rate. A more general model indicating in detail the various areas where reactive oxygen species might play a role in aging is shown in FIG. 12.

These data briefly reviewed here have suggested the working hypothesis shown in TABLE 11 that has guided much of our recent experimental work. Most recently, an extension of the dysdifferentiation model has been proposed. It is now recognized that small changes in the proper differentiated state of cells may have their greatest impact in certain areas of the brain involved in regulating homeostatic functions.[25a] Such tissues are represented by the various areas of the pituitary gland and the hypothalamus. Specific areas of the brain such as those noted could be under high oxidative stress and often consist of a relatively few number of cells. Thus, alterations of regulatory genes in regulatory tissues are predicted to be the most important targets in the dysdifferention model of aging.

Many tissues of the body are in a constant cell renewal process. Tissues made up of nondividing cells are constantly renewing themselves through endogenous degradation-resynthesis processes and tissues made up of dividing cells are constantly being renewed through cell turnover. Such renewal processes are called

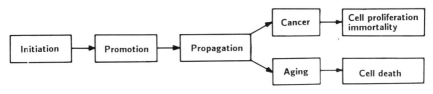

FIGURE 11. Multistep model of aging and cancer. This model represents the proposed multistep phenomena of both cancer and aging in their progress to increasing stages of dysdifferentiation. Ultimate end result of transformed cancer cell is cell proliferation immortality and of the aging process (other than cancer) is cell death. (From Cutler and Semsei.[21] Reprinted by permission from the *Journal of Gerontology*.)

TABLE 11. The Working Hypothesis Being Tested in Recent Experimental Work

1. Aging is in part a result of changes in proper gene expression and regulation. This process has been called dysdifferentiation.
2. Active oxygen species contribute to the dysdifferentiation process.
3. Mechanisms that act to reduce the dysdifferentiative effects of active oxygen species prolong the proper state of differentiation and thus the longevity of the animal.
4. Human longevity is a result of unusually high efficiency of these stabilizing mechanisms.
5. Aging and cancer are a result of the same dysdifferentiation process.

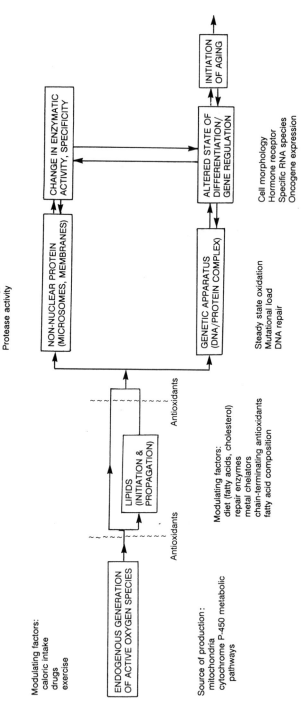

FIGURE 12. Model of oxidative initiation of aging.

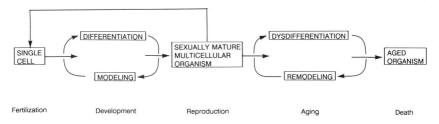

FIGURE 13. Dysdifferentiative and remodeling nature of aging.

remodeling, and it is proposed that dysdifferentiation of cells might influence proper remodeling kinetics as well as the qualitative aspects of tissue remodeling. This model is shown in FIGURE 13 and could explain some of the qualitative age-dependent changes found in bone and skin and how small changes of dysdifferentiation can be greatly amplified through remodeling kinetics.

Testing the Dysdifferentiative Hypothesis of Aging

Details will not be presented in this paper of our work testing the dysdifferentiation hypothesis of aging.[6] Briefly, we have conducted some experiments to determine if increased improper gene expression does occur with age.[26] These results are summarized in TABLE 12. More recent experiments in our laboratory have shown an age-dependent increase in the c-*myc* proto-oncogene in apparently normal tissues[27] (FIG. 14). Because of evidence that an increase of c-*myc* expression may be caused by genetic alterations (perhaps via reactive oxygen species), it appears possible that such genetic alterations may also be accumulating with age in normal-appearing tissue, increasing the probability of transformation of every cell in the organ.[27]

Testing the Role Reactive Oxygen Species May Have in Aging

Our first approach in testing the concept that aging may in part be caused by reactive oxygen species was carried out by determining if longer-lived species had superior defense mechanisms (antioxidants). According to our hypothesis,

TABLE 12. Summary of Investigation of Possible Age-Dependent Changes of Specific Genes

No change with age (brain, liver, kidney):
    1. Alpha-fetoprotein (mouse)
    2. Casein (mouse)
    3. Alpha and beta hemoglobin (human WI-38 cells)
Increase with age (brain, liver, kidney):
    1. Alpha and beta hemoglobin, quantitative (mouse and human)
    2. Mouse leukemia virus (MuLV), qualitative (mouse)
    3. Mouse mammary tumor virus (MMTV), qualitative (mouse)
    4. c-*myc* oncogene, quantitative (3rd Extron, mouse)

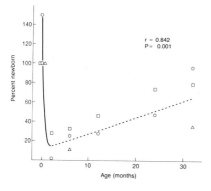

FIGURE 14. Relative c-*myc* proto-oncogene RNA levels in liver of mice as a function of age as determined by both Northern and slot blot data. The points are from three independent experiments (○, slot blot; □△, Northern). Newborn RNA is used as internal standard in all experiments and assigned 100%. (From Semsei et al.[27] Reprinted by permission from *Oncogene*.)

longer-lived species would not be predicted to have different types of protective mechanisms (a qualitative difference) but rather more of the same type of protective mechanisms (a quantitative difference) resulting from genetic changes occurring in regulatory genes.[19,28]

Results of some of these experiments are summarized in TABLE 13 and shown specifically for superoxide dismutase in FIGURE 15.[29] These data generally indicate that longer-lived species, particularly human, do indeed have higher levels of antioxidants per amount of reactive oxygen species produced endogenously.[30] A

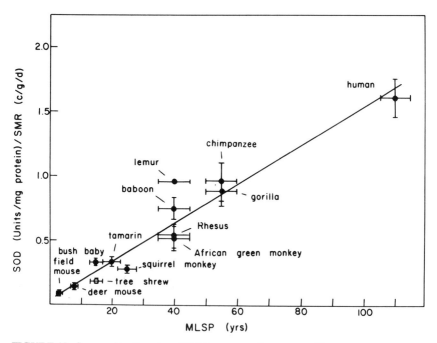

FIGURE 15. Superoxide dismutase (SOD) concentration per specific metabolic rate (SMR) in liver of mammals as a function of maximum lifespan potential (MLSP). (From Cutler.[31] Reprinted by permission from Plenum Press.)

TABLE 13. Summary of Antioxidant Comparison Results

Positive Correlation	No Correlation	Negative Correlation
1. Cu/Zn SOD	1. Ascorbate	1. Catalase
2. Mn SOD	2. Retinol	2. Glutathione
3. Carotenoids		3. Glutathione peroxidase
4. Alpha tocopherol		
5. Urate		
6. Ceruloplasmin		

simple experiment supporting this conclusion was carried out by comparing the spontaneous autoxidation rate in air of whole tissue homogenates taken from animals having different life spans. Rate of autoxidation was determined by measuring the amount of peroxides being produced (TBA assay). A typical result is shown in FIGURE 16, indicating an increased resistance of autoxidation with increasing life span. Thus, in this experiment, human brain tissue was found to be the most resistant to spontaneous autoxidation. The mechanism for this resistance is not yet understood but could involve less peroxidative substances (unsaturated fatty acids) as well as higher levels of antioxidants. These data are supported by the recent publication of a series of papers indicating positive results of antioxidant vitamins and beta carogene in disease prevention.[30a]

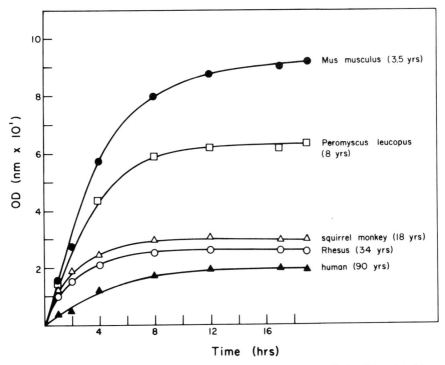

FIGURE 16. Kinetics of autoxidation of brain homogenate. (From Cutler.[30] Reprinted by permission from the National Academy of Sciences.)

If antioxidant protection is indeed higher in tissues of longer-lived species, then it would be expected that these same tissues should have a lower steady state level of oxidative damage. Since our model predicts the genetic apparatus of cells to be a key target to oxidative damage, we have compared the steady state oxidative damage level in DNA as a function of age and aging rate in different species.

FIGURE 17 shows the chemical structures of some of the more common oxidative products of nucleic acid bases that might be expected to be found *in vivo*.[32] The experiments to be described were made possible by taking advantage of the high sensitivity of the electrochemical detector (ECD) in detecting the oxidative products of deoxyguanosine (dG). One product is 8-OHdG and can be measured at femtomole levels using an HPLC/ECD instrument. Typical results for liver DNA are shown in FIGURE 18, indicating that DNA from longer-lived species does appear to have a lower steady state level of oxidative damage, at least for 8-OHdG, as compared to short-lived species.

After the repair of oxidative damage by excision of the oxidized nucleotide, the nucleoside appears later in the urine of an organism. By this pathway, a 24-hr urine sample would be expected to contain the total body level of excised products of 8-OHdG. This procedure allows the assessment of total body level of repair of oxidative DNA damage. Furthermore, if we assume that all oxidative products are repaired, then the amount of 8-OHdG detected could reflect rate of DNA damage as well as rate of repair.

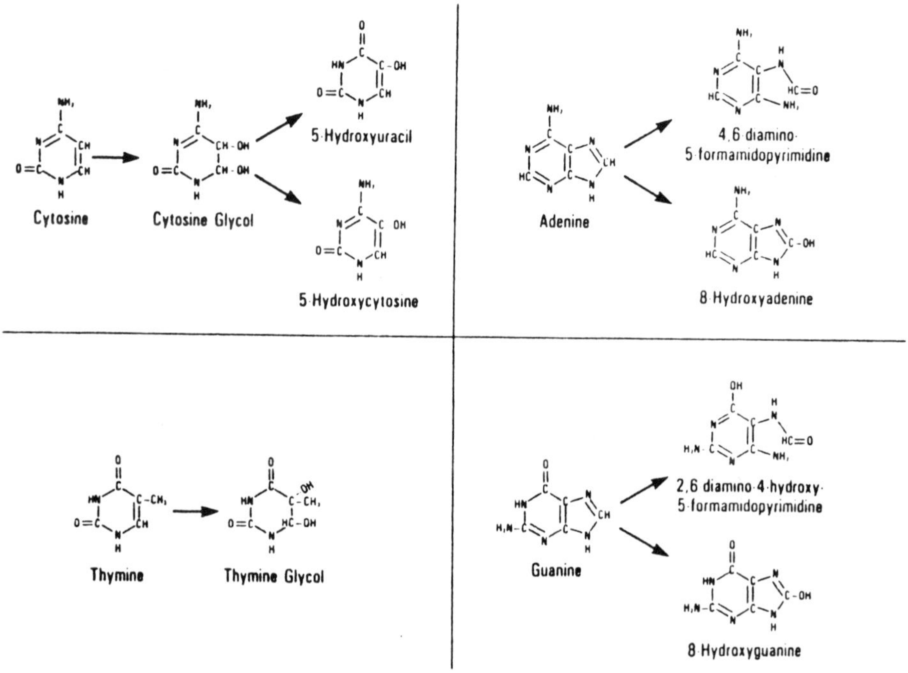

FIGURE 17. Major modifications of nucleic acid bases formed by the superoxide radical. (From Jackson *et al.*[32] Reprinted by permission from the *Journal of Clinical Investigation*.)

FIGURE 18. Steady state level of 8-OHdG per dG in liver DNA in species having different life spans (MLSPs).

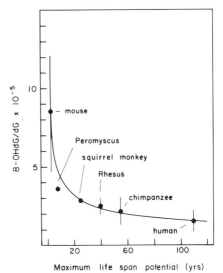

Preliminary results of such experiments are shown in FIGURE 19, where the amount of 8-OHdG per creatinine or lean body mass was found to decrease with increasing life span. These results suggest that the low levels of 8-OHdG found in human urine are likely to be the result of less 8-OHdG in the DNA needed to be repaired. The reason for the low level of oxidative damage in human DNA may in turn be the result of the unusually high levels of antoxidants that have been found in human tissue. Thus, the comparative results of antioxidant levels in tissues, DNA damage in tissues and urine levels of oxidized nucleosides are mutually complementary and together support the importance of oxidative damage as a cause of aging and of antioxidants in governing aging rate. These results are summarized in FIGURE 20.

Experimental Results from Other Laboratories Supporting the Longevity Determinant Gene Hypothesis

An important argument demonstrating the potential feasibility of effective intervention in human aging processes is the demonstration in laboratory animals that relatively simple processes can significantly increase life span. Below is a brief list of such experiments.

1. It is now well established that food or calorie restriction can dramatically decrease aging rate in experimental animals (mice and rats) as compared to ad libitum-fed controls.[33] The mechanism of how food restriction works is now being actively explored, but it does not appear to be a result of food restriction itself. Instead, a popular hypothesis is that food restriction stimulates through a few key regulatory mechanisms a change in hormonal status and/or a neuroendocrine response that in turn acts to slow down the aging rate of most physiological systems of the organism. Thus, food restriction experiments support the view that aging rate is coordinately governed by a few key regulatory processes.[33,34]

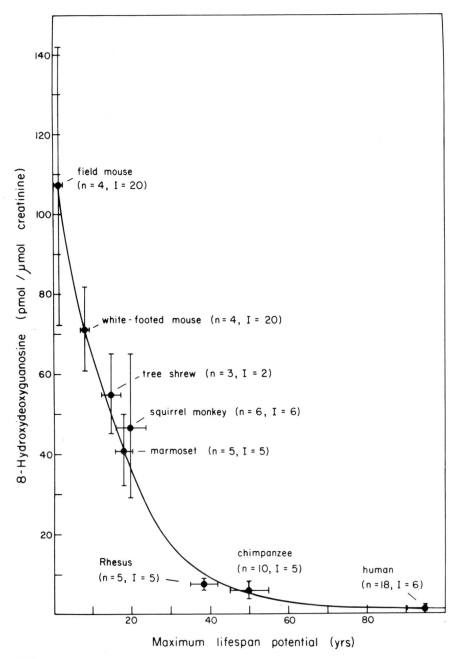

FIGURE 19. Relative amount of 8-OHdG per creatinine in urine samples taken from species having different life spans (MLSPs).

2. Experiments designed to select for long-lived strains of Drosophila and nematodes have been remarkably successful. Preliminary results indicate that some of the long-lived Drosophila strains have enhanced levels of antioxidant protection.[35-38] More impressive are the results in nematodes, where substantial increase of life span was found to be due to a change in activity of a single gene called AGE-1.[39,40] These experiments demonstrate that life span can be significantly increased by changes in one or a few genes.

3. Transgenic Drosophila strains carrying extra gene dosages of the protein system elongation factor EL-1 have been found to have a life span about twice as long as controls.[41] This result again demonstrates that life span can be increased by changing the expression of a single gene.

4. Hormone replacement therapy using human growth hormone, both in human and experimental animals, has been found to have remarkable rejuvenative results in terms of thickness of skin and the mass ratio of lean muscle to body fat.[8,9]

5. Topical application of retinoic acid to skin has been found to have antiaging effects and appears to reverse cellular changes in the skin that seem to be dysdifferentiated. Retinoic acid, known to effect states of differentiation of a cell, may actually be capable of reversing many of the characteristics of aging.[42]

SUMMARY AND CONCLUSION

A brief overview has been given of the biological nature of human aging processes, where it has been emphasized that, in addition to the diseases of aging, there is also great economic loss as a result of human aging processes that began many years before medical costs related to aging begin to escalate. Because of the ubiquitous nature of aging, reducing the function of essentially all physiological processes, it appears that the only long-term solution to human aging problems is to decrease uniformly the aging rate of the entire body.

Although the uniform decrease of aging rate has usually been considered impossible, where emphasis has consequently been placed on diseases of aging by the medically-oriented investigator, there is now at least one theoretical argument, accompanied by some experimental data, that suggests that progress can be made in achieving this goal. This progress has been based on the longevity determinant gene hypothesis predicting the existence of a relatively few key regulatory factors governing aging rate of the entire organism. If this hypothesis is not true, then indeed the prospect for significant intervention into human aging would appear impossible in the near future.

Experiments have been briefly reviewed testing the longevity determinant gene hypothesis, the possibility that aging may be a result of dysdifferentiation and if aging rate is determined by mechanisms acting to stabilize the differentiated state of cells. In testing the dysdifferentiation hypothesis of aging, there is not yet much data one way or the other. It is evident, however, that changes in gene expression do occur with age, sometimes involving endogenous retroviruses or oncogenes. Other morphological evidence shows an increase with age in unusual cell type such as metaplasia cells.

However, there is considerably more evidence indicating that aging may be a result of genetic instability (as it is in cancer) and that longer-lived species appear to have a more stable genetic apparatus and superior protective mechanisms against reactive oxygen species. There is a striking similarity in this model of

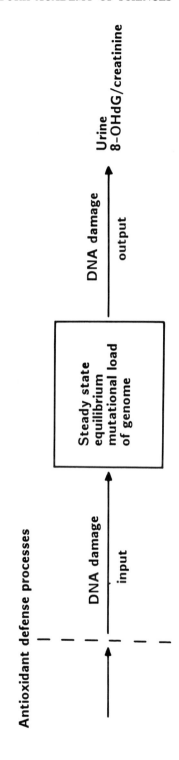

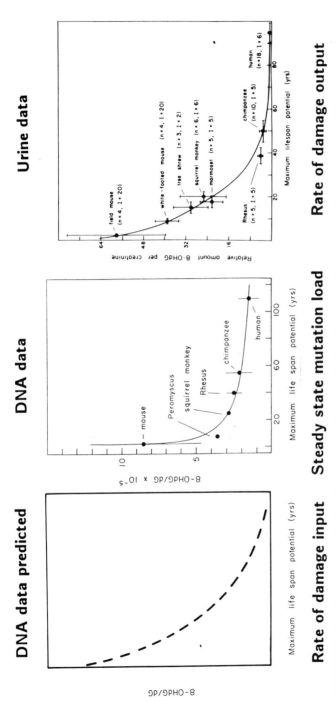

FIGURE 20. Model showing the relationship of oxidative damage in DNA with that of oxidative damage found in the urine. The conclusion is that antioxidant defense mechanisms have played a major role in accounting for the decrease in DNA damage in longer-lived species rather than DNA repair processes.

TABLE 14. Summary and Conclusion

1. Evidence indicates aging to be a result of genetic instability (dysdifferentiation) and aging rate to be governed by processes acting to stabilize the differentiated state of cells.
2. Evidence also indicates cancer to be a result of genetic instability leading to altered states of differentiation.
3. Aging rate and onset frequency of cancer appear to be correlated in different mammalian species.
4. Age-dependent increase in expression of endogenous viruses (MuLV, MMTV, 4-1 human endogenous virus) and oncogenes (c-*myc*) are found to occur in apparently normal noncancerous tissues.
5. Methods known to decrease aging rate (food restriction) also are effective in decreasing cancer incidence and those increasing aging rate (ionizing radiation) increase cancer rate.

TABLE 15. Knowledge and Knowledge Gaps

Knowledge	Knowledge Gaps
Aging is associated with dysdifferentiation.	But to what extent does this association occur? Can dysdifferentiation cause aging?
Oxyradicals can cause dysdifferentiation (genetic alterations).	But, do oxyradicals actually cause sufficient genetic alterations *in vivo* to contribute to aging?
Aging is associated with oxyradical generation and defense/protective mechanisms.	But, is the association of aging, oxyradicals and dysdifferentiation a cause-and-effect relationship?

aging and models of cancer, and much might be gained in bringing together these two fields of research.

Taking all of these data together, as summarized in TABLE 14, it appears we may be on the right track and that mechanisms acting to protect DNA against oxidative damage may be one class of longevity determinant mechanisms. There is of course much work remaining to be done, some of which is listed in TABLE 15 in terms of our knowledge and our gaps of knowledge in this field.

REFERENCES

1. SCHNEIDER, E. L. & J. M. GURALNIK. 1990. The aging of America. Impact on health care costs. J. Am. Med. Assoc. **263:** 2335–2340.
2. FRIES, J. F. & L. M. CRAPO. 1981. Vitality and Aging. W. H. Freeman & Co. San Francisco, CA.
3. MARSH, R. P. 1989. Ethical implications of life extension. Age **12:** 103–106.
4. CUTLER, R. G. 1976. Nature of aging and life maintenance processes. *In* Interdisciplinary Topics in Gerontology. R. G. Cutler, Ed. Vol. 9: 83–133. S. Karger. Basel.
5. CUTLER, R. G. 1976. Evolution of longevity in primates. J. Hum. Evol. **5:** 169–202.
6. CUTLER, R. G. 1982. Longevity is determined by specific genes: Testing the hypothesis. *In* Testing the Theories of Aging. R. Adelman & G. Roth, Eds. 25–114. CRC Press. Boca Raton, FL.

7. CUTLER, R. G. 1984. Evolutionary biology of aging and longevity. *In* Aging and Cell Structure. J. E. Johnson, Ed. Vol. 2: 371–428. Plenum Press. New York, NY.
8. EVERITT, A. & J. MEITES. 1989. Aging and anti-aging effects of hormones. J. Gerontol. **44**: B139–B141.
8a. MEITES, J. 1990. Aging: hypothalamic catecholamines, neuroendocrine-immune interactions, and dietary restriction. Proc. Soc. Exp. Biol. Med. **195**: 304–311.
9. RUDMAN, D., A. G. FELLER, H. S. NAGRAJ, G. A. GERGANS, P. Y. LALITHA, A. F. GOLDBERG, R. A. SCHLENKER, L. COHN, I. W. RUDMAN & D. E. MATTSON. 1990. Effects of human growth hormone in men over 60 years old. N. Engl. J. Med. **323**: 1–6.
10. CUTLER, R. G. 1975. Evolution of human longevity and the genetic complexity governing aging rate. Proc. Natl. Acad. Sci. USA **72**: 4664–4668.
10a. WILSON, A. C. 1976. Gene regulation in evolution. *In* Molecular Evolution. F. J. Ayala, Ed. 225–234. Sinauer Associates, Inc.
11. COMFORT, A. 1978. The Biology of Senescence. Elsevier. New York, NY.
12. ACSÁDI, G. & J. NEMESKÉRI. 1970. History of Human Lifespan and Mortality, Akadémiai Kiadó. Budapest.
13. STREHLER, B. L. 1978. Time, Cells and Aging. Academic Press. New York, NY.
14. SAGAN, L. A. 1987. The Health of Nations. Basic Books, Inc. New York, NY.
15. KOHN, R. R. 1978. Principles of Mammalian Aging. Prentice-Hall, Inc. Englewood Cliffs, NJ.
15a. KOHN, R. R. 1982. Cause of death in very old people. J. Am. Med. Assoc. **247**: 2793–2797.
15b. OLSHANSKY, S. J., B. A. CARNES & C. CASSEL. 1990. In search of Methuselah: estimating the upper limits to human longevity. Science **250**: 634–640.
16. SCHNEIDER, E. L. & J. W. ROWE, EDS. 1990. Handbook of the Biology of Aging. 3rd edit. Academic Press. New York, NY.
17. BAFITIS, H. & F. SARGENT. 1977. Human physiological adaptability through the life sequence. J. Gerontol. **32**: 402–410.
18. National Center of Health Statistics, USPHS & U.S. Bureau of the Census, "Some Demographic Aspects of Aging in the United States." Feb. 1973.
19. CUTLER, R. G. 1986. Aging and oxygen radicals. *In* Physiology of Oxygen Radicals. A. E. Taylor, S. Matlon & P. Ward, Eds. Clinical Monograph Series. 251–285. Am. Physiol. Soc. Bethesda, MD.
19a. SACHER, G. A. 1975. Maturation and longevity in relation to cranial capacity in hominid evolution. *In* Primate Functional Morphology and Evolution. R. Tuttle, Ed. 417–441. Mouton. The Hague.
19b. SCHNEIDER, E. L. & J. D. REED. 1985. Modulations of aging processes. *In* Handbook of the Biology of Aging. C. E. Finch & E. L. Schneider, Eds. 45–76. Van Nostrand Reinhold. New York.
19c. KIRKLAND, J. L. 1989. Evolution and ageing. Genome **31**: 398–405.
20. CUTLER, R. G. 1983. Superoxide dismutase, longevity and specific metabolic rate. Gerontology **29**: 113–120.
20a. HARMAN, D. 1981. The aging process. Proc. Natl. Acad. Sci. USA **78**: 7124–7128.
20b. HALLIWELL, B. & J. M. C. GUTTERIDGE. 1989. Free Radicals in Biology and Medicine. Clarendon Press. Oxford.
20c. SAUL, R. L., P. GEE & B. N. AMES. 1987. Free radicals, DNA damage, and aging. *In* Modern Biological Theories of Aging. H. R. Warner, R. N. Butler, R. L. Sprott & E. L. Schneider, Eds. 113–129. Raven Press. New York.
20d. ANISIMOV, V. N. 1989. Dependence of susceptibility to carcinogenesis on species life span. Arch. Geschwulstforsch. **59**: 205–213.
21. CUTLER, R. G. AND I. SEMSEI. 1989. Development, cancer and aging: Possible common mechanisms of action and regulation. J. Gerontol. **44**: 25–34.
22. AMES, B. N. 1983. Dietary carcinogens and anticarcinogens. Science **221**: 1256–1264.
23. CERUTTI, P. A. 1985. Prooxidant states and tumor promotion. Science **227**: 375–381.
24. CUTLER, R. G. 1985. Dysdifferentiation and aging. *In* Molecular Biology of Aging: Gene Stability and Gene Expression. R. S. Sohal, L. Birnbaum & R. G. Cutler, Eds. 307–340. Raven Press. New York, NY.

25. RÖHME, D. 1981. Evidence for a relationship between longevity of mammalian species and life spans of normal fibroblasts in vitro and erythrocytes in vivo. Proc. Natl. Acad. Sci. USA **78:** 5009–5013.

25a. FINCH, C. E. 1984. Recent findings in the neurobiology of aging. *In* Frontiers in Medicine. Implications for the Future. R. J. Morin & R. J. Bing, Eds. 264–283. Human Sciences Press, Inc. New York.

26. ONO, T. & R. G. CUTLER. 1978. Age-dependent relaxation of gene repression; increase of globin and endogenous murine leukemia virus related RNA in brain and liver of mouse. Proc. Natl. Acad. Sci. USA **75:** 4431–4435.

27. SEMSEI, I., S. MA & R. G. CUTLER. 1989. Tissue and age specific expression of the *myc* protooncogene family throughout the life span of the C57BL/6J mouse strain. Oncogene **4:** 465–470.

28. CUTLER, R. G. 1984. Antioxidants, aging, and longevity. *In* Free Radicals in Biology. W. A. Pryor, Ed. Vol. 6: 371–428. Academic Press. New York, NY.

29. TOLMASOFF, J. M., T. ONO & R. G. CUTLER. 1980. Superoxide dismutase: correlation with life span and specific metabolic rate in primate species. Proc. Natl. Acad. Sci. USA **77:** 2777–2781.

30. CUTLER, R. G. 1985. Peroxide-producing potential of tissues: correlation with the longevity of mammalian species. Proc. Natl. Acad. Sci. USA **82:** 4798–4802.

30a. SLATER, T. F. & G. BLOCK. 1991. Antioxidant vitamins and β-carotene in disease prevention. Am. J. Clin. Nutr. **53**(Suppl.): 189S–396S.

31. CUTLER, R. G. 1985. Antioxidants and longevity of mammalian species. *In* Molecular Biology of Aging. A. D. Woodhead, A. D. Blackett & A. Hollaender, Eds. 15–73. Plenum Press. New York, NY.

32. JACKSON, J. H., E. GAJEWSKI, I. U. SCHRAUFSTATTER, P. A. HYSLOP, A. F. FUCIARELLI, C. G. COCHRANE & M. DIZDAROGLU. 1989. Damage to the bases in DNA induced by stimulated human neutrophils. J. Clin. Invest. **84:** 1644–1649.

33. WEINDRUCH, R. & R. L. WALFORD. 1988. The Retardation of Aging and Disease by Dietary Restriction. C. C. Thomas, Pub. Springfield, IL.

34. YU, B. P., D. W. LEE, C. G. MARLER & J.-H. CHOI. 1990. Mechanism of food restriction: protection of cellular homeostasis. Proc. Soc. Exp. Biol. Med. **193:** 13–15.

35. LUCKINBILL, L. S., J. L. GRAVES, A. H. REED & S. KOETSAWANG. 1988. Localizing genes that defer senescence in Drosophila melanogaster. Heredity **60:** 367–374.

36. ARKING, R. & S. P. DUDAS. 1989. Review of genetic investigations into the aging processes of Drosophila. J. Am. Geriatr. Soc. **37:** 757–773.

37. PHILLIPS, J. P., S. D. CAMPBELL, D. MICHAUD, M. CHARBONNEAU & A. J. HILLIKER. 1989. Null mutation of copper/zinc superoxide dismutase in Drosophila confers hypersensitivity to paraquat and reduced longevity. Proc. Natl. Acad. Sci. USA **86:** 2761–2765.

38. SETO, N. O. L., S. HAYASHI & G. M. TENER. 1990. Over expression of Cu-Zn superoxide dismutase in Drosophila does not affect life-span. Proc. Natl. Acad. Sci. USA **87:** 4270–4274.

39. FRIEDMAN, D. B. & T. E. JOHNSON. 1987. A mutation in the *age-1* gene in *Caenorhabditis elegans* lengthens life and reduces hermaphrodite fertility. Genetics **118:** 75–86.

40. JOHNSON, T. E. 1988. Genetic specification of life span: processes, problems, and potentials. J. Gerontol. **43:** B87–B92.

41. SHEPHERD, J. C., U. WALLDORF, P. HUG & W. J. GEHRING. 1989. Fruit flies with additional expression of the elongation factor EF-1a live longer. Proc. Natl. Acad. Sci. USA **86:** 7520–7521.

42. KLIGMAN, A. M., G. L. GROVE, R. HIROSE & J. J. LEYDEN. 1986. Topical tretinoin for photoaged skin. J. Am. Acad. Dermatol. **15:** 836–859.

Electroimmunology: Membrane Potential, Ion-Channel Activities, and Stimulatory Signal Transduction in Human T Lymphocytes from Young and Elderly

SANDOR DAMJANOVICH AND CARLO PIERI[a]

Department of Biophysics
University Medical School of Debrecen
H-4012 Debrecen, Hungary

and

[a]Centro Citologia
Dipartimento Ricerche Gerontologiche e Geriatriche
Italian National Research Center on Aging (INRCA)
Via Birarelli, 8
60100 Ancona, Italy

INTRODUCTION

A flexible responsiveness of plasma membrane elements and changes in the concentrations of inorganic ions at the two sides of the plasma membrane of excitable cells has been in the focus of interest for many decades. Although lymphocytes are classified as nonexcitable cells, they have membrane potential and similar channel activities, specific for particular ions of different charge and size.[1,2] Earlier attempts to determine lymphocyte membrane potentials by using intracellular microelectrodes had not yielded correct data.[2] The advent of the chemical synthesis of fluorescent dyes, carrying net negative or positive charge and having a distribution in and outside the cells according to their electrical gradient and solubility, opened a new world in the last decade. Similarly, new techniques in electrophysiology like patch clamp and the variations of this elegant method, which is based upon sealing a small part of the plasma membrane and measuring the pico-amper level activity of individual channels, helped to explore at least in part the existence and role of ion channels in lymphocyte membranes.[1-6]

Lymphocytes, like nerve or muscle cells, have voltage-, ligand-, and G-protein-gated channels. These channels are integral membrane proteins having a virtual channel, specific for certain types of hydrophylic ions, like Na^+, K^+, Ca^{2+}, Cl^-, etc. Voltage gating means the functional opening or closing a channel upon changing transmembrane potential. Ligand gating is also a regulatory possibility through the binding of a specific ligand to a channel or its immediate vicinity, thereby influencing the passage of ions through steric hindrance or evoked conformational changes. G-protein gating is a complex regulatory circle where channel opening or closing depends upon the binding of the di- or triphosphorylated forms of guanosine nucleotides to specific proteins. Recent advances in this field succeeded in detecting structural differences between active and inactive forms of protooncogenic ras protein when it is in GTP (active), or GDP (inactive) complexed form, by high resolution X-ray diffraction.[7-9]

29

There is general agreement on the average levels of membrane potentials of resting lymphocytes, but many contradictory data appeared concerning the changes in membrane potential and the real causative role of channel activities in case of activated lymphocytes.[2,7,8] The importance of these questions is accentuated by the fact that cell activation processes may serve as models for normal cell proliferation and differentiation as well as oncogenic transformations.[10]

Not much effort has been expended yet on studying such delicate mechanisms during aging, although the more refined an investigation is, the higher the hope is of finding an explanation for the difference, e.g., between the immunological behavior of young and elderly.[11]

Here we shall confine our attention to the biophysical events during activation and regulation of immunologically competent cells in general, and the possibilities offered by these processes in gerontological research in particular.

Recent reviews permit us to focus our interest on the latest events in this field, and restrict the presentation and discussion of known facts and correlations to the bare minimum, yet without impairing the readability of the paper by those who are interested, but do not work in this area of science.[1,2,7,8]

Ion Transport and Membrane Potential Changes in Lymphocyte Activation Processes

The discovery of K^+, Ca^{2+}, Na^+ and also anionic channels in lymphocyte membranes practically coincided with the suggestion that they have an active role in T-cell activation. Less convincing and also much less numerous are the data on B cell functions. The potassium channels, both the calcium-activated and voltage-gated ones, were described in the first part of the 1980s, detected by membrane potential sensing dyes and also patch and whole cell clamp techniques.[1-4,7,8] Fukushima and Hagiwara studied the calcium channels of different cell lines of lymphocytic origin by patch clamp techniques.[12,13]

The occurrence rate of Na^+ channels and their participation in the cell activation processes are far less studied questions. In this communication an attempt has been made to compile some new data, obtained principally, but not exclusively by us, on the nature and biological significance of Na^+ and K^+ channels in the plasma membrane of human T lymphocytes, in resting and activated state, and also in young and elderly.

Recently we discovered that a known sodium channel opener, a quaternary ammonium ion, bretylium tosylate (BT), may influence cellular stimulatory events at more than one site. Flow cytometric and patch clamp measurements have been carried out in parallel, the latter with the so-called whole cell clamp variation of the patch clamp, where channel activities of the whole cell as well as membrane potential can be determined. The majority of the experiments were carried out on human peripheral blood lymphocytes, but in a number of cases murine T and B lymphocytes were also investigated.[14-16] BT helped us to explore a voltage- and ligand-gated type of Na^+ channels, which seem to occur in human as well as rodent T and B lymphocytes. It was immediately suggested that these channels may play a role in the lymphocyte activation processes. Flow cytometric membrane potential measurements with bis-oxonol, a membrane potential sensing dye, which carries negative charge, showed an increase in the plasma membrane potential of partially depolarized human and rodent T and B lymphocytes in a dose-dependent fashion upon addition of BT.[14,15] Neither the Na^+/H^+ exchange nor any change in the intracellular pH was involved, although the effect was amiloride sensitive. Direct measurements with bis-carboxy-ethyl carboxy fluorescein, a pH sensitive fluorescent dye, did not show a change upon BT treatment. On the other hand the phenomenon was ten-fold more sensitive to amiloride than the Na^+/H^+ antiporter, a membrane protein that changes protons and sodium ions between the extra and intracellular space and thereby alters intracellular pH values.

The effect of BT was inhibited by oubain, and tetrodotoxin, known inhibitors of Na^+-K^+ ATP-ase and Na^+ channels, respectively. The lack of Na^+ in the extracellular fluid or decreased temperature were also inhibitory to the hyperpolarization. The slight (10–15 mV) depolarization prior to addition of BT was essential for obtaining its repolarizing or hyperpolarizing effect. Our obvious conclusion was that the sodium influx, initiated by the BT, activated the electrogenic sodium-potassium pump, i.e., the Na^+-K^+ ATP-ase, and that was the reason for the re-, or hyperpolarization of the lymphocytes. Thus, since the mitogenic lectins are known to increase intracellular Na^+ and also Na^+-K^+ ATP-ase, the next plausible step was to look for the interaction of the observed effect and lectin-induced T lymphocyte activation.

This interest was further justified by the fact that mitogenic activation of T cells can also serve as a general model of induced cell proliferation and differentiation.

Phytohemagglutinin (PHA), a plant lectin, was selected for stimulation, which stimulates T cells by binding particular oligosaccharide moieties of glycoproteins in the cell membrane. PHA increases the intracellular calcium level and initiates a cascade of events which lead to the activation of protein kinase C enzyme and to phosphorylation of specific proteins, and finally the cells will proliferate as a consequence of a number of yet unknown steps leading to DNA synthesis and mitosis.[10]

Stimulation of human peripheral blood lymphocytes, treated simultaneously with PHA and BT, was blocked by BT in a dose-dependent fashion (Pieri et al., submitted). The BT proved to be nontoxic and reversibly removable, and did not change either the intracellular Ca^{2+} level or the expression of IL-2 and transferrin receptors. Addition of rIL-2 did not suspend the blocking effect of BT, which was completely reversible even after 6 hours of incubation with the PHA-stimulated cells. When both PHA and BT were removed by washing the cells with medium, the cells recovered, and reached the state of proliferation without significant impairment, as compared to the controls. On the other hand, about 80% of the cells were confined to the G_1 phase of the cell cycle when the BT was not removed. Both direct and indirect evidence indicated that BT was not impairing the major steps of PHA stimulation at such concentrations as caused sustained hyperpolarization of the lymphocytes. It has been concluded that the sustained hyperpolarization itself was the reason for the suspension of cell proliferation. This statement seems to be in direct conflict with those observations which show that lectin stimulation itself may cause changes in the membrane potential, and also increases the intracellular Na^+ and membrane ATP-ase activity.[1,18] Let us investigate first the effect of plant lectins upon the plasma membrane potential of T lymphocytes. Authors applying PHA or Con A (another plant lectin) to stimulate murine or human lymphocytes obtained hyperpolarization with the negatively charged fluorescent dye, bis-oxonol, using either spectrofluorimetric or flow cytometric membrane potential determination.[19–21] Early data by others, applying the positively charged carbocyanine dyes obtained depolarization.[22,23] Consistent data with the patch clamp method have not been presented yet to our knowledge. One comment is that positively charged fluorescent dyes are better indicators of depolarization, while the negatively charged oxonol is highly sensitive for hyperpolarization. These facts can be derived from the mode of action by which these dyes monitor the polarization degree of the cells. In our earlier studies we found that the well-known immunosuppressive drug, cyclosporin A, which is indispensable for solid organ (kidney, heart) transplantation, has a very early effect on the cell membranes. In our first experiments carried out at that time with carbocyanine dyes, we always obtained depolarization.[24–26] Other authors confirmed our data both with oxonol and carbocyanine based fluorescent indicators.[27] Recently, we observed that the effect is biphasic, and a quick hyperpolarizing effect is followed by a slower depolarization (Damjanovich *et al.*, submitted). Thus, being aware of the possible artifacts, we also investigated the effect of PHA on plasma membrane potential using bis-oxonol and human lymphocytes in a flow cytometer (Pieri *et al.*, submitted). Incubation of lymphocytes with stimulatory doses of PHA for three minutes generally hyperpolarized the human peripheral blood lymphocytes. Longer, approximately 10 minutes, incubation increased the probability to hyperpolarization.

When lymphocytes were slightly depolarized by isotonic increase of the extracellular [K^+] before adding the PHA, it quickly and effectively hyperpolarized the cells. This effect was not sensitive to potassium channel blockers like 4-aminopyridine or quinine, but was eliminated by oubain and lack of extracellular sodium. It also proved to be temperature sensitive. Our suggestion is that, without excluding an effect at more than one site, the PHA opens the same voltage and ligand-gated sodium channels as BT, and thus activates the electrogenic Na^+-K^+-ATP-ase. An important difference between the effect of BT and PHA is that the former initiates a sustained hyperpolarization while the latter is internalized in a reasonably short time.

Herewith we offer a model that may provide a general explanation for the known experimental facts from a different point of view: The transient dipoles of the cell membrane (*i.e.*, lipid and protein molecules stretched by the electric field and their own charge distribution across the plasma membrane), generated by the membrane potential, regulate intramembrane molecular interactions. The recently discovered similarities between the cells of the nervous and immune systems, and the ever accumulating evidence that proximity and dynamic behavior of membrane proteins and their lipid-domain dependent conformational changes can significantly influence, up or down regulate, membrane functions underline this statement.[1,2,7–9,28] Thus, only a relatively narrow potential window is optimal for those intermolecular interactions which dominate the initiation and propagation of transmembrane signaling at the plasma membrane level. Any significant and sustained deviation from this optimum may dramatically change the efficiency of the signaling processes (Pieri *et al.*, submitted). The permanent activation of the Na^+-K^+ ATP-ase by an agent which is not internalized in a reasonably short time results in a sustained repolarized state that influences the flexible responsiveness of plasma membrane molecules to extracellular signals. This new kind of regulatory role of Na^+ accentuates that the cell activation processes are influenced not only by potassium, but also by sodium channels and by the membrane potential. Thus, alongside the Na^+/H^+ exchange and Na^+-metabolite co-transport possibilities, the Na^+ influx can regulate the Na^+-K^+ ATP-ase activity and thereby cell activation.

Existence, Types, and Suggested Functional Significance of Cell Surface Patterns

Membrane potential and ion channel activities are per se highly dependent on the molecular interactions of cell membrane elements. Thus, it is not a distraction of our attention from our main goal to deal also with those biophysical methods and biological realities which may enhance the probability of obtaining useful information about the difference in lymphocyte plasma membranes from old and young human beings.

The great success of the Singer-Nicolson fluid mosaic membrane model overshadowed some facts for a considerably long period. Namely, that the authors of the model themselves never thought of it as an absolute dogma, that every membrane constituent is completely independent in its movement. Co-capping phenomena, successful crosslinking experiments of functionally cooperating elements, like receptor subunits, in the membranes signaled very early that the cell surface elements, although mobile in general, do not have an absolute, independent freedom of mobility.

An earlier suggestion by us predicted the existence of a "two-dimensional" pattern of lipid and protein elements in plasma membrane. Furthermore, we also predicted that any significant changes in this pattern may have functional consequences.[28] Cells are capable of responding to external signals in specific ways, and these capabilities include practically all the known immunological defense mechanisms. The specific response, being a highly complex phenomenon, is generally preceded by a number of steps, partially confined to the cell membrane. The activation at the level of the nuclei is less clear.[29,30]

Among the phenomena at the level of plasma membrane, the best understood is the redistribution of receptors or other membrane constituents which occur frequently inside, or rather in the plane of the membrane. Ligands having bound to their respective receptors often induce local aggregations following a relatively slow dynamics. At the same time the altered plasma membrane offers a different target to the external world, with a new "pattern" of ligand binding capacity and reactivity.[31,32] In order to obtain topological information on such alterations in these patterns, one has to have refined methods revealing distance relationships, the proximity of cell surface elements at a nm level.

Beyond the chemical crosslinking of nearby elements, a novel biophysical method was introduced by us in the late seventies and early eighties, the flow cytometric energy transfer measurement, or briefly FCET.[33–40] The method was described in detail; thus here we merely summarize it. Specific labeling of cell surface elements by suitably selected pairs of fluorescent dyes offers the possibility of applying the Foerster type fluorescence resonance energy transfer. This means that the energy, absorbed by one of the dyes (donor) is transferred to, and emitted by the other dye (acceptor) if they are close enough at the angstrom level. A number of other conditions are to be fulfilled as well, but finally the distance relationship of the two specific labels can be determined from relatively easily measurable spectroscopic parameters. The flow cytometric application by us could overcome the difficulties caused by the biological variability in cell populations, since measurements can be carried out on a cell-by-cell basis. Furthermore, a great number of cells can be studied in a reasonably short time.[33–35,37] The mathematical and physical problems of cell surface measurements have been solved, and the method was successfully applied to obtain precise data on cell surface pattern changes in a number of cases.[33–42]

The consistent application of the method by us and also by others revealed that many elements are interdependent in the membrane. The murine H2-K^k antigen and the Con A receptors showed a nonrandom codistribution without having any covalent molecular connection.[33] A new subunit of the IL-2 receptors was confirmed by flow cytometric energy transfer.[38] An unexpected molecular proximity of the HLA class I and II antigens was recently also reported.[40] The ligand binding induced colocalization of the CD-4 and Ti-CD-3 receptor was elegantly described by application of flow cytometric energy transfer method.[41] Another, independent biophysical approach of such questions was the application of fluorescence recovery after photobleaching in studying comobilities of functional elements in membranes.[8,40] Similar, generally sophisticated ways of studying cell surface phenomena are more and more readily available.[8,9]

Now it is generally accepted that colocalizations in the plasma membrane are not only beyond a chance occurrence, but are predetermined at the level of protein synthesis at the surface of the rough endoplasmic reticulum.[43,44]

Phenomenologically, but not without some indications of functional importance the following types of cell surface patterns may be described:

a. *Nonrandom codistribution of membrane elements in the plasma membrane.* Such a topological arrangement can be elicited, *e.g.,* by the lipid domains, which may preferentially accommodate functionally unrelated protein elements in close proximity.[33]

b. *Evoked redistribution in the plane of the membrane.* A type of this was demonstrated when a physical association of T-cell receptor and CD-4 antigen was induced by antigen receptor ligation and the proximity was followed by flow cytometric energy transfer measurement.[41]

c. *Evoked redistribution of proteins and lipids perpendicular to the membrane.* Endocytosis and de novo synthesis of membrane elements offer examples. Experimentally, *e.g.,* a change in the plasma membrane potential can also influence the accessibility of cell surface elements, even atomic groups.[32]

d. *Functional nonrandom codistribution of membrane proteins facilitated by their preferential accommodation in a particular type of lipid domain.* The orientation of eukaryotic membrane spanning proteins, *e.g.,* can be predicted from their amino acid sequences.[45]

e. *Assembly of functional subunits by the presence of ligands.* A likely example of this type of pattern is the IL-2 receptor complex.[38,39]

f. *Turnover of membrane elements caused by internalization or the appearance of newly synthetized elements by intracellular vesicle fusion with plasma membrane.* This is supposed to be a physiologic phenomenon, which may reflect actual metabolic activities. Such a pattern, or rather changes in this pattern, could be likely and very sensitive targets of gerontologic research.

g. *Conformational change induced accessibility alterations of functional groups evoked by perturbations during interactions with the changing environment.* Cell surface patterns are more likely targets of age related changes than those in the number of, *e.g.,* cell surface antigens, which characterize subsets of lymphocytes.[11]

Changes in Dynamic Responsiveness of Lymphocyte Plasma Membranes with Aging

Membrane potential and channel activities are sensitive indicators of the accommodating capability of human immunocompetent cells. Herewith we present data which show a significant difference in the responsiveness of peripheral blood lymphocytes from old and young to environmental perturbations.

TABLE 1 compares data indicating the responses of lymphocytes from old and young. The first phenomenon, which also supports our earlier preliminary data, is that elderly lymphocytes have the same membrane potential values as those from young. However, their response to the depolarizing effect of the isotonic increase in extracellular potassium concentrations is less.[11] A probing of the responses of the so-called calcium-activated potassium channels served a dual purpose. Ionomycin, a specific ionophore for calcium ions, merges into the lipid phase of the plasma membrane and shuttles calcium ions alongside to their concentration gradients. Thus, any changes in the structure of the lipid domains which alter diffusibility of the ionophore (*e.g.*, viscosity) may be reflected by a kinetic change in the calcium traffic. Another aspect of the same mechanism is that an increase in intracellular calcium is supposed to activate the "calcium-activated potassium channels." Changes in the calcium traffic could also be indicated by this second phase of the effect. The calcium influx, as an increase in the intracellular positive charges, has a depolarizing effect on the lymphocytes. In the second phase the

TABLE 1. Response of Calcium-Activated Potassium Channels to Ionomycin by T-Lymphocytes from Young and Elderly[a]

	Mean Values of Flow Cytometric Histograms Channel Numbers		
	Before	After	
		Addition of Ionomycin	
		Immediately	After Incubation
Young controls	31.4	90.18	30.7
Elderly	34.25	88.34	89.57
Young controls[b]	79.70	60.48	58.36
Elderly[b]	72.29	89.17	88.64

[a] Peripheral blood lymphocytes were prepared from young and old healthy volunteers and kept in RPMI-1640 medium with 10% fetal calf serum for 2–3 hours, at 37°C. The cells were then transferred to phosphate buffered saline (PBS) solution at pH 7.4. 10^6 cells in 1 ml PBS were treated with 150 nM oxonol (Molec.Probes Eugene, OR). The fluorescence of the cells was determined in the absence and presence of Ca^{2+} and also before and after addition of 2 μM ionomycine. Fluorescence of individual cells was measured in a flow cytometer (Coulter Epics V.Hialeah, FL) after 1 minute and 20 minutes incubation at 37°C as described before.[14] The table shows the mean (a weighted average of the membrane potential over the cell population) values of the fluorescence histograms obtained in the flow cytometer. Data represent a typical experiment with lymphocytes of elderly (85 ± 6 year) and appropriate young controls measured in the same series of experiments. Each series had two elderly and one young sample and five such series were investigated so far. No contradictory data were obtained, and the experiments showed a remarkable reproducibility also from quantitative point of view. The SD values were within 7–8%, while the differences were in the order of 30–50% when data were normalized to internal control.

[b] The lymphocytes were partially depolarized by 35 mM extracellular K^+.

outwardly directed potassium flow increases the intracellular negativity, thereby hyperpolarizing the cells. Of course, this second phase depends, on the one hand, on the calcium influx, and on the other hand, on the responsiveness and availability of potassium channels. Thus, upon addition of ionomycin these two separate aspects of the behavior of the membrane can be observed simultaneously. In the case of the young controls the addition of the ionophore increased the membrane potential, depending upon the degree of polarization of the membrane. As the mean values (a weighted average of the membrane potential over the cell population) of the flow cytometric membrane potential measurements show, the response of the calcium-activated potassium channels was retarded when the cells were not previously partially depolarized. The decrease in the mean value represents a depolarization first, caused by the Ca^+ influx. Hyperpolarization follows this first effect only after several minutes. When depolarization is initiated by an isotonic increase of the extracellular potassium, an immediate hyperpolarization, a decrease in the mean values was observed, signaling the quick response of the Ca^+-activated K^+ channels.

The response of the peripheral blood lymphocytes from elderly was quite different. In an overwhelming majority of cases, the response of the potassium channels was not observed among the same conditions when the lymphocytes of young origin responded unconditionally with the opening of the suitable class of potassium channels. Similar differences, *e.g.,* the lack of response of the old lymphocytes, were observed when the sodium channel opener BT was added among conditions where the young lymphocytes were unconditionally hyperpolarized.

A plausible explanation could be physicochemical. The altered membrane viscosity that was detected by several authors in connection with aging could be responsible for the observed effect.

However, the immediate depolarization of cells from both old and young indicates the capability of ionomycine to increase the intracellular calcium level. The lack of extracellular calcium, or appropriate doses of the calcium chelator EGTA, added prior to the ionomycin, could also eliminate the depolarization. A more likely cause of the phenomenon, *e.g.,* the missing response of the calcium-activated potassium channels, may be an altered responsiveness due to age-related changes in protein flexibility or a new type of interaction between the changed lipid and protein moieties. Of course, a further in-depth analysis is necessary, since the above-offered explanations are far from being proven. An equally possible cause could be a down regulation of the number of channels during aging. Electrophysiological experiments are in progress to obtain data on this possibility. Changes in the kinetics of such responses as well as their magnitude may reveal a number of differences between young and elderly at this level. As pointed out above, one cannot really expect a large difference in average parameters between old and young, since there are broad scales of such parameters for both. A more likely difference may be found in the dynamic responsiveness of cellular or molecular systems. As was demonstrated above, one readily available target of such investigations is offered by the newly opened possibilities of electroimmunology. In this field the complicated cellular regulatory mechanisms though readily accessible for measurements, are also very likely to suffer some alterations during aging. At present it is very difficult to define aging by exact parameters, due to the broad scale of processes, where the alterations are highly optional and show a high degree of individual variations.

However, it has long been observed that elderly are more vulnerable to extracorporal infections than young; thus the investigation of the immune system at such a sophisticated level can be rewarding.

SUMMARY

There are conflicting data on the functional role and direction of the changes in membrane potential and ion currents accompanying lymphocyte stimulation. Recently, we discovered that a known sodium channel opener, bretylium tosylate (BT), may influence the stimulatory processes of lymphocyte activation at more than one site. Parallel flow cytometric and electrophysiological measurements with patch clamp techniques showed that BT quickly repolarizes previously slightly depolarized human peripheral blood as well as splenic murine lymphocytes. The repolarization occurred through opening ligand- and voltage-gated, hitherto unknown sodium channels, and the sodium influx activated Na^+-K^+-dependent, electrogenic ATP-ase activity. A comparison of the flexible responsiveness of the membrane potential was carried out between lymphocytes from young and elderly using the above mechanism and a number of combinations of channel blockers and ionophores in order to obtain information on the alleged changes in immunological behavior. A significant difference has been found between lymphocytes from human young and elderly volunteers in the readiness to respond to channel-activating perturbations. An explanation is offered, based upon known physicochemical changes in the plasma membrane during aging.

REFERENCES

1. LEWIS, R. S. & M. D. CAHALAN. 1988. The plasticity of ion channels: parallels between the nervous and the immune system. Trends Neurosci. **11:** 214–218.
2. GRINSTEIN, S. & J. S. DIXON. 1989. Ion transport, membrane potential, and cytoplasmic pH in lymphocytes: changes during activation. Physiol. Rev. **69**(2): 417–481.
3. MATTESON, D. R. & C. DEUTSCH. 1984. K^+ channels in T lymphocytes: a patch clamp study using monoclonal antibody adhesion. Nature (London) **307:** 468–471.
4. DeCOURSEY, T. E., K. G. CHANDY, S. GUPTA & M. D. CAHALAN. Voltage-gated K^+ channels in human T lymphocytes: a role in mitogenesis. Nature (London) **307:** 465–468.
5. FUKUSHIMA, Y., S. HAGIWARA & M. HENKART. 1984. Potassium current in clonal cytotoxic T lymphocytes from the mouse. J. Physiol. (London) **351:** 645–656.
6. FUKUSHIMA, Y. & S. HAGIWARA. 1985. Currents carried by monovalent cations through calcium channels in mouse neoplastic B lymphocytes. J. Physiol. (London) **358:** 255–284.
7. SZOLLOSI, J., S. DAMJANOVICH, S. A. MULHERN & L. TRON. 1987. Fluorescence energy transfer and membrane potential measurements monitor dynamic properties of cell membranes: a critical review. Prog. Biophys. Molec. Biol. **49:** 65–87.
8. MATKO, J., J. SZOLLOSI, L. TRON & S. DAMJANOVICH. 1988. Luminescence spectroscopic approaches in studying cell surface dynamics. Quart. Rev. Biophys. **21:** 479–544.
9. MILBURN, M. V., L. TONG, A. M. DeVOS, A. BRUNGER, Z. YAMAIZUMI, S. NISHIMURA & S-H. KIM. 1990. Molecular switch for signal transduction: structural differences between active and inactive forms of protooncogenic ras protein. Science **247:** 939–945.
10. CRABTREE, G. R. 1989. Contingent genetic regulatory events in T lymphocyte activation. Science **243:** 355–361.
11. VARGA, ZS., N. BRESSANI, A-M. ZAIA, L. BENE, A. LEOVEY, N. FABRIS & S. DAMJANOVICH. 1990. Cell surface markers, inositol phosphate levels and membrane potential of lymphocytes from young and old human patients. Immunol. Lett. **23:** 275–280.
12. FUKUSHIMA, Y. & S. HAGIWARA. 1983. Voltage gated Ca^{2+} channel in mouse myeloma cells. Proc. Natl. Acad. Sci. USA **80:** 2240–2242.
13. FUKUSHIMA, Y., S. HAGIWARA & R. E. SAXTON. 1984. Variation of calcium current during the cell growth cycle in mouse hybridoma lines secreting immunoglobulins. J. Physiol. (London) **355:** 313–321.
14. PIERI, C., R. RECCHIONI, F. MORONI, L. BALKAY, T. MARIAN, L. TRON & S. DAMJANOVICH. 1989. Ligand and voltage gated sodium channels may regulate electrogenic pump activity in human, mouse and rat lymphocytes. Biochem. Biophys. Res. Commun. **160:** 999–1002.
15. TRON, L., C. PIERI, T. MARIAN, L. BALKAY, M. EMRI & S. DAMJANOVICH. 1990.

Bretylium causes a Na^+/H^+ exchange independent activation of Na^+-K^+ pump of rodent and human lymphocytes. Mol. Immunol. In press.

16. PIERI, C., R. RECCHIONI, F. MORONI, F. MARCHESELLI, M. FALASCA & S. DAM-JANOVICH. 1990. A sodium channel opener inhibits stimulation of human peripheral T-lymphocytes. Submitted.

17. L'ALLEMAIN, G., A. FRANCHI, E. CRAGOE, JR. & J. POUYSSEGUR. 1984. Blockade of the $Na+/H+$ antiport abolishes growth factor induced DNA synthesis in fibroblasts. J. Biol. Chem. **259:** 4313–4319.

18. AVERDUNK, R. & P. K. LAUF. 1975. Effect of mitogens on Na^+-K^+ transport, ^3H-oubain binding, and adenosin triphosphatase activity in lymphocytes. Exp. Cell Res. **93:** 331–342.

19. TATHAM, P. E. & P. J. DELVES. 1984. Flow cytometric detection of membrane potential changes in murine lymphocytes induced by Concanavalin A. Biochem. J. **221:** 137–146.

20. TATHAM, P. E., K. O'FLYNN & D. C. LYNCH. 1986. The relationship between mitogen induced membrane potential changes and intracellular free calcium in human T lymphocytes. Biochim. Biophys. Acta **856:** 201–211.

21. TSIEN, R. Y., T. POZAN & T. J. RINK. 1982. T-cell mitogens cause early changes in cytoplasmic free Ca^{2+} and membrane potential in lymphocytes. Nature (London) **295:** 68–71.

22. SHAPIRO, H. M., P. J. NATALE & L. A. KAMENTSKY. 1979. Estimation of membrane potentials of individual lymphocytes by flow cytometry. Proc. Natl. Acad. Sci. USA **70:** 5728–5730.

23. MONROE, J. G. & J. C. CAMBIER. 1983. B-cell activation. I. anti-immunoglobulin induced receptor cross-linking results in a decrease in the plasma membrane potential of murine B-lymphocytes. J. Exp. Med. **157:** 2073–2086.

24. DAMJANOVICH, S., A. ASZALOS, S. A. MULHERN, M. BALAZS & L. MATYUS. 1986. Cytoplasmic membrane potential of mouse lymphocytes is decreased by cyclosporins. Mol. Immunol. **23:** 175–180.

25. MATYUS, L., M. BALAZS, A. ASZALOS, S. A. MULHERN & S. DAMJANOVICH. 1986. Cyclosporin A depolarizes cytoplasmic membrane potential and interacts with Ca^{2+} ionophores. Biochim. Biophys. Acta **886:** 353–360.

26. DAMJANOVICH, S., A. ASZALOS, S. A. MULHERN, J. SZOLLOSI, M. BALAZS, L. TRON & M. J. FULWYLER. 1987. Cyclosporin depolarizes human lymphocytes: earliest observed effects on cell metabolism. Eur. J. Immunol. **17:** 763–768.

27. GELFAND, E. W., R. K. CHEUNG & G. B. MILLS. 1987. The cyclosporins inhibit lymphocyte activation at more than one site. J. Immunol. **138:** 1115–1120.

28. DAMJANOVICH, S., B. SOMOGYI & L. TRON. 1981. Macromolecular dynamics and information transfer. *In* Adv. Physiol. Sci. G. Szekely, E. Labos & S. Damjanovich, Eds. Vol. **30:** 9–21.

29. CUETRECASAS, P. 1986. Hormone receptors, membrane phospholipids and protein kinases. Harvey Lect. **80:** 89–128.

30. BERRIDGE, M. J. & R. F. IRVINE. 1989. Inositol phosphates and cell signalling. Nature (London) **341:** 197–202.

31. ZIDOVETZKY, R., Y. YARDEN, J. SCHLESSINGER & T. M. JOVIN. 1981. Rotational diffusion of epidermal growth factor complexed to cell surface receptors reflects rapid microaggregation and endocytosis of occupied receptors. Proc. Natl. Acad. Sci. USA **78:** 6981–6985.

32. BALAZS, M., J. MATKO, J. SZOLLOSI, L. MATYUS, M. J. FULWYLER & S. DAM-JANOVICH. 1986. Accessibility of cell surface thiols in human lymphocytes is altered by ionophores or OKT-3 antibody. Bichem. Biophys. Res. Commun. **140:** 999–1006.

33. DAMJANOVICH, S., L. TRON, J. SZOLLOSI, R. ZIDOVETZKI, W. L. C. VAZ, F. REGA-TEIRO, D. J. ARNDT-JOVIN & T. M. JOVIN. 1983. Distribution and mobility of murine histocompatibility H-2Kk antigen in the cytoplasmic membrane. Proc. Natl. Acad. Sci. USA **80:** 5985–5989.

34. TRON, L., J. SZOLLOSI, S. DAMJANOVICH, S. H. HELLIWELL, D. J. ARNDT-JOVIN &

T. M. JOVIN. 1984. Flow cytometric measurements of fluorescence resonance energy transfer on cell surfaces. Biophys. J. **45:** 939–946.

35. SZOLLOSI, J., L. TRON, S. DAMJANOVICH, S. H. HELLIWELL, D. J. ARNDT-JOVIN & T. M. JOVIN. 1984. Energy transfer measurements on cell surfaces. Cytometry **5:** 210–216.

36. TRON, L., J. SZOLLOSI & S. DAMJANOVICH. 1987. Proximity measurements of cell surface proteins by fluorescence energy transfer. Immunol. Lett. **16:** 1–9.

37. SZOLLOSI, J., L. MATYUS, L. TRON, M. BALAZS, I. EMBER, M. J. FULWYLER & S. DAMJANOVICH. 1987. Flow cytometric measurements of fluorescence energy transfer using single laser excitation. Cytometry **8:** 120–128.

38. SZOLLOSI, J., S. DAMJANOVICH, C. K. GOLDMAN, M. J. FULWYLER, A. ASZALOS, G. GOLDSTEIN, P. RAO, M. A. TALLE & T. A. WALDMANN. 1987. Flow cytometric resonance energy transfer measurements support the association of a 95-kD termed T27 with the 55-kD Tac peptide. Proc. Natl. Acad. Sci. USA **84:** 7246–7250.

39. EDIDIN, M., A. ASZALOS, S. DAMJANOVICH & T. A. WALDMANN. 1988. Lateral diffusion measurements give evidence for association of the Tac peptide of IL-2 receptor with T27 peptide in the plasma membrane of HUT-102-B2 T cells. J. Immunol. **141:** 1206–1210.

40. SZOLLOSI, J., S. DAMJANOVICH, M. BALAZS, P. NAGY, L. TRON, M. J. FULWYLER & F. M. BRODSKY. 1989. Physical association between MHC class I and class II molecules detected on the cell surface by flow cytometric energy transfer. J. Immunol. **143:** 208–213.

41. MITTLER, R. S., S. J. GOLDMAN, G. L. SPITALNY & S. J. BURAKOFF. 1989. T-cell receptor-CD4 physical association in a murine T-cell hybridoma: induction by antigen receptor ligation. Proc. Natl. Acad. Sci. USA **86:** 8531–8535.

42. GORVEL, J-P., Z. MISHAL, F. LIEGEY, A. RIGAL & S. MAROUX. 1989. Conformational change of rabbit aminopeptidase N into erythrocyte plasma membrane domains analysed by flow cytometry fluorescence energy transfer. J. Cell Biol. **108:** 2193–2200.

43. COX, J. H., J. W. YEWDELL, L. C. EISENLOHR, P. R. JOHNSON & J. R. BENNINK. 1990. Antigen presentation requires transport of MHC class I molecules from the endoplasmic reticulum. Science **247:** 715–747.

44. HARTMANN, E. T., A. RAPOPORT & H. F. LODISH. 1989. Predicting the orientation of eukaryotic membrane spanning proteins. Proc. Natl. Acad. Sci. USA **86:** 5786–5790.

Age Changes in Chromatin: Accumulative or Programmed?

ZHORES A. MEDVEDEV AND
MARGARITA N. MEDVEDEVA

Genetics Division
National Institute for Medical Research
The Ridgeway, Mill Hill
London NW7 1AA, Great Britain

INTRODUCTION

Before 1980, when only low-resolution gel electrophoresis of histones was available, no age- or tissue-specific changes in the pattern of the main nucleosomal core histones (H2A, H2B, H3 and H4) were observed by this technique. Later however, when it became possible by new high-resolution methods of polyacrylamide gel electrophoresis to resolve each of the histones except H4 into the families of individual histone variants or subtypes, the existence of tissue- and age-specific changes in the composition of histone variants became apparent.[1,2] We also recently found definite age-related changes in the composition of histone variants in mouse tissues and suggested that these changes may reflect the programmed alteration of the expression of histone genes.[3,4]

The studies of the composition of histone variants in different species and tissues made it possible to identify two main groups; more abundant DNA replication-dependent histone variants which are actively synthesized only during the S-phase of the cell cycle, and the second, less prominent, group represented by the replication-independent or replacement histone variants which are synthesized more slowly, but throughout the whole cell cycle.[1,5–7] The existence of replacement histones, which are more easily identified in nondividing differentiated cells was originally explained as probably linked to differentiation, or the necessity for the repair of the nucleosomal units. Chromosomal DNA is also synthesized only during the S-phase of the cell cycle and the integrity of DNA in postmitotic cells depends on the existence of DNA repair systems. Inaccuracy of DNA repair enzymes in nondividing cells and their inability to remove all damage, were often considered as possible causes of ageing due to the gradual deterioration of genetic information.[8,9] Replacement histones are also probably not able to provide the accurate repair of nucleosomal histone octamers because the patterns of the DNA-dependent and the replacement histones are quite different. But if accurate repair of nucleosomal units is impossible this can open the way for the accumulation of changes in the character of the interaction between DNA and histones, which could lead to age-related deterioration of accuracy of transcription.

It has been shown that the half-lives of histones in the highly differentiated cells of mouse liver and brain (average 117 and 159 days for total histone) is much shorter than the half-life of the DNA in the same tissues (318 and 593 days respectively).[10] If the synthesis of the main histone variants is indeed entirely inhibited in nondividing cells, the major fraction of histones in aged cells should therefore be represented by the replication-independent variants, which are coded by randomly located single copy genes. (Replication-dependent histones are encoded by reiterated, intronless genes clustered together and transcribed into non-polyadenylated mRNAs.[5,11]) In our previous study, which was the first attempt to analyse the pattern of the histone variants in senescent mice, no significant proportion of replacement histone variants was found in tissues with low proliferating activity (kidney and liver) even in 29-month-old animals.[3] This suggests that the main DNA replication-dependent nucleosomal core histones are either more stable than reported earlier or have some, probably only highly reduced, basal turnover because their genes are not completely inhibited. In this case the appearance of specific age-related new histone variants, even minor, may indicate primarily the signs of a genetic program, but not nucleosomal repair. In order to test this possibility, it was necessary not only to analyze the age-related pattern of histone variants in different tissues, but also to study the rate of their synthesis and turnover.

MATERIALS AND METHODS

Animals and Labelling

Groups of 2.5-, 12- and 29–30-month-old male CBA mice were used for experiments. In the old, male CBA mice, about 50% of the animals had hepatocarcinomas in various stages of growth. High incidence of spontaneous age-related and slow-growing hepatocarcinomas in CBA mice is well known,[12] but despite this, the CBA strain is widely used for research on ageing because of its very high maximum life span potential of up to 35–36 months. Only normal livers in the old group were analyzed. Ten mice in the young and twelve in the old groups were selected for intraperitoneal administration of [^{3}H] L-amino acid mixture (DuPont, Boston, MA) which contained 15 individual labelled amino acids. 0.5 mCi was administered to each mouse. The animals were killed 24 hours after administration of the labelled amino acids. Only 8 mice in the old group had normal livers.

Isolation of Nuclei and Chromatin and Protein Extraction

Livers, spleens, kidneys, thymuses and brains from labelled and nonlabelled groups of mice in different experiments were removed, immediately frozen and stored at $-80°C$ until required for analysis. Nuclei were isolated by the method of Schibler and Weber[13] which minimizes possible proteolytic degradation by working at $-20°C$. Protease inhibitor (PMSF, 1.0 mM) was added to all media used during homogenization and different stages of extraction. Chromatin was obtained by repeatedly blending nuclei in a Dounce homogenizer with 0.025 M EDTA in 0.07 M NaCl, pH 7.5. All the extracts, including the initial homogenate, were tested for levels of radioactivity, calculated per 1 g of fresh tissue, in order to compare the differences of the distribution of labelled amino acids in different tissues and in young and old animals. All loosely bound nonhistone chromatin proteins, including acid-soluble high mobility group (HMG proteins), were removed by repeated ($\times$ 3) 0.35 M NaCl extraction of chromatin. H1 histones (H1A, H1B and H1°) were extracted with 5% (w/v) perchloric acid ($\times$ 3). Nucleosomal core histones were then extracted from H1-free chromatin with 0.25 M HCl ($\times$ 4). Liver-specific acid-soluble nonhistone proteins (LSP1 and 2) usually are co-extracted with the core histones but are located well above histones during electrophoresis due to their higher molecular weight.[14]

Gel Electrophoresis, Fluorography and Measurements of Radioactivity

High resolution acetic acid-urea-Triton X-100 gel electrophoresis was carried out by the method of Zweidler[1] with some modifications. The resolving gel contained 15% acrylamide and slab gels were used rather than the tube gels of the original method. This made it possible to receive more narrow bands and to use gels for subsequent fluorography. Normally each slab gel contained two identical sets of lanes, one set was stained with Coomassie Brilliant blue and the duplicate set was soaked with autoradiography enhancer (EN³HANCE, DuPont, Boston) dried and exposed to X-ray film (X-OMAT, Kodak Diagnostic Film, Eastman Kodak Co., Rochester, NY) at −80°C. The time of exposure was rather long, and varied from 4 to 8 months because the administration of labelled amino acids to live animals cannot produce the same high levels of specific radioactivity of proteins which is usual in experiments with tissue cultures. Stained gels also were sometimes used for fluorography. Additionally the radioactivity of individual histone bands was estimated quantitatively by scintillation counting of solubilized slices of stained gels, using the Beckman LS6800 Liquid Scintillation System.

Classification of Histone Variants

There is not yet a universally accepted classification system for histone variants, mainly because rather wide differences in the numbers of bands and spots which were identified using several modifications of one-dimensional and two-dimensional gel electrophoresis, long or short slabs and tubes, etc. It also is not easy to distinguish nonallelic histone variants from histone postsynthetic modifications (phosphorylation and acetylation) without extensive additional study of protein from each band. For the purpose of this investigation it was sufficient just to number each extra band in the main histone family (from top to bottom). We consider this as a tentative but more simple approach. Other authors, who also identified more bands than in the Zweidler's classification, used for designation of extra variants either letters (e.g., H2A.X, H2A.Z)[15] or extra numbers (H2A.2.1, H2A.2.3, etc.).[16]

RESULTS

Tissue-Specific Differences in the Composition and in the Rate of Synthesis of Histone Variants

FIGURE 1 shows the tissue-specific pattern of histone variants in four organs of young mice to which were administered labelled amino acids, and the fluorographs from the duplicate set of lanes. Mitotic activity was maximal in the thymus, and this was reflected in the high rate of synthesis of DNA replication-independent histone variants. All major bands of histones in the thymus, which show a high level of incorporation of [³H] amino acids, should therefore be considered as DNA replication-dependent. The pattern of histone variants in liver and kidney differed in all of the groups, except H4 and the rate of their synthesis was much lower, apparently due to the low level of cellular proliferation.

It is important to mention that differences in the levels of incorporation of labelled amino acids into different histones were primarily linked to their rates of synthesis, but not to the unequal distribution of administered [³H] mixture of

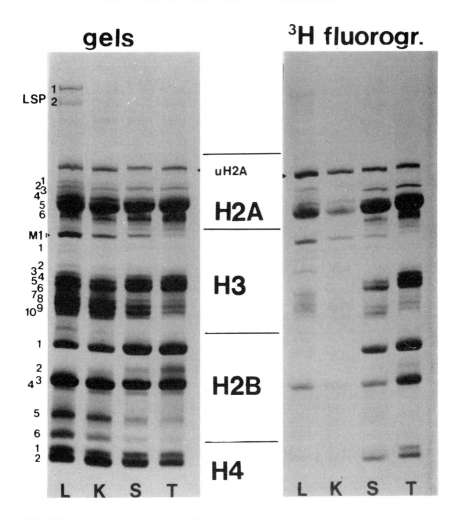

FIGURE 1. Comparison of the core histone variants composition in young mouse tissues and fluorographs of the identical duplicate gel showing the histone variants synthesis pattern. 100 μg of protein were used for each gel lane. Abbreviations: LSP, liver-specific nonhistone proteins; L, liver; K, kidney; S, spleen; T, thymus. Numbers on the *left side* of the gel note individual histone variants or histone modifications. An unidentified DNA replication-independent variant is labelled as MI.

amino acids among tissues. In experiments with live animals the factor of tissue-specific distribution of any injected substances should always be taken into account. In this experiment the presence of labelled amino acids per g of tissue was rather close in liver and spleen (9.24 and 9.89 × 10⁶ cpm, respectively) and slightly lower in kidney and thymus (6.89 and 5.09 × 10⁶ cpm, respectively). In nuclear sap, or material released during blending purified nuclei with 0.025 M EDTA in 0.07 M NaCl, liver, kidney and spleen also showed the presence of very similar amounts of labelled amino acids (1.95, 2.08 and 2.17 × 10⁵ cpm per g of tissue, respectively), while in thymus the level of activity was lower (1.18 × 10⁵ cpm per g of wet tissue).

If all of the actively synthesized histone variants in thymus are considered as DNA replication-dependent, the most obvious differences in the rate of synthesis between the high and the low-proliferating tissues were visible in the H4 group and in the ubiquitinated H2A (uH2A). There were no DNA replication-independent histone variants in the H4 group as identified earlier[7] and the rate of turnover of H4 histones in liver and kidney was minimal. Ubiquitinated H2A, which has maximal rate of synthesis in liver and rather high rates in other tissues as well, however, should be treated as a special case. Incorporation of labelled amino-acids into this unique semi-histone molecule in nondividing cells was mostly due to the independent turnover of ubiquitin and not the H2A histone part of the molecule.[17] Histone indicated as M1 by Zweidler[1] (because it was not clear to which family it belongs) is apparently a replication-independent or replacement variant. It was nearly absent in thymus and most prominent in liver, and it had a much higher rate of synthesis in liver than any individual H2B or H4 histones. Within the H2A family, which on this gel was separated into 6 dominant variants, those histones which are numbered as bands 5 and 6 and a minor variant 3 can be identified as DNA replication-dependent. Among variants of H3 group, those which are labelled as bands 3, 4 and 5 also are replication-dependent—they showed a high rate of synthesis in thymus and did not incorporate labelled amino acids in kidney and liver. Two major histone variants, H2B.1 and H2B.3 also showed only replication-dependent synthesis. The same was the case for H4 histone.

Discussion: On the basis of composition of histone variants, those which are more prominent in kidney and liver than in thymus (M1, H2A.4, H3.2, H3.7, H3.8, H3.9, H3.10, H2B.5 and H2B.6) cannot yet be definitely considered as DNA replication-independent. This difference in young mice may reflect the changes during tissue-specific morphogenesis. Only M1 and H3.2 can be treated as replication-independent variants, because their rate of synthesis is higher in liver than in thymus. H2B.3, which is apparently a DNA replication-dependent histone in thymus, is nevertheless more actively synthesized in liver than the replacement variants H2B.5 and H2B.6. The same is true for H2A.5, the most prominent histone in thymus and also the most prominent in liver and kidney as well. This is true also of their rate of synthesis. Liver has a complex cellular composition and specific groups of cells in liver (or in kidney) apparently have specific patterns of histone variants. However, it is difficult to attribute the high rate of H2A.5 synthesis in liver or kidney only to the presence of some mitotically active cells, because this would not explain the absence of synthesis of the major H3.3, H3.4, H3.5 and H2B.1 histone variants in the same tissues. This may mean that histones like H2A.5 and H2B.3, which are replication-dependent in proliferating tissues, continue to be synthesized and undergo turnover in nonproliferating tissues as well.

Age-Related Differences in the Composition and the Rate of Turnover of Histone Variants

The half-life of total histone in young adult mouse liver was found to be about 117 days.[10] This means that all the replication-dependent histone variants which were synthesized during active growth are still present in liver and kidney in young, 2.5-month-old, mice. For kidney, the half-life of total histone was not measured, but it is probably intermediate between brain histones (average about 159 days) and liver. Therefore, if the gradual replacement of DNA-replication-dependent variants by an entirely new set of histones really takes place, the composition and the synthesis of histones in tissues of 29-month-old mice should be markedly different.

FIGURE 2 shows the extent of the age-related changes in the composition of histone variants in different tissues. The results do not support the theory of substantial replacement of nucleosomal histones throughout the life span. Only two minor variants of the H2A and H2B groups show age-related increases in liver (H2A.8 and H2B.4), and none shows a decrease. (Sequence numbers of histone variants in this experiment do not always correspond to the same numbers in FIG. 2 because of the higher resolution of electrophoresis and the presence of brain-specific variants. Variations in resolution are usual for this method, due to various factors, and this explains some confusion among different designations of histone variants in the literature.) However, there is an obvious age-related replacement of slow moving major variants of H3 histone (H3.5 and H3.6) with more rapidly moving major variants H3.8 and H3.9. The disappearance of the slow-moving H3 histone variants is most visible in brain chromatin, probably due to the stability of cellular composition in most parts of the brain. No visible age-related changes in the pattern of histone variants occur in spleen chromatin, except in two very minor faster moving proteins in H2B group. Two H2B variants can be considered as brain-specific. Age-related increases of liver-specific acid-soluble nonhistone proteins (LSP) which is also visible, were reported earlier.[18] The presence of all the major replication-dependent histone variants and subtypes of H2A, H2B and H4 families in 29–30-month-old mouse nonproliferating tissues might indicate that they are either very stable and have much longer half-lives than earlier reported on the basis of total histone turnover rates,[10] or that they continue to be synthesized, probably at a very low rate in postmitotic nondividing cells.

FIGURE 3 shows the rate of synthesis of histone variants in different tissues of young and old mice. Some increase of the total rate of synthesis of chromatin proteins in spleen in older animals is probably linked with the known increase of the spleen proliferation activity in old animals. While the thymus undergoes atrophy in older animals, the spleen often shows signs of hypertrophy. At the same time, all of the tested tissues contained at least 20–30% lower concentrations of [³H] amino acids per g of tissue in the old group as compared with the young. The pattern of synthesis of histone variants in spleen therefore can be considered as related mostly to the replication-dependent variants. The pattern of synthesis of histone variants in liver and kidney of old mice is very similar to spleen, despite a very low rate of synthesis. Incorporation of labelled amino-acids into nucleosomal histones of liver chromatin was only about 10% of that in spleen. In brain chromatin, the incorporation of [³H] amino acids into the core histones was much lower than in liver or kidney and most of it was due to the high level of turnover of uH2A. Earlier, we found that the tissue and age-related increase of the incorporation of [³H] methionine into u2HA was linked mainly with the ubiquitin part of the molecule.[17] Among the nucleosomal histones, very low levels of synthesis were registered for H2A.1, H2A.5 and H2A.6, all of which are replication-dependent variants. Histone designated as M1 also showed low incorporation, and this is the only replication-independent protein (it is practically absent in thymus) which can be identified on the fluorographs. Incorporation of [³H] amino acids into replication-dependent histone variants in H2B and H4 groups in liver and kidney might

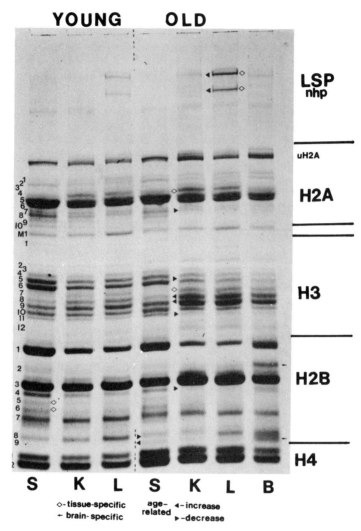

FIGURE 2. The age-related and tissue-specific variations of the composition of the core histone variants. The location of tissue-specific and age-decreasing or increasing variants and modifications are marked with special symbols. 100 μg of protein were used for each gel lane. Proteins were stained with Commassie Brilliant blue. Abbreviations: LSP, liver-specific nonhistone proteins; S, spleen; K, kidney; L, liver; B, brain. Young mice were 2.5 months old, old mice were 29 months old. Histone variants and histone modifications in each main histone groups are noted with figures on the *left side* of the gel. These figures are introduced for convenience of this study and they do not correspond to Zweidler's classification of histone variants.[1]

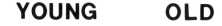

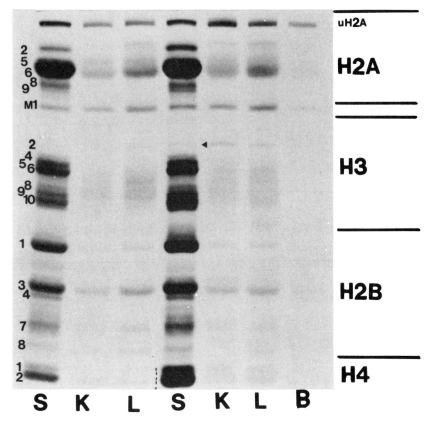

FIGURE 3. ³H fluorographs from the duplicate high resolution gel electrophoresis shown in FIGURE 2. The results show the histone variants synthesis patterns in 2.5- and 29-month-old mice. Abbreviations: S, spleen; K, kidney; L, liver; B, brain. Only one minor histone variant, H3.2, shows age-related increase of the rate of synthesis in nonproliferating tissues, kidney and liver. Fluorograph negatives show a low level synthesis of the same H2A variants in brain as in liver and kidney and synthesis of M1 and H3.2 variants. Other histone variants in brain have too low a level of incorporation of [³H] amino-acids to be visible on fluorographs even after 12 months' exposure.

be related to a few cell divisions in these tissues. In the H3 histone family, the incorporation of labelled amino-acids into the faster moving H3 variants, H3.8, H3.9 and H3.10 remained higher in older tissues than the incorporation into the slow-moving replication-dependent variants H3.5 and H3.6. This change in the

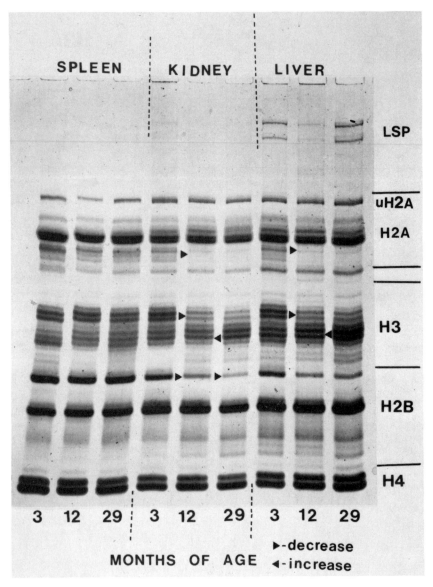

FIGURE 4. The age-related and tissue-specific variations of the composition of the core histone variants in 2.5-, 12- and 29-month-old mice. 50 μg of protein were used for each gel lane.

pattern of synthesis in the H3 histone group is the only one which reflects the replacement histone variants in the nucleosomal cores typical for young tissues with the new combination of histone variants which occurs during aging.

It was, however, important to relate these changes more clearly to senescence by comparing the composition of histone variants in young and very old mice with mice of adult mature age. FIGURE 4 shows the results of the experiment in which a comparison of the composition of histone variants in three tissues was made between young, middle age and old mice. There were no visible age-related alterations in the pattern of histone variants in spleen. Most of the histone variants in spleen and thymus apparently belong to the DNA replication-dependent group, because of high cellular proliferation activity in these tissues. FIGURE 4 shows clearly that the changes in the family of H3 histone variants starts early but also continues during the second half of the mouse life cycle (between 12 and 29 months of age). There were obvious increases of several major fast moving H3 variants in old kidney and liver. There is also an increase of the upper slow moving variant of H2B histone which continues throughout the whole life. However, this H2B variant is much more prominent in spleen and apparently belongs to the DNA replication-dependent group.

DISCUSSION AND HYPOTHESIS

The formation of highly specialized and terminally differentiated cells is related to the loss of their capability to undergo further cell division. However, cellular proliferation provides tissues not only with regeneration capacities, but also with a selective cellular turnover which allows the replacement of damaged or aged cells. In very short-lived organisms, like nematodes or insects, there are no processes of cellular replacement in adult tissues. The life span of the whole organism in such systems practically depends on aging and the death of the most sensitive groups of cells, because all cells are irreplaceable. In vertebrates, most tissues are able to replace their senescent and defective cells, either from the pool of embryonic nondifferentiated stem cells, or by the process of de-differentiation of functional cells. In the liver of some mammalian species, replacement of aged or functionally defective hepatocytes is provided by the polyploidization of the more viable remaining hepatocytes.[19,20] Regeneration and periodic replacement of some tissues and organs, such as hairs, nails, feathers, skin surface or leaves of plants, also represent the evolutionary designs and inventions which are necessary to increase the life-span potentials of individual organisms and to provide adaptation to the adverse seasonal changes. A long life span in certain species is necessary for their evolutionary survival. The possibilities of cellular turnover, regeneration, creation of redundancies of most essential functional systems or the periodic replacement of organs or tissues represent essential methods to keep individual organisms viable for many years or decades. However, there are some forms of cellular differentiation which serve functions incompatible with cellular replacement or regeneration because the loss of cells also means the loss of essential and vital information necessary for survival. Neurons are the most obvious examples of such irreplaceable cells even in long-lived organisms. The maximum life span of such cells is the same as the maximum life span of the whole organism.[21] The evolution which created cellular proliferation to keep the functional integrity of liver function, also created some still unknown molecular mechanisms of maintaining the integrity of some highly differentiated cells throughout the whole life span of individual organisms.

Similar situations exist in nondividing differentiated cells at the molecular level as well. Most macromolecules, particularly enzymes, mRNAs and tRNAs, are easily replaceable and their genes are active throughout the whole of life. Some protein and RNA molecules have shorter life spans and others are more durable, and regulation of molecular turnover rates is essential for the functional integrity of differentiated cells. However, some structural proteins in cytoplasm and nuclei, such as ribosomal proteins and nucleosomal proteins (histones and HMG proteins), probably can be replaced only together with the ribosomes and nucleosomes, but not as individual molecules. Only DNA, which stores the information necessary for cellular function and the coded messages which maintain the accuracy of the interaction and turnover of all the other molecular systems in the cells, is currently considered as irreplaceable. Damage to DNA, which is inevitable, has therefore to be repaired. But such repair in nondividing cells cannot be entirely accurate and error-free. Before a special group of replication-independent histone variants was discovered, nucleosomal histones were also often considered as proteins which can be synthesized only once, during the S-phase of the cell cycle. Highly reiterated, sequentially clustered and intronless histone genes were clearly shown to be activated only during DNA replication. At the same time many reliable studies carried out in the 1960s and 1970s showed slow turnover of histones in nondividing differentiated cells, including nerve cells. The controversy seemed to be solved by the discovery of the entirely separate and random set of individual histone genes which contain introns and are active independently of DNA replication.[5,6,11] It was assumed that these histone genes were responsible for histone turnover in nondividing cells and that the main function of this turnover is the replacement of the previously synthesized replication-dependent histone molecules, either as a type of nucleosomal repair, or as a part of the differentiation process. However, there was then no study of the pattern of histone variants and their turnover in different tissues in mature and senescent animals.

Our results, reported here, show that there is no complement of replacement histones for the original, S-phase linked set of nucleosomal core histones. Only the H3 histone group shows extensive age-related substitution of the S-phase dominant variants by the new variants. At the same time, the postmitotic turnover of histones is not restricted by the replacement variants. This suggests that there is no complete inhibition of DNA replication-dependent histone genes, and even in neurons, a very low basal level of synthesis of a few such histone variants can take place. When we started this study, our working hypothesis was based on the attempt to link age changes in chromatin to the possible inability of replacement histones to substitute for the original set of nucleosomal core histones formed only during the S-phase of the cell cycle.[22] The evolutionary conservation of the core histones and their unique clustered gene structure indicate that the DNA-histone octamer unit was designed to serve germ-cell lines from generation to generation, not just somatic cells. Switching off their synthesis in postmitotic cells and switching on the new set of genes for replication-independent histone variants looked like a possible signal for transition from morphogenesis to somatic aging. In this case, a longer life span potential could correlate with a replacement of the DNA replication-dependent histones in the nucleosomal octamer. In cells in which damaged nucleosomes are not repaired, defects in transcription should start to accumulate. The results of current studies do not seem to support this hypothesis. The replacement histones which are increasing in senescent cells are represented only by very minor variants. The main age-related transition from one group of histones (slowly moving H3 variants) to another (more rapidly moving H3 variants) occurs only in one family of histones and both groups seem to contain the replication-dependent variants. This transition occurs in all three nonproliferating tissues. This picture strongly suggests that the age-related changes in the pattern of histones which continue throughout the whole life span in nonproliferating cells are programmed. It is, however, not yet certain that this program is actually the program of aging, nor is it certain that it is relevant to the deterioration of cellular functions. The possibility, that one or another histone variant, which shows an increase in older cells, distorts or inhibits transcription, is a separate problem and requires studies with more complex experimental methods.

REFERENCES

1. ZWEIDLER, A. 1984. Core histone variants of the mouse: primary structure and differential expression. *In* Histone Genes. Structure, Organization and Regulation. G. S. Stein, J. L. Stein & W. F. Marzluff, Eds. 339–369. John Wiley & Sons. New York, NY.
2. URBAN, M. K. & Z. ZWEIDLER. 1983. Changes in nucleosomal core histone variants during chicken development and maturation. Dev. Biol. **95:** 421–428.
3. MEDVEDEV, ZH. A. & M. N. MEDVEDEVA. 1989. Changes in the composition of nucleosomal histone variants in mouse liver and other tissues related to ageing and hepatocarcinogenesis. *In* The Liver Metabolism and Ageing. K. W. Woodhouse, C. Yelland & O. F. W. James, Eds. 203–213. Eurage. Topics in Aging Research in Europe. Vol. 13. Rijswijk.
4. MEDVEDEV, ZH. A. & M. N. MEDVEDEVA. 1990. Age-related changes of the H1 and H1° histone variants in murine tissues. Exp. Gerontol. **25:** 189–200.
5. MARZLUFF, W. F. & R. A. GRAVES. 1984. Organization and expression of mouse histone genes. *In* Histone Genes. Structure, Organization and Regulation. G. S. Stein, J. L. Stein & W. F. Marzluff, Eds. 281–315. John Wiley & Sons. New York, NY.
6. WU, R. S., M. H. P. WEST & W. M. BONNER. 1984. Pattern of histone gene expression in human and other mammalian cells. *In* Histone Genes. Structure, Organization and Regulation. G. S. Stein, J. L. Stein & W. F. Marzluff, Eds. 457–483. John Wiley & Sons. New York, NY.
7. WU, R. S., H. T. PANUSZ, CH. L. HATCH & W. M. BONNER. 1986. Histones and their modifications. CRC Crit. Rev. Biochem. **20:** 210–263.
8. GENSLER, H. L. & H. BERNSTEIN. 1981. DNA damage as the primary cause of aging. Quart. Rev. Biol. **56:** 279–303.
9. MEDVEDEV, ZH. A. 1989. DNA-information and aging: the balance between alteration and repair. *In* Gerontology. D. Platt, Ed. 3–29. Springer-Verlag. Berlin, Heidelberg.
10. COMMERFORD, S. L., A. L. CARSTEN & E. P. CRONKITE. 1982. Histone turnover within non-proliferating cells. Proc. Natl. Acad. Sci. USA **79:** 1163–1165.
11. HENTSCHEL, CH. C. & M. L. BIRNSTIEL. 1981. The organization and expression of histone gene families. Cell **25:** 301–313.
12. STORER, J. B. 1966. Longevity and gross pathology at death in 22 inbred mouse strains. J. Gerontol. **21:** 404–409.
13. SCHIBLER, U. & R. A. WEBER. 1974. A new method for isolation of undergraded nuclear and cytoplasmic RNA from liver of *Xenopus laevis*. Anal. Biochem. **58:** 225–230.
14. MEDVEDEV, ZH. A., J. H. BUCHANAN, M. N. MEDVEDEVA & H. M. CROWNE. 1982. The characterisation of non-histone protein whose amounts increase in chromatin from mouse hepatocarcinomas. Int. J. Cancer **30:** 87–92.
15. WEST, M. H. P. &. W. M. BONNER. 1980. Histone 2A, a heteromorphous family of eight protein species. Biochemistry **19:** 3238–3245.
16. PLESKO, M. & R. CHALKLEY. 1986. Figure 10-14. *In* Darnell, J., H. Lodish & D. Baltimore. 1986. Molecular Cell Biology. Scientific American Books, W. H. Freeman & Company. New York, NY.

17. MEDVEDEV, ZH. A. & M. N. MEDVEDEVA. 1987. The turnover rates of the histone ubiquitin conjugates uH2A and uH2B: tissue specificity and age-related changes. Biochem. Soc. Trans. **15:** 1066–1067.
18. MEDVEDEV, ZH. A., M. N. MEDVEDEVA & H. M. CROWNE. 1984. Changes in the pattern of mouse and rat liver chromatin proteins related to ageing and development of hepatocarcinomas. *In* Pharmacological, Morphological and Physiological Aspects of Liver Aging. C. F. A. van Beooijen, Ed. 41–47. Eurage. Rijswijk.
19. BRODSKY, W. YA. & J. V. URYVAEVA. 1977. Cell polyploidy: its relation to tissue growth and function. Int. Rev. Cytol. **50:** 275–332.
20. MEDVEDEV, ZH. A. 1986. Age-related polyploidization of hepatocytes: the cause and possible role. Exp. Gerontol. **21:** 277–282.
21. CRESPO, D., B. B. STANFIELD & W. M. COWAN. 1986. Evidence that late-generated granule cells do not simply replace earlier formed neurons in the rat dentate gyrus. Exp. Brain Res. **62:** 541–548.
22. MEDVEDEV, ZH. A., M. N. MEDVEDEVA & H. M. CROWNE. 1989. Switching on synthesis of replication-independent histone variants may signal the transition from morphogenesis to somatic aging. (Abstract). *In* Book of Abstracts of the XIV International Congress of Gerontology. June 18–23, 1989. 198. Acapulco, Mexico.

DNA Processing, Aging, and Cancer

The Impact of New Technology[a]

JAN VIJG, JAN A. GOSSEN, WILJO J. F. DE LEEUW,
ERIK MULLAART,[b] P. ELINE SLAGBOOM,[b]
AND ANDRÉ G. UITTERLINDEN

Medscand Ingeny
P.O. Box 376
2280 AJ Rijswijk, The Netherlands

[b]Department of Molecular Biology
TNO Institute for Experimental Gerontology
P.O. Box 5815
2280 HV Rijswijk, The Netherlands

INTRODUCTION

DNA sequence variation, as a consequence of error-prone processing of (damaged) DNA, has been implicated in the etiology of both aging and cancer.[1-3] In this regard DNA sequence changes in both the germ line and the soma are important. For example, associations between germinal and somatic mutations are considered to play important roles in the pathogenesis of retinoblastoma and other human tumors.[4] For aging, the situation is less clear. Two-step mutations leading to homozygous deficiencies could, of course, occur at various autosomal loci in humans[5] and hence contribute to the aging phenotype. In general, it has been postulated that the accumulation in the germ line of late-acting deleterious mutations could underly the genetic component of age-related disorders, such as Alzheimer's disease.[6]

In order to obtain more fundamental insight in intrinsic mutagenesis as a significant factor in aging and cancer it is necessary to study the composition of the genome on a large scale. In this respect the rapid pace at which new techniques in molecular biology continue to emerge lend confidence that such deeper insight is within reach. We have recently initiated two new experimental approaches for studying DNA sequence variation in genomic DNA from higher animals. The first approach involves the construction of transgenic mice harboring a number of tandemly integrated shuttle vectors, each with a lacZ bacterial gene as a target for mutagenesis. Using this system we have assessed both spontaneous and induced mutation frequencies in various organs and tissues.

The second approach concerns a two-dimensional electrophoretic separation system for the analysis of restriction enzyme-digested genomic DNA from humans or experimental animals. The system uses size-separation in neutral gels, followed by denaturing gradient polyacrylamide gel separation on the basis of sequence content. Hybridization analysis using repetitive sequence probes results in high-resolution two-dimensional spot patterns. By using this system we were

[a] This work was supported by grants from the North Atlantic Treaty Organization, Senetek plc, the Dutch Ministry of Welfare and Health Affairs and the Netherlands Organization for Advancement of Pure Research.

able to follow transmission of large numbers of alleles simultaneously in human pedigrees. The use of these two novel experimental systems in studying the molecular basis of aging and cancer will be discussed.

Transgenic Mice as a Model to Study DNA Mutations

In order to be able to study induced and age-related DNA sequence changes in all cells of the body of an experimental animal, a system is required in which mutant genes can be rescued and selected among nonmutant genes from the DNA of various organs and tissues. In recent years methods have been developed to study mutagenesis in mammalian cells.[7,8] Most of these methods are limited to the *in vitro* situation and therefore do not allow comparative studies on mutation induction in various organs and tissues in the intact organism. The main difficulty in studying mutagenesis in endogenous genes of higher organisms is the lack of techniques to identify and isolate mutated DNA sequences with a high efficiency. A mammalian gene that has been used extensively as a target for both *in vivo* and *in vitro* mutagenesis studies is the gene coding for hypoxanthine phosphoribosyl transferase (HPRT). Cells mutated in this gene can be selected on the basis of their β-thioguanine resistance. The results obtained with this method suggest that the spontaneous mutation frequency in human T-lymphocytes is about 10^{-5} and increases with age.[9,10] However, the HPRT assay is laborious, limited to one or a few cell types, and may not always reflect the mutation frequency in the tissue of origin.[11]

A promising category of short-term mutagenicity assays is based on the use of so-called shuttle vectors (for a review see REF. 12). These are vectors containing a marker gene which can be introduced into mammalian cells and then retrieved ("shuttled") to bacteria to select between mutated and nonmutated marker genes. Most of the shuttle vectors described are extrachromosomally located in the nucleus,[12] although shuttle vectors which integrate in the genome have also been used.[13] The latter situation has the advantage that it more closely resembles the natural environment of mammalian endogenous genes, but widespread application has been effectively constrained by the fact that rescue of vectors integrated in the genome was very inefficient.[13]

The disadvantage of shuttle vectors for mutation analysis in mammalian cells is the often high background mutation frequency, caused by changes in the vector during transfer via the cytoplasm to the nucleus (see REF. 12 and references cited therein). In order to avoid such high background mutation levels and simultaneously extend the shuttle vector principle to the *in vivo* situation, we proposed to microinject a bacteriophage lambda shuttle vector, which contains the LacZ gene as a target for mutagenesis, into the male pronucleus of fertilized mouse oocytes.[14] LacZ encodes the enzyme β-galactosidase. Upon rescuing the vectors by *in vitro* packaging in lambda heads, the phages can be analyzed by propagation in *E. coli* LacZ in the presence of the chromogenic β-galactosidase indicator X-Gal. Mutants can be scored on the basis of absence of β-galactosidase activity (colorless plaques). The strategy as a whole is schematically depicted in FIGURE 1 and has been described previously.[14]

Accordingly, we initiated a series of experiments aimed at establishing an *in vivo* mouse model system for mutation detection in relation to aging. Thus far our attempts have resulted in a number of transgenic mouse strains harbouring the bacteriophage lambda vector gt10LacZ in one to about eighty copies in a head-to-tail arrangement in their genome.[15] This head-to-tail organization allowed us to rescue the integrated phage with high frequency by using *E. coli* C-derived packaging extracts and propagation of the phages with *E. coli* C.[16,15] By applying *in vitro* packaging using *E. coli* C, the background mutation frequency was determined in vectors isolated from genomic DNA of brain and liver of transgenic mice. The results obtained with transgenic mouse strain 20.2 indicated background mutation frequencies lower than 10^{-5}, while intraperitoneal injection of the animals with the strong mutagenic agent ethyl nitrosourea (ENU) resulted in higher mutation frequencies, that increased with the dose up until about 7×10^{-5}

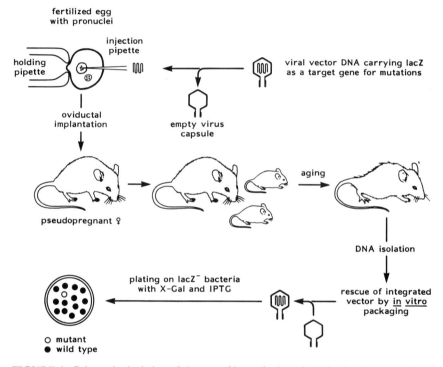

FIGURE 1. Schematic depiction of the use of bacteriophage lambda shuttle vectors integrated in the genome of (transgenic) mice for mutation analysis *in vivo*. (From Vijg and Uitterlinden.[14] Reprinted by permission from *Mechanisms of Ageing and Development*.)

for the brain at a dose of 250 mg ENU per kg bodyweight.[15] Nucleotide sequencing learned that all these mutations were G.C → A.T transitions.[15]

An important observation made during the course of this study concerns the spontaneous mutation frequency which appeared to differ among transgenic mouse strains. In strain 35.5 far higher background mutation frequencies were observed than in the other 2 strains thus far tested (TABLE 1). This phenomenon can be explained by integration of the vector-cluster in this specific strain at a site which is highly susceptible to spontaneous mutagenesis. Assuming that integration after microinjection occurs randomly, the chromosomal location of the vector-cluster, which will be different for each strain, may be an important determinant for mutation susceptibility. Alternatively, the possibility should be taken into account that integration of the vector-cluster in the genome of the founder animal of this specific strain has inactivated a gene involved in mutagenesis, for example, a DNA repair gene.

As yet our data do not allow to rule out either of these possibilities. However, an interesting observation that may help to explain the phenomenon is that all crosses among these animals resulted in female but never in male homozygous animals. This indicates that the vector-cluster in strain 35.5 is located on the X-chromosome. In addition, while Southern analysis of the vector-clusters in all other strains has thus far indicated that during mendelian inheritance rearrangement events do not occur, in 35.5 such recombinatorial activity was clearly present. FIGURE 2 shows the results of Southern analysis of a number of offspring from heterozygous 35.5 males and female mice. In about 15% of the offspring deletions of specific 3'-fragments were observed. Since in no case vector fragments were detected in the "empty" males (males that had no vector-cluster on their X-chromosome) these rearrangements probably result from pre-meiotic recombination events.

The above described phenomenon indicates that greatly enhanced mutation frequencies can occur in higher animals *in vivo*. As yet, the relevance of such high

TABLE 1. Spontaneous Mutation Frequencies in Different Transgenic Mouse Strains[a]

Strain (Organ)	Spontaneous Mutation Frequency ($\times 10^{-5}$)		
	40.6	20.2	35.5
Liver	<0.6* (4)	<0.5* (8)	10.3 ± 6.9 (14)
Brain	<0.7* (4)	<0.5* (8)	4.2 ± 3.6 (14)

[a] Mutation frequencies were measured as the ratio of colorless versus colored plaques 15. *Numbers between brackets* indicate the total number of animals tested.
* No mutants detected.

mutation frequencies for the animals in terms of survival and aging rate remains unclear until there is more insight in the underlying cause of the phenomenon. With respect to the type of the spontaneous mutations detected in the brain and liver of 35.5 mice, some preliminary data are available. In contrast to the ENU-induced mutations, the spontaneous mutations in strain 35.5 were predominantly transversions and deletions varying from 1 to about 900 bp. Thus far we have no clue as to their origin.

Whatever the precise explanation for the dramatic interstrain variations in spontaneous mutation frequencies will turn out to be, we anticipate that this newly developed transgenic mouse model system will provide new insight in both spontaneous and induced mutation in different organs and tissues in relation to aging and cancer. Indeed, DNA damage, repair and mutagenesis can now be studied in the same *in vivo* model system that will ultimately undergo the biological endpoints of this chain of molecular events.

Two-Dimensional DNA Typing

The possibility to scan large areas of the genome for DNA sequence heterogeneity is of major importance for the analysis of genetic diseases and genomic

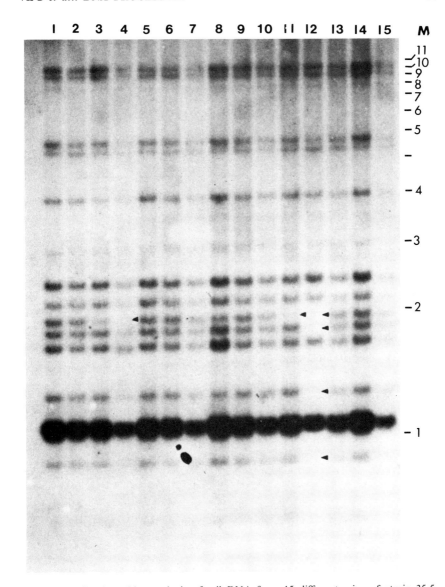

FIGURE 2. Southern blot analysis of tail DNA from 15 different mice of strain 35.5. Genomic tail DNA was digested with the restriction enzyme Dra I and subsequently subjected to agarose gel electrophoresis, alkaline blotted and hybridized to a radioactively labelled 3' bacteriophage lambda DNA fragment. In addition to the fragment containing 1.2 kb cos-site (visible as a strong band in all lanes in the autoradiogram) a number of other fragments are visible. Such fragments, which are characteristic for the integration site area in every transgenic mouse, are due to rearrangements and duplications near the 3' site of the transgene. *Arrowheads* indicate fragments that are absent in mice born from crosses between heteroxygous 35.5 males and females. (Submitted for publication.)

instabilities. Such analyses require probes that detect variable sites distributed over all chromosomes and high-resolution electrophoretic separation techniques for studying DNA restriction fragments. A recently discovered set of suitable markers are the minisatellite sequences.[17] Large numbers of highly polymorphic minisatellite or V(ariable) N(umber) of T(andem) R(epeats) are present in the genome and can be detected by Southern blot analysis. It has been demonstrated that so-called core probes derived from minisatellites can be used to simultaneously detect a large number of hyperpolymorphic VNTR loci, dispersed throughout the genome, to provide genetic "fingerprints" of human individuals.[17] Core sequences have been successfully applied in the analysis of tumours for genetic instability.[18] Such applications rely on the resolution of Southern blot hybridization analysis, which is based on the gel electrophoretic separation of genomic DNA restriction fragments according to size.[19] The limiting factor in the presently available techniques for the detection of DNA sequence variation in the human genome is the low resolution of Southern blot analysis. One-dimensional separation of DNA fragments allows only about 30 hypervariable minisatellite fragments to be resolved.[17,20]

Recently, a protocol for two-dimensional DNA typing has been developed in our laboratory with a resolution high enough to analyse virtually all VNTR loci in the genome of an individual within a limited amount of experimental time.[20] This technique is based on the separation in two dimensions of restriction enzyme digests of genomic DNA.[21] The first dimension consists of a separation according to size in a neutral polyacrylamide gel and the second dimension involves a separation according to base pair composition in a polyacrylamide gel containing a gradient of denaturants. After electrophoresis, the separation patterns are transferred to nylon membranes and hybridized using one or more minisatellite core sequences as probe(s). We anticipate that this protocol will be useful in two major areas of the molecular genetics of aging: (a) the identification and isolation of aging and longevity genes and (b) the study of somatic DNA instabilities in relation to aging and cancer. The latter application was discussed earlier.[22] Here we shall mainly focus on the potential application of this technique in studying the hereditary component of aging and age-related disorders.

Genetics of Aging and Disease

Molecular biological research on aging is severely hindered by the lack of information with respect to the identity of aging and longevity genes. The identification, isolation and characterization of such genes is important to reveal primary aging and anti-aging processes.[23] Unfortunately, due to the multifactorial nature of aging and the relatively large size of the human genome there is as yet no other than circumstantial evidence for the existence of aging and longevity genes in the human population (see, for example, REF. 24). Even in the case of lower organisms, which with their relatively small genomes and short life spans are easy to manipulate, it is only very recently that some progress has been made in showing the importance of genes in modulating life span.[25] For humans, with a haploid genome of about 3 billion base pairs of DNA, there is no firm evidence with respect to genes that influence intrinsic aging processes. The situation is slightly better for genes that are involved in diseases associated with the aging process, such as Alzheimer's disease. With respect to this disease, neither its precise relationship with the aging process, nor its level of genetic heterogeneity is known. There is, however, abundant evidence that a gene near the centromere of chromosome 21 is involved.[26] On the basis of genetic syndromes characterized by dementia and/or certain types of degenerative neuropathology, Martin calculated that as many as 2350 genes could be involved in brain aging alone.[27]

In principle, allelic variations in the human population that predispose to age-related disease or accelerate or retard intrinsic aging processes can be mapped by linkage analysis (for a review, see REF. 28). Linkage analysis has been successfully applied to map monogenic disorders by using well defined pedigrees. Unfortunately, the application of such an approach to map genes involved in multifactorial diseases or, for that matter, the genes involved in aging and longevity is not feasible with the technology currently available. A great leap forward is the present attempt to generate detailed linkage maps of the human genome.[29,30] In

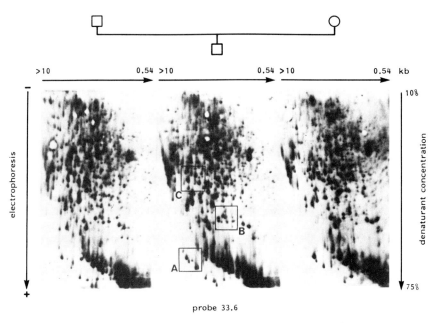

probe 33.6

FIGURE 3A. Two-dimensional DNA fingerprint analysis of Hae III digested genomic DNA from three members of a human pedigree, using probe 33.6.[20] (From Uitterlinden *et al.*[20] Reprinted by permission from the National Academy of Sciences.)

addition, new strategies have recently been proposed to increase mapping efficiency for determining the location and number of genes that condition quantitative traits.[31,32]

In combination with such new developments in evaluating large amounts of genetic information, methods are required that allow the simultaneous analysis of large numbers of polymorphic genetic loci. It occurred to us that two-dimensional DNA typing could be extremely useful for that purpose. The suitability of 2-D DNA analysis in genetic studies on humans is demonstrated in FIGURE 3, showing the results of the analysis of 3 members of a pedigree (mother, father and a son). For optimal comparisons a 30 cm-wide version of the gel apparatus originally described by Fischer and Lerman[21] was constructed and used in these experi-

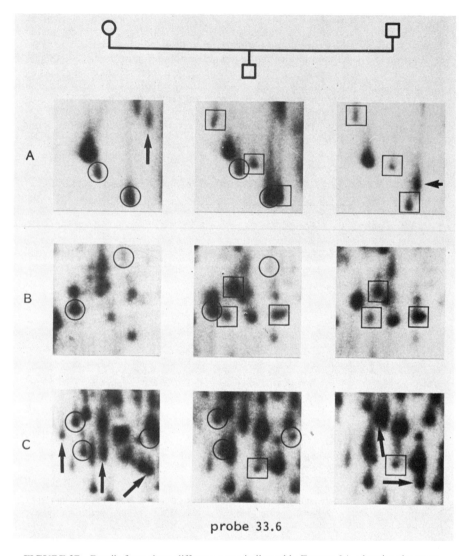

probe 33.6

FIGURE 3B. Details from three different areas indicated in FIGURE 3A, showing the transmission of particular spot polymorphisms. O mark maternal fragments and [ ] mark paternal fragments. *Arrows* indicate nontransmitted polymorphic fragments. (From Uitterlinden *et al.*[20] Reprinted by permission from the National Academy of Sciences.)

ments so that up to 6 individuals could be compared on one denaturing gradient gel. Close inspection and comparison of individual spot patterns of the two parents obtained with probe 33.6 (FIG. 3A) revealed a total number of 569 spots for the father, 607 for the mother and 625 for the son. Between the two parents 150 spot polymorphisms were observed, 105 (= 70%) of which were transmitted to the son (52 of maternal and 53 of paternal origin). Details of the separation pattern are shown in FIGURE 3B. For a more extensive discussion of these results, see REF-ERENCE 20.

An important aspect of the above described 2-D DNA typing system is that DNA fragments that migrate into a denaturing gradient gel start melting at the region containing the lowest-melting domain. Since most minisatellite sequences (and many other repeats as well) contain relatively many stable G and C base-pairs, the lowest melting domain of the DNA fragments resolved in this system is likely to be in the regions that flank the tandem repeats detected by the core probes. Indeed, from experiments in which Hinf I-digested genomic DNAs from a number of randomly selected human individuals were subjected to electrophoresis in denaturing gradient gels followed by hybridization with locus-specific VNTR probes, it became clear that in spite of the large allelic size-differences (see SBA in FIG. 4) all fragments had migrated to the same isotherm (see DGGE in FIG. 4). This phenomenon can be explained by assuming that the lowest melting domain in the genomic DNA fragments generated by Hinf I is not the minisatellite

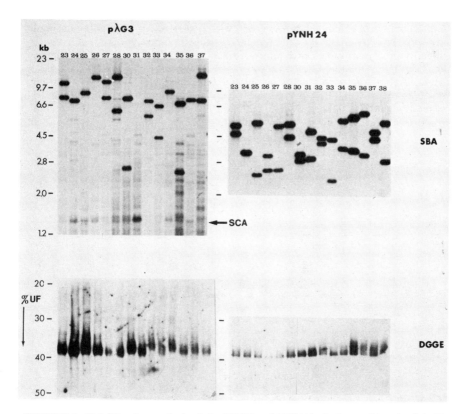

FIGURE 4. Hybridization analysis of the D7S22 and D2S44 loci, detected by plambdaG3 and pYNH24, respectively, in genomic DNA from 14 unrelated individuals. Genomic DNA was digested with Hinf I and separated in a neutral agarose gel (SBA) and in a denaturing gradient gel (DGGE). Results for pYNH were obtained by rehybridizing the filters used for the plambdaG3 hybridization. SCA = short common allele detected by plambdaG3. (From Uitterlinden and Vijg.[33] Reprinted by permission from *Electrophoresis*.)

part, but one of the flanking sequences, which are identical among different individuals.[33]

The locus-specific migration of VNTR alleles in denaturing gradient gels could become an important factor in the identification of the different (polymorphic) spots in a 2-D DNA separation pattern as alleles from specific loci. Such identification is important for the use of the system in linkage analysis. Indeed, it may ultimately become possible to generate 2-D DNA patterns that consist of polymorphic marker loci at regularly spaced intervals. Information as to the loci of origin of the different spots can be stored in the computer and used as reference values in large-scale linkage studies.[34] Automatic comparison can be realized by image analysis of the spot patterns.[34]

Before such "total genome scanning" can become reality it is necessary to first assure complete coverage of the genome by polymorphic markers. In this respect polymorphic minisatellites are not sufficient as sole sources of markers, since these repeat families are clustered at the telomeres. However, besides 33.6, 33.15 and other minisatellite core sequences other polymorphic repeats can be used, such as simple sequence motifs.[35] FIGURE 5 shows a 2-D DNA separation pattern of human genomic DNA digested with Hae III and probed with the simple sequence motif (CAC)n. As can be seen, hybridization patterns are much comparable to the ones obtained with minisatellite core probes, while simple sequences are even more polymorphic.[36]

A different approach employing the highly repeated element Alu as a marker, involves the use of PCR (polymerase chain reaction) amplification. When 2-D separation patterns of human total genomic DNA are directly probed with Alu the result is a smear, which is probably due to the large number of copies (about

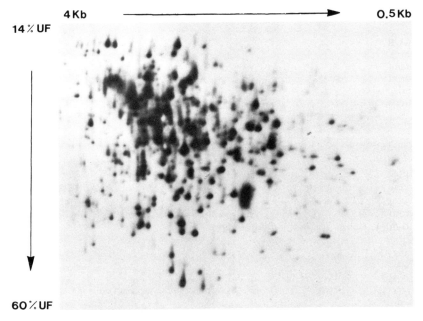

4 Kb ──────────────────────────▶ **0.5 Kb**

14 % UF

60 % UF

FIGURE 5. Hybridization analysis of a 2-D separation pattern of Hae III-digested human total genomic DNA, using the simple sequence motif (CAC)n as a core probe.

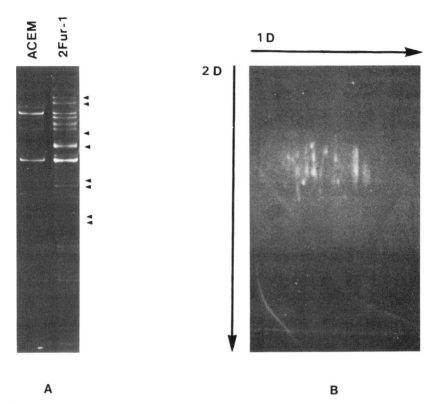

FIGURE 6. (A) One-dimensional size separation by PAAGE of inter-Alu PCR products from 2 hybrid cell lines ACEM and 2Fu^r-1 using primer TC65.[37] By comparison of the banding patterns of the 2 hybrids, specific inter-Alu fragments could be regionally mapped (indicated by *arrowheads*). **(B)** Two-dimensional separation of inter-Alu PCR products from hybrid cell line 7253X6, containing 21q, Yp and a small portion of chromosome 5 (Dr. D. Patterson, Denver, CO, personal communication).

1,000,000) and/or the unfavourable separation characteristics of Alu-containing DNA fragments (unpublished results). However, by using Alu-specific primers it is possible to amplify so-called inter-Alu regions, that is, regions that lie in between 2 Alu repeat elements in reverse or direct orientation. By applying this principle, which was first described by Nelson *et al.*,[37] we were able to generate chromosome 21-specific 2-D DNA separation patterns. FIGURE 6 shows one- and two-dimensional separation patterns of the products obtained from inter-Alu PCRs on human-hamster hybrid cell lines, containing parts of the human chromosome 21. The primers used in the reaction do not cross-hybridize with hamster DNA and were chosen in a way that only those regions in between 2 Alu's in inversed orientation were amplified. We now have evidence that the inter-Alu fragments detected are polymorphic in the human population, which is in agreement with recent data from Economou *et al.*[38]

The above results provide ample evidence that genome coverage by 2-D DNA typing is within reach by using selected probes for repetitive sequence elements.

By using the inter-Alu approach it should even be possible to generate chromo-some-specific 2-D DNA separation patterns of total human genomic DNA.

ACKNOWLEDGMENTS

We thank Mr. A. Verwest and Ms. I. Meulenbelt for technical assistance, and Dr. D. Patterson (Denver, CO) for generously providing the human-hamster hybrid cell line DNAs.

REFERENCES

1. BURNET, F. M. 1974. Intrinsic Mutagenesis: A Genetic Approach to Aging. MTP Medical and Technical Publishing. Lancaster.
2. HANAWALT, P. C. & A. SARASIN. 1986. Cancer prone hereditary diseases with DNA processing abnormalities. Trends Genet. 2: 124–129.
3. VIJG, J. & D. L. KNOOK. 1987. DNA repair in relation to the aging process. J. Am. Geriatr. Soc. 35: 532–541.
4. HANSEN, M. F. & W. K. CAVENEE. 1988. Tumor suppressors: Recessive mutations that lead to cancer. Cell 53: 172–173.
5. HAKODA, M., K. NISHIOKA & N. KAMATANI. 1990. Homozygous deficiency at autosomal locus aprt in human somatic cells in vivo induced by two different mechanisms. Cancer Res. 50: 1738–1741.
6. KIRKWOOD, T. B. L. 1989. DNA, mutations and aging. Mutat. Res. 219: 1–7.
7. LEHMAN, A. R. 1985. Use of recombinant DNA techniques in cloning DNA repair genes and in the study of mutagenesis in mammalian cells. Mutat. Res. 150: 61–67.
8. VIJG, J. 1990. DNA sequence changes in aging: How frequent, how important? Aging 2: 105–123.
9. ALBERTINI, R. J., J. P. O'NEILL, J. A. NICKLAS, N. H. HEINTZ & P. C. KELLEHER. 1985. Alterations of the HPRT gene in human in vivo-derived 6-thioguanine-resistant T lymphocytes. Nature (London) 316: 369–371.
10. TRAINOR, K. J., D. J. WIGMORE, A. CHRYSOSTOMOU, J. L. DEMPSEY, R. SESHADRI & A. A. MORLEY. 1984. Mutation frequency in human lymphocytes increases with age. Mech. Ageing Dev. 27: 83–86.
11. FEATHERSTONE, T., P. D. MARSHALL & H. J. EVANS. 1987. Problems and pitfalls in assessing human T-lymphocyte mutant frequencies. Mutat. Res. 179: 215–230.
12. DUBRIDGE, R. B. & M. P. CALOS. 1988. Recombinant shuttle vectors for the study of mutation in mammalian cells. Mutagenesis 3: 1–9.
13. GLAZER, P. M., S. N. SARKAR & W. C. SUMMERS. 1986. Detection and analysis of UV-induced mutations in mammalian cell DNA using a lambda phage shuttle vector. Proc. Natl. Acad. Sci. USA 83: 1041–1044.
14. VIJG, J. & A. G. UITTERLINDEN. 1987. A search for DNA alterations in the aging mammalian genome: An experimental strategy. Mech. Ageing Dev. 41: 47–63.
15. GOSSEN, J. A., W. J. F. DE LEEUW, C. H. T. TAN, E. C. ZWARTHOFF, F. BERENDS, P. H. M. LOHMAN, D. L. KNOOK & J. VIJG. 1989. Efficient rescue of integrated shuttle vectors from transgenic mice: A new model for studying mutations in vivo. Proc. Natl. Acad. Sci. USA 86: 7971–7975.
16. GOSSEN, J. A. & J. VIJG. 1988. E. coli C: A convenient host strain for rescue of highly methylated DNA. Nucleic Acids Res. 16: 9343.
17. JEFFREYS, A. J., V. WILSON & S. L. THEIN. 1985. Hypervariable 'minisatellite' regions in human DNA. Nature (London) 314: 67–73.
18. THEIN, S. L., A. J. JEFFREYS, H. C. GOOI, F. COTTER, J. FLINT, N. T. J. O'CONNOR, O. J. WEATHERALL & J. S. WAINSCOAT. 1987. Detection of somatic changes in human cancer DNA by DNA fingerprint analysis. Br. J. Cancer 55: 353–356.

19. SOUTHERN, E. M. 1975. Detection of specific sequences among DNA fragments separated by gel electrophoresis. J. Mol. Biol. **98:** 503–517.
20. UITTERLINDEN, A. G., P. E. SLAGBOOM, D. L. KNOOK & J. VIJG. 1989. Two-dimensional DNA fingerprinting of human individuals. Proc. Natl. Acad. Sci. USA **86:** 2742–2746.
21. FISCHER, S. G. & L. S. LERMAN. 1979. Length-independent separation of DNA restriction fragments in two-dimensional gel electrophoresis. Cell **16:** 191–200.
22. VIJG, J., J. A. GOSSEN, P. E. SLAGBOOM & A. G. UITTERLINDEN. 1990. New methods for the detection of DNA sequence variation: Applications on molecular genetic studies on aging. *In* Molecular Biology of Aging. C. E. Finch & T. E. Johnson, Eds. UCLA Symposia on Molecular and Cellular Biology New Series. Vol. **123:** 103–119. Wiley-Liss. New York, NY.
23. VIJG, J. & J. PAPACONSTANTINOU. 1990. Aging and longevity genes: strategies for identifying DNA sequences controlling life span. J. Gerontol. **45:** B179–182.
24. SACHER, G. A. 1982. Evolutionary theory in gerontology. Perspect. Biol. Med. **25:** 339–353.
25. JOHNSON, T. E. 1987. Aging can be genetically dissected into component processes using long-lived lines of Caenorhabditis elegans. Proc. Natl. Acad. Sci. USA **84:** 3777–3781.
26. TANZI, R. E., P. H. ST GEORGE-HYSLOP & J. F. GUSELLA. 1989. Molecular genetic approaches to Alzheimer's disease. TINS **12:** 152.
27. MARTIN, G. M. & E. M. BRYANT. 1988. Genetics of aging and of disease models. *In* Aging and the Brain. R. D. Terry, Ed. Raven Press. New York, NY.
28. WHITE, R. & C. T. CASKEY. 1988. The human as an experimental system in molecular genetics. Science **240:** 1483–1488.
29. WHITE, R., M. LEPPERT, D. T. BISHOP, D. BARKER, J. BERKOWITZ *et al.* 1985. Construction of linkage maps with DNA markers for human chromosomes. Nature **313:** 101–105.
30. DONIS-KELLER, H. and 32 others. 1987. A genetic linkage map of the human genome. Cell **51:** 319–337.
31. PATERSON, A. H., E. S. LANDER, J. D. HEWITT, S. PETERSON, S. E. LINCOLN & S. D. TANKSLEY. 1988. Resolution of quantitative traits into Mendelian factors by using a complete linkage map of restriction fragment length polymorphisms. Nature **335:** 721–726.
32. LANDER, E. S. & D. BOTSTEIN. 1989. Mapping Mendelian factors underlying quantitative traits using RFLP linkage maps. Genetics **121:** 185–199.
33. UITTERLINDEN, A. G. & J. VIJG. 1990. Denaturing gradient gel electrophoretic analysis of minisatellite alleles. Electrophoresis. In press.
34. UITTERLINDEN, A. G. & J. VIJG. 1989. Two-dimensional DNA typing. Tibtech **7:** 336–341.
35. TAUTZ, D., M. TRICK & G. DOVER. 1986. Cryptic simplicity in DNA is a major source of genetic variation. Nature **322:** 652–656.
36. NÜRNBERG, P., L. ROEWER, H. NEITZEL, K. SPERLING, A. POPPERL, J. HUNDRIESER, H. PÖCHER, C. EPPLEN, H. ZISCHLER & J. T. EPPLEN. 1989. DNA fingerprinting with the oligonucleotide probe (CAC)5/(GTG)5: somatic stability and germline mutations. Hum. Genet. **84:** 75–78.
37. NELSON, D. L., S. A. LEDBETTER, L. CORBO, M. F. VICTORIA, R. RAMIREZ-SOLIS, T. D. WEBSTER, D. H. LEDBETTER & C. T. CASKEY. 1989. Alu polymerase chain reaction: A method for rapid isolation of human-specific sequences from complex DNA sources. Proc. Natl. Acad. Sci. USA **86:** 6686–6690.
38. ECONOMOU, E. P., A. W. BERGEN, A. C. WARREN & S. E. ANTONARAKIS. 1990. The polydeoxyadenylate tract of Alu repetitive elements is polymorphic in the human genome. Proc. Natl. Acad. Sci. USA **87:** 2951–2954.

The Effect of Aging on Constitutive mRNA Levels and Lipopolysaccharide Inducibility of Acute Phase Genes[a]

DAVID J. POST,[b,c] KENNETH C. CARTER,[b,d] AND
JOHN PAPACONSTANTINOU[b,e,f]

[b]Department of Human Biological Chemistry and Genetics
University of Texas Medical Branch

and

[e]Shriners Burns Institute
Galveston Unit
Galveston, Texas 77550

INTRODUCTION

Current theories invoke that aging consists of many intrinsic processes characterized by progressive declines in tissue functions and that these age-associated characteristics occur in the absence of disease.[1] Although evidence supports the concept of intrinsic aging as a natural process, it has been difficult to clearly separate the natural intrinsic processes of aging from disease or toxic response due to environmental factors, that enhance the characteristics of aging. Eukaryotic organisms possess natural defence mechanisms associated with their responses to injury, inflammation and pollutants. One of these, the acute phase host response, is characterized by a series of hepatic physiological reactions triggered by factors released as a result of inflammation or tissue injury and is believed to be the mechanism by which cells and tissues are protected against further damage and injury.[2–4] We propose that the acute phase response represents a series of intrinsic processes and interactions that may be affected by aging. More specifically it is our hypothesis that components of eukaryotic gene regulatory processes may be intrinsic processes affected by aging and that this could be the basis for either reduced or increased gene expression associated with aging. On the basis of this hypothesis we have initiated studies to assess the acute phase response as a potential model system to determine how intrinsic processes involving gene regulation might be affected by aging. Because the regulatory processes

[a] This research supported by grants to John Papaconstantinou from the Shriners Burns Institute, Galveston Texas Unit, Galveston, Texas 77550, and from the National Institutes of Health.
[c] Present address: Department of Chemistry, Texas A & M University, College Station, Texas 77843.
[d] Present address: Department of Cell Biology, University of Massachusetts Medical School, Worcester, Massachusetts.
[f] Address for correspondence: John Papaconstantinou, Ph.D., Department of H.B.C. & G., F-43, The University of Texas Medical Branch, Galveston, Texas 77550.

66

of the acute phase response have been extensively studied this system facilitates studies of how aging may affect the regulation of a diverse family of genes that carry out vital functions. Furthermore, this gene family exhibits a high degree of tissue specificity (*i.e.,* liver specificity) which facilitates studies of the effect of aging on the regulation of gene expression in a differentiated tissue. In these studies we have examined the effect of aging on the constitutive mRNA levels of α_1-acid glycoprotein (AGP), α_1-antitrypsin (AT), and albumin. We have also examined the effect of aging on the ability of these genes to respond to bacterial lipopolysaccharide (LPS). The regulation of these acute phase protein genes involves gene activation and repression, as well as the stabilization of mRNA. Furthermore, protein factors that interact with cis-acting sequences to regulate transcription or mRNA levels (potential stabilization factors) have been reported. In this study we present preliminary data to indicate that aging may affect the constitutive level of expression as well as the regulatory processes that mediate either positive or negative responses to inflammatory agents.

MATERIALS AND METHODS

Total liver RNA was isolated by the method of Chirgwin *et al.*[5] Isolated RNA was electrophoresed (12 μg/lane) in formaldehyde agarose gels[6] and transferred to nitrocellulose filters.[7] Filters were hybridized with ^{32}P-labelled RNA probes prepared from cDNA clones in T7, T3 RNA polymerase vectors.[8,9] Filters were audioradiographed and hybridized bands were cut out and analyzed by liquid scintillation spectrometry. Data are reported as a percentage of a noninduced control included on every filter.

RESULTS

The relationship of aging and its effects on the expression of the acute phase reactant genes has been of considerable interest to us because of the role that the products of these genes have in wound healing, *i.e.,* protection against damage and injury due to inflammation. Since genes of the acute phase reactant family exhibit both positive and negative regulatory responses to mediators of the inflammation response, and since some of their mRNAs exhibit high levels of stability, we believe that these genes provide models for specific regulatory processes and how these processes may be affected by aging. Furthermore, many of the genes exhibit strict tissue specificity so that they also serve as excellent models to study how aging may affect factors that regulate tissue-specific gene expression. Thus, within the acute phase reactant family we find genes that respond to a variety of signals that mediate the acute phase response as well as liver-specific gene expression.

Male Balb/c mice of four different ages were injected with LPS to induce inflammation. At specific time intervals following injection the mice were sacrificed and the AT, AGP, and albumin mRNA levels were determined. The amount of constitutive and inflammation-induced mRNA for each gene was then compared between the mice of various ages. Additionally, the time course of induction for each gene was compared between young (2 month) and old (24 month) animals. The pattern of expression for each mRNA is discussed below.

Effect of Aging on α_1-AT mRNA Levels

The marked decrease in constitutive AT mRNA levels in older animals (FIG. 1A), is the most striking and perhaps the most physiologically relevant age-associated change in the liver because of the potential damaging effects reduced AT levels may have on the ability of the lung to respond to inflammation or pollution. AT, which is a principle protease inhibitor, is essential for the control of elastase activity in the alveoli of the lungs during inflammation.[10] AT deficiency is associated with both lung[11] and liver[12] diseases and the genetic AT deficiency is known to be the major cause of emphysema in humans.[13,14] During acute inflammation in

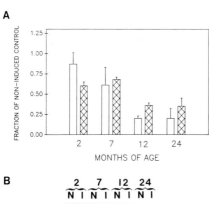

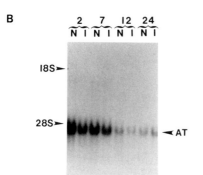

FIGURE 1. A comparison of the α_1-antitrypsin mRNA levels in the livers of 2-, 7-, 12-, and 24-month-old Balb/c mice. (**A**) The *open bars* represent the constitutive levels of AT mRNA. The *cross-hatched bars* represent the levels of AT mRNA 24 hours after treatment with LPS. (**B**) A Northern analysis showing the levels of AT mRNA in control (N) and LPS-induced (I) mouse livers. The LPS-induced samples were prepared 24 hours after the administration of LPS.

humans and rats, AT levels in serum increase two- to fourfold,[13,15] but corresponding increases in mRNA levels have not been reported. In this study, constitutive mRNA levels which are abundant in the mouse liver were reduced in 2-month-old mice by LPS injection, an effect that has not been reported previously and which we also observed in other mouse strains (data not shown). Constitutive levels of AT mRNA were reduced 77 percent between 2 and 12 months of age, but were unchanged between 12 and 24 months. No significant change in mRNA levels occurred with LPS treatment of 7- or 24-month-old animals, and a slight increase was observed following LPS injection of 12-month-old animals (FIG. 1A and B). The time course of AT mRNA expression during LPS treatment of 2-month-old mice shows a significant repression as early as 3 hours after injection (FIG. 2) with return to normal levels by 48 hours (data not shown). Expression of AT in 24-month-old mice was not significantly changed by LPS treatment (FIG. 2).

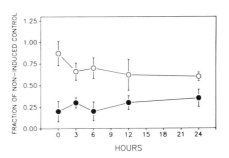

FIGURE 2. The effect of LPS on the α_1-antitrypsin mRNA levels in the livers of 2- and 24-month-old Balb/c mice. mRNA samples were prepared at 0, 3, 6, 12, and 24 hours after LPS injection from 2- (-○-) and 24-month-old (-●-) mice.

The significant reduction in AT mRNA levels in the livers of aged animals could result in reduced serum AT levels (not tested) and the availability of AT in the alveolar areas of the lung. If this is the case, then the ability of aged animals to respond to lung inflammation or respiratory pollutants may be severely impaired and may be a factor in the "increased sensitivity" of aged animals and humans to insults to the lung.

Effect of Aging on AGP mRNA Levels

Although the biological function of AGP is not clearly understood, several investigators have suggested that this serum glycoprotein may function in suppression of the immune response during the early stages of the acute phase response.[16,17] AGP has a relatively low level of constitutive expression in the young adult, but the mRNA and protein levels are strongly induced by acute phase stimulation in humans, rats, and mice.[15,18–20] In the young adult mouse (2 months old), constitutive mRNA levels are very low and the gene is strongly and rapidly induced (10- to 100-fold) by LPS and other acute phase stimulants (FIG. 3A and

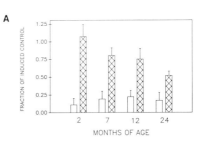

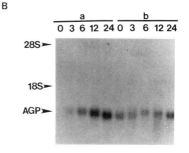

FIGURE 3. A comparison of the α_1-acid glycoprotein mRNA levels in the livers of 2-, 7-, 12-, and 24-month-old Balb/c mice. The RNA samples are the same as those used for the AT mRNA analyses shown in FIGURE 1A and 1B.

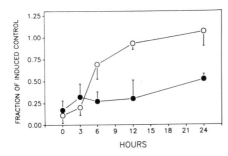

FIGURE 4. The effect of LPS on the induction of the α_1-acid glycoprotein mRNA levels in the livers of 2- and 24-month-old Balb/c mice. The mRNA samples are the same as those used for the AT mRNA analyses shown in FIGURE 2.

B). However, it was observed in older mice that the gene exhibits a significantly reduced level of induction by LPS and by 24 months the ability to respond was reduced by 50 percent. The time course of induction indicates that the lag period was significantly extended and that the peak of mRNA level, normally reached by 12 hours after stimulation was not achieved even after 24 hours (FIG. 4). It has been reported that constitutive AGP protein levels increase in elderly humans[21] and constitutive mRNA levels increase slightly in rats.[22] The data presented in our studies indicate an increasing trend in the constitutive AGP mRNA pool although it is minimal.

Effect of Aging on Albumin mRNA Levels

Analysis of the constitutive levels of albumin mRNA pool in aged mice revealed that as with AT, there is a marked age-associated decrease. The constitu-

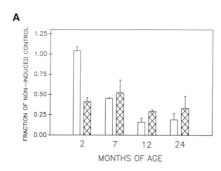

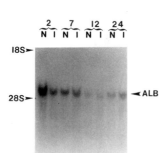

FIGURE 5. A comparison of the albumin mRNA levels in the livers of 2-, 7-, 12-, and 24-month-old Balb/c mice. The mRNA samples are the same as those used for the AT mRNA analyses shown in FIGURE 1A and 1B.

tive levels of albumin mRNA in the livers of young adult mice (2 months) are highly abundant, and in aged animals the mRNA levels are sharply reduced (FIG. 5). Similar observations were made for AT mRNA levels (reported above), which is another high abundance liver specific mRNA. There are, therefore, several regulatory mechanisms that could account for this reduction in albumin (and AT) mRNA levels. These include a reduction in the rate of transcription, alteration or defective processing of the primary transcript, or the change in stability of mRNA. Further analyses to localize the site of regulation affected by aging are in progress.

Albumin is a negatively regulated acute phase protein because its constitutive mRNA and protein levels are reduced during acute phase stimulation.[15,19,23,24] In this study, injection of LPS caused a 60-percent reduction in mRNA levels at 24 hours in 2-month-old mice; however, at 7,12, and 24 months in addition to the significant drop in constitutive mRNA levels no negative response or down regulation was observed (FIG. 5) as indicated by reduced mRNA levels. A comparison of the time courses of induction in 2- versus 24-month-old mice again indicated a decrease in albumin mRNA in 2-month-old mice, but no effect in aged animals (24 months) (FIG. 6). In rats, constitutive albumin and mRNA levels are reported to

FIGURE 6. The effect of LPS on the negative regulation of the albumin mRNA levels in the livers of 2- and 24-month-old Balb/c mice. The mRNA samples are the same as those used for the AT mRNA analyses shown in FIGURE 2.

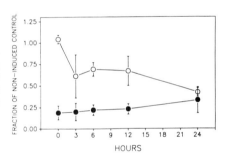

increase with age;[29] however, protein levels in humans have been reported to decrease with age.[21] According to the data presented here, aged mice not only have reduced constitutive levels of albumin mRNA, but have also lost the ability to repress or downregulate albumin mRNA levels during acute phase stimulation. This does not necessarily mean that the level of transcription has changed, since a similar effect could result from alterations in either processing or changes in mRNA stability. Further identification of the regulatory site affected by aging depends upon the measurement of both rates of transcription and mRNA stability. These experiments are in progress.

DISCUSSION

Our studies and those from other laboratories indicate that age-associated changes of gene expression can affect both the constitutive level of gene expression as well as the regulation of gene(s) by various hormonal and growth factors.[22,25-35] Although there are many indications of the age-associated deregulation of gene expression in various tissues, in this discussion we shall limit ourselves to these events in aged liver cells (for references to other tissues see REFS. 36–41).

The Effect of Aging on the Constitutive mRNA Levels

The first point we wish to discuss is the effect of aging on the constitutive level of tissue-specific gene expression as indicated by changes in the levels of mRNA pools. In the young adult mouse (2 months) the constitutive levels of both AT and albumin mRNAs are of high abundance, whereas in the aged animal these mRNA levels are severely reduced. These observations indicate that transcription, mRNA processing, or mRNA stability may be the regulatory sites affected by aging and an alteration of either of these regulatory processes could account for the establishment of a new steady state level of each mRNA. Alteration of transcription could be due to age-associated changes in chromatin structure, and more specifically in the function or levels of trans-acting factors. Recent studies have clearly demonstrated that both albumin[42,43] and AT[44,45] promoters have binding sites for several of the same liver-specific trans-acting factors. Therefore, if the reduced albumin and AT levels are due to altered levels of transcription, one possible mechanism could involve an alteration of the binding capacity of one or more of the trans-acting factors that bind to the promoters and/or enhancers of these genes. If this occurs with a factor shared by both promoters, this would explain the reduced level of both mRNAs, and would also point to the possibility that other genes that share these factors may be affected by aging. Recent studies in our laboratory indicate that the trans-acting factor C/EBP is reduced in aged nuclear extract (Alam and Papaconstantinou, in preparation). Furthermore, both albumin and AT promoters are known to have C/EBP binding sites.[42–45] Whether this affects the transcription of these genes in aged animals is presently being investigated. Another important point to stress here is that an age-associated change in either positive or negative trans-acting factors that are shared by several genes, whose only common characteristic is tissue specificity, may be the basis for an age-associated increase or decrease in the constitutive level of expression of various tissue-specific genes.

Alternatively, the level of these mRNAs may be regulated in aged liver cells by factors associated with mRNA processing or stability of mRNA. There are studies which indicate that the stability of mRNAs is mediated by proteins that bind to the mRNA.[46–49] mRNAs *in vivo* are associated with specific proteins to form ribonucleoprotein complexes (mRNPs). It has been suggested that these RNA-binding proteins may function to modulate aspects of mRNA stability or translation. Recent studies have indicated that the poly(A)-binding protein is a positive regulator of translation.[47] There are, however, other proteins of the mRNP particles that bind to various regions of the mRNA whose function may involve the stability of mRNAs.

It is well known that labile mRNAs such as those that code for cytokines and various oncogenes contain an AU-rich sequence in the 3' untranslated region that confers instability *in vivo*.[50–52] These sites are recognition signals for specific, rapid mRNA degradation. Thus, labile mRNAs possess structural features that confer instability. Since mRNPs are complex structures it is possible that there are proteins that may confer stability on specific mRNAs.

The alternative situation is seen in mRNAs such as β-globin or albumin which are very stable. These mRNAs do not contain the AU-rich instability sequences. The question that is relevant to our observations on age-effects is whether there are mRNA-binding proteins that confer stability on these stable mRNAs. In general, therefore, an important aspect of understanding new steady state levels of mRNAs (and proteins) associated with aging may revolve around understanding the roles of specific structures or sequences in the mRNA and mRNA-binding proteins in controlling mRNA turnover. If aging affects the levels of these proteins, then it would be expected that the turnover of the mRNA may be altered, and new steady state levels are established. Furthermore, if the gene(s) of this (these) protein(s) is affected by aging, then the mRNAs that contain the binding sites would be "singled out" for age-associated changes in their steady state levels.

The AGP, AT, and albumin mRNAs in our studies, as well as T-kininogen mRNA levels in studies elsewhere are examples of the age-associated changes in constitutive tissue specific mRNA levels. Both the T-kininogen and AGP genes which are expressed solely in liver and macrophages are positive acute phase reactants whose mRNA levels accumulate dramatically during an acute phase response,[3,19,53] and return to their normal constitutive levels within 48 hours of the stimulus. In aged animals the T-kininogen constitutive mRNA level increases significantly in the absence of an acute phase stimulus (approximately 8-fold). The constitutive level of mouse AGP mRNA also increases, albeit slightly (approx. 1.5-fold), in aged animals. These observations indicate that constitutive mRNA levels of certain genes increase in the apparent absence of signals involved in the acute phase response. Furthermore, there is ample documentation from other studies that aging can effect either an increase (or decrease as discussed below) in the steady state levels of various specific mRNAs. These specific effects can be explained by alterations in regulatory events that affect transcription, RNA processing and/or stability of mRNA. In the case of T-kininogen and AGP, there is evidence that aging results in an increase in the endogenous level of transcription.[30] Furthermore, they strongly suggest that the molecules that are involved in these various regulatory processes may be the intrinsic factors whose functions may be altered by aging. It is interesting that the constitutive level of both mRNAs is very low (compared to AT and albumin) and that in the aged animal these levels have the tendency to increase. The increase is especially dramatic in the case of the T-kininogen mRNA in aged rat liver.[30] The fact that these genes show very low constitutive levels indicate that they may interact with a repressor whose function is lost in aged cells. These data, as well as the reports that c-myc mRNA levels increase with age, indicate a possible "relaxation" or regulation of the constitutive mRNA level due to chromatin structure changes.[54,55] Wareham *et al.*[34] also showed a similar effect with ornithine carbamoyl transferase (OCT) which is X-linked. Their studies showed that there is an age-related decrease in the stability of the X-inactivation as indicated by the appearance of OCT activity in liver of aged mice. Whether this is related to dysdifferentiation or the age-associated decrease in the stability of chromatin structure is discussed below.

The Effect of Aging on the Inducibility of Liver-Specific–Acute Phase Protein Genes

The acute phase response is defined as the molecular response of the liver to tissue injury due to chemical, mechanical or biological insults. Upon stimulation the liver responds by coordinately increasing the synthesis of a family of serum proteins whose functions are related to protection of the organism against further injury.[2-4] However, there are also some serum proteins such as albumin, transthyretin and α_{2u}-globulin whose synthesis is reduced during the acute phase response. These are referred to as the negative acute phase reactants. In these studies we asked whether the regulatory processes, both positive and negative, are affected by aging, using AGP as positive reactant and albumin as a negative reactant. In the young adult mouse the AGP gene is rapidly and strongly induced by LPS and other acute phase stimulants. However, the kinetics of induction of the AGP gene are significantly altered in aged animals. A time course of the induction indicated that the lag period was significantly extended from 3 hours in young adults to 12 hours or more in aged animals and that the peak of mRNA level, normally reached by 12 hours after stimulation was not achieved even after 24 hours. On the other hand, the induction of T-kininogen was not affected by aging. The failure of the AGP gene to be induced efficiently and to reach maximal mRNA levels may be due to an age-associated reduction in the level of transcription which in turn may be due to changes in the levels of transcription factors or mediators of the response. Our preliminary data clearly show a significant decrease in the binding of trans-acting factors to the AGP promoter (Alam & Papaconstantinou, in preparation). The specificity of the age-associated effect on the inducibility of one gene (AGP) and not the other (T-kininogen) could be explained on the basis of the availability of their specific trans-acting factors.

Albumin, on the other hand, is one of several negatively regulated acute phase proteins whose mRNA levels are the most abundant in the normal liver. During the acute phase response, the albumin mRNA pool is significantly reduced and transcription of the gene is repressed.[23,24] In aged animals the constitutive mRNA pool shows a significant decrease as was described above. When young mice (2 months) are treated with LPS the level of transcription of the albumin gene is turned off and the albumin mRNA level is significantly reduced. After several days the gene is reactivated and the mRNA pool level returns to its normal level of abundance. In aged animals, however, in addition to a reduction in the constitutive level of albumin mRNA, the LPS-treated animals do not exhibit the expected reduction in the mRNA pool. These data indicate that the negative regulation of the albumin gene as measured by mRNA levels, during the acute phase response does not occur in aged liver cells. Although no trans-acting factors have been identified for this negative regulation, analyses are now in progress to define the DNA-protein interactions of the albumin promoter in the young and aged liver nuclei, during the LPS-mediated acute phase response.

It has been observed in many laboratories that aging is accompanied by an overall deregulation in gene activity and the above discussions dealt with the deregulation of tissue-specific gene expression in its homologous tissue or environment. Another question that arises is whether aging affects tissue-specific gene expression in heterologous tissues, a phenomenon which has been described as dysdifferentiation.[38,56,57] Expression of the AGP, AT, albumin and T-kininogen genes is essentially confined to the liver and macrophages.[30] In aging animals, tissue specificity of expression of all of these genes appears to be fully retained. However, longer autoradiographic exposure reveals a significant low level of expression of the T-kininogen gene in the lungs.[30] This may be an example of dysdifferentiation or alternatively may be due to the presence of more alveolar macrophages in lungs of older animals. The possibility that tissue specificity and inducibility of the T-kininogen gene breaks down in aging was not tested, but is nonetheless an interesting concept. For example, can nonresponsive tissues of young animals exhibit an age-associated response to LPS stimulus? It is possible therefore that in aged animals, some APR genes may be activated in tissues that are nonresponsive in young adults. This raises the question of whether this is dysdifferentiation. Furthermore, is this an indication of chromatin destabilization in response to an age-associated state of chronic "stress." Thus it is important that in studying the tissue-specific characteristics in aging that the products of these genes be sought in other tissues.

Finally, in many cases, transcriptional activity is reduced during aging because of the dependence of some genes on hormonal control. One such example is the extinction of expression of the α_{2u}-globulin gene in aging animals.[33] It has been shown that this gene is turned off not only because of a diminishing level of several controlling hormones but also because the receptors for these hormones appear to diminish with age.[32] In addition a recent report has shown that in aging animals, the α_{2u}-globulin gene is detached from the nuclear matrix,[58] which may be an important structural prerequisite for its expression. These studies clearly point to the importance of both regulatory molecules and chromatin structure in the level of regulation of expression in aging.[59] Recently it has been shown that factors such as IL-6 alone or in combination with other cytokines is involved in the transcriptional activation of the positive AP genes.[23,60] Also it has been shown that TGF-β inhibits the accumulation of negative acute phase reactant transcripts such as albumin and ApoA-I mRNA.[60] The data indicate that TGF-β causes an increase in the degradation of the two mRNAs. These very interesting studies point to the specific role of factors in the regulation of gene expression at transcriptional and posttranscriptional levels. It is the balance of these factors and their complex interactions that are important in aging. These processes and interactions may indeed be the normal intrinsic processes that are affected by aging in the absence of disease.

SUMMARY

Eukaryotic organisms possess natural defense processes associated with their response to injury, inflammation and pollutants. One of these, the acute phase (AP) host response, is characterized by a series of hepatic physiological reactions triggered by factors released as a result of bacterial infection, inflammation or tissue injury and is believed to be the mechanism by which cells and tissues are protected against further damage and injury. The capacity to respond to these physiological insults is known to be affected by aging. We propose that the AP response represents a series of intrinsic processes and interactions that may be affected by aging. Furthermore, we propose that this may be due to the progressive failure of the acute phase response. In this study we examine the relationship between aging and the expression of both positive and negative acute phase reactants, *i.e.*, acute phase serum proteins whose levels are increased or decreased in response to systemic injury and infection. The mRNA levels of the positive acute phase reactants, α_1-acid glycoprotein (AGP), α_1-antitrypsin (AT), and the negative acute phase reactant, albumin were measured in both normal and inflammation-induced mice of ages 2, 7, 12, and 24 months. A significant decrease in the constitutive levels of AT and albumin mRNAs occurred as a function of increased age. Furthermore, aging decreased the ability of the AGP and albumin genes to respond to inflammation. Our studies indicate that aging may affect the transcription of these genes, processing of their mRNA or stability of the mRNA levels.

ACKNOWLEDGEMENT

We thank Marg Hillesheim for her assistance during the preparation of the manuscript.

REFERENCES

1. BUTLER, R. N. 1987. Aging in Today's Environment. National Academy Press. Washington, DC.
2. KUSHNER, I. 1982. Ann. N.Y. Acad. Sci. **389:** 39–48.
3. BAUMAN, H. 1989. In Vitro Cell. Dev. Biol. **25:** 115–126.
4. ROY, A. & A. H. GORDON. 1985. The acute phase response to injury and infection. Research monographs in cell and tissue physiology, Vol. 10. Elsevier. North Holland, New York.
5. CHIRGWIN, J. M., A. E. PRZYBYLA, R. J. MACDONALD & W. J. RUTTER. 1979. Biochemistry **18:** 5294–5299.
6. PAPACONSTANTINOU, J., J. A. STEWART, J. P. RABEK, P. R. McCLINTOCK & E. Y. WONG. 1983. Arch. Biochem. Biophys. **227:** 542–551.
7. THOMAS, P. S. 1980. Proc. Natl. Acad. Sci. USA **77:** 5201–5205.
8. MIFFLIN, R. C., P. C. MOLLER & J. PAPACONSTANTINOU. 1988. Somatic Cell Mol. Genet. **14:** 553–566.
9. KRAUTER, K. S., B. A. CITRON, M.-T. HAU, D. POWELL & J. E. DARNELL, JR. 1986. DNA **5:** 29–36.
10. SENIOR, R. & E. T. AL. 1977. Am. Rev. Resp. Dis. **116:** 469–475.
11. ERIKSSON, S. 1964. Acta Med. Scand. **175:** 197–205.
12. SHARP, H. L. 1971. Hosp. Pract. **6**(5): 83–96.
13. CARRELL, R. W., J.-O. JEPPSSON, C.-B. LAURELL, S. O. BRENNAN, M. C. OWEN, L. VAUGHAM & D. R. BOSWELL. 1982. Nature **28:** 329–334.
14. LAURELL, C.-B. & S. ERIKSSON. 1963. Scand. J. Clin. Lab. Invest. **15:** 132–140.
15. SCHREIBER, G., G. HOWLETT, M. NAGASHIMA, A. MILLERSHIP, H. MARTIN, J. URBAN & L. KOTLER. 1982. J. Biol. Chem. **257:** 10271–10277.
16. CHIU, K. M., R. F. MORTENSEN, A. P. OSMAND & H. GEWURZ. 1977. Immunology **32:** 997–1005.
17. BENNETT, M. & K. SCHMID. 1980. Proc. Natl. Acad. Sci. USA **77:** 6109–6113.
18. COOPER, R. & J. PAPACONSTANTINOU. 1986. J. Biol. Chem. **261:** 1849–1853.
19. SCHREIBER, G., A. R. ALDRED, T. THOMAS, H. E. BIRCH, W. G-F. DICKINSON, C. HEINRICH, W. NORTHEMANN, G. F. HOWLETT, F. A. DEJONG & A. MITCHELL. 1986. Inflammation **10:** 59–66.
20. CARTER, K. C., D. J. POST & J. PAPACONSTANTINOU. 1991. Biochim. Biophys. Acta. In press.
21. PACIFICI, G. M., A. VIANI, G. TADDEUCCI-BRUNELLI, G. RIZZO, M. CARRAI & H-U. SCHULZ. 1986. Ther. Drug Monit. **8:** 259–263.
22. RUTHERFORD, M. S., C. S. BAEHLER & A. RICHARDSON. 1986. Mech. Ageing Dev. **35:** 245–254.
23. CARTER, K. C., R. COOPER, J. PAPACONSTANTINOU & D. G. RITCHIE. 1988. J. Biol. Chem. **264:** 515–519.
24. DARLINGTON, G. J., D. R. WILSON & L. B. LACHMAN. 1986. J. Cell Biol. **103:** 787–793.
25. RICHARDSON, A. & H. T. CHENG. 1982. Life Sci. **31:** 605–613.
26. RICHARDSON, A., M. C. BIRCHENALL-SPARKS, J. L. STAECKER, J. P. HARDWICH & D. S. H. LIU. 1982. J. Gerontol. **37:** 666–672.
27. BIRCHENALL-SPARKS, M. C., M. S. ROBERTS, M. S. RUTHERFORD & A. RICHARDSON. 1985. Mech. Ageing Dev. **32:** 99–111.
28. RICHARDSON, A., M. S. ROBERTS & M. S. RUTHERFORD. 1985. Aging and gene expression. *In* Review of Biological Research in Aging. M. Rothstein, Ed. Vol. 2: 395–419. Alan R. Liss, Inc. New York.
29. RICHARDSON, A., J. A. BUTLER, M-S. RUTHERFORD, I. SEMSEI, M-Z. GU, G. FERNANDES & W-H. CHIANG. 1987. J. Biol. Chem. **262:** 12821–12825.
30. SIERRA, F., G. H. FEY & Y. GUIGOZ. 1989. Mol. Cell. Biol. **9:** 5610–5616.
31. ROY, A. K. & B. CHATTERJEE. 1985. Mol. Aspects Med. **8:** 1–88.
32. ROY, A. K., W. F. DEMYAN, C. V. R. MURTY, D. MAJUMDAR & B. CHATTERJEE. 1984. Age-dependent changes in the androgen sensitivity of rat liver. *In* Proceedings

of the 57th Nobel Symposium on Steroid Hormone Receptors. J. A. Gustaffson & H. Eriksson, Eds. Elsevier/North-Holland Biomedical Press. Amsterdam.

33. ROY, A. K., T. S. NATH, N. M. MOTWANI & B. CHATTERJEE. 1983. J. Biol. Chem. **258:** 10123–10127.
34. WAREHAM, K. A., M. F. LYON, P. H. GENISTER & E. D. WILLIAMS. 1987. Nature **327:** 725–727.
35. WELLINGER, R. & Y. GUIGOZ. 1986. Mech. Ageing Dev. **34:** 203–217.
36. FLEMING, J. E., J. K. WALTON, R. DUBITSKY & K. G. BENSCH. Proc. Natl. Acad. Sci. USA **85:** 4099–4103.
37. KUCK, U., H. D. OSIEWACZ, U. SCHMIDT, B. KAPPELHOFF, E. SCHULTE, U. STAHL & K. ESSER. 1985. Curr. Genet. **9:** 373–382.
38. ONO, T., R. G. DEAN, S. K. CHATTOPADHYAY & R. G. CUTLER. 1985. Gerontology **31:** 362–372.
39. RYAN, R. F., J. P. HANCOCK, J. J. MCDONALD & P. J. HORNSBY. 1989. Exp. Cell Res. **180:** 36–48.
40. SHAIN, S. A., J. K. HILLIARD & C. DELEON. 1983. Endocrinology **113:** 1292–1298.
41. WEBSTER, G. C. & S. L. WEBSTER. 1984. Mech. Ageing Dev. **24:** 335–342.
42. LIEHTSTEINER, S., J. WUARIN & U. SCHIBLER. 1987. Cell **51:** 963–973.
43. IZBAN, M. G. & J. PAPACONSTANTINOU. 1989. J. Biol. Chem. **264:** 9171–9179.
44. DESIMONE, V., G. CILIBERTO, E. HARDON, G. PAONESSA, F. PALLA, L. LUNDBERG & R. CORTESE. 1987. EMBO J. **6:** 2759–2766.
45. MONTGOMERY, K. T., J. TARDIFF, L. M. REID & K. S. KRAUTER. 1990. Mol. Cell. Biol. **10:** 2625–2637.
46. BERNSTEIN, P. & J. ROSS. 1989. TIBS **14:** 373–377.
47. HARGROVE, J. L. & F. H. SCHMIDT. 1989. FASEB J. **3:** 2360–2370.
48. MALTER, J. S. 1989. Science **264:** 664–666.
49. SACHS, A. B. & R. W. DAVIS. 1989. Cell **58:** 857–867.
50. CAPUT, D., B. BEUTLER, K. HARTOG, R. THAYER, S. BROWN-SHIMER & A. CERAMI. 1986. Proc. Natl. Acad. Sci. USA **83:** 1670–1674.
51. SHAW, G. & R. KAMEN. 1986. Cell **46:** 659–667.
52. BREWER, G. & J. ROSS. 1989. Mol. Cell. Biol. **9:** 1996–2006.
53. ANDERSON, K. P., A. D. MARTIN & E. C. HEATH. 1984. Arch. Biochem. Biophys. **233:** 624–635.
54. MATOCHA, M. F., J. W. COSGROVE, J. R. ATACK & S. I. RAPOPORT. 1987. Biochem. Biophys. Res. Commun. **147:** 1–7.
55. WAGGONER, S., M-Z. GU, W-H. CHIANG & A. RICHARDSON. 1990. The effect of dietary restriction of the expression of a variety of genes. *In* Genetic Effects of Aging II. D. E. Harrison, Ed. 255–273. The Telford Press. Caldwell, NJ.
56. ONO, T. & R. G. CUTLER, 1978. Proc. Natl. Acad. Sci. USA **85:** 4431–4435.
57. ZS.-NAGY, I., R. G. CUTLER & I. SEMSEI. 1988. Ann. N.Y. Acad. Sci. **521:** 215–225.
58. MURTY, C. V. R., M. A. MANCINI, B. CHATTERGEE & A. K. ROY. 1988. Biochim. Biophys. Acta **949:** 27–34.
59. MEDVEDEV, Z. A. 1984. Mech. Ageing Dev. **28:** 139–154.
60. MORRONE, G., G. CILIBERTO, S. OLIVIERO, R. ARCONE, L. DENTE, J. CONTENT & R. CORTESE. 1988. J. Biol. Chem. **263:** 12554–12558.

Longevity and Heredity in Humans

Association with the Human Leucocyte Antigen Phenotype[a]

A. M. LAGAAY,[b] J. D'AMARO,[c] G. J. LIGTHART,[b]
G. M. Th. SCHREUDER,[c] J. J. van ROOD,[c]
AND W. HIJMANS[b]

[b]Section of Gerontology and
[c]Department of Immunohematology
University of Leiden
P.O. Box 9603
2300 RC Leiden, The Netherlands

INTRODUCTION

It is still not understood why some people live to be very old while others die at an earlier age from natural causes. There are several arguments supporting the hypothesis that genetic factors are important in this respect. Both average and maximum life span are fixed for each species. Between species and also between different strains within a species, average life span differs, as, for example, in different strains of mice reared under identical laboratory conditions. Smith and Walford[1] have demonstrated that in mice the major histocompatibility complex (MHC) exerts a significant influence on life span. In mice, MHC is also associated with premature tumor incidence, a low immune response, less effective DNA-repair and autoimmune disease.[2-4] These observations could be an indication of the existence of a "biological clock" which is governed by genetic factors.

Common knowledge has it that in the human species familial differences in longevity do exist and that these are at least partially accounted for by genetic factors: "longevity runs in the family." Scientifically this has been studied by Abbott et al.[5] who compared the parental age at death of subjects who died at different ages. There was a weak but significant trend for survival to increase with increasing age at death of the parent. This trend was more marked for the maternal age at death and more evident for males than for females. Palmore in the Dukes longitudinal study[6] partly confirmed these observations. He found an influence of the father's age at death and again this was more evident in males. The mother's age at death had no influence.

An important study from Sorensen et al. in Denmark[7] includes 960 individuals who had been separated from their biologic parents in early childhood and had been reared by adoptive parents. In those who died prematurely, that is between 16 and 58 years of age, there was a significant correlation with the death of one of the biologic parents before the age of 50 (relative risk (RR) 1.71). There was no correlation with a premature death of one of the adoptive parents. The relative risk was higher regarding infectious (RR 5.8) or vascular (RR 4.5) causes of death. These findings may be interpreted as evidence for a genetic effect on the immune

[a] Supported by National Institutes of Health Grant AG 06354.

system, or of a genetic influence on premature atherosclerosis. It is of interest that death from cancer of an adoptive parent before the age of 50 increased the rate of mortality among the adoptees fivefold. Death from cancer of a biologic parent had no detectable effect on the mortality of the adoptees.

The MHC in man is called the human leucocyte antigen (HLA) system. The HLA region is located on the short arm of the sixth chromosome. It codes for the immunological repertoire in its broadest sense. A characteristic property is its extreme polymorphism. In man several associations between HLA antigens and disease exist with a relative risk which varies from 1.3 to 358.[8] Therefore, we studied the HLA system for genes associated with longevity.

Age-related differences in HLA antigen frequencies will be more difficult to detect in the human species than in mice, since humans are an outbred population with an inherent genetic heterogeneity. In addition, there is no possibility to control other exogenous variables that may influence longevity. Even if ethnic and geographic matching between the study population and the control group is assured, a considerable genetic heterogeneity persists so that HLA types cannot be compared against a common background. For these reasons Walford *et al.*[9] stated that it would be a more fruitful approach to do HLA typing in family studies or to determine the segregation of certain traits with haplotypes.

The number of studies comparing the HLA phenotype between young and old age groups is limited and their results are not uniform. It is essential that the study population and the young control group share the same genetic and geographic background and that both groups consist of large enough numbers for statistical analysis. The age difference between the two groups must be adequate, or age-brackets should be provided. Only some of the previous studies fulfill these requirements. In the following we will briefly review the most important findings from the literature.

Brief Literature Review

Recently, the Japanese group of Takata *et al.*[10]—reporting on the oriental population of Okinawa, Japan—mentioned an extremely low frequency of HLA-DRw9 in nona- and centenarians as compared to younger age groups, and also a frequency of HLA-DR1 of 10.0 and 6.1% in the nona- and centenarians, respectively, while DR1 was absent in the younger age groups. Since HLA-B40 is linked to DRw9 in the Japanese population, its frequency was decreased as well.

Macurova *et al.* in Prague,[11] described a marked difference in many antigens: a 50% decrease in HLA-A1, a threefold increase in HLA-B40, a 30% decrease in HLA-B8 and a more than 50% decrease in HLA-B27 in the old age group.

In a well designed study, Yarnell *et al.* in Wales,[12] also found a higher frequency of HLA-B40 in the old population. On the other hand, three studies in caucasoid populations[13-15] reported a slight decrease of HLA-B40 in the elderly.

Greenberg[16] reported a decreased prevalence of HLA-B8 in women over 70 years of age as compared to men of the same age. He also found a decreased prevalence of the A1-B8 haplotype in this group as compared to both the young ages and men of the same age. Thompson *et al.*[17] noted an increase of the phenotypic frequencies HLA-A29, B7 and B35 in 17 healthy centenarians in Kentucky, USA. One study[20] mentions a higher frequency of the A1/Cw7/B8/DR3 haplotype in highly aged males.

An increase in heterozygosity, mostly at the HLA-B locus, in older age groups has been reported,[11,18,19] but other studies have not confirmed this observation.

In the authoritative book *HLA and Disease Associations,*[21] in the chapter on "miscellaneous diseases" a paragraph is devoted to the subject of "age" in the context of association with HLA antigens. A meta-analysis on HLA-B40 was performed with the combined data of eight independent studies. The result was a marginally significant increase in the frequency of B40. This increase in the old group was primarily a consequence of the data of Macurova[11] and Yarnell.[12] Critical remarks were made concerning some of the studies, and we quote: "The increased frequency of B40 in the old group may be an artifact of classification criterion, sample size, HLA serology, and typing techniques".

These discrepancies prompted us to reinvestigate the association of HLA antigens with survival. We performed a study of the HLA phenotypes of all available inhabitants, that is, 964 persons, aged 85 years and over of the community of Leiden, the Netherlands. The frequencies of HLA antigens were compared with a control group, consisting of 2444 blood donors, 20–35 years of age, with an identical ethnic (Dutch caucasoid) and geographic background. Also, control groups of different age brackets were used from the same region.

SUBJECTS AND METHODS

Subjects

85-Plus Group

On the entry date of December 1st, 1986, the total cohort of inhabitants of Leiden, aged 85 years and over comprised 1259 subjects. From January 1987 until March 1989, 977 individuals of this age group were visited at their place of residence. After appropriate informed consent was obtained, a medical history was taken and blood was drawn by venipuncture for HLA typing. A total of 222 persons had died before they could be visited and 60 persons did not cooperate. Blood samples for HLA typing were obtained from 964 persons.

Young Control Group: 20–35 Years of Age

A large database was available with HLA typings of blood donors of different ages from the same geographical district. We chose the age group of 20–35 because the mortality rate is lowest at these ages. These subjects have survived the diseases of childhood and have yet to encounter diseases of middle age: malignancies, cardiovascular disorders and autoimmune diseases. The database of HLA typings of the blood bank was also used to generate control groups of different age-brackets from identical ethnic and geographic background.

Ethnic Homogeneity

To obtain an ethnically homogeneous sample, nine elderly subjects of non-caucasoid parentage (data obtained during personal visit or from family) were excluded. Four of these excluded subjects were of Indonesian (oriental) parentage, four of Surinamese (negroid, or mixed oriental/negroid) and one of Chinese parentage.

People with names suggesting a noncaucasoid parentage (n = 35) were excluded from the young control group. This method is not successful in recognizing people from the former Dutch colonies with a Dutch name, but with negroid or oriental parentage.

These selection and exclusion procedures resulted in 964 HLA typings of subjects of 85 years and older, and 2444 of 20–35 years of age. The number of HLA typings of the different age groups are: newborns n = 476; 20–29 years n = 1311; 30–39 years n = 2143; 40–49 years n = 1477; 50–59 years n = 354; 60–84 years n = 38.

Methods

HLA Typing

Typing for the HLA-A, B and C (class I) antigens was performed with the standard lymphocytotoxicity test, and typing for HLA-DR and DQ (class II) antigens with a two-color fluorescence test using a set of highly selected alloantisera to class II antigens.

Statistical Analysis

The relative risk was calculated with the following formula:

$$RR = \frac{(\text{pat. with AG}) \times (\text{contr. without AG})}{(\text{pat. without AG}) \times (\text{contr. with AG})}$$

pat. = patient; contr. = control; AG = HLA antigen.

The phenotype frequencies of the antigens were compared using Fisher's χ^2 test for 2×2 contingency tables.

The ages of the subjects for the analysis were taken as their ages at the time of collection of the blood sample for HLA typing.

RESULTS

The results of HLA typing of 48 antigens are listed in TABLE 1. The distribution of HLA antigens in the study population was in good general agreement with that in the control group with two exceptions: the frequency of HLA-B40 was lower and that of HLA-DR5 was higher in the age group of 85 years and over. After correction for the number of antigens tested, these differences were statistically significant in females only (TABLES 2 and 3). The changes appeared gradually with age, as shown in FIGURE 1.

The percentages of homozygotes were not different between the young and old age groups (data not shown).

TABLE 1. Phenotype Frequency of HLA Antigens (%)

Age Phenotype	20–35 N = 2444	85+ N = 964	RR	χ^2	p Value[a]
A1	30.6	30.8	1.009	0.012	0.877
A2	52.7	49.5	0.890	2.359	0.121
A3	28.7	27.2	0.937	0.581	0.453
A9	19.3	21.8	1.148	2.171	0.137
A10	6.9	9.2	1.382	5.627	0.017
A11	11.5	10.4	0.877	1.132	0.287
A28	10.0	9.2	0.918	0.441	0.514
AW19	20.6	23.5	1.185	3.465	0.059
B5	11.9	12.9	1.091	0.585	0.451
B7	27.4	28.0	1.032	0.140	0.708
B8	22.8	22.5	0.989	0.016	0.869
B12	25.3	27.4	1.131	2.072	0.146
B13	4.4	4.8	1.116	0.383	0.544
B14	2.9	3.5	1.268	1.303	0.252
B15	15.8	15.7	0.968	0.096	0.751
B16	7.2	7.0	0.972	0.038	0.825
B17	6.6	8.0	1.236	2.176	0.136
B18	6.5	8.2	1.297	3.315	0.065
B21	2.2	2.8	1.242	0.828	0.366
BW22	5.8	4.5	0.800	1.644	0.197
B27	6.4	7.7	1.206	1.642	0.197
B35	17.5	16.0	0.908	0.891	0.348
B37	4.1	3.4	0.876	0.441	0.514
B40	17.8	13.2	0.703	10.5	0.002
BW4	55.2	59.8	1.202	5.695	0.016
BW6	87.8	87.6	0.983	0.023	0.851
CW1	4.8	6.0	1.265	2.053	0.148
CW2	9.9	9.3	0.921	0.398	0.535
CW3	32.8	28.6	0.819	5.731	0.016
CW4	21.0	20.6	0.986	0.022	0.854
CW5	12.9	16.0	1.311	6.469	0.011
CW6	16.5	16.7	1.033	0.092	0.755
CW7	49.3	51.4	1.078	0.939	0.334
DR1	19.7	20.6	1.072	0.548	0.466
DR2	28.7	28.3	0.960	0.230	0.637
DR3	25.1	23.1	0.898	1.439	0.228
DR4	28.3	25.0	0.856	3.188	0.071
DR5	19.0	23.4	1.318	8.953	0.003
DRW6	33.7	31.8	0.913	1.216	0.270
DR7	19.2	22.1	1.204	3.943	0.044
DRW8	5.3	7.5	1.457	6.118	0.013
DR9	2.4	2.7	1.127	0.257	0.619
DRW10	4.3	2.5	0.588	5.493	0.018
DRW52	69.1	72.6	1.196	4.428	0.033
DRW53	46.1	47.0	1.049	0.379	0.546
DQW1	71.2	68.8	0.896	1.740	0.184
DQW2	37.5	36.7	0.965	0.202	0.658
DQW3	50.4	53.0	1.111	1.589	0.205

[a] p values uncorrected for number of antigens tested.

TABLE 2. Phenotype Frequency of HLA-B40 and its Splits: Bw60 and Bw61 (%)

Age Phenotype	25–35	85+	RR	χ^2	p Value[a]
Male + female					
B40	17.8	13.2	0.703	10.5	0.002
Bw60	14.7	11.3	0.732	7.1	0.008
Bw61	3.0	1.9	0.662	2.6	0.10
n	2444	964			
Males					
B40	17.1	16.2	0.944	0.106	0.74
Bw60	13.6	14.4	1.083	0.179	0.67
Bw61	3.5	1.8	0.558	1.756	0.18
n	1277	278			
Females					
B40	18.5	12.0	0.601	13.4	0.001
Bw60	16.0	9.9	0.580	13.2	0.001
Bw61	2.5	2.1	0.827	0.353	0.56
n	1167	686			

[a] p values uncorrected for number of antigens tested.

TABLE 3. Phenotype Frequency of HLA-DR5 and its Splits: DRw11 and DRw12 (%)

Age Phenotype	20–35	85+	RR	χ^2	p Value[a]
Male + female					
DR5	19.0	23.6	1.318	8.953	0.003
DRw11	14.4	18.4	1.349	8.694	0.004
DRw12	4.6	4.9	1.067	0.131	0.72
n	2381	954			
Males					
DR5	19.3	21.3	1.141	0.650	0.43
DRw11	14.9	18.2	1.080	0.180	0.68
DRw12	4.3	4.9	1.160	0.233	0.64
n	1261	273			
Females					
DR5	18.7	24.5	1.416	8.814	0.003
DRw11	13.8	19.5	1.519	10.45	0.002
DRw12	4.9	4.9	0.998	0.000	0.94
n	1120	681			

[a] p values uncorrected for number of antigens tested.

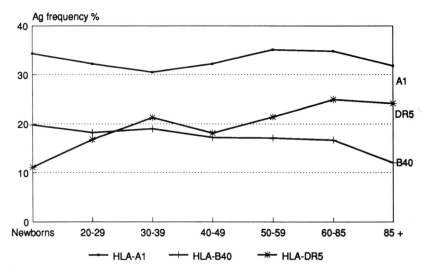

FIGURE 1. The distribution of HLA-B40 and HLA-DR5 in the Dutch-caucasoid population of Leiden, The Netherlands, in seven age groups, in females. HLA-A1 is shown as an example of an antigen that does not change in frequency with age.

DISCUSSION

A difference was found in two HLA antigens: the frequency of HLA-B40 was lower and that of HLA-DR5 was higher in the age group of 85 years and over. No major disease associations with HLA-B40 or with DR5 have been reported. The possibility remains that either of these antigens is in linkage disequilibrium with gene systems, as yet obscure to us, which are involved in controlling life span or which may be associated with diseases or aging processes. Both Dawkins in Australia (personal communication) and Kramer et al. in Hungary[22] have mentioned the possible association of HLA-B40 with gene duplication of the fourth component of complement. This could be relevant in the light of our results and it indicates the need for further studies on linkage of the different HLA classes.

Concerning HLA-DR5, no data about age-related differences in class II antigens in caucasoids have been reported. HLA-B40, on the other hand, has repeatedly been found to differ between young and old age groups (FIG. 2). Macurova et al.[11] mentioned a marked increase with age, but this study should be regarded critically, as mentioned above. Since then, one study reported an increase[12] and two studies found a decrease of HLA-B40 with age.[13,14,23] We have not yet succeeded in finding a plausible explanation for this variance in direction of the difference in HLA-B40.

Walford[24] predicted an enhanced survival chance in HLA-B40 positive—caucasoid—individuals, and HLA-B40 is officially listed as being associated with aging.[8] Since in our study, the frequency of HLA-B40 is lower in subjects aged 85 years and over, especially in females, it is clear that our data do not support this conclusion.

The percentage of HLA-B40 in the control group, 20–35 years of age, in the present study is higher than in the other studies published on caucasoid populations (FIG. 2). It is well known that within the same race, a considerable variation in HLA antigen frequencies can exist between different populations, for example, between neighboring countries. For the region of Leiden, we have checked this percentage in six other Dutch caucasoid control groups of the same region and of the same age, containing 101 up to 5490 subjects. The percentage of HLA-B40-positive subjects in these control groups was of the same order of magnitude as in the present study, ranging from 16.8 to 18.0 percent.

The general similarity of the pattern of HLA frequencies in the different age groups provides evidence that we are looking at two generations of the same population. Some of the previous studies reported differences in nearly all antigens tested at that time;[11] while in other studies[10] the age-related differences appeared abruptly. This generates questions about the historic background and similarity of the study population and the control group, as Wainscoat *et al.*[25] have pointed out. We have no indication that major demographic changes have occurred in our population during this century. This is illustrated by the gradual growth of the population and of the percentage of people over 85 years of age (FIG. 3). Neither did we find an abrupt or disproportionally large difference in HLA frequencies between different age groups (FIG. 2).

Gerkins *et al.*,[18] Macurova *et al.*[11] and Converse and Williams[19] report a significant increase in heterozygosity in the old age group. This was not confirmed in other studies,[12–15,20,22,26] In our study the heterozygosity was not different in the old as compared to the young age group.

The fact that the differences in HLA frequency both in B40 and in DR5 are more evident in females is intriguing. Can we take this as a key to the understanding of the difference in life expectancy between the sexes? It is clear that we cannot answer this question without further studies. This also brings us to the

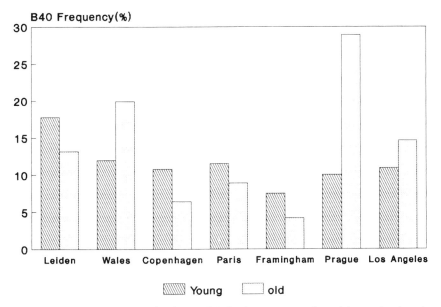

FIGURE 2. The frequency (%) of HLA-B40 in the present study and in previously published studies, in young and old age groups.

option of "longevity genes" being located outside the HLA region. With the association of the maternal age of death and the higher life expectancy for contemporary women in mind, the sex chromosome and even mitochondrial DNA could be proposed as a possible site. It has been postulated that the double X-chromosome is favorable for an extended length of life.[27] This advantage can act through hormonal influence or by an overcapacity of the immune system, the latter provided by nature in order to ensure maximum reproductive success for the human female gender.

Our study did not detect a significant decrease in the frequency of established disease-associated HLA antigens, *e.g.*, B27, B8, DR4, in the oldest age group. The following arguments should be considered in this respect:

Firstly, our control group consists of blood donors who are selected on the basis of health criteria. This selection can cause the frequency of disease-associ-

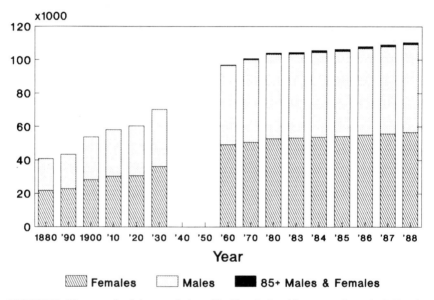

FIGURE 3. The growth of the population of Leiden during this century is gradual. For the total population the number of males and females are plotted separately. For the inhabitants of 85 years and over males and females are pooled.

ated HLA antigens to be lower than in the total population. In other words our control group could be "too healthy." The fact that in this particular age group the prevalence of disorders leading to rejection as blood donor will be low, and that relatives of diseased subjects can be expected to be especially motivated to enlist as blood donor, counters the argument that the control group may be too healthy. Moreover, we have checked the HLA frequencies of 134 cornea donors, 20–35 years of age, who can be considered a random sample of the population. The HLA pattern of the blood donors and the cornea donors did not differ (data not shown).

The *second* explanation is that most of the known associations between HLA and diseases are weak, and that the prevalence of these diseases is also low. For example: insulin-dependent diabetes mellitus (IDDM) is associated with HLA-DR3 or DR4. Individuals with those antigens, have a relative risk to develop IDDM which is 4 to 10 times higher than those lacking these antigens. The prevalence of IDDM in the population has been estimated to be approximately 0.26 percent. A population-based study such as the present is not suitable to detect such minimal differences.

Thirdly, these HLA associated disorders do not necessarily lead to an early death. In the present study this is exemplified by subjects with well documented rheumatoid arthritis, who apparently survived while, or because, the disease process was burnt out.

On the other hand, this negative finding could emphasize the postulated advantage of these disease-associated HLA antigens. After all, according to the principles of Darwin, these disease-associated HLA antigens would have become extinct, had they not been beneficial for the maintenance of the species.

Referring again to the article of Takata *et al.:*[10] they explicitly mention that in their study both the adult controls and the nona- and centenarians were healthy. This is remarkable in the light of the first point mentioned above: one would not expect a difference in autoimmune disease-associated HLA antigens if both young and old age groups are selected on health criteria. The fact that the difference is found casts a doubt on the significance of the Okinawa results, or alternatively, on the strictness of the health criteria employed. To illustrate this critical remark, it is noteworthy that in the present population 54 (5.5%) out of 977 persons aged 85 years or over were considered healthy according to the criteria described in the SENIEUR-protocol.[28]

It is not clear at what age the hypothetised differences in HLA frequencies would show. Is it at middle age, when diseases like cancer, cardiovascular disorders and rheumatoid arthritis take their toll? Or is it in the oldest age group, where the protecting, beneficial ''longevity genes'' would become manifest, as could be exemplified by the results of Takata *et al.*[10] We are presently in the process of integrating the life expectancy curve into the data of HLA phenotype.

The idea of the existence of longevity genes is difficult to understand in the light of Darwin's theory of evolution. We can hardly expect an extension of life span after 85 years of age to be advantageous for the preservation of the species. Hayflick,[29] however, has recently proposed an interesting theory on this topic:

> In order to insure maximum parental fitness for survival of slowly maturing human progeny, there would be a selective advantage for parents to maintain their physiological vigor after sexual maturation. The reserve capacity, present in virtually all organs, is the essential element in determining postdevelopmental longevity.

CONCLUSION

The finding of a statistically significant decrease of the frequency of HLA-B40 and an increase of HLA-DR5 in the oldest old is fascinating. Its biological meaning or impact is not yet understood and therefore it encourages further investigations, for example by family studies, or by techniques of molecular biology used to identify the neighboring DNA sequence.

The age-related differences in HLA antigens should however never distract us from the importance of prevention, life style and other nongenetic factors which contribute to reach an active, healthy and independent old age.

SUMMARY

Several arguments support the idea of a link between longevity and heredity, both in experimental animals and in the human species. In mice, genes in the major histocompatibility complex (MHC) are associated with a significant effect on life span. Results of analogous studies in man are confusing and contradictory.

We have therefore investigated the question of an association of the human leucocyte antigen (HLA) and longevity in a large and ethnically homogeneous population. Our study population consisted of all 964 available inhabitants aged 85 years and over in the Dutch community of Leiden (pop. 104,000). Our control group comprised 2444 young inhabitants, aged 20–35 years, with an identical ethnic and demographic background. In addition, control groups of different age-brackets from the same region were used.

Two antigens differed in frequency: HLA-B40 was lower and HLA-DR5 was higher in the group of 85 years and over, as compared to the control group, aged 20–35 years. Both differences were more evident in females. No major disease associations with HLA-B40 or HLA-DR5 have been reported. It is unlikely that these results are a chance observation: the overall similarity of the HLA pattern of the old and young age groups is a confirmation of their identical ethnic and demographic background and the changes as observed in the different age-groups were gradual. The biological meaning of these results is still unclear.

ACKNOWLEDGMENTS

We thank Professor J. Vandenbroucke for valuable and indispensable epidemiologic advice; Mrs. E. P. J. M. Mudde-Hoogveld for collecting the demographic data; Mr. Jipje Krebbers for correction of the English text; Mrs. M. den Hollander-Numans for the preparation of the manuscript; and all participants of the 85-plus project in Leiden, both active and passive, who were, and will be, a source of inspiration.

REFERENCES

1. SMITH, G. S. & R. L. WALFORD. 1977. Influence of the main histocompatibility complex on ageing in mice. Nature **270:** 727–729.
2. SMITH, G. S. & R. L. WALFORD. 1978. Influence of the H2 and H2 histocompatibility systems upon life span and spontaneous cancer incidence in congenic mice. *In* Genetic Effects on Ageing. D. Bergsma and D. E. Harrison, Eds. 281–312. National Foundation–March of Dimes. Alan R. Liss. New York.
3. MEREDITH, P. & R. L. WALFORD. 1977. Effect of age on response to T and B cell mitogens in mice congenic at the H-2 region. Immunogenetics **5:** 109.
4. YUNIS, E. J., G. FERNANDES, P. O. TEAGUE, O. SUTMAN & R. A. GOOD. 1972. The thymus, autoimmunity and the involution of the lymphoid system. *In* Tolerance, Autoimmunity and Aging. M. M. Sigel, Ed. 62–119. Charles C. Thomas. Springfield.
5. ABBOTT, M. H., E. A. MURPHY, D. R. BOLLING & H. ABBEY. 1974. The familial component of longevity, a study of offspring of nongenarians. II. Preliminary analysis of the completed study. Hopkins Med. J. **134:** 1–16.
6. PALMORE, E. B. 1982. Predictors of the longevity difference: a 25-year follow-up. Gerontologist **22:** 513–518.
7. SORENSEN, T. I. A., G. G. NIELSEN, P. K. ANDERSEN & T. W. TEASDALE. 1988. Genetic and environmental influences on premature death in adult adoptees. N. Engl. J. Med. **318:** 727–732.

8. TIWARI, J. L. & P. I. TERASAKI, Eds. 1985. *In* HLA and disease associations. 32–48. Springer-Verlag Inc. New York.

9. WALFORD, R. L., G. S. SMITH, P. J. MEREDITH & K. E. CHENEY. 1978. Immunogenetics of Aging. *In* The Genetics of Aging. E. L. Schneider, Ed. 383–401. Plenum Publishing Corporation. New York.

10. TAKATA, H., M. SUZUKI, T. ISHI, S. SEKIGUCHI & H. IRI. 1987. Influence of major histocompatibility complex region genes on human longevity among Okinawan-Japanese centenarians and nonagenarians. Lancet ii: 824–826.

11. MACUROVA, H., P. IVANYI, H. SAJDLOVA & J. TROJAN. 1975. HL-A antigens in aged persons. Tissue Antigens **6**: 269–271.

12. YARNELL, J. W. G., A. S. ST. LEGER, I. C. BALFOUR & R. B. RUSSELL. 1979. The distribution, age effects and disease associations of HLA antigens and other blood group markers in a random sample of an elderly population. J. Chron. Dis. **32**: 555–561.

13. HANSEN, H. E., J. V. SPARCK & S. O. LARSEN. 1977. An examination of HLA frequencies in three age groups. Tissue Antigens **10**: 49–55.

14. BENDER, K., A. MAYEROVA, B. KLOTZBUCHER, K. BURCKHARDT & C. H. HILLER. 1976. No indication of postnatal selection at the HL-A loci. Tissue Antigens **7**: 118–121.

15. BLACKWELDER, W. C., K. K. MITTAL, P. M. McNAMARA & F. J. PAYNE. 1982. Lack of association between HLA and age in an aging population. Tissue Antigens **20**: 188–192.

16. GREENBERG, L. J. 1979. Aging and immune function in man: influence of sex and genetic background. *In* Aging and Immunity. S. K. Singhal, M. R. Sinclair & C. R. Stiller, Eds. 43–59. Elsevier, North Holland Inc. Amsterdam.

17. THOMPSON, J. S., D. R. WEKSTEIN, J. L. RHOADES, C. KIRKPATRICK, S. A. BROWN, T. ROSZMAN, R. STRAUS & N. TIETZ. 1984. The immune system of healthy centenarians. J. Americ. Geriatr. Soc. **32**: 274–281.

18. GERKINS, V. R., A. TING, H. T. MENCK, J. T. CASSAGRANDE, P. I. TERASAKI & M. C. PIKE. 1974. HL-A heterozygozity as a genetic marker of long term survival. J. Natl. Cancer Inst. **52**: 1909–1911.

19. CONVERSE, P. J. & D. R. R. WILLIAMS. 1978. Increased HLA-B heterozygosity with age. Tissue Antigens **12**: 275–278.

20. PROUST, J., R. MOULIAS, F. FUMERON, F. BEKKHOUCHA, M. BUSSON, M. SCHMID & J. HORS. 1982. HLA and longevity. Tissue Antigens **19**: 168–173.

21. TIWARI J. L. & P. I. TERASAKI, Eds. 1985. *In* HLA and disease associations: 445–446. Springer-Verlag New York, Inc.

22. KRAMER, J., E. GYODI & G. FUST. 1989. Usefulness of densitometry in typing of human complement component C4. Immunogenetics **29**: 121–123.

23. PANDEY, J. P., H. H. FUDENBERG & C. B. LOADHOLT. 1977. HLA antigens in different age groups. Ric. Clin. Lab. **7**: 220–223.

24. WALFORD, R. L. 1987. MHC Regulation of aging: an extension of the immunologic theory of aging. *In* Modern Biological Theories of Aging. H. R. Warner *et al.*, Eds. 722–726. Raven Press. New York.

25. WAINSCOAT, J. S., T. E. A. PETO & A. WASWO. 1987. HLA genes and longevity (letter). Lancet ii: 1399.

26. HODGE, S. E. & R. L. WALFORD. 1980. HLA distribution in aged normals. *In* Histocompatibility Testing P. I. Terasaki, Ed. 722–726. UCLA. Los Angeles.

27. SMITH, D. W. E. & H. R. WARNER. 1989. Does genotypic sex have a direct effect on longevity? Exp. Gerontol. **24**: 277–288.

28. LIGTHART, G. J., J. X. CORBERAND, C. FOURNIER, P. GALANAUD, W. HIJMANS, B. KENNES, H. K. MULLER-HERMELINK & G. S. STEIMANN. 1984. Mech. Ageing Dev. **28**: 47–55.

29. HAYFLICK, L. 1989. Antecedents of cell aging research. Exp. Gerontol. **24**: 355–365.

In Vivo Probing of the Brain Cholinergic System in the Aged Rat

Effects of Long-Term Treatment with Acetyl-L-Carnitine

ASSUNTA IMPERATO, MARIA G. SCROCCO,
ORLANDO GHIRARDI,[a] MARIA T. RAMACCI,[a] AND
LUCIANO ANGELUCCI

Istituto di Farmacologia Medica 2nda Cattedra
Università "La Sapienza"
Piazzale A. Moro, 2
00185 Rome, Italy

and

[a]Istituto di Ricerca sulla Senescenza
Sigma-Tau
Via Pontina, km 30.400
00040 Pomezia, Italy

INTRODUCTION

The aging of the brain is a complex phenomenon characterized by many morphological and biochemical alterations which lead to functional modifications in the central nervous system.

On the basis that the amount of neurotransmitter released is the most direct index of neuronal activity, we have investigated the effect of aging on the release of ACh from the hippocampus of awake freely-moving Fischer rats from 3 up to 31 months by means of brain microdialysis.

It is well known that cholinergic activity is regulated via various types of receptors. With regards to the muscarinic receptors many subtypes have been recently identified;[1-4] among them the involvement of the M3 type in the regulation of ACh release in the striatum in vivo has been recently suggested.[5]

The aim of this study was to investigate whether or not ACh release is affected by age, and also to assess the functional responsiveness of the cholinergic synapse through different ages, probing the receptor-mediated release response by the use of preferential antagonists for the M1, M2 and M3 types. Moreover, rats treated for 6 months with acetyl-l-carnitine (ALCAR) were also evaluated. This compound is a naturally occurring substance involved in the mitochondrial transport and utilization of fatty acids and it has been shown to possess a variety of metabolic actions able to restore some energetic processes in the aged brain.[6-8] We

90

have recently shown that ALCAR is able to increase the *in vivo* release of ACh, possibly through an increase of ACh synthesis.[9]

MATERIALS AND METHODS

Animals

Male Fischer and Sprague-Dawley rats (Charles River) (200–250 g) were housed in groups of three per cage for at least 10 days prior to use. Food and water were freely available and animals were maintained under an artificial 7 a.m.–7 p.m. light-dark cycle. Experiments were carried out between 9 a.m. and 7 p.m.

Microdialysis Implantation and HPLC Assay

Rats were anesthetized with chloralhydrate (0.4 gr/kg i.p.) and implanted with dialysis tubes (O.D. = 150 μm; Hospal-Dasco, Bologna, Italy) at the level of the dorsal hippocampus, according to König and Klippel atlas. Surgery was carried out as previously described.[9] Ringer solution (KCl 4 mM; NaCl 147 mM; CaCl$_2$ 1.5 mM) was pumped through the dialysis tubes at a constant rate of 2 μl/min and neostigmine (10^{-7}M) was added to it for ACh determination. ACh was estimated in 20 min samples of dialysate (40 μl) using an enzyme-coupled high performance liquid chromatography with electrochemical detection according to the techniques described previously.[9,10]

Experiments were performed 24 hours after the implantation of the dialysis tubes. The basal output (picomoles/20 min) of ACh in the hippocampus (mean ± S.E.M. of at least seven rats) was 11 ± 0.65.

Drugs

Atropine-sulfate, pirenzepine-HCl, 4-DAMP methiodide and AF-DX 116 were dissolved in saline and injected intraperitoneally, or dissolved in the Ringer solution and perfused locally in the hippocampus.

ALCAR was dissolved in the drinking water (1.72 gr/lit) to which the rats were exposed for six months.

Statistics

The statistical significance of the difference between the groups was evaluated with the ANOVA followed by Duncan Multiple Comparisons using the individual undercurve area of response.

RESULTS

FIGURE 1 shows that basal release of ACh in the hippocampus was significantly reduced in 18-, 26-, and 31-month-old rats as compared to 3-month-old rats.

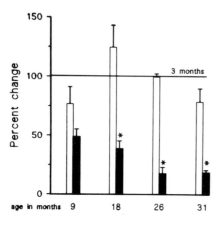

FIGURE 1. Age-induced modifications of ACh hippocampal concentration (*empty columns*) and release (*filled columns*). Data are expressed as % changes in respect to 3 month age. *p <0.1 versus 3 months. ACh hippocampal concentration (mean ± S.E.M. of 4 rats) was 249.57 ± 35 pmol/mg protein. ACh release in the hippocampus (mean ± S.E.M. of 4 rats) was 10.31 ± 2.2 pmol/40 μl.

However, it was unexpectedly found that tissue levels of ACh were substantially unchanged in aged rats.

It was hypothesized that this uncoupling between concentration and release could be due to age-dependent changes in the muscarinic receptors regulating ACh release. Therefore, the functional responsiveness of the cholinergic synapse, by probing the various muscarinic receptor subtypes with specific blockers, was investigated.

FIGURE 2 shows that atropine (10 μmol/kg) induced a remarkable increase of ACh release in the hippocampus of young rats (+ 400% over basal values), while the effect was drastically reduced in old rats (+ 200% over basal values). Moreover, the increase of ACh release in old rats pretreated with ALCAR was much higher than in control old rats (+ 300% over basal values).

Because atropine is antagonist for several subtypes of muscarinic receptors, the effects of more selective antagonists were studied. FIGURE 3 shows that AF-DX 116, preferentially active at the M2 cardiac type, is much less potent than atropine in stimulating ACh release. The dose of 50 μmol/kg increased ACh release of up to + 150% over basal values, and the effect was similar in young

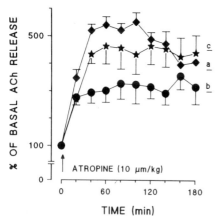

FIGURE 2. Effects of atropine 10 μmol/kg i.p. on *in vivo* ACh release from the hippocampus of 3-month- (*diamonds*, n = 5), 24-month- (*circles*, n = 3) and 24-month-old Fischer rats pretreated with ALCAR (*stars*, n = 5). Undercurve-areas (UCA) *a* versus *b:* p <0.01; *b* versus *c:* n.s.; *a* versus *c:* n.s.

FIGURE 3. Effects of AF-DX 116 50 μmol/kg i.p. on *in vivo* ACh release from the hippocampus of 3-month- (*diamonds,* n = 5), 24-month- (*circles,* n = 4) and 24-month-old Sprague-Dawley rats pretreated with ALCAR (*stars,* n = 5). Undercurve-areas (UCA) *a* versus *b:* n.s.; *b* versus *c:* n.s.; *a* versus *c:* n.s.

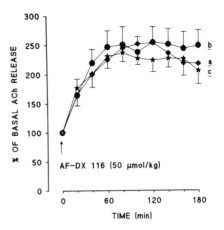

rats, in old rats and in old rats pretreated with ALCAR. The dose of 10 μmol/kg (the same used for atropine) had almost no effect on ACh release (not shown).

FIGURE 4 shows that also pirenzepine, a selective M1 antagonist, was much less potent than atropine. The dose of 50 μmol/kg increased ACh by about + 30% over basal values in young rats, but surprisingly enough the effect was greater in old rats (+ 100% over basal values). As was the case after atropine, the effect of pirenzepine in old rats pretreated with ALCAR was in between that of young and old rats (+ 50 over basal values).

These results show that the selective blockade of the M1 or M2 receptors has a much smaller effect on ACh release than that observed after the blockade by atropine. Whether or not the stronger potency of atropine (10 μmol/kg) was due to a cooperation between M1 and M2 receptors was studied. Consequently, the possibility that the effect of AF-DX 116 10 μmol/kg + pirenzepine 10 μmol/kg injections could resemble the effect of atropine 10 μmol/kg was also tested.

It was found that the injections of these drugs, at these doses, did not significantly stimulate ACh release. Only the administration of AF-DX 116 50 μmol/kg

FIGURE 4. Effects of pirenzepine 50 μmol/kg i.p. on *in vivo* ACh release from the hippocampus of 3-month- (*diamonds,* n = 3), 24-month- (*circles,* n = 3) and 24-month-old Sprague-Dawley rats pretreated with ALCAR (*stars,* n = 5). Undercurve-areas (UCA) *a* versus *b:* p < 0.01; *b* versus *c:* p <0.05; *a* versus *c:* n.s.

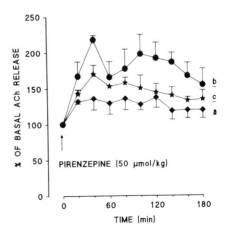

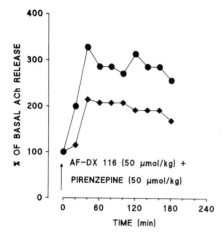

FIGURE 5. Effects of AF-DX 116 50 μmol/kg i.p. + pirenzepine 50 μmol/kg i.p. on *in vivo* ACh release from the hippocampus of 3-month- (*diamonds*, n = 3) and 24-month-old Fischer rats (*circles*, n = 3).

+ pirenzepine 50 μmol/kg stimulated ACh release (FIG. 5). However, the entity of the stimulation was just the sum of the stimulatory effect of each drug suggesting that the greater potency of atropine was due to another factor which was beyond M1 and M2 receptors, namely, M3 receptors; therefore, the effects of a preferential M3 antagonist were tried.

The M3 antagonist 4-DAMP 10^{-7} M dissolved in the Ringer solution perfusing the hippocampus enhanced the release of ACh by about 100% over basal values in young rats, while having no effects on old rats (not shown). FIGURE 6 shows that 4-DAMP 10^{-6} M stimulated ACh release by about + 200% over the basal values in young rats and had small effects in old rats (+ 50%). In old rats pretreated with ALCAR the effect was greater than in untreated old rats (+ 100% over basal values).

TABLE 1 shows the potency of 4-DAMP, atropine, AF-DX 116 and pirenzepine, all dissolved in the Ringer solution perfusing the hippocampus in stimulating ACh release in young and old rats. These results confirm those obtained after i.p. injections, showing that pirenzepine and AF-DX 116 are much less potent than atropine and 4-DAMP which, on the other hand, are approximately equipotent in enhancing ACh release from the hippocampus of young rats. Moreover, while in

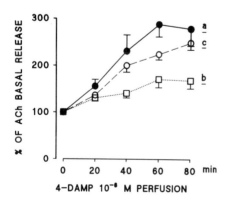

FIGURE 6. Effects of perfusion with 4-DAMP 10^{-6} M on *in vivo* ACh release from the hippocampus of 3-month- (*filled circles*, n = 7), 24-month- (*squares*, n = 7) and 24-month-old Sprague-Dawley rats pretreated with ALCAR (*open circles*, n = 7). Undercurve-areas (UCA) *a* versus *b:* n.s.; *b* versus *c:* n.s.; *a* versus *c:* n.s.

young rats pirenzepine and AF-DX 116 showed the same potency as in old rats, atropine and 4-DAMP were much less potent.

DISCUSSION

This study in freely-moving rats shows that the endogenous release of ACh in the hippocampus declines during aging. This finding is in line with the *in vitro* findings showing that electrically-evoked release of ACh, from cortical slices, undergoes a decline which is maximum in 24-month-old rats;[11] moreover, it was also shown *in vivo* that the K+-stimulated release of ACh declines within aging.[12]

The regulation of ACh release by muscarinic receptors has been the subject of several *in vitro* studies using different preparations. Ono *et al.*[13] used muscarinic agonists to study the release of ACh from hippocampal synaptosomes and release of ACh. The release of ACh from striatal slices seems also to be regulated by an M2 type of muscarinic receptor.[14,15]

Our data demonstrate that the release of ACh in the hippocampus of freely-moving animals can be enhanced by both i.p. or local infusion of muscarinic

TABLE 1. Effects of Perfusion with Atropine, 4-DAMP, AF-DX 116, and Pirenzepine on *In Vivo* ACh Release from the Hippocampus of 3-Month- and 24-Month-Old Fischer Rats

	% Over Basal Values	
	Young	Old
4-DAMP 10^{-6} M	+ 200	+ 70
Atropine 10^{-6} M	+ 250	+ 50
AF-DX 116 10^{-5} M	+ 70	+ 70
Pirenzepine 10^{-5} M	+ 80	+ 100

antagonists in the following order of potency: atropine $\geq$ 4-DAMP > AF-DX 116 > pirenzepine.

This order of potency compares with the activity of these compounds at M3 receptor because this receptor has a high affinity for atropine and 4-DAMP and low affinity for pirenzepine and AF-DX 116.[4,16]

Our findings are in agreement with those of De Boer *et al.*[5] showing the involvement of an M3 rather than M2 muscarinic autoreceptor in the regulation of ACh release in the striatum of freely-moving rats.

We have also shown that pirenzepine which is preferentially acting at M1 (with a potency 150 and 100 times greater than at M2 and M3 receptors) and AF-DX 116 which is preferentially acting at M2 (with a potency about 10 times greater than at M1 and M3 receptors),[4] stimulated ACh release in old rats with no reduction compared to young ones, suggesting that M1 and M2 muscarinic receptors are not damaged in aging. Instead, both atropine and 4-DAMP, which are equipotent at the three receptor subtypes, are by far more potent in young than in old rats therefore suggesting that the M3 receptor is the muscarinic receptor more involved in the aging process.

Therefore, it appears that the function of the cholinergic synapse in the hippocampus of the old rat could be impaired as a consequence of altered biochemical properties of the neuronal membrane involving the functional impairment of M3 receptors.

The finding that old rats pretreated with ALCAR respond to the atropine- and 4-DAMP-challenge with an increase of ACh release higher than in control old rats, suggests that this compound might preserve the biochemical properties of the neuronal membrane and consequently the functional expression of the existing receptors. The basis of this effect can be envisaged in the amelioration by ALCAR of the energetic processes in the aging brain.[6-8]

The ability of long-term treatment with ALCAR to reduce the significant differences between young and old rats in the receptor-mediated functional release of ACh candidates ALCAR as an ameliorative agent of receptor functionality in the aging brain.

SUMMARY

The regulation of acetylcholine (ACh) release by the different subtypes of muscarinic (M) receptors in the hippocampus of freely-moving Fischer and Sprague-Dawley rats, was investigated. Atropine (10 μmol/kg i.p.) induced a pronounced increase of ACh release (+ 400% over basal values) in the hippocampus of young rats (3 months) while the effect was drastically reduced (+ 100% over basal values) in old rats (24 months). The preferential M2 antagonist AF-DX 116 (50 μmol/kg i.p.) showed similar effects in young and old rats being, furthermore, 10 times less potent than atropine. The preferential M1 antagonist pirenzepine (50 μmol/kg i.p.) was even less potent than AF-DX 116 in enhancing ACh release in young rats, while the effect was more pronounced in the old ones. Therefore, the effect of the preferential M3 antagonist 4-DAMP was studied. 4-DAMP 10^{-6} M, dissolved in the Ringer solution perfusing the hippocampus, induced an enhancement of ACh release (+ 200% and + 70% over basal values, in young and old rats, respectively) which was comparable to that obtained after atropine at the same concentration. AF-DX 116 and pirenzepine, on the other hand, were by far less potent.

Six months' pretreatment with acetyl-l-carnitine (ALCAR) reduced the significant differences between young and old rats in the release response after M1 and M3 receptor antagonists.

Taken all together, these findings indicate that the regulation of ACh release, at least in the hippocampus, is mainly through the M3 receptors subtype of muscarinic receptors and that this subtype is the most involved in the aging process. Moreover, the ability of ALCAR to preserve the receptor-mediated functional ACh release response with respect to old animals suggests that ALCAR could be utilized in the amelioration of receptor functionality in the aging brain.

REFERENCES

1. GILLARD, M., M. WAELBROECH & J. CHRISTOPHE. 1987. Muscarinic receptor heterogeneity in the rat central nervous system. Mol. Pharmacol. **32:** 100–108.
2. HOSS, W. & W. MESSER, JR. 1986. Multiple muscarinic receptors in the CNS. Significance and prospects for future research. Biochem. Pharmacol. **35**(22): 3895–3901.
3. WAELBROECK, M., M. GILLARD, P. ROBBERECHT & J. CHRISTOPHE. 1987. Muscarinic receptor heterogeneity in the rat central nervous system. Finding of four selective antagonists to the three muscarinic receptor subclasses: a comparison with M2 cardiac muscarinic receptors of the C type. Mol. Pharmacol. **32:** 91–99.

4. HULME, E. C., N. J. M. BIRDSALL & N. J. BUCKLEY. 1990. Muscarinic receptor subtypes. *In* Annual Review of Pharmacology and Toxicology. R. George, A. K. Cho & T. F. Blaschke, Eds. Vol. **30:** 633–673.
5. DE BOER, P., B. H. C. WESTERINK, H. ROLLEMA, J. ZAAGSMA & A. S. HORN. 1990. An M3-like muscarinic autoreceptor regulates the *in vivo* release of acetylcholine in the rat striatum. Eur. J. Pharmacol. **170:** 167–171.
6. CURTI, D., F. DAGANI, M. R. GALMOZZI & F. MARZATICO. 1989. Effects of aging and acetyl-l-carnitine on energetic and cholinergic metabolism in the rat brain. Mech. Ageing Dev. **47:** 39–45.
7. GADALETA, M. N., V. PETRUZZELLA, M. RENIS, F. FRACASSO & P. CANTATORE. 1990. Reduced transcription of mitochondrial DNA in the senescent rat. Tissue dependence and effect of acetyl-l-carnitine. Eur. J. Biochem. **187:** 501–506.
8. RUGGIERO, F. M., F. CAFAGNA, M. N. GADALETA & E. QUAGLIARIELLO. 1990. Effect of aging and acetyl-l-carnitine on the lipid composition of rat plasma and erythrocytes. Biochem. Biophys. Res. Commun. **170**(2): 621–626.
9. IMPERATO, A., M. T. RAMACCI & L. ANGELUCCI. 1989. Acetyl-l-carnitine enhances ACh release in the striatum and hippocampus of awake freely-moving rats. Neurosci. Lett. **107:** 251–255.
10. DAMSMA, G., B. H. C. WESTERINK, P. DE BOER, J. B. DE VRIES & A. S. HORN. 1988. Basal acetylcholine release in freely moving rats detected on-line trans-striatal dialysis: pharmacological aspects. Life Sci. **43:** 1161–1168.
11. PEDATA, F., J. SLAVIKOVA, A. KOTAS & G. PEPEU. 1982. Acetylcholine release from cortical slices during postnatal development and aging. Neurobiol. Aging **4:** 31–35.
12. TAKEI, N., I. NIHONMATSU & H. KAWAMURA. 1989. Age-related decline of acetylcholine release evoked by depolarizing stimulation. Neurosci. Lett. **101:** 182–186.
13. ONO, S., Y. SAITO, N. OHGANE, G. KAWANISHI & F. MIZOBE. 1988. Heterogeneity in muscarinic autoreceptors and heterogeneity in the brain: effects of a novel M1 antagonist, AF102B. Eur. J. Pharmacol. **155:** 4–10.
14. JAMES, M. K. & L. X. CUBEDDU. 1987. Pharmacological characterization and the functional role of muscarinic autoreceptors in the rabbit striatum. J. Pharmacol. Exp. Ther. **240**(1): 203–209.
15. SCHOFFELMEER, A. N. M., B. J. VAN VLIET, G. WARDEH & A. H. MULDER. 1986. Muscarinic receptor mediated modulation of [3H]dopamine and [14C]acetylcholine release from rat neostriatal slices: selective antagonism for gallamine but not pirenzepine. Eur. J. Pharmacol. **128:** 291–299.
16. BIRDSALL, N. J. M. & E. C. HULME. 1985. Multiple muscarinic receptors: further problems in receptor classification. Trends Auton. Pharmacol. **3:** 17–34.

Reactive Capacities of the Central Nervous System in Physiological Aging and Senile Dementia of the Alzheimer Type

CARLO BERTONI-FREDDARI, PATRIZIA FATTORETTI,
TIZIANA CASOLI, WILLIAM MEIER-RUGE,[a]
AND JURG ULRICH[a]

Center for Surgical Research
INRCA Gerontological Research Department
Via Birarelli 8,
60121 Ancona, Italy

and

[a]Division of Gerontological Brain Research
Pathology Department
University of Basel
CH-4003 Basel, Switzerland

INTRODUCTION

Dementing illnesses in elderly people represent the largest constituent of social and medical care in the aged in most developed countries. An awareness of this fact has multiplied scientific efforts in studying physiological and pathological aspects of brain aging in human beings, since the percentage of the population older than 65 is expected to further increase. Senile dementia of the Alzheimer type (SDAT) has been reported to have a very high incidence among age-related neurological diseases even when, due to its subtle onset, it is often undiagnosed until a clear symptomatology becomes evident. Loss of memory and a subsequent progressive cognitive decline are the classic behavioral impairments at the basis of SDAT diagnosis. However, especially at the very beginning of the disease, the symptoms are similar to those found in physiological brain aging and may lead to an underestimation of the severity of forthcoming pathological conditions. Associated with these behavioral symptoms, dysfunctions and eventual neuron cell death in discrete areas of the central nervous system (CNS), such as cerebral cortex, hippocampus and basal forebrain, have been shown to occur in the SDAT brain. Histopathology has demonstrated that demented CNS shows increased amounts of neuritic plaques (NP), neurofibrillary tangles (NFT) and Hirano bodies (HB) which are also found, to a lesser extent, in the normal old brain.[1,2] Despite the wealth of studies on changes of the demented CNS, the pattern of histological and cytological alterations is incomplete and the primary causes of this devastating disease are still unknown. The present paper reports the results of a computer-assisted morphometric investigation on synaptic and mitochondrial ultrastructure in the human brain during normal aging and SDAT: we undertook this study in order to verify whether morphological changes can contribute to SDAT pathogenesis and progression.

CNS Potentialities for Neural Plasticity

Some years ago it was commonly assumed that the adult mammalian central nervous system was "hard wired," structurally static and incapable of growth. Repair processes in severed neurites did not occur and any function recovery was thought to depend on the brain's use of alternative pathways. Only peripheral nerves were known to be capable of regeneration, thus much scientific interest in neuronal plasticity was directed at the very simple nervous system of lower animals and at developing and peripheral nerves. Recently, mainly as a consequence of the improvement in research methodologies, it has been clearly shown that, if properly stimulated, the mature CNS can modify its wiring diagram in order to give the best response.[3] Different kinds of stimuli have been reported to elicit recovery phenomena and they include environmental factors such as stress, trauma and dietary manipulation or learning and memory trials. Restorative events involve both axons and synaptic terminals and since they have been documented in several areas of the CNS, it is widely accepted that they have a ubiquitous character. Axonal sprouting, that is, the growth of new branches from axons of intact neurons, and synapse turnover, that is, the loss and replacement of contacts, have been demonstrated to represent ongoing processes in the adult CNS. However, so far, it is not well proven if they have a positive functional significance or are detrimental to normal brain performances. To restore the lost functions new contacts should be equivalent to the originals, conversely the overproduction of abnormal connectivities may constitute a serious drawback to reestablishing the lost circuitries. The detailed mechanisms at the basis of the abovementioned ongoing CNS plastic processes, are still unknown. However, some insights into clarifying the basic steps leading to functional recovery have been provided by lesioning fibers, innervating discrete areas of the rodent hippocampal formation.[4] Axonal growth and the subsequent restoration of the number of synapses begin very early (48–96 hours after the lesion has been made) despite the presence of degenerating products in the reactive zone: a fact which supports the CNS's promptness to repair the damaged circuits. The environment where rebuilding of new connections takes place also appears important: it has been shown *in vitro* that a specific substrate and neurotrophic and growth factors can play a crucial role once the process of functional recovery has been triggered.[5]

Among biological models tested to check CNS potentialities for regeneration and repair, aging has been taken into account by many investigators and it has been clearly demonstrated that the reactive capacities of old nerve cells are impaired, probably due to some of the factors mentioned above. In particular, old lesioned rats recover lost functions later than young animals, but restoration is complete.[6] Thus, it seems to be clearly ascertained that mature CNS has a large potential for recovering lost functions through retained mechanisms also during aging, although to a lesser extent.

Morphological Reactive Capacities of Old and Demented CNS

As mentioned above, loss of memory and impairment to cognitive functions are the very early, and mostly misunderstood, symptoms of SDAT pathogenesis.

Although still under debate among neurobiologists, the recently proposed hypotheses concerning the anatomical basis of learning and memory support the fact that major structural modifications occur in the brain's basic wiring diagram and that these changes take place in synaptic regions.[7-9] In agreement with these concepts and in the searching for subcellular alterations of the senile and demented brain, we wanted to investigate the ultrastructural features of synaptic terminal areas by means of computer-assisted morphological methods recently set up in our laboratory.[10] Qualitative ultrastructural changes, if not extreme, are not detectable and statistical comparisons among the different groups are not permitted; thus, to obtain reliable information on several parameters regarding specific nerve cell structures, quantitative evaluations must be performed. A few years ago, Weibel[11] elaborated mathematical equations in order to carry out measurements from sectioned tissue; in addition, he stated some morphometrical criteria which are still valid, and what is more, may be transferred to the modern automatized and semiautomatized computer assisted image analysers. Specifically with regard to nervous tissue, a major task for the researcher involved in quantitative morphological studies is to find out anatomical models which fulfill Weibel's morphometric principles. In this context, since the brain is a very anisotropic organ, great care should be taken in looking for anatomical regions suitable for investigating biological problems by means of morphometric methods.

Discrete areas of the CNS appear to be selected targets for SDAT pathology, whereas some regions are reported to be completely unaffected by histopathological changes, such as NP, NFT and HB, which are closely related to the demented state. Although the majority of neurotransmitter systems have been documented to be involved in SDAT pathogenesis, cholinergic fibers seem to suffer the earliest and most dramatic alterations.[12,13]

Taking into account these points, we first decided to investigate the dentate gyrus supragranular layer and second, the cerebellar glomerulus, for opposite reasons. The former is reported to be a very sensitive area both to aging and age-related disorders of memory and cognitive functions, since it is a crossroads of important connections between enthorinal cortex and other structures within the limbic system. This area of the hippocampal formation is innervated by cholinergic inputs arising in the septum: these fibers do not overlap and therefore we were able to sample synaptic terminals using acetylcholine as neurotransmitter. The latter is a cell-free island in the granular layer of the cerebellar cortex, which besides being devoid of any histopathological SDAT hallmark, receives mixed fibers using many compounds as transmitters:[14] therefore, in our study, the cerebellar glomerulus represented a suitable "control" area as compared with each patient's more SDAT-vulnerable hippocampus. Due to its well-defined anatomical structure, the glomerulus also served as a good model to perform quantitative studies on mitochondrial ultrastructural features. In the glomerular area of the cerebellar granular layer, the mossy fiber swells up and establishes synaptic contacts with the dendrites of the surrounding granular cells and Golgi axons; thus, the mitochondria present in this zone directly subserve synaptic functions and are referred to as synaptic mitochondria.

Patients and the staining procedure we sampled and employed are reported in detail elsewhere.[15,16] Here is a brief summary of the main steps of our study: hippocampal and cerebellar samples were collected at autopsy from 5 SDAT patients and 5 age-matched controls. Tissue pieces were immediately processed for synaptic junctions by means of the ethanol phosphotungstic acid (E-PTA) preferential staining technique, according to our previous papers.[10,16,17] Cerebellar samples for mitochondrial investigation were processed according to conven-

TABLE 1. Morphometry of the Human Dentate Gyrus: Synapses and Granular Cells (Mean ± SEM)[a]

Parameters	Adult	Old	Demented
Sv (μm^2/μm^3)	0.1798 ± 0.0097	0.1399 ± 0.0025	0.1083 ± 0.0081*
S (μm^2)	0.1149 ± 0.0041	0.1756 ± 0.0096	0.1780 ± 0.0098*
Nv (syn./μm^3)	1.599 ± 0.1331	0.8308 ± 0.0424	0.6270 ± 0.0270*
Nvg (× 10^3/mm^3)	135.40 ± 8.31	92.19 ± 8.13	102.16 ± 9.10
Syn./Neur. (× 10^3/mm^3)	11.81 ± 0.83	9.96 ± 0.31	6.14 ± 0.58*

[a] Statistical comparisons: All the values in the old group are statistically significant when compared to the adult ones, respectively. * = p <0.01 vs old, age-matched group.

tional electron microscopic methods. We measured numerical density (Nv), surface density (Sv) and the average size (S) of the synaptic junctional zones in both the CNS areas considered. In the hippocampus we also evaluated the numerical density of dentate gyrus granular cells (Nvg) in order to relate this parameter to the synaptic numerical density (Nv). In the cerebellum, the following mitochondrial parameters were investigated: volume density (Vv), numerical density (Nvm) and the average volume of the single organelle (V). The results of our study are shown in TABLES 1, 2, and 3.

In the hippocampus of old patients, as compared with adult values, we found a significant decrease in Sv, Nv, Nvg and in the number of synapses per neurone (−15%), whereas the average size of the junctional areas (S) appeared to be significantly increased. The demented hippocampi, as compared with the age-matched controls, showed a significant decrease of Sv and Nv and in the number contacts/granular cells (−39%), whereas no significant difference was shown with regard to S and Nvg.

During physiological aging the cerebellar glomeruli undergo a significant decrease in synaptic Nv; Sv decreased, but not to a significant extent, and S increased. Mitochondrial Vv and Nv significantly decreased, whereas V increased. In senile demented cerebella, as compared to age-matched controls, we found significant decreases of Sv and Nv, whereas S was unchanged. Mitochondrial Vv and Nv decreased and V increased.

TABLE 2. Morphometry of the Human Cerebellar Glomerulus: Synapses (Mean ± SEM)[a]

Parameters	Adult	Old	Demented
Sv (μm^2/μm^3)	0.2095 ± 0.0136	0.1831 ± 0.0155	0.1231 ± 0.0118■
S (μm^2)	0.0132 ± 0.0040	0.1646 ± 0.0137*	0.1526 ± 0.0066*
Nv (syn./μm^3)	2.0286 ± 0.0834	1.1294 ± 0.0370*	0.8303 ± 0.1033●

[a] Statistical comparisons: * = p <0.001 vs the adult group; ■ = p <0.02 and ● = p <0.05 vs the old, age-matched group.

TABLE 3. Morphometry of the Human Cerebellar Glomerulus: Mitochondria (Mean ± SEM)[a]

Parameters	Adult	Old	Demented
Vv ($\mu m^3/\mu m^3$)	0.1381 ± 0.0036	0.1123 ± 0.0035	0.0888 ± 0.0029
Nvm (no.mit./μm^3)	1.207 ± 0.0311	0.533 ± 0.018	0.372 ± 0.013
V (μm^3)	0.114 ± 0.006	0.211 ± 0.004	0.239 ± 0.003

[a] Statistical comparisons: $p < 0.001$ when the data are compared with each other, respectively.

In the light of the above-mentioned updated concepts on CNS potentialities for neuronal plasticity, we interpret the present findings as documentation of morphofunctional rearrangements of synaptic terminals in aging and disease. In particular, the increase in synaptic S would seem to support a reactive phenomenon, countercting the reduced Sv found in aging and to a higher extent, in SDAT.[16] The close similarity of the alterations observed in both areas investigated demonstrates a ubiquitous character of synaptic ultrastructural impairment. With regard to the results obtained on the mitochondrial population in cerebellar glomeruli, (TABLE 3) it would seem that changes in the morphology of these organelles may be associated and/or contribute to reported alterations in metabolic processes related to energy production during aging and SDAT.[18,19] In particular, we interpret the decrease in Vv and Nv as reduced potentiality to produce energy and to cope with increased energy demands, conceivably the increase in V would seem to show a progressive impairment of the mitochondria to split into smaller organelles.

In the search for possible explanations of our present findings, we must consider that, although the causative events leading to the morphological synaptic rearrangements here documented are actively investigated, no evidence has been so far presented to single out a unique factor which determines these changes. Conversely, the reported age-dependent metabolic imbalance,[19,20] the vulnerability of synaptic terminal regions to oxidative stress[21] and decreased axonal flow in aging[22] support the idea that the wiring diagram of the old and demented brain is the final result of ongoing multifactorial influences. With specific consideration of synaptic contact zones, we propose that from a morphofunctional standpoint, nerve cells can better meet the functional demands of fewer enlarged junctions than those of many small synapses over the same dendritic domain. In this context, the reduction in the number of contacts may be considered as a physiological process of aging, although the fine tuning of neuronal circuitries is lost.

To conclude, old and demented CNS are both capable of morphological adaptive response at synaptic junctional regions. Consciousness of the retention of such reactive capacities during aging and senile dementia should multiply the efforts of neurobiologists and neurologists to look for proper strategies and compounds to strengthen these processes and hopefully, to prevent the cascade of events leading to SDAT.

REFERENCES

1. TOMLINSON, B. E. 1980. The structural and quantitative aspects of the dementias. *In* Biochemistry of Dementia. P. J. Roberts, Ed. 15–52. John Wiley. London.

2. ULRICH, J., A. PROBST, B. H. ANDERTON & J. KAHN. 1986. Dementia of Alzheimer type (DAT)—a review of its morbid anatomy. Klin. Wochenschr. **64:** 103–114.

3. COTMAN, C. W., N. NIETO-SAMPEDRO & E. V. HARRIS. 1981. Synapse replacement in the nervous system of adult vertebrates. Physiol. Rev. **61:** 684–784.

4. COTMAN, C. W. & N. NIETO-SAMPEDRO. 1984. Cell biology of synaptic plasticity. Science **255:** 1287–1294.

5. AGUAYO, A. J., M. VIDAL-SANZ, M. P. VILLEGAS-PEREX, S. A. KEIRSTEAD, M. RASMINSKY & G. M. BRAY. 1986. Axonal regrowth and connectivity from neuron in the adult rat retina. *In* Retinal Signal Systems, Degeneration and Transplants. E. Agardh & B. Ehinger, Eds. 257–270. Elsevier. New York, NY.

6. COTMAN, C. W. & C. PETERSON. 1989. Aging in the nervous system. *In* Basic Neurochemistry. G. Siegel, B. Agranoff, R. W. Albers & P. Molinoff, Eds. 523–540. Raven Press. New York, NY.

7. LYNCH, G. & M. BAUDRY. 1984. The biochemistry of memory: a new and specific hypothesis. Science. **224:** 1057–1063.

8. CARLIN, R. K. & P. SIEKEVITZ. 1983. Plasticity in the central nervous system: do synapses divide? Proc. Natl. Acad. Sci. USA **80:** 3517–3521.

9. PETIT, T. L. 1988. Synaptic plasticity and the structural basis of learning and memory. *In* Neuronal Plasticity: a Lifespan Approach. T. L. Petit & G. O. Ivy, Eds. 201–234. Alan R. Liss, Inc. New York, NY.

10. BERTONI-FREDDARI, C., W. MEIER-RUGE & J. ULRICH. 1988. Quantitative morphology of synaptic plasticity in the aging brain. Scanning Microsc. **2:** 1027–1034.

11. WEIBEL, E. R. 1979. Stereological methods. *In* Practical Methods for Biological Morphometry. E. R. Weibel, Ed. Vol. 1: 100–120. Academic Press. New York.

12. BARTUS, R. T., R. L. DEAN III, B. BEER & A. S. LIPPA. 1982. The cholinergic hypothesis of geriatric memory dysfunction. Science **217:** 408–417.

13. COYLE, J. T., D. L. PRICE & M. R. DeLONG. 1983. Alzheimer's disease: a disorder of cortical cholinergic innervation. Science **219:** 1184–1190.

14. SCHULMAN, J. A. 1983. Chemical neuroanatomy in the cerebellar cortex. *In* Chemical Neuroanatomy. P. C. Emson, Ed. 209–228. Raven Press. New York, NY.

15. BERTONI-FREDDARI, C., P. FATTORETTI, W. MEIER-RUGE & J. ULRICH. 1989. Computer-assisted morphometry of synaptic plasticity during aging and dementia. Pathol. Res. Pract. **185:** 799–802.

16. BERTONI-FREDDARI, C., P. FATTORETTI, T. CASOLI, W. MEIER-RUGE & J. ULRICH. 1990. Morphological adaptive response of the synaptic junctional zones in the human dentate gyrus during aging and Alzheimer's disease. Brain Res. **517:** 69–75.

17. BERTONI-FREDDARI, C., C. GIULI, C. PIERI & D. PACI. 1986. Quantitative investigation of the morphological plasticity of synaptic junctions in rat dentate gyrus during aging. Brain Res. **366:** 187–192.

18. MEIER-RUGE, W. 1985. Neurochemistry of the aging brain and senile dementia. *In* Aging 2000: Our Health Care Destiny. C. M. Gaitz & T. Samorajski, Eds. 101–112. Springer-Verlag, New York, NY.

19. SMITH, C. B. 1984. Aging and changes in cerebral energy metabolism. Trends Neurol. Sci. 203–208. Elsevier Science Publishers. Amsterdam.

20. SIESJO, B. K. & S. REHNCRONA. 1980. Adverse factors affecting neuronal metabolism: relevance to the dementias. *In* Biochemistry of Dementia. P. J. Roberts, Ed. 91–120. John Wiley and Sons, Ltd. New York, NY.

21. BERTONI-FREDDARI, C. 1989. Synaptic plasticity in the cerebellar glomeruli of rats: effects of aging and vitamin E deficiency. *In* Handbook of Free Radicals and Antioxidants in Biomedicine. J. Miquel, A. T. Quintanilha and H. Weber, Eds. pp. 255–267. CRC Press, Inc. Boca Raton, FL.

22. GEINISMAN, Y., W. BONDAREFF & A. TELSER. 1977. Diminished axonal transport of glycoproteins in senescent rat brain. Mech. Ageing Dev. **6:** 363–378.

Senile Dementia: a Threshold Phenomenon of Normal Aging?

A Contribution to the Functional Reserve Hypothesis of the Brain

W. MEIER-RUGE, O. HUNZIKER, AND P. IWANGOFF

Division of Gerontological Brain Research
Department of Pathology
University Medical School
Schönbeinstrasse 40
CH 4003 Basel, Switzerland

INTRODUCTION

The term senile dementia of the Alzheimer type, often used synonymous with Alzheimer's disease, is not well defined. Senile dementia which develops in later life, i.e. over the age of 70, is possibly much more a syndrome than a clearly defined disease.[1,2] In contrast, Alzheimer's disease as an early onset dementing disease (presenile dementia) represents a separate entity. It is a hereditary disease with genetic abnormalities in chromosome 21.[3-5]

Many of the senile demented who develop the disease in later life have much more a secondary or a vascular dementia than a hereditary one. Secondary dementias are at the onset often forms of benign senile forgetfulness aggravated by pneumonia, head trauma, bone fracture with fat embolism, intoxications etc.[6-8] The observation that the degree of the development of neuritic plaques, neurofibrillary tangles and a cholinergic cortical deficit are directly correlated with the severity of the dementia[9-12] supports the hypothesis that the primary or secondary syndrome of dementia is a threshold phenomenon.[13]

This may explain why it is not possible to identify one of the many parameters as the major key factor, which is changed in dementia.[1,2] Gottfries[2] therefore postulated that the many neurochemical changes in senile dementia of Alzheimer's type are secondary phenomena or epiphenomena of a more fundamental metabolic process. The fact that neurochemical and morphological changes in old age and senile dementia show many more quantitative than qualitative differences[6,7,14-16] could be an indication that the development of a dementia syndrome is a threshold phenomenon in a continuous process of declining brain performance partially accelerated by diseases which have secondary effects on brain performance.[1,17]

The aim of this study was to investigate normal brain aging and old age dementia from the viewpoint of the functional reserve hypothesis of senile dementia.

MATERIAL AND METHODS

A total of 82 autoptic brains were investigated: 59 neurochemically and 23 morphometrically. Fifty-six brains were normal aging and 26 brains had a senile dementia. The individuals investigated were between 20 and 92 years of age. The time which elapsed between death and the freezing of the brain tissue at $-80°C$ varied between 4 and 20 hours.

The normal aging brains were from subjects free of metabolic, neurologic and psychiatric diseases. These brains had from a neuropathological point of view no major morphological changes. The brains investigated are distributed as shown in TABLE 1.

Morphometric Methods

The nerve cell measurements on cerebral cortex were done on five sections per brain area, selected at random from 10 serial 14 μm frozen sections. The randomized sampling procedure for selecting sections was described by Sandoz and Meier-Ruge.[18] The nerve cells were stained with cresyl violet. The basic stereologic parameters, measured with an optic electronic image analysis system (ASBA Leitz), have been described in several papers.[19–21] The effect of postmortem delay in the morphometric parameters of nerve cells[22] and the capillary network[23] have also been evaluated in previous studies.[24]

Brain cortex from the medial frontal, parietal, medial temporal gyrus and putamen was investigated.

TABLE 1. Brains Investigated

		Neurochemically Investigated	Morphometrically Investigated
Normal aging brains	20–69 years	n = 26	
	70–92 years	n = 19	n = 11
Brains with senile dementia of the Alzheimer type	75–86 years	n = 14	n = 12

Neurochemical Methods

The neurochemical investigations were carried out in cortex areas (and putamen) identical with the brains investigated morphometrically. The tissue was frozen in dry ice and stored at $-80°$. The glycolytic enzymes were investigated according to methods described by Bücher *et al.*[25] Carbonic anhydrase was measured according to McArmstrong *et al.*[26] and acetylcholinesterase according to Ellman *et al.*[27] Protein kinase was studied as described by Reichlmeier.[28] All enzymatic investigations were carried out with homogenates or the supernatant fraction centrifuged from homogenates of brain cortex samples.

The influence of the cause of death and the duration of agony was investigated by Iwangoff *et al.*[29] It was shown that the duration of agony is of greater significance than the time interval between death and autopsy.

RESULTS

Neurochemical Findings in Normal Aging and Senile Dementia

To gain a better insight into the changes in *normal aging* brains, the enzymes of the glycolytic pathway were investigated. First changes of the glycolytic path-

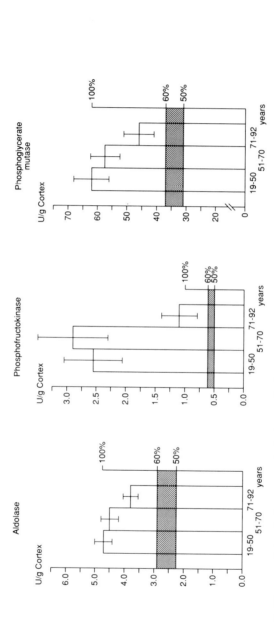

FIGURE 1. Changes of glycolytic enzymes in the human brain cortex which are in the range of −20 to −30% in normal aging up to 92 years of age. (From Meier-Ruge.[13] Reprinted by permission from *Excerpta Medica*.)

way were observed in only a few key enzymes. At ages exceeding 70 years a significant decrease of glycolytic turnover could be demonstrated with soluble hexokinase, phosphofructokinase, aldolase (FIG. 1) and pyruvate kinase.

Soluble hexokinase shows age-dependent increases in activity in the cytosol. The lower turnover of glucose is associated with a decrease in carbonic anhydrase activity in the brain (FIG. 2).

Since it has been shown that a decrease in glycolytic turnover results in a lower rate of pyruvate production, a lower synthetic rate of acetylcoenzyme A could be predicted (FIG. 3).

Acetylcoenzyme A is the rate limiting key substrate for the synthesis of acetylcholine. Therefore, a lower synthetic rate of acetylcoenzyme A should result in a decreased synthesis of acetylcholine which in turn induces a decrease of acetyl-

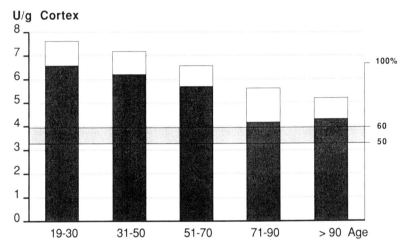

FIGURE 2. Age-related changes of carbonic anhydrase in human brain cortex. The decrease in carbonic anhydrase activity may be a consequence of a lower pCO_2 due to a decreased glycolytic turnover. (Based on Iwangoff *et al.*[36])

cholinesterase activity in the brain. In fact, at ages over 70 years, a decrease in acetylcholinesterase activity is observed (FIG. 4).

cAMP-dependent protein kinase activity decreases with age which becomes significant for ages over 72 years. The decrease of protein kinase activity is, in contrast to acetylcholinesterase, much more pronounced in the cortex than in the putamen. This decrease of cAMP activated protein kinase is mainly limited to the membrane-bound cortex fraction and less in the soluble fraction. Between 70 and 79 years of age protein kinase activity decreases about 25%; between 79 and 94 years the enzyme activity declines a further 35% (FIG. 5).

In senile dementia phosphofructokinase, hexokinase and pyruvate kinase are significantly decreased. In addition, aldolase, triosephosphate-isomerase, phosphoglyceratemutase, carbonic anhydrase (but not cAMP-stimulated protein kinase), are significantly decreased in comparison to age-matched controls (FIG. 6).

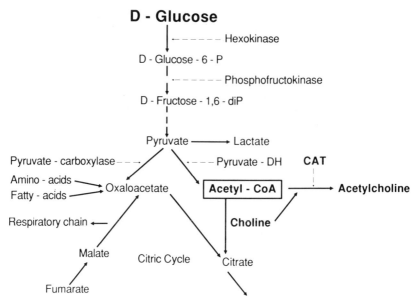

FIGURE 3. Schematic representation of the glycolytic pathway and its links to Acetyl-CoA synthesis.

Morphometric Results in Normal Brain Aging and Senile Dementia

Age-dependent nerve cell changes were studied in the brain cortex and in the putamen. Investigations of the nerve cell size demonstrated a clear trend towards smaller nerve cells in brains older than 85 years. In layers II–V of the medial

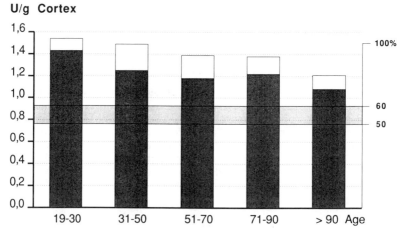

FIGURE 4. Age-induced decrease in acetylcholinesterase activity in the human brain cortex. (Based on Iwangoff *et al.*[36])

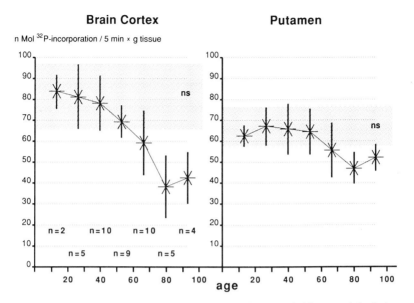

FIGURE 5. Age-dependent decrease of cAMP-dependent protein kinase activity in human brain cortex. (Based on Reichlmeier.[28])

frontal gyrus an average nerve cell shrinkage of 31.9%, compared with young adults of 19–45 years, is observed. Similar morphometric measurements demonstrated a shrinkage of 21% in the precentral gyrus and of 16% in the medial temporal gyrus (FIG. 7).

The comparison of the morphometric parameters of the capillary net of the normal aging brains showed no significant differences (TABLE 2).

The comparison of age-matched controls and senile demented brains demonstrates a significant nerve cell shrinkage in the brain cortex (FIG. 8) which is accompanied by a significant decrease of brain cortex volume.

These volume changes can be clearly correlated with the changes of the stereological parameters of the brain capillaries (FIG. 9).

The cortex shrinkage is characterised by an increase in the total capillary length, the capillary volume and a decrease in the intercapillary distance.

The changes in volume of the nerve cells (−58.6%) and of capillaries (+72.1%) in the brain cortex exceed the limits of a 40% redundancy (FIG. 10). The capillary diameters, however, remain unchanged.

TABLE 2. Stereological Parameters of the Capillary Net of Normal Aging Brains

Age Group (Years)	Capillary Volume (%)	Minimal Intercapillary Distance (μm)	Total Capillary Length (cm/mm³)	Capillary Diameter (μm)
18–44	2.23 ± 0.46	55.85 ± 4.25	21.58 ± 4.35	6.35 ± 0.45
85–94	2.26 ± 0.46	56.20 ± 3.32	21.10 ± 3.82	6.55 ± 0.24

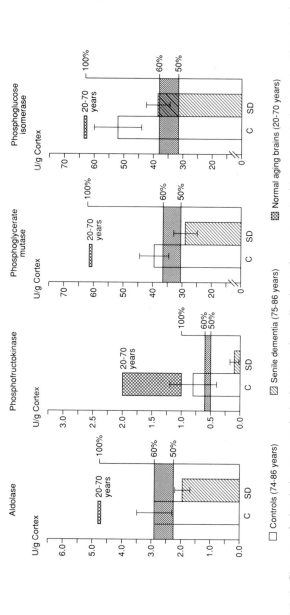

FIGURE 6. Changes of glycolytic enzymes in brain cortex in senile dementia compared with age-matched controls. (From Meier-Ruge.[13] Reprinted by permission from *Excerpta Medica.*)

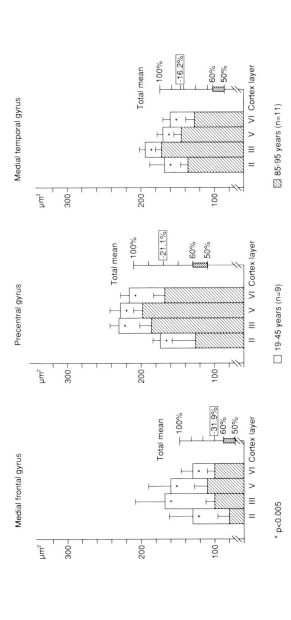

FIGURE 7. Changes in neurone size in the normal aging brain. The mean shrinkage of cortical nerve cell size is between 31.9 and 16.2% in the medial frontal, precentral and medial temporal gyrus. (From Meier-Ruge.[13] Reprinted by permission from *Excerpta Medica*.)

DISCUSSION

The results show that *senile dementia* in subjects of 82 years or older is characterized by a significant decrease in the turnover rates of key enzymes in the glycolytic pathway. The glycolytic turnover drops below the critical threshold of 40–50% of the functional reserve capacity.[36–38]

Even stereological investigations of the brain cortex show that nerve cells in senile dementia show a 58.6% decrease in mean size compared with age-matched controls. With the aid of the morphometric investigations of the net of brain cortex capillaries a significant shrinkage of the brain cortex can be shown,[14,30,31] which is in agreement with findings of an age dependent loss of synapses.[32–35]

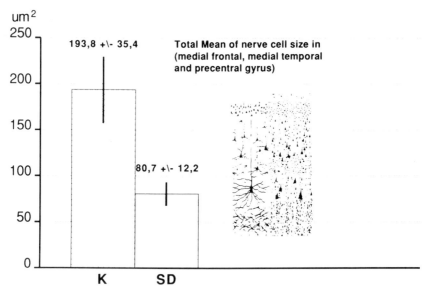

FIGURE 8. Nerve cell shrinkage in senile dementia (age 82 ± 5 years) compared with age-matched controls (age 82 ± 8 years). The nerve cell shrinkage is in the range of −58.3%.

The stereological change in the capillary network is a secondary phenomenon of the nerve cell change in the brain cortex and not a specific phenomenon of the degenerative process of senile dementia.[30–31]

With reference to *normal brain aging* the first symptoms of aging are a significant decrease in the enzyme activity of key enzymes of the glycolytic pathway[39–41] starting at about 70 years of age.[7,42] After a delay of 10–15 years a significant shrinkage (−20%) of the nerve cells in the brain cortex can be demonstrated.[43] A major loss of nerve cells could not be observed.[31,44]

Normal aging of the brain shows neurochemical and stereological changes in the range 20–30%[45] which are within the reserve capacity of the brain. Similar findings in the nucleus basalis Meynert complex of the basal forebrain were reported by Bigl *et al.*[46] Our comparative neurochemical and morphometrical stud-

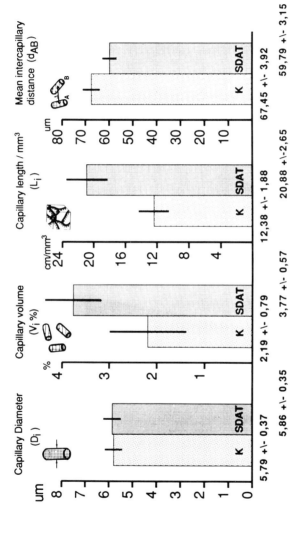

FIGURE 9. Morphometric results of the capillaries in the brain cortex which demonstrate the shrinkage of the brain cortex in senile dementia compared with age-matched controls. The values represent the total mean of medial frontal, medial temporal and precentral gyrus, characterized by a significant increase in capillary volume and capillary length, and a decrease in intercapillary distances.

ies in normal aging brains have shown that the earliest aging phenomenon is a metabolic decline, followed by a secondary moderate nerve cell atrophy.[47]

By correlating cognitive performance and synthetic rate of acetylcholine Perry et al.[10] have shown that a decrease of acetylcholine synthesis of more than 50% results in a psycho-organic defect syndrome or senile dementia. That senile dementia is characterised by a decrease of choline acetyl transferase activity has also been established by other authors.[48–52]

Coleman and Flood[53] observed that it is almost impossible to find a single marker characteristic for senile dementia of Alzheimer's type.[1] They routinely observed an overlap between normal aging and senile dementia.

With the exception of the fact that certain patients with old age dementia may have some genetic defects which are of importance for the abnormal phosphoryl-

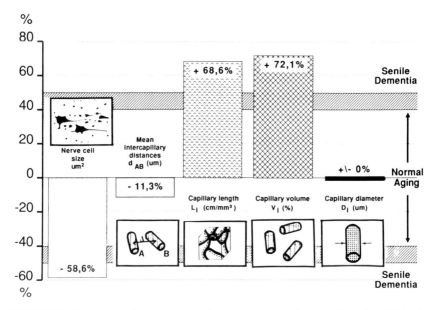

FIGURE 10. Percentage changes in stereologic parameters of nerve cells and capillaries in senile dementia and age-matched controls.

ation of cytoskeletal proteins or neurofilaments, it is clear that many dementia syndromes are simply nothing more than an exhaustion of the functional reserve capacity of the brain.[1,17,54] In the pathogenesis of this syndrome vital brain structures (hippocampus, nucleus basalis Meynert, cingulate gyrus etc.) often are involved which need for their normal function a minimum level of performance.[15,16,41,46,55]

The question of a continuity of benign senile forgetfulness in a dementia syndrome due to aging is also supported by the exponential increase of dementia with age.[1,41,56]

Gottfries[1] has extensively discussed whether it is possible to differentiate between a dementia syndrome of Alzheimer's type and a dementia as consequence of a cumulative destruction of the functional reserve capacity of the brain.

This could be of great importance for an effective therapy. Up to the present, it has not been possible to differentiate between the different forms of dementia.

In summary the task of further investigation is to clearly differentiate between a genetic linked form of Alzheimer's disease and an age-induced exhaustion of the functional reserve of the brain. Head injuries, respiratory disease, cardiac insufficiency, a collapse during general anaesthesia, electrolyte imbalance or intoxication are all pace-makers of a dementia syndrome in old age. The practical consequence of the prevention of secondary dementia could be a prophylactic therapy with drugs such as codergocrine mesylate[57–62] which compensate for a pathological decline of brain glucose turnover or for a neurotransmitter deficit. The aim of such therapy is to avoid an exhaustion of the resting reserve capacity of the brain.

In conclusion there are indications that a part of the senile dementia syndrome, from a pathogenetic point of view, is similar to a multiinfarct dementia and are secondary dementias due to hypoxic, toxic, traumatic or electrolyte induced disturbances of brain function. The development of major cognitive dysfunction in old age is much more a threshold phenomenon, even for classical Alzheimer cases, than a defect of a single, functional important parameter as is the case in Parkinson's disease.[1,2,17,41,45,54]

SUMMARY

Neurochemical investigations with *normal aging* brains show that in the first 70 years of life no major changes of the glycolytic pathway can be observed. Only in the following decades does a significant decrease of brain metabolic turnover occur. Changes in nerve cell size, one of the most relevant parameters in evaluating a diffuse nerve cell atrophy, appear in the brain cortex not earlier than between 85 and 94 years of age; a 21% nerve cell shrinkage is the mean. The results demonstrate that a significant decrease in turnover of the glycolytic pathway is followed by a significant but moderate shrinkage of the nerve cells after a delay of 10–15 years. Similar investigations in brains from *senile demented* subjects demonstrate that the change in glycolytic turnover is much more a quantitative than a qualitative phenomenon. In comparison with age-matched controls a decrease in glycolytic turnover of more than 60% is observed. Morphometric investigations of the nerve cell sizes in the brain cortex of senile demented subjects showed a decrease of 45–55% when compared with age-matched controls. When normal aging is compared with senile dementia it seems that old age dementia is a threshold phenomenon which starts if the glycolytic turnover drops below 50% of its value in young healthy adults. Physiological aging, however, stays within the range of the reserve capacity of normal brain performance.

In conclusion, it seems that the exhaustion of the functional reserve capacity may shift an aging brain into a dementia syndrome.

REFERENCES

1. GOTTFRIES, C. G. 1985. Alzheimer's disease and senile dementia: Biochemical characteristics and aspects of treatment. Psychopharmacology **86:** 245–252.
2. GOTTFRIES, C. G. 1990. Neurochemical aspects of dementia disorders. Dementia **1:** 56–64.
3. ST. GEORGE-HYSLOP, P. H., R. E. TANZI, R. J. POLINSKY, J. L. HAINES, L. NEE, P. C. WATKINS, R. H. MYERS, R. G. FELDMAN, D. POLLEN, D. DRACHMAN, J.

GROWDEN, A BRUNI, J.-F. FONCIN, D. SALMON, P. FROMMELT, L. AMADUCCI, S. SORBI, S. PLACENTINI, G. D. STEWART, W. J. HOBBS, P. M. CONNEALLY & J. F. GUSELLA. 1987. The genetic defect causing familial Alzheimer's disease maps on chromosome 21. Science **235:** 885–890.

4. VAN BROECKHOVEN, C. L. 1989. Molecular genetic analysis of early onset familial Alzheimer's disease. Neurobiol. Aging **10:** 437–438.

5. SELKOE, D. J. 1989. Molecular pathology of amyloidogenic proteins and the role of vascular amyloidosis in Alzheimer's disease. Neurobiol. Aging **10:** 387–395.

6. SORBI, S., S. PLACENTINI & L. AMADUCCI. 1984. Energy metabolism in aging and dementia. *In* Senile Dementia: Outlook for the Future. J. Wertheimer & M. Marois, Eds. 21–25. Alan R. Liss, Inc. New York, NY.

7. MEIER-RUGE, W. 1987. Introduction to the pathogenetic mechanisms of senile dementia and its therapeutic approaches. Excerpta Med. Asia Pacific Congr. Ser. **79:** 1–8.

8. PASCHALIS, C., P. POLYCHRONOPOULUS, N. P. LEKKA, M. J. G. HARRISON & T. PAPAPETROPOULUS. 1990. The role of head injury, surgical anaesthesia and family history as aetiological factors in dementia of Alzheimer type. Dementia **1:** 52–55.

9. TOMLINSON, B. E. 1977. The pathology of dementia. *In* Dementia. C. E. Wells, Ed. Vol. 2: 113–153. F. A. Davic Co. Philadelphia, PA.

10. PERRY, E. K., B. E. TOMLINSON, G. BLESSED, K. BERGMANN, P. H. GIBSON & R. H. PERRY. 1978. Correlation of cholinergic abnormalities with senile plaques and mental test scores in senile dementia. Br. Med. J. **2:** 1457–1459.

11. PRICE, D. L., P. J. WHITEHOUSE, R. G. STRUBLE, J. T. COYLE, A. W. CLARK, M. R. DELONG, L. C. CORK & J. C. HEDREEN. 1982. Alzheimer's disease and Down syndrome. Ann. N.Y. Acad. Sci. **396:** 145–164.

12. ULRICH, J. & H. B. STÄHELIN. 1984. The variable topography of Alzheimer type changes in senile dementia and normal old age. Gerontology **30:** 210–214.

13. MEIER-RUGE, W. 1990. Senile dementia—a disease of exhaustion of functional brain reserve capacity. Excerpta Med. Current Clin. Pract. Ser. **59:** 371–375.

14. MEIER-RUGE, W., J. ULRICH & H. B. STÄHELIN. 1985. Morphometric investigation of nerve cells, neuropil and senile plaques in senile dementia of the Alzheimer type. Arch. Gerontol. Geriatr. **4:** 219–229.

15. BRIZEE, K. R. 1987. Neuron numbers and dendritic extent in normal aging and Alzheimer's disease. Neurobiol. Aging **8:** 579–580.

16. JELLINGER, K. 1987. Quantitative changes in some subcortical nuclei in aging, Alzheimer's disease and Parkinson's disease. Neurobiol. Aging **8:** 556–561.

17. BRAYNE, C. & P. CALLOWAY. 1988. Normal aging, impaired cognitive function, and senile dementia of Alzheimer's type: a continuum? Lancet **1:** 1265–1267.

18. SANDOZ, P. & W. MEIER-RUGE. 1977. Age-related loss of nerve cells from the human inferior olive, and unchanged volume of its gray matter. IRCS Med. Sci. **5:** 376.

19. HUNZIKER, O., U. SCHULZ, CH. WALLISER & J. SERRA. 1976. Morphometric analysis of neurons in different depths of the cat's brain cortex after hypoxia. Natl. Bureau of Standards (NBS) Spec. Publ. Nr. 431: 203–206.

20. SCHULZ-DAZZI, U., O. HUNZIKER & CH. WALLISER. 1976. Quantitative investigations on neurons in the cerebral cortex of hypoxic cats. Z. Anal. Chem. **279:** 98–99.

21. MEIER-RUGE, W. 1988. Morphometric methods and their potential value for gerontological brain research. Interdiscip. Top. Gerontol. **25:** 90–100.

22. SCHULZ, U., O. HUNZIKER, H. FREY & A. SCHWEIZER. 1980. Postmortem changes in stereological parameters of cerebral neurons. Pathol. Res. Pract. **166:** 260–270.

23. HUNZIKER, O. & A. SCHWEIZER. 1977. Post-mortem changes in stereological parameters of cerebral capillaries. Beitr. Pathol. **161:** 244–255.

24. WIEDERHOLD, K.-H., W. BIELSER, JR., U. SCHULZ, M.-J. VETEAU & O. HUNZIKER. 1976. Three-dimensional reconstruction of brain capillaries from frozen serial sections. Microvasc. Res. **11:** 175–180.

25. BÜCHER, TH, W. LUTZ & D. PETTE. 1964. Einfache und zusammengesetzte optische Tests mit Pyridinnukleotiden. *In* Handbuch der physikalischen und pathologisch-chemischen Analyse. Vol. VI/A: 293–339. Hoppe-Seyler/Thierfelder, Springer. Berlin.

26. McArmstrong, J. D., D. V. Myers, J. A. Verpoorte & J. T. Edsall. 1966. Purification and properties of human erythrocyte carbonic anhydrase. J. Biol. Chem. **241:** 5137–5149.
27. Ellman, G. L., K. D. Coastney, V. Andres, Jr. & R. M. Featherstone. 1961. A new and rapid colorimetric determination of acetylcholinesterase activity. Biochem. Pharmacol. **7:** 88–95.
28. Reichlmeier, K. D. 1976. Age related changes of cyclic AMP-dependent protein kinase in bovine brains. J. Neurochem. **27:** 1249–1251.
29. Iwangoff, P., R. Armbruster, A. Enz & P. Sandoz. 1978. Influence of ageing, post-mortem delay and agonal state of phosphofructokinase (PFK) in human brain tissue obtained at autopsy. IRCS Med. Sci. **6:** 83.
30. David, M., A. Mann, N. R. Eaves, B. Marcyniuk & P. O. Yates. 1986. Quantitative changes in cerebral cortical microvasculature in ageing and dementia. Neurobiol. Aging **7:** 321–330.
31. Meier-Ruge, W., S. Abdel-Al & U. Schulz. 1983. Etudes stéréomorphométriques des capillaires et des cellules nerveuses du cerveau normal chez le sujet âgé et dans la maladie d'Alzheimer. Presse Méd. (Paris) **12:** 3115–3118.
32. Bertoni-Freddari, C. & C. Giuli. 1980. A quantitative morphometric study of synapses of rat cerebellar glomeruli during aging. Mech. Aging **12:** 127–136.
33. Bertoni-Freddari, C., C. Giuli, C. Pieri & D. Paci. 1986. Quantitative investigations of the morphological plasticity of synaptic junctions in rat dentate gyrus during aging. Brain Res. **366:** 187–192.
34. Adams, I. 1987. Plasticity of the synaptic contact zone following loss of synapses in the cerebral cortex of aging humans. Brain Res. **424:** 343–351.
35. Casey, M. A. & M. L. Feldman. 1988. Age-related loss of synaptic terminals in the rat medial nucleus of the trapezoid body. Neuroscience **24:** 189–194.
36. Iwangoff, P., K. Reichlmeier, A. Enz & W. Meier-Ruge. 1979. Neurochemical findings in physiological aging of the brain. Interdiscip. Top. Gerontol. **15:** 13–33.
37. Hoyer, S. 1988. Glucose and related brain metabolism in dementia of Alzheimer type and its morphological significance. Age **11:** 158–166.
38. Hoyer, S., K. Oesterreich & O. Wagner. 1988. Glucose metabolism as the site of the primary abnormality in early-onset dementia of Alzheimer type. J. Neurol. **235:** 143–148.
39. Iwangoff, P., R. Armbruster, A. Enz & W. Meier-Ruge. 1980. Glycolytic enzymes from human autoptic brain cortex: normal aged and demented cases. Mech. Ageing Dev. **14:** 203–209.
40. Hoyer, S. 1985. The effect of age on glucose and energy metabolism in brain cortex of rats. Arch. Gerontol. Geriatr. **4:** 193–203.
41. Hoyer, S. 1988. Glucose and related brain metabolism in normal aging. Age **11:** 150–156.
42. Svanborg, A., S. Landahl & D. Mellström. 1983. New perspectives on old age. A message to decision makers. *In* Thomas, H. & G. L. Maddox. Eds. 31–52. Springer Publ. Comp. New York, NY.
43. Meier-Ruge, W., O. Hunziker, U. Schulz, H. J. Tobler & A. Schweizer. 1980. Stereologic changes in the capillary network and nerve cells of the aging human brain. Mech. Ageing Dev. **14:** 233–243.
44. Haug, H. 1985. Are neurons of the human cerebral cortex really lost during aging? A morphometric study. *In* Senile Dementia of the Alzheimer Type. J. Traber & W. G. Gripsen, Eds. 150–163. Springer. Berlin, Heidelberg, New York.
45. Lowes-Hummel, P., H.-J. Gertz, R. Ferszt & J. Cervos-Navarro. 1989. The basal nucleus of Meynert revised: the nerve cell number decreases with age. Arch. Gerontol. Geriatr. **8:** 21–27.
46. Bigl, V., T. Arendt, S. Fischer, S. Fischer, M. Werner & A. Arendt. 1987. The cholinergic system in aging. Gerontology **33:** 172–180.
47. Bondareff, W. 1987. Changes in the brain in aging and Alzheimer's disease assessed by neuronal counts. Neurobiol. Aging **8:** 562–563.
48. Rossor, M., J. Fahrenkrug, P. Emson, C. Mountjoy, L. Iversen & M. Roth.

1980. Reduced cortical choline acetyltransferase activity in senile dementia of Alzheimer type is not accompanied by changes in vasoactive intestinal polypeptides. Brain Res. **201:** 249–253.

49. WHITEHOUSE, P. J., D. L. PRICE, A. W. CLARK, J. T. COYLE & M. R. DELONG. 1981. Alzheimer disease: evidence for selective loss of cholinergic neurons in the nucleus basalis. Ann. Neurol. **10:** 122–126.

50. WHITEHOUSE, P. J., D. L. PRICE, R. G. STRUBLE, A. W. CLARK, J. T. COYLE & M. R. DELONG. 1982. Alzheimer's disease and senile dementia: loss of neurons in the basal forebrain. Science **215:** 1237–1239.

51. NEARY, D., J. S. SNOWDEN, D. M. A. MANN, D. M. BOWEN, N. R. SIMS, B. NORTHEN, P. O. YATES & A. N. DAVISON. 1986. Alzheimer's disease: a correlative study. J. Neurol. Neurosurg. Psychiatr. **49:** 229–237.

52. DECKER, M. W. 1987. The effects of aging on hippocampal and cortical projections of the forebrain cholinergic system. Brain Res. **434:** 423–438.

53. COLEMAN, P. D. & D. G. FLOOD. 1987. Neuron numbers and dendritic extent in normal aging and Alzheimer's disease. Neurobiol. Aging **8:** 521–545.

54. BOWEN, D. M., P. WHITE, J. A. SPILLANE, M. J. GOODHARDT, G. CURZON, P. IWANGOFF, W. MEIER-RUGE & A. N. DAVISON. 1979. Accelerated ageing or selective neuronal loss as an important cause of dementia? Lancet **1:** 11–14.

55. MESULAM, M. M., E. J. MUFSON & J. ROGERS. 1987. Age-related shrinkage of cortically projecting cholinergic neurons: a selective effect. Ann. Neurol. **22:** 31–36.

56. KATZMAN, R. 1988. Alzheimer's disease as an age-dependent disorder. *In* Research and the Ageing Population. 69–85. Ciba Foundation Symposium 134. Wiley. Chichester.

57. LOEW, D. M., J. M. VIGOURET & A. L. JATON. 1980. Effects of dihydroergotoxine (Hydergine) on cerebral synaptic transmission. Interdiscip. Top. Gerontol. **15:** 85–103.

58. MARKSTEIN, R. 1983. Dopamine receptor profile of co-dergocrine (Hydergine®) and its components. Eur. J. Pharmacol. **86:** 145–155.

59. MARKSTEIN, R. 1985. Hydergine®: Interaction with neurotransmitter systems in the central nervous system. J. Pharmacol. (Paris) **16:** 1–17.

60. MARKSTEIN, R. 1989. Pharmacological approaches in the treatment of senile dementia. Eur. Neurol. **29**(Suppl. 3): 33–41.

61. MEIER-RUGE, W. 1986. Effects of prolonged co-dergocrine mesylate (Hydergine®) treatment on local cerebral glucose uptake in aged Fischer 344 rats. Arch. Gerontol. Geriatr. **5:** 65–77.

62. BERTONI-FREDDARI, C., C. GIULI, C. PIERI, D. PACI, L. AMADIO, M. ERMINI & A. DRAVID. 1987. The effect of chronic Hydergine® treatment on the plasticity of synaptic junctions in the dentate gyrus of aged rats. J. Gerontol. **42:** 482–486.

Behavioral and Electrocortical Spectrum Power Effects after Microinfusion of Lymphokines in Several Areas of the Rat Brain

GIUSEPPE NISTICÒ AND GIOVAMBATTISTA DE SARRO

Institute of Pharmacology
Faculty of Medicine
University of Reggio Calabria
Via T. Campanella
88100 Cantanzaro, Italy

INTRODUCTION

There exists considerable evidence that the growth of glial cells can be influenced by T-cell-derived lymphokines and monokines.[1] Lymphokines and monokines are not found in any quantity in normal brain. When they do occur because of infiltration by activated T-cells and macrophages or when endogenous proteins similar or identical to lymphoid factors are produced by activated astrocytes or microglia, brain cells including oligodendroglia and neurons may be affected. Such redundancies allow for safeguarding repair and homeostatic mechanisms in response to trauma and disease in the central nervous system (CNS).[1-4] Brain tissues have receptors for and can respond directly to interleukins.[5-8] The evidence indicates that not only some of the actions involve the CNS, but that they are initiated on the brain side of the blood-brain barrier.[7,9-11]

Interleukin-1 (IL-1) seems to be an important mediator of the inflammatory and fever responses to infection and injury[12] while interleukin-2 (IL-2) affects differentiation of brain cells through enhanced gene expression[1,13] and interleukin-3 (IL-3) acts as a growth factor for microglia cells.[14] We have recently described some typical changes in behavior and bioelectrical activity following IL-2 and other lymphokines.[15,16] These changes may well represent the reason for the potent central nervous system side effects reported to occur in man after the administration of high systemic doses of interferons and interleukins.[17]

The effects of interferons and interleukins on seizure activity is not clearly understood. In some previous studies performed by our group we reported a spiking activity in the cortical and hippocampal recordings after α-interferon or IL-2 injection into the third cerebral ventricle of the rat.[16]

The present experiments aimed to characterize and compare the behavioral, body temperature and electrocortical (ECoG) activity of IL-1-β, IL-2 and IL-3 after their intracerebral microinfusion. In addition, the possible epileptic activity of these lymphokines was studied. The results of the present experiments could give us some information on the most sensitive areas of the brain through which the central effects of IL's are mediated. In addition, they could show analogies and differences among the different interleukins as far as their central effects are concerned.

119

METHODS

Animals and Surgery

Adult male Wistar rats (200–250 g) were purchased from Morini (San Polo d'Enza, Reggio Emilia) and maintained on a 12-hr light-dark cycle (lights on 6:00–18:00 hr, off 18:00–6:00 hr). The animals were stereotaxically implanted with stainless steel guide cannulae, under chloral hydrate anaesthesia (400 mg/Kg i.p.), according to the atlas coordinates of Paxinos and Watson,[18] to permit intracerebroventricular infusion (i.c.v.) or a unilateral or a bilateral injection into the locus coeruleus or into other areas of the brain, *i.e.,* the caudate nucleus, dorsal hippocampus, substantia nigra (pars compacta) or ventromedial hypothalamus. The steel guide cannulae were chronically implanted with the tips 2 mm away from each area of the brain studied. After surgery, a minimum of 48 hr was allowed for recovery before experiments were carried out. All experiments were performed, beginning at approximately 10:00 hr. Freely-moving rats were injected through an injector cannula, which extended approx 2 mm below the tip of the guide cannula. *Postmortem* histological examination confirmed the location of the guide cannulae.

Body Temperature Changes and Statistical Analysis

Body temperature was recorded on a Grant temperature recorder by means of a thermistor implanted beneath the skin of the interscapular region as previously described.[19]

Values are presented as a means $\pm$ SEM. Statistical analysis between control and drug-treated groups was performed with ANOVA or Student t test for unpaired data and was considered significant when p was <0.05 (two-tailed analysis).

Electrocortical Activity and Statistical Analysis

Electrocortical (ECoG) activity was recorded (8 channel ECoG machine OTE Biomedica, Florence) through 4 chronically-implanted steel screw electrodes, inserted bilaterally onto the fronto-parietal and the fronto-occipital area. The ground electrode was implanted epidurally over the nasal bone. At least 3 rats for each group were implanted with bipolar electrodes in the hippocampus (AP = 4.3 posterior to the bregma, L = 3.5, H = 3.5 mm ventral to the skull surface) and amygdala (AP = 2.8 posterior the bregma, L = 5.1, H = 7.5 mm ventral to the skull surface). For statistical purposes, the bipolar signals from each cortical area were integrated by means of a Berg-Fourier analyser (OTE Biomedica, Florence, Italy) according to Bricolo *et al.*[20] In particular, the ECoG changes were continuously (every 5 min) computerized as previously described,[21] in order to obtain continuous information on the total voltage power as well as on preselected bands of ECoG frequency (0.25–3; 3–6; 6–9; 9–12 and 12–16 Hz or 0.5–3; 3–7; 8–12; 12–16 and 14–32 Hz). The time constant (0.03) was short enough to reduce the number of artifacts (HF cut-off was 5.3 Hz). The spectrum power was plotted and the integrated energy signals were expressed as μV^2 per second.

In order to quantify the changes of total voltage power and of preselected bands of frequency induced by lymphokines, the area (expressed in mm²) under the curve corresponding to plotted total voltage values, during periods of 30 min after each compound, was integrated by means of a Commodore computer, and the percentage changes of the integrated area, in comparison to the same interval during the pretreatment period, were calculated according to the "trapezoidal rule."[22] In addition, in order to reduce possible interanimal variations of the baseline electrocortical activity and of a single frequency band existing in the same group, the percentage changes after treatment with drugs were compared to the values for the corresponding period before treatment, using paired Student t test. Statistical analysis between groups treated with interleukins or vehicle (in the same volume) was performed using the Mann-Whitney U test.

Infusion of the same volume of the vehicle (0.5 μl or 2,0 μl for the specific area of brain studied, or intraventricular injection, respectively) lacked effects on behavior and electrocortical activity.

Gross analgesic changes were noted and quantified but not statistically analysed, using the tail immersion assay, with 49.5 C water as the nociceptive stimulus or the tail-flick method in the rat.

Drugs

The following compounds were used: human-recombinant interleukin-1 beta (hr-IL-1-β, Eurogenetics, Torino, Italy), human interleukin-2 (h-IL-2) and rat interleukin-2 (rat-IL-2) (Sigma, St. Louis, MO), human-recombinant interleukin-2 (hr-IL-2, Janssen, Beerse, Belgium) and human-recombinant interleukin-3 (hr-IL-3) (Omnia res, Cinisello Balsamo, Milano, Italy).

All drugs were easily dissolved in 67 mM sodium phosphate buffer, containing 5 mg of serum albumin for 1 ml.

RESULTS

Interleukin-1

Intracerebroventricular Administration

hr-IL-1 (0.89, 2.67 and 8.01 pmol) possesses behavioral and electrocortical sedative properties when administered intracerebroventricularly in rats. These effects appeared within 10–20 min after the infusion and lasted from 40 to 150 min depending on the dose (at least n = 4 rats for each dose). When sedative behavior was evident this was associated with ECoG synchronization and an increase in total voltage power as well as in 0–3 and 3–6 Hz frequency bands (FIG. 1). The dose of 2.67 pmol of hr-IL-1 induced an increase in body temperature within 20 min after injection, reached the maximum increase after 70–120 min and remained elevated for approx 180 min, while the dose of 8.01 of hr-IL-1-β elicited a higher increase in body temperature which was also longer lasting (FIG. 2).

Intra-Locus Coeruleus Administration

Much lower doses of hr-IL-1 (0.2 and 0.3 pmol, at least 6 rats for each dose) were necessary in order to observe similar behavioral and electrocortical sedative

LOCUS   COERULEUS

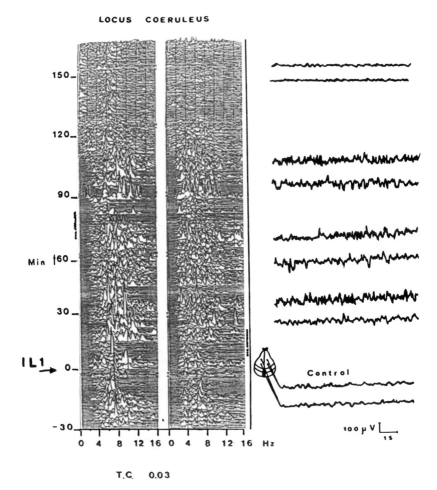

T.C.   0.03

FIGURE 1. Sequential spectral analysis and ECoG activity in a rat, illustrating the effects on cortical electrical activity after microinjection of hr-IL-1 (2.67 pmol) into the third cerebral ventricle. The ECoG activity, evaluated at various times after hr-IL-1 administration, shows cortical synchronization. The ECoG activity was characterized by a power increase, with a shift in 0–3 and 3–6 Hz frequency bands. No major alterations in cortical recordings were observed 80 min after hr-IL-1.

TABLE 1. Soporific Potency and ECoG Changes of Interleukins after Their Microinjection into the Third Cerebral Ventricle (ivt) or into the Locus Coeruleus (ilc)

Lymphokine	Minimum Soporific Dose (pmol)ivt	Minimum Soporific Dose (pmol)ilc
hr-IL-1	0.89	0.2
h-IL-2	2.67	0.89
rat-IL-2	2.67	0.89
hr-IL-3	1.34	0.3
hr-IL-2	2.67	0.4

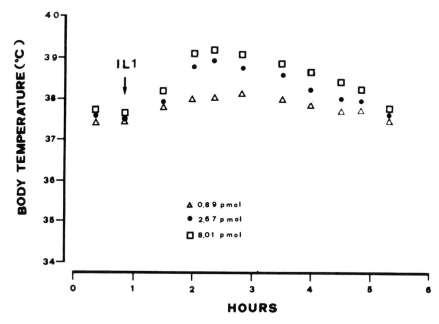

FIGURE 2. Body temperature changes after intraventricular administration of hr-IL-1 (0.89, 2.67 and 8.01 pmol). Each point represents the mean of at least 5 animals.

effects to those seen after its intracerebroventricular administration of hr-IL-1. The sedative behavior was associated with ECoG synchronization and an increase in total voltage power as well as in 0–3 and 3–6 Hz frequency bands and lasted 80 to 130 min depending on the dose. No ECoG epileptiform discharges or changes in body temperature were observed when hr-IL-1 was injected into the locus coeruleus.

Intrahippocampal Administration

In comparison to the locus coeruleus administration, equimolar doses of hr-IL-1 (0.2 and 0.3 pmol) injected into the dorsal hippocampus were ineffective in inducing behavioral and ECoG slow-wave sleep (at least 4 experiments for each dose). No significant changes in locomotor activity or in ECoG pattern were observed.

TABLE 2. Pyrogenic Potency of Interleukins after Intracerebroventricular Administration

Lymphokine	Minimum Pyrogenic Dose (pmol)	Mean Duration ± SEM of Pyrogenic Activity
hr-IL-1	2.67	162 ± 24
hr-IL-2	not pyrogenic up to 13.35	
hr-IL-3	8.01	137 ± 22

Interleukin-2

Intracerebroventricular Administration

h-IL-2 (2.67–13.35 pmol), rat-IL-2 (2.67–13.35 pmol) and hr-IL-2 (2.67, 8.01 and 13.35 pmol), after injection into the third cerebral ventricle, induced typical behavioral sedation and/or sleep, associated with ECoG synchronization and an increase in total voltage power (at least 5 animals for each dose). The sedative effects appeared within 5–10 min, depending on the dose and with the largest dose of h-IL-2 and r-IL-2 were preceded by spiking in cortical and hippocampal activity, sometimes associated with episodes of wet-dog shakes. No spiking activity was observed in animals treated with 2.67 and 8.01 pmol of hr-IL-2. The sedative effects, induced by IL-2 or rat-IL-2 lasted between 25 and 140 min, depending on the dose. During the sedative state an increase in 3–6 and 6–9 Hz frequency bands was recorded at the cortical level.

TABLE 3. Epileptogenic Potency and ECoG Discharges of Interleukins after Intracerebroventricular Administration

Lymphokine	Minimum Epileptogenic Dose (pmol)	Predominant Type of ECoG Discharges
hr-IL-1	12	spike-waves or sharp waves
h-IL-2 or rat-IL-2	13.35	single or polyspikes spike-waves
hr-IL-2	24.03	single or polyspikes
hr-IL-3	16.02	spike-waves

Intra-Locus Coeruleus Administration

Smaller doses of h-IL-2 or rat-IL-2 (0.89–2.67 pmol) and hr-IL-2 (0.30–1.34 pmol) microinfused into the locus coeruleus (n = 6) induced behavioral and ECoG sedative activity similar to that observed after intraventricular injection. These sedative behavioral and ECoG effects lasted from 40 to 120 min depending on the dose. No spiking activity was observed when h-IL-2, rat-IL-2 or hr-IL-2 were infused into the locus coeruleus. Bilateral injection of h-IL-2, rat-IL-2 (0.15 and 0.45 pmol) or hr-IL-2 (0.15 and 0.30 pmol) into the locus coeruleus was as effective as unilateral injection of 1.34 pmol of both recombinant and not recombinant IL-2 in producing behavioral and ECoG slow wave sleep (n = 4).

Microinjection into Other Brain Areas

In comparison to the locus coeruleus, equimolar doses of h-IL-2 or rat-IL-2 (0.30, 1.34, 0.89 and 2.67 pmol) and hr-IL-2 (0.89–2.67 pmol) given into the dorsal hippocampus, caudate nucleus, substantia nigra and ventromedial hypothalamus, were ineffective in inducing behavioral and ECoG slow wave sleep (at least 3 experiments for each dose and area of brain studied). However, h-IL-2, rat-IL-2 and hr-IL-2 injected into the caudate nucleus and substantia nigra (pars compacta) elicited an asymmetric body posture, with ipsilateral turning behavior and periodic ipsilateral circling, lasting from 25 to 60 min, depending on the dose. These effects were longer lasting in animals injected in the substantia nigra than in those injected in the caudate nucleus.

Animals treated with h-IL-2, rat-IL-2 or hr-IL-2 (0.89–2.67 pmol) into the dorsal hippocampus or ventromedial hypothalamus showed an increase in locomotor and exploratory activity lasting 20–65 min depending on the dose.

Interleukin-3

Intracerebroventricular Administration

hr-IL-3 (1.34, 2.67–8.01 and 13.35 pmol) induced behavioral and electrocortical sedative effects when injected intracerebroventricularly (FIG. 3, at least 5 rats for each dose). These effects were observed from 5 to 10 min after the infusion and lasted 30 to 190 min depending on the dose. When sedative behavior was observed the spectral analysis revealed an increase in total voltage power and a significant increase in 9–12 and 12–16 Hz frequency bands. The dose of 8.01 and 13.35 pmol of hr-IL-3 induced an increase in body temperature within 10 min and reached the maximum increase 60–90 min after injection and remained elevated for 150–210 min depending on the dose (FIG. 4).

Intra-Locus Coeruleus Administration

Much lower doses of hr-IL-3 (0.4 and 0.6 pmol) were necessary in order to induce a reduction in locomotor activity and behavioral and electrocortical sedative changes which seemed to be similar to those observed after intracerebroventricular administration (n = 4 for each dose). Sedative behavior was associated with ECoG synchronization and an increase in total voltage power; however, the spectral analysis revealed an increase in 3–6 and 6–9 Hz frequency bands, whereas after intracerebroventricular injection of hr-IL-3 there was a predominant increase in 9–12 and 12–16 Hz power. These sedative behavioral and ECoG changes lasted from 30 to 80 min depending on the dose.

No ECoG epileptiform discharges or changes in body temperature were observed when hr-IL-3 was administered into the locus coeruleus.

Intrahippocampal Administration

In comparison to the locus coeruleus injections, equimolar doses of hr-IL-3 (0.4 and 0.6 pmol) injected into the dorsal hippocampus were unable to significantly affect behavior and electrocortical activity (n = 4 for each dose).

Behavioral and Epileptic Electrocortical Changes after Intracerebroventricular or Intrahippocampal Administration of High Doses of Interleukins

Following hr-IL-1 (0.89–2.67 and 8.01 pmol), h-IL-2 (2.67, 8.01 and 13.35), rat-IL-2 (2.67, 8.01 and 13.35 pmol), hr-IL-2 (2.67 and 8.01 pmol) and hr-IL-3 (2.57, 8.01 and 13.35 pmol) usually produced a cortical synchronization, characterized by slow waves of high voltage associated with sedative behavior. All interleukins

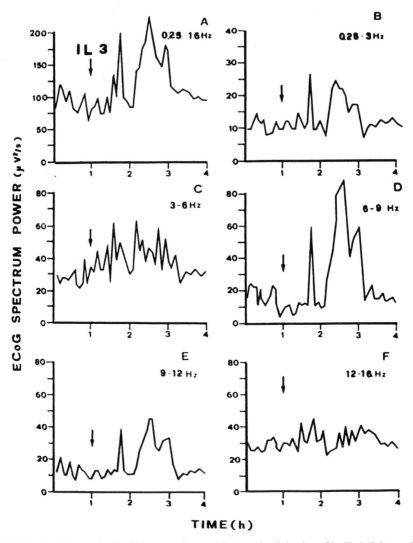

FIGURE 3. Effects of a single intracerebroventricular microinjection of hr-IL-3 (8.01 pmol) on electrocortical spectrum power. *Ordinates* show the voltage power expressed in μV^2 per sec; *abscissae* show the time (hr). The ECoG activity was characterized by a power increase in total voltage as well as a predominant increase with in 3–6, 6–9, and 9–12 Hz frequency bands. No major alterations were observed 120 min after hr-IL-3.

studied at higher doses induced epileptiform activity, which showed a different ECoG pattern depending on the lymphokine injected. Spiking activity induced by hr-IL-1 (12 and 13.35 pmol) began within 1–3 min from the injection and occurred periodically for about 40 min. It was characterized by medium amplitude (300–400 μV) bouffées of sharp-waves or spike-waves which had an irregular frequency of 1–5 spikes for 15 to 40 sec duration and recurring at 6–10-min intervals (FIG. 5).

No spiking activity was observed when hr-IL-1 (2.67 and 8.01 pmol) was microinfused into the dorsal striatum.

Rat-IL-2 (13.35, 16.02 and 24.03 pmol) and h-IL-2 (13.35 and 16.02 pmol) induced electrocorticographic epileptiform activity within 1 min from the injection and these recurred periodically for 40 to 180 min depending on the dose. On the contrary, hr-IL-2 was less epileptogenic in comparison to the nonrecombinant IL-2 since almost a double dose (24.03 pmol) was required to induce epileptogenic discharges.

Typically, each episode of spiking activity following h-IL-2 or rat-IL-2 lasted 30 to 60 sec and occurred at 4–10-min intervals. When high amplitude (400–500 μV) bouffées of polyspikes or polyspike waves occurred, these had an irregular frequency of 3–7 spikes and sometimes were associated with episodes of wet-dog shake or more frequently with episodes of frozen immobility (FIG. 6). In addition, after microinfusion of all three types of IL-2 studied (2.67 and 8.01 pmol) into the dorsal hippocampus electrocorticographic epileptiform activity was observed. These ECoG discharges were characterized by single or polyspikes of high amplitude, 300–450 μV, which lasted 20 to 40 sec and occurred at 3–8-min intervals. When spiking activity occurred this had an irregular frequency of 3–7 spikes/s and was associated with episodes of frozen immobility.

hr-IL-3 (16.02 and 24.03 pmol) after intracerebroventricular microinjection produced within 5 min from the infusion an ECoG epileptic activity characterized by spike-waves occurring (3–5 Hz) which were associated with episodes of frozen immobility or more rarely with wet-dog shake episodes. The electrocortical epileptic discharges lasted 15–35 min depending on the dose and were followed by

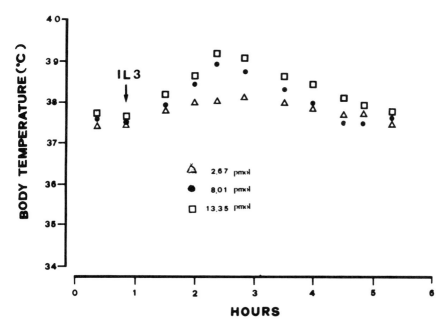

FIGURE 4. Body temperature changes after intraventricular administration of hr-IL-3 (2.67, 8.01 and 13.35 pmol). Each point represents the mean of at least 5 animals.

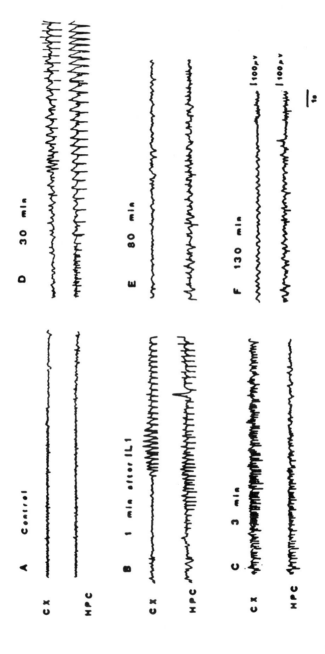

FIGURE 5. Electrographic recordings illustrating the effects of intracerebroventricular microinjection of hr-IL-1-β (12 pmol). **(A)** Pre-drug control electrographic (EEG) recording. **(B)** The EEG activity 1 min after hr-IL-1-β microinjection shows bouffées of spike-waves. **(C,D)** The EEG activity 3 and 30 min after hr-IL-1-β microinjection shows bouffées of spikes or spike-waves. **(E,F)** EEG recordings demonstrating EEG activity occurring 80 and 130 min after hr-IL-1-β. CX, cortex; HPC, hippocampus.

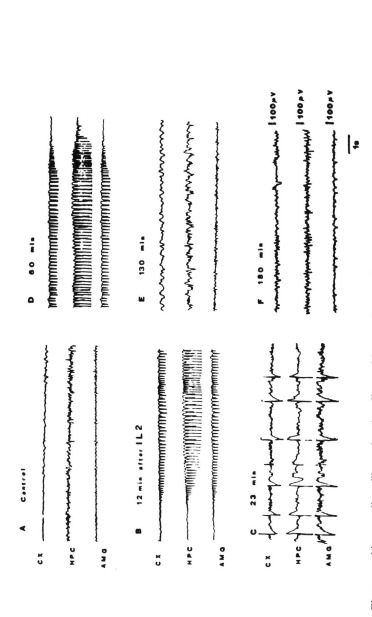

FIGURE 6. Electrographic recordings illustrating the effects of intracerebroventricular microinjection of H-IL-2 (16.02 pmol). **(A)** Pre-drug control electrographic (EEG) recording. **(B)** The EEG activity 12 min after h-IL-2 microinjection shows bouffées of spike-waves. **(C,D)** The EEG activity 23 and 60 min after h-IL-2 microinjection shows bouffées of spikes or spike-waves. **(E,F)** EEG recordings demonstrating EEG activity occurring 130 and 180 min after h-IL-2. CX, cortex; HPC, hippocampus; AMG, amygdala.

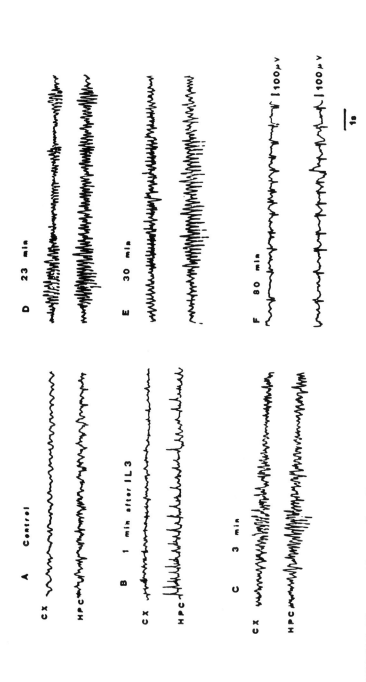

FIGURE 7. Electrographic recordings illustrating the effects of intracerebroventricular microinjection of hr-IL-3 (16.02 pmol). **(A)** Pre-drug control electrographic (EEG) recording. **(B)** The EEG activity 1 min after hr-IL-3 microinjection shows spikes. **(C,D)** The EEG activity 3 and 23 min after hr-IL-3 microinjection shows bouffées of spikes or spike-waves. **(E,F)** EEG recordings demonstrating EEG discharges occurring 30 and 80 min after hr-IL-3. CX, cortex; HPC, hippocampus.

ECoG synchronization with slow waves of high voltage and behavioral sedation lasting 100–160 min (FIG. 7).

No spiking activity occurred when hr-IL-3 (2.67 and 8.01 pmol) was microinfused into the dorsal striatum.

However, animals never showed generalized convulsions after interleukin microinjection.

DISCUSSION

The present experiments show that IL-1, IL-2 and IL-3 produced specific and marked behavioral and ECoG changes. Thus, it is not surprising that more frequently or occasionally, according to the lymphokine used, after systemic administration in man several central nervous system disorders, including confusion, fatigue and lethargy, have been described to occur.[17]

The sedative effects observed after intracerebroventricular administration of interleukins confirm previous studies showing that all interleukins studied possess sleep-promoting effects.[16,23,24]

Recently, it was reported that IL-1 and IL-2 are able to cross the blood-brain barrier thereby entering the central nervous system from the blood.[25,26] Other evidence based on newer, more sensitive techniques has shown that many substances assumed to be excluded by the blood-brain barrier because of size, including peptides and proteins, enter the CNS by saturable and nonsaturable processes.[27,28] Furthermore, peptides and other compounds may enter the brain at the level of circumventricular organs where the blood-brain barrier is absent, with subsequent leakage to nearby structures.

Banks and co-workers[25] showed that the hypothalamus possesses a higher concentration of IL-1 than other brain areas. The hypothalamus seems to be important in mediating the activity of some interleukins; in fact, this area, where the thermoregulatory centers are located, is easily reached from the third cerebral ventricle and most likely mediates sensitive body temperature changes of IL-1 and IL-3. Moreover, no fever responses were evoked by IL-1 and IL-3 when microinfused into the hippocampus or into the locus coeruleus.

In addition, other effects of circulating IL-1 and IL-2 might be mediated through the hypothalamic neurons such as the release of hypothalamic peptides, anorexia, analgesia and changes in monoamines and amino acids in the brain.[29,30,31] From the present experiments, it seems that IL-3 possesses similar central effects to IL-1.

The reason for nonpyrogenic action of h-IL-2, IL-2 and hr-IL-2 is not known, but similar results have already been observed in rabbits.[32]

Furthermore, in the present experiments evidence has been provided showing that the sleep-inducing effects of interleukins are likely to be mediated through the locus coeruleus. This area was the most or the only sensitive one in mediating behavioral and ECoG sleep, and sleep was not obtained after direct infusion of interleukins into other brain structures.

The locus coeruleus is the area containing the largest clusters of noradrenaline-containing cell bodies in the CNS.[33] Evidence exists that α2-adrenoceptors and opiate receptors are located at the soma and dendrites of neurones in the locus coeruleus and that clonidine and opioid peptides produce behavioral and ECoG sleep, when injected directly into this area in rats.[21,34]

The finding that interleukin-2's produced the same behavioral and ECoG effects after infusion into the locus coeruleus indicates that these lymphokines may influence the firing of neurones in the locus coeruleus, through an increase in K^+ conductance, as with $\alpha2$-adrenoceptor agonists[35,36] or opioid peptides.[37] The different potency of interleukins studied may depend both on the number of specific receptors for these lymphokines and on their intrinsic potency.

Of course, the fact that neurones in the locus coeruleus are also activated by glutamate, substance P, muscarinic acetylcholine and corticotropin-releasing factor[37] suggests that the influences of interleukins on such neurotransmitters needs to be further investigated.

The higher convulsant properties of IL-2 when injected directly into the dorsal hippocampus in comparison to other interleukins studied may well be due to the higher density of specific receptors for IL-2 in this brain area,[38] while the higher density of specific receptors for IL-1 in the CNS was observed in the hypothalamus.[29,39] No similar data are yet available for IL-3. The higher epileptogenic activity of r-IL-2 and h-IL-2 in comparison to hr-IL-2 suggests that such phenomena may be in part related to presence of some contaminating compounds which are not present in the latter preparation.

In conclusion, the present experiments show that all interleukins studied possess soporific effects and produce EcoG epileptic discharges, the most powerful being IL-1-β followed by IL-3 and IL-2. The site through which the soporific effects are mediated seems to be represented by the locus coeruleus. In addition, from the present results it is evident that only IL-1-β and IL-3 at higher doses than the soporific ones produce hyperthermic effects. Further experiments are necessary in order to ascertain the possible mechanisms of action of ILs at the receptor level.

REFERENCES

1. MERRILL, J. E. 1988. Lymphokines, monokines and glial cells. PNEI **1:** 13–14.
2. BENVENISTE, E. N. & J. E. MERRILL. 1988. Stimulation of oligodendroglial proliferation and maturation by interleukin-2. Nature **321:** 610–613.
3. NIETO-SAMPEDRO, M. & M. A. BERMAN. 1987. Interleukin-1-like activity in rat brain: sources, targets and effect of injury. J. Neurosc. Res. **17:** 214–219.
4. GIULIAN, D., R. ALLEN, T. J. BAKER & Y. J. TOMOZAWA. 1986. Brain peptides and glial growth. 1. Glia-promoting factors as regulators of gliogenesis in the developing and injured central nervous system. Cell. Biol. **102:** 803–811.
5. GIULIAN, D., J. WOODWARD, D. G. YOUNG, J. F. KREBS & L. B. LACJMAN. 1988. Interleukin-1 injected into mammalian brain stimulates astrogliasis and neovascularization. J. Neurosci. **8:** 2485–2490.
6. HORI, T., M. SCHIBATA, T. NAKASHIMA, M. YAMASAKI, A. ASAMI, T. ASAMI & H. KOGA. 1988. Effects of interleukin-1 and arachidonate on the preoptic and anterior hypothalamic neurons. Brain Res. Bull. **20:** 75–82.
7. KATSUURA, G., P. E. GOTTSCHALL & A. ARIMURA. 1988. Identification of a high-affinity receptor for interleukin-1 beta in rat brain. Biochem. Biophys. Res. Commun. **156:** 61–67.
8. YAMAMOTO, K., T. MIWA, R. UENO & O. HAYAISHI. 1988. Muramyl dipeptide-elicited production of PGD2 from astrocytes in culture. Biochem. Biophys. Res. Commun. **156:** 882–888.
9. HASHIMOTO, M., T. BANDO, M. INKI & K. HASHIMOTO. 1988. Effect of indomethacin on febrile response to recombinant human interleukin-1 in rabbits. Am. J. Physiol. **255:** R527–R533.
10. NAKAMURA, H., K. NAKANISHI, A. KITA & T. KADOKAWA. 1988. Interleukin-1 induces analgesia in mice by a central action. Eur. J. Pharmacol. **149:** 49–54.
11. PLATA-SALAMAN, C. R., Y. OOMURA & Y. KAI. 1988. Tumor necrosis factor and

interleukin-1 beta: suppression of food intake by direct action in the central nervous system. Brain Res. **448:** 106–114.

12. DINARELLO, C. A. 1986. Multiple biological properties of recombinant human interleukin-1 (beta). Immunology **178:** 301–315.

13. MERRILL, J. E. 1987. Macroglia: neural cells responsive to lymphokines and growth factors. Immunol. Today **8:** 146–150.

14. FREI, K., S. BODMER, C. SCHWERDEL & A. FONTANA. 1986. Astrocyte-derived interleukin-3 as a growth factor for microglia cells and peritoneal macrophages. J. Immunol. **137:** 3521–3527.

15. DE SARRO, G. B., C. ASCIOTI, M. G. AUDINO, V. RISPOLI & G. NISTICÒ. 1989. Behavioural and ECoG spectrum changes induced by intracerebral microinfusion of interferons and interleukin-2 in rats are antagonized by naloxone. *In* Interactions among Central Nervous System, Neuroendocrine and Immune Systems. 351–356. Pythagora Press. Rome and Milan.

16. DE SARRO, G. B., Y. MASUDA, C. ASCIOTI, M. G. AUDINO & G. NISTICÒ. 1990. Behavioural and ECoG spectrum changes induced by intracerebral infusion of interferons and interleukin-2 in rats are antagonized by naloxone. Neuropharmacology **29:** 167–179.

17. FENT, K. & G. ZBINDEN. 1987. Toxicity of interferon and interleukin. Trends Pharmacol. Sci. **8:** 100–105.

18. PAXINOS, F. & C. WATSON. 1982. The Rat Brain in Stereotaxic Coordinates. Academic Press. London.

19. NISTICÒ, G., D. ROTIROTI, F. NACCARI, G. B. DE SARRO & E. MARMO. 1980. Effects of intraventricular beta-endorphin and D-ala-methionine-enkephalinamide on behaviour, spectrum power of electrocortical activity and body temperature in rats. Res. Commun. Chem. Pathol. Pharmacol. **28:** 295–308.

20. BRICOLO, A., S. TURAZZI, F. FACCIOLI, F. ODORIZZI, C. SCIARRETTA & P. ERCULIANI. 1978. Clinical application of compressed spectral array in long-term EEG monitoring of comatose patients. Electroencephalogr. Clin. Neurophysiol. **45:** 211–225.

21. DE SARRO, G. B., C. ASCIOTI, F. FROIO, V. LIBRI & G. NISTICÒ. 1987. Evidence that locus coeruleus is the site where clonidine and drugs acting at alpha-1 and alpha-2-adrenoceptors affect sleep and arousal mechanisms. Br. J. Pharmacol. **90:** 675–685.

22. TALLARIDA, R. J. & R. B. MURRAY. 1981. Manual of Pharmacological Calculations with Computer Programs. Springer. Berlin.

23. KRUEGER, J. M., C. WALTER, C. A. DINARELLO, S. M. WOLFF & L. CHEDID. 1984. Sleep-promoting effects of endogenous pyrogen (interleukin-1). Am. J. Physiol. **246:** R994–R999.

24. MCCANN, S. M., V. RETTORI & L. MILENKOVIC. 1989. Effects of monokines and anterior pituitary hormone release by hypothalamic and pituitary actions. *In* Interactions Among Central Nervous System, Neuroendocrine and Immune Systems. J. W. Hadden, K. Masek & G. Nisticò, Eds. 93–106. Pythagora Press. Rome and Milan.

25. BANKS, W. A., A. J. KASTIN & D. A. DURHAM. 1989. Bidirectional transport of interleukin-1 alpha across the blood-brain barrier. Brain Res. Bull. **23:** 433–437.

26. SARIS, S. C., S. A. ROSENBERG, R. B. FRIEDMAN, J. T. RUBIN, D. BARBA & E. H. OLDFIELD. 1988. J. Neurosurg. **69:** 29–34.

27. BANKS, W. A. & A. J. KASTIN. 1989. Quantifying carrier-mediated transport of peptides from the brain to the blood. Methods Enzymol. **168:** 652–660.

28. FISHMAN, J. B., J. B. RUBIN, J. V. HANDRAHAN, J. R. CONNOR & R. E. FINE. 1987. J. Neurosci. Res. **18:** 299–304.

29. DINARELLO, C. A. 1988. Biology of interleukin 1. FASEB J. **2:** 108–115.

30. DUNN, A. J. 1988. Systemic interleukin-1 administration stimulates hypothalamic norepinephrine metabolism paralleling the increased plasma corticosterone. Life Sci. **43:** 429–435.

31. BINDONI, M., V. PARCIAVALLE, F. BEUTTA, N. BELLUARDO & T. DIAMASTSTEIN. 1980. Interleukin-2 modifies the bioelectric activity of some neurosecretory nuclei in the rat hypothalamus. Brain Res. **462:** 10–14.

32. MIER, J. M., M. S. LARRY, M. ALLEGRETTA, T. BOONE, H. A. BERNHEIM & C. A. DINARELLO. 1985. Dissimilarities between purified human interleukin-1 and recombinant human interleukin-2 in the induction of fever, brain prostaglandin, and acute-phase protein synthesis. J. Biol. Response Modif. **4:** 35–45.
33. DAHLSTROM, A. & K. FUXE. 1964. Evidence for the existence of monoamine containing neurons in the central nervous system. I. Demonstration of monoamine in the cell bodies of brain stem neurons. Acta Physiol. Scand. **232:** 1–55.
34. DE SARRO, G. B., S. SAKURADA, G. BAGETTA, C. ASCIOTI, M. G. AUDINO, V. RISPOLI & G. NISTICO. 1988. Behavioural and ECoG spectrum power effects induced by microinfusion of compounds acting at different opioid receptors into the locus coeruleus. Neurosci. Lett. **33:** 74S.
35. NORTH, A. R. 1986. Opioid receptor types and membrane ion channels. Trends Neurol. Sci. **9:** 114–117.
36. PEPPER, C. M. & G. HENDERSON. 1980. Opiates and opioid peptides hyperpolarize locus coeruleus neurons *in vitro*. Science **209:** 394–396.
37. AGHAJANIAN, G. K. & C. P. VANDER-MAELEN. 1982. Alpha-2-adrenoceptor mediated hyperpolarization of locus coeruleus: intracellular studies *in vivo*. Science **215:** 1394–1396.
38. ARAUJO, D. M., P. A. LAPCHAK, B. CALLIER & R. QUIRON. 1989. Localization of interleukin-2 immunoactivity and interleukin-2 receptors in the rat brain. Interaction with the cholinergic system. Brain Res. **498:** 257–266.
39. BREDER, C. D., C. A. DINARELLO & C. B. SAPER. 1988. Interleukin-1 immunoreactive innervation of the human hypothalamus. Science **240:** 321–324.

Enkephalin-Induced Stimulation of Humoral and Cellular Immune Reactions in Aged Rats[a]

BRANISLAV D. JANKOVIĆ AND DRAGAN MARIĆ

Immunology Research Center
Vojvode Stepe 458
11221 Belgrade, Yugoslavia

INTRODUCTION

Numerous systemic studies have led to the notion that aging of the immune system is the consequence of microenvironmental changes of different tissue/organ systems. Although the thymus and its hormonal activity may play a critical role in immune function development during age,[1-3] other systems may also be as significant. Several lines of evidence have indicated that, in senescence, there is a general inability of the organism to maintain the homeostatic balance of the endocrine and nervous systems, which leads to altered hormone and neurotransmitter responsiveness[4-6] and impaired immune system function.[7-11] Homeostatic imbalance with age may also be related to function of the opioid system.[12] There is a large body of evidence suggesting a very potent *in vitro* regulating influence of the opioids on the immune responses.[13-20] However, we have previously shown that *in vivo* administered opioid peptides, the enkephalins, exert a dual and dose-dependent immunomodulating activity in young adult rats.[21-25] In this study we describe immunorestorative functions of the opioid pentapeptide, methionine-enkephalin, in senescent rats.

MATERIALS AND METHODS

Animals

Experiments were performed on 8-week-old (200–250 g) and 20-month-old (500–600 g) female Wistar rats. Animals were housed, in groups of 3, in conventional plexiglass cages, and supplied food pellets and tap water *ad libitum*. Experimental and control groups consisted of 20–24 rats, each.

Antigens

Sheep red blood cells (SRBC) and five times crystalized bovine serum albumin (BSA) served as antigens. SRBC, stored in Alsever's solution, were washed three times with physiological saline before use. BSA was purchased from ICN Pharmaceuticals (lot no. 9218; Cleveland, OH) and dissolved in apyrogenic saline, *ex tempore*. BSA and old tuberculin were employed in skin hypersensitivity tests.

[a] This work was supported by the Republic of Serbia Research Fund, Belgrade.

Immunization

One group of rats was sensitized with 5×10^9 SRBC in 1 ml of saline injected intraperitoneally (i.p.), and another group was immunized, into the left hind footpad, with 0.5 mg BSA in 0.1 ml of complete Freund's adjuvant (CFA).

Enkephalin

Methionine-enkephalin (Met-Enk) was obtained from Serva (Heidelberg, F.R.G.). The pentapeptide was stored at $-20°C$ and dissolved in apyrogenic physiological saline before use.

Treatment

Animals received i.p. injections of Met-Enk (0.2 mg/kg b.w.) according to the following schedules: (a) 1 injection every 24 hours, 1 day before and 4 days after immunization with SRBC; and (b) 1 injection every 48 hours for a period of 14 consecutive days after sensitization with BSA-CFA. Controls were treated with saline in an identical manner.

Plaque-Forming Cell (PFC) Assay

Rats immunized with SRBC were sacrificed on day 4 after sensitization, and their spleens extirpated and processed for direct PFC microassay in Cunningham's chambers using normal guinea pig serum as a source of complement. The PFC response was ascertained by counting hemolysin-producing cells.

Antibody Determinations

Serum samples, obtained by heart puncture 4 days after immunization with SRBC and 14 days after inoculation of BSA-CFA, were examined for hemagglutinin titers using direct and passive microhemmaglutination reactions, respectively. In the former reaction fresh SRBC were used, whereas formalinized SRBC coated with BSA were employed in the latter.

Evaluation of Inflammatory Foot Swelling

The degree of inflammatory enlargement of the foot injected with BSA-CFA was evaluated on day 12. Using a micrometer gauge, diameters (mm) of ankle, tarsus, metatarsus and toe region of the injected and diameters of the contralateral noninjected foot were measured. The average difference between the two groups of diameters was taken as an indicator of the foot inflammatory swelling.

Evaluation of Foot Necrosis

Necrosis of the immunized foot was measured 15 days after injection of BSA-CFA into the toe-pad. Mean score of necrosis was defined as a numerical score reflecting an overall intensity of necrosis: $0 = 0$, no necrosis; $+ = 1$, mild necrosis

($<$10% of foot); $++$ = 2, moderate necrosis (11–30% of foot); $+++$ = 3, severe necrosis (31–50% of foot); and $++++$ = 4, very severe necrosis ($>$50% of foot).

Evaluation of Inflammatory Lymph Node Enlargement

On the day of sacrifice, *i.e.*, 15 days after immunization with BSA-CFA, inguinal lymph nodes of the adjuvant-inoculated leg and those of the contralateral noninjected leg were carefully dissected free and weighed on a Sartorius analytic balance. The average difference between the injected and noninjected legs was taken as the degree of node enlargement.

Evaluation of Nonspecific Inflammation

Two weeks after immunization with BSA-CFA, rats were injected intracutaneously in the depilated flank with 0.05 ml turpentine (diluted 1 : 20 in olive oil). Skin reactions were read at 20 minutes, and 2, 6 and 24 hours and mean diameters (mm) calculated for each group.

Hypersensitivity Skin Reactions

Animals sensitized with BSA-CFA were skin-tested on day 14 after immunization. Thirty μg of BSA and 1 : 10 diluted old tuberculin in 0.1 ml of saline were injected into the skin of depilated flank. Arthus and delayed hypersensitivity reactions were read at 4 and 24 hours respectively. The mean diameter, severity (mean score) and incidence of positive reactions were calculated for each group. Mean score was defined as a numerical score reflecting the overall intensity of skin reaction based on degree of edema (Arthus reaction) and induration (delayed reaction): 0 = 0; + = 1; $++$ = 2; $+++$ = 3; and $++++$ = 4. The highest possible mean score was 4.

Body and Organ Weights

Animals were weighed on a small animal scale. After sacrifice, thymus and spleen weights were measured, using an analytical balance. Results were expressed as mg of organ weight/g of body weight. The organs were embedded in paraffin. The tissue sections were stained with hematoxylin and eosin, and methyl green and pyronin, for histological examination.

Statistical Analysis

Statistical significance was determined by Student t test. Differences between groups were considered significant if the p values were less than 0.05.

RESULTS

Plaque-Forming Cell Response and Antibody Production

There was a striking depletion of splenic hemolysin-releasing cells and a decrease of circulating hemagglutinins in senescent saline-treated Wistar rats immu-

TABLE 1. Effect of Methionine-Enkephalin (Met-Enk) on Plaque-Forming Cell (PFC) Response and Hemagglutinin Production in 8-Week-Old and 20-Month-Old Wistar Rats Immunized with Sheep Red Blood Cells[a]

Rats Treated with	N	Humoral Immune Response	
		No. of PFC/10^6 Cells	Hemagglutinin Titer (Log_2)
8-week-old rats			
Saline	20	2114 ± 367^b	5.8 ± 0.5^b
Met-Enk	20	3090 ± 512^c	6.9 ± 0.6^c
20-month-old rats			
Saline	20	1036 ± 371	4.0 ± 0.6
Met-Enk	20	2187 ± 543^d	6.1 ± 0.7^d

[a] Dose of Met-Enk: 0.2 mg/kg bw. Values represent mean $\pm$ SD. Statistically significant differences were determined by Student t test:

[b] $p < 0.001$, saline-treated group (8-week-old) vs saline-treated group (20-month-old).

[c] $p < 0.001$, Enk-treated group (8-week-old) vs saline-treated group (8-week-old).

[d] $p < 0.001$, Enk-treated group (20-month-old) vs saline-treated group (20-month-old).

nized with SRBC compared to sensitized 8-week-old controls (TABLE 1). Met-Enk increased significantly the humoral immune responses both in young adult and aged rats. However, the immunopotentiating effect of enkephalin was much more pronounced in senescent rats. Met-Enk also elevated the titers of precipitating anti-BSA antibody in 8-week-old and 20-month-old animals immunized with BSA-CFA (TABLE 2).

Inflammatory Response of Adjuvant-Injected Foot

In young, 8-week-old rats, the inflammatory enlargement of the foot inoculated with BSA-CFA was evident on day 12 after antigen challenge (TABLE 3). Significantly weaker inflammatory response was observed in 20-month-old rats. Treatment with Met-Enk, however, augmented the inflammatory reaction of in-

TABLE 2. Effect of Met-Enk on Anti-BSA Antibody Titers in 8-Week-Old and 20-Month-Old Wistar Rats Sensitized to Bovine Serum Albumin[a]

Rats Treated with	N	Serum Anti-BSA Antibody Titer (Log_2)
8-week-old rats		
Saline	21	6.3 ± 0.6^b
Met-Enk	21	7.8 ± 0.8^c
20-month-old rats		
Saline	21	5.4 ± 0.7
Met-Enk	21	7.2 ± 0.8^d

[a] Dose of Met-Enk: 0.2 mg/kg bw. Values represent mean $\pm$ SD. Statistically significant differences:

[b] $p < 0.001$, saline-treated group (8-week-old) vs saline-treated group (20-month-old).

[c] $p < 0.001$, Enk-treated group (8-week-old) vs saline-treated group (8-week-old).

[d] $p < 0.001$, Enk-treated group (20-month-old) vs saline-treated group (20-month-old).

TABLE 3. Effect of Met-Enk on Inflammatory Enlargement of the Foot Injected with BSA-CFA in 8-Week-Old and 20-Month-Old Wistar Rats[a]

| Rats Treated with | N | Mean Diameter of the Foot (mm ± SD) | | |
		Injected Leg	Noninjected Leg	Mean Difference
8-week-old rats				
Saline	21	12.6 ± 1.5	4.7 ± 0.5	7.9 ± 1.8[b]
Met-Enk	21	15.0 ± 2.3	4.6 ± 0.6	10.4 ± 2.5[c]
20-month-old rats				
Saline	21	11.4 ± 1.1	5.9 ± 0.5	5.5 ± 0.9
Met-Enk	21	17.2 ± 1.0	6.0 ± 0.8	11.2 ± 0.8[d]

[a] Dose of Met-Enk: 0.2 mg/kg bw. Statistically significant differences:
[b] $p < 0.001$, saline-treated group (8-week-old) vs saline-treated group (20-month-old).
[c] $p < 0.001$, Enk-treated group (8-week-old) vs saline-treated group (8-week-old).
[d] $p < 0.001$, Enk-treated group (20-month-old) vs saline-treated group (20-month-old).

jected foot in both 8-week-old and 20-month-old rats. The latter responded much more to Met-Enk than did the former.

The foot inoculated with BSA-CFA exhibited signs of necrosis 15 days after sensitization. Both incidence and degree of necrosis were greater in 8-week-old than in 20-month-old animals (TABLE 4). Rats treated with 0.2 mg/kg Met-Enk showed significantly larger necrotic lesions. The exacerbation of necrosis by Met-Enk was more pronounced in senescent rats.

Inflammatory Response of Inguinal Lymph Nodes

There was a considerable increase of the inguinal lymph node weight of the leg injected with BSA-CFA, 15 days after inoculation (TABLE 5). This is an event which always appears after inoculation of mycobacterial adjuvant into the foot pad. The extent of inflammatory response of lymph nodes was greater in 8-week-old saline-treated animals than in 20-month-old controls. However, Met-Enk

TABLE 4. Effect of Met-Enk on Necrosis of the Foot Injected with BSA-CFA in 8-Week-Old and 20-Month-Old Wistar Rats[a]

| Rats Treated with | N | Severity of Necrosis of Injected Foot | | | | | Mean Score | Incidence of Foot Necrosis (%) |
		0	+	++	+++	++++		
8-week-old rats								
Saline	21	1	6	8	3	3	2.0 ± 1.1[b]	75
Met-Enk	21	0	0	5	9	7	3.1 ± 0.8[c]	100
20-month-old rats								
Saline	21	4	8	6	2	0	1.3 ± 0.9	60
Met-Enk	21	0	3	5	10	2	2.6 ± 0.9[d]	100

[a] Dose of Met-Enk: 0.2 mg/kg bw. Values represent mean ± SD. Statistically significant differences:
[b] $p < 0.05$, saline-treated group (8-week-old) vs saline-treated group (20-month-old).
[c] $p < 0.01$, Enk-treated group (8-week-old) vs saline-treated group (8-week-old).
[d] $p < 0.001$, Enk-treated group (20-month-old) vs saline-treated group (20-month-old).

TABLE 5. Effect of Met-Enk on Inguinal Lymph Nodes in 8-Week-Old and 20-Month-Old Wistar Rats Challenged with BSA-CFA[a]

Rats Treated with	N	Mean Weight of Inguinal Lymph Nodes (μg/g Body Weight)		
		Injected Leg	Noninjected Leg	Mean Difference
8-week-old rats				
Saline	21	455.5 ± 86.7	65.2 ± 15.6	390.3 ± 72.5[b]
Met-Enk	21	718.9 ± 92.4	60.8 ± 18.1	658.1 ± 79.8[c]
20-month-old rats				
Saline	21	408.9 ± 78.9	117.2 ± 24.7	291.7 ± 61.6
Met-Enk	21	679.6 ± 81.2	136.4 ± 19.7	543.2 ± 70.9[d]

[a] Dose of Met-Enk: 0.2 mg/kg bw. Values represent mean ± SD.
[b] $p < 0.001$, saline-treated group (8-week-old) vs saline-treated group (20-month-old).
[c] $p < 0.001$, Enk-treated group (8-week-old) vs saline-treated group (8-week-old).
[d] $p < 0.001$, Enk-treated group (20-month-old) vs saline-treated group (20-month-old).

markedly augmented the weights of the lymph nodes both in senescent and young adult rats. Again, the potentiating activity of enkephalin was more pronounced in aged animals.

Inflammatory Skin Reaction to Turpentine

In Met-Enk-treated rats, there was a progressive increase of local nonspecific inflammation to turpentine, 20 minutes, and 2, 6 and 24 hours after intradermal challenge (TABLE 6). The effect of Met-Enk was similar in 8-week-old and 20-month-old rats.

Hypersensitivity Skin Reactions to BSA

Arthus (TABLE 7) and delayed (TABLE 8) skin hypersensitivity reactions to BSA and old tuberculin were sharply reduced in saline-treated senescent rats

TABLE 6. Effect of Met-Enk on Local Nonspecific Skin Inflammation to Turpentine in 8-Week-Old and 20-Month-Old Wistar Rats[a]

Rats Treated with	N	Mean Diameter of Skin Reaction (mm ± SD) Time after Skin Injection			
		20 min	2 h	6 h	24 h
8-week-old rats					
Saline	21	15.0 ± 3.2[b]	15.4 ± 3.0[b]	16.1 ± 2.5[b]	15.9 ± 2.2[b]
Met-Enk	21	18.1 ± 2.4[c]	19.5 ± 2.1[c]	20.3 ± 3.3[c]	21.0 ± 3.5[c]
20-month-old rats					
Saline	21	11.4 ± 2.1	11.5 ± 2.2	12.5 ± 1.6	12.8 ± 0.7
Met-Enk	21	13.8 ± 1.6[d]	14.4 ± 1.4[d]	15.4 ± 1.8	15.5 ± 1.0[d]

[a] Dose of Met-Enk: 0.2 mg/kg bw. Statistically significant differences:
[b] $p < 0.001$, saline-treated group (8-week-old) vs saline-treated group (20-month-old).
[c] $p < 0.001$, Enk-treated group (8-week-old) vs saline-treated group (8-week-old).
[d] $p < 0.001$, Enk-treated group (20-month-old) vs saline-treated group (20-month-old).

TABLE 7. Effect of Met-Enk on Arthus Skin Hypersensitivity Reactions to Bovine Serum Albumin (BSA) and Old Tuberculin (OT) in 8-Week-Old and 20-Month-Old Wistar Rats Immunized with BSA-CFA[a]

Rats Treated with	N	Arthus Reactions to BSA			Arthus Reactions to OT		
		Mean Diameter (mm)	Severity of Reaction (Mean Score)	Positive Reaction (%)	Mean Diameter (mm)	Severity of Reaction (Mean Score)	Positive Reaction (%)
8-week-old rats							
Saline	21	14.1 ± 3.0^b	2.2 ± 0.6^b	100	10.1 ± 1.9^c	0.9 ± 0.5	88
Met-Enk	21	18.0 ± 2.7^d	2.8 ± 0.7^e	100	13.0 ± 2.0^d	1.9 ± 0.5^d	100
20-month-old rats							
Saline	21	10.3 ± 2.8	1.2 ± 0.6	90	7.2 ± 1.7	0.6 ± 0.5	65
Met-Enk	21	15.8 ± 3.4^f	2.0 ± 0.7^f	100	11.5 ± 2.1^f	1.2 ± 0.7^g	85

[a] Dose of Met-Enk: 0.2 mg/kg bw. Values represent mean ± SD. Statistically significant differences:
[b] $p < 0.001$, [c] $p < 0.01$, saline-treated group (8-week-old) vs saline-treated group (20-month-old).
[d] $p < 0.001$, [e] $p < 0.01$, Enk-treated group (8-week-old) vs saline-treated group (8-week-old).
[f] $p < 0.001$, [g] $p < 0.01$, Enk-treated group (20-month-old) vs saline-treated group (20-month-old).

TABLE 8. Effect of Met-Enk on Delayed Skin Hypersensitivity Reactions to Bovine Serum Albumin (BSA) and Old Tuberculin (OT) in 8-Week-Old and 20-Month-Old Wistar Rats Immunized with BSA-CFA[a]

Rats Treated with	N	Delayed Reactions to BSA			Delayed Reactions to OT		
		Mean Diameter (mm)	Severity of Reaction (Mean Score)	Positive Reaction (%)	Mean Diameter (mm)	Severity of Reaction (Mean Score)	Positive Reaction (%)
8-week-old rats							
Saline	21	20.6 ± 2.9[b]	3.1 ± 0.7[b]	100	13.3 ± 1.5[b]	1.8 ± 0.7[b]	100
Met-Enk	21	25.5 ± 3.1[c]	3.7 ± 0.8[c]	100	16.1 ± 2.1[c]	2.4 ± 0.6[d]	100
20-month-old rats							
Saline	21	12.4 ± 3.1	1.7 ± 0.8	95	8.4 ± 1.7	0.9 ± 0.7	80
Met-Enk	21	18.9 ± 3.4[f]	2.8 ± 0.8[f]	100	12.8 ± 1.5[f]	1.8 ± 0.5[f]	100

[a] Dose of Met-Enk: 0.2 mg/kg bw. Values represent mean ± SD. Statistically significant differences:
[b] $p < 0.001$, saline-treated group (8-week-old) vs saline-treated group (20-month-old).
[c] $p < 0.001$, [d] $p < 0.01$, and [e] $p < 0.05$, Enk-treated group (8-week-old) vs saline-treated group (8-week-old).
[f] $p < 0.001$, Enk-treated group (20-month-old) vs saline-treated group (20-month-old).

immunized with BSA-CFA, in comparison to saline-treated young adult rats. On the other hand, animals repeatedly injected with 0.2 mg/kg Met-Enk showed a marked increase of both Arthus and delayed responses. This immunoenhancing activity of enkephalin was particularly evident in 20-month-old rats.

Organ Weight and Histology

The weight of the thymus, but not spleen, significantly decreased with age (TABLE 9). Intraperitoneal administration of 0.2 mg/kg Met-Enk produced a striking increase of both thymus and spleen weight in senescent rats. In 8-week-old animals, this pentapeptide increased only the thymus weight. Body weights of adolescent and senescent rats were not affected by enkephalin-treatment. Histologically, Met-Enk induced an enlargement of the cortical and medullary areas, and a pronounced pyroninophilia in the subcortical zone of the thymus and thymus-dependent areas of the spleen.

TABLE 9. Effect of Met-Enk on Thymus and Spleen Weights in 8-Week-Old and 20-Month-Old Wistar Rats Immunized with BSA-CFA[a]

Rats Treated with	N	Organ Weight (mg/g Body Weight)	
		Thymus	Spleen
8-week-old rats			
Saline	21	0.93 ± 0.11^b	2.97 ± 0.76
Met-Enk	21	1.18 ± 0.10^c	3.15 ± 0.62
20-month-old rats			
Saline	21	0.34 ± 0.07	2.81 ± 0.63
Met-Enk	21	0.67 ± 0.19^d	3.79 ± 0.55^d

[a] Dose of Met-Enk: 0.2 mg/kg bw. Values represent mean $\pm$ SD. Statistically significant differences:
[b] $p < 0.001$, saline-treated group (8-week-old) vs saline-treated group (20-month-old).
[c] $p < 0.001$, Enk-treated group (8-week-old) vs saline-treated group (8-week-old).
[d] $p < 0.001$, Enk-treated group (20-month-old) vs saline-treated group (20-month-old).

DISCUSSION

Immunosenescence can be defined as the alteration of immune function which occurs in all aged organisms, and which is distinguishable from the immunodeficiency secondary to underlying disease, malnutrition, toxic exposure, distress, etc. The increased incidence of malignancy, infectious diseases, autoimmune disorders and monoclonal gammopathies with age are thought to be linked with the decline of immunocompetence.[26–28] However, the immune system is not uniformly affected by the aging process. Thus, total number of white blood cells, lymphocytes and granulocytes, as well as phagocytic function of neutrophils, and the complement system do not change appreciably with age.[29–31] The most significant decrement occurs in cellular immunity, in such functions as delayed type hypersensitivity,[32] resistance to tumor cells,[33] resistance to viruses and protozoa,[26,27] primary allograft rejection, and graft-versus-host disease.[34] On the other hand, the humoral type of immune reactions seems to increase during senescence, as shown in different animal models, and in elderly humans with elevated titers of autoantibodies and circulating immune complexes.[35,36] This dysregulation of immune homeostasis may be attributed to changes in the immune cells themselves and their secretory products, as well as to alterations in the cellular milieu in which they are situated. Since the total number of immune cells does not significantly change with age,[37] one may assume that the reduced efficiency of these cells plays an important role in immunosenescence.

Besides, the damaged function of the immune system during aging may be due to the dysfunction of several other systems which directly or indirectly control the immune system, *e.g.*, impairment of the thymus gland and thymus-associated structures,[1-3] alterations of the nervous system and its neurohumoral activity,[34,38,39] and deviations of the endocrine system function.[40-46]

The role of opioids in senescence has been the subject of several recent studies. It has been shown that levels of opioids and their receptors diminish significantly in the aging brain.[12,47-51] Furthermore, it appears that during senescence there are marked changes in posttranslational processing of opioids in the nervous system,[52] and an imbalance of mu and delta opioid receptors.[53] The possibility that similar changes of the opioids may occur in the immune system with age suggested the present study. The results described here clearly show that a low dose of the simplest form of an opioid peptide, methionine-enkephalin, exerts a significant immunostimulatory effect in young adult rats and marked immunorestorative influence in senescent rats. These observations are in agreement with our earlier findings on the enkephalin-induced modulation of humoral and cellular immune reactions in adolescent animals.[21-25] It seems, however, that the immunoenhancing activity of Met-Enk influenced more cellular immune-inflammatory reactions, such as delayed type of skin hypersensitivity, and inflammatory reactions of the foot and inguinal lymph nodes to CFA, than humoral immune responses, such as the plaque-forming cell response, antibody production and the Arthus skin reaction. Thus it appears that in senescence, Met-Enk exerts a selective (greater) effect on cellular immunity. This contention is supported by the observations that precursors of Met-Enk which are present in T-helper cells[54,55] may be down-regulated in senescence.[53] Furthermore, the thymus gland itself has been shown to produce opioid peptides,[56] and these peptides as well as thymic hormones may decline during age-related thymic involution. It is well documented that different thymic hormones can restore, at least in part, cellular immunity and related structural and functional components in the thymus and other lymphoid tissues.[3,57-61] The present study provides the first evidence that Met-Enk may act as a "replacement hormone" and ameliorate the immunodeficient state caused by physiological aging.

In conclusion, the results imply that the complex structural and functional alterations of the immune microenvironment and neuroendocrine functions in aged animals can be restored by exogenous administration of methionine-enkephalin. The mechanisms underlying the immunoreconstitutive activity of this opioid peptide are poorly understood.

SUMMARY

Twenty-month-old Wistar rats received intraperitoneal injections of the opioid pentapeptide, methionine-enkephalin (Met-Enk) in periods before and after immunization with cellular and soluble antigens. Animals were treated with 0.2 mg of Met-Enk/kg b.w., a dose previously found to increase immune capacity in young adult rats. Saline-treated 20-month-old, and Met-Enk-treated rats and saline-treated 8-week-old controls were set up for each experimental group. Immune performance was evaluated by plaque-forming cell response, antibody production and various immunoinflammatory reactions. At autopsy, thymus and spleen were weighed and processed for histological examination. The results showed that 0.2 mg dose of Met-Enk produced significant enhancement of both humoral and cellular immune responses in senescent rats. Methionine-enkephalin treatment also induced a significant increase in thymus and spleen weights in these animals. Analysis of the cellular make up of these organs revealed the enlargement of cortical and medullary areas, and pronounced pyroninophilia in the subcortical zone of the thymus and thymus-dependent areas of the spleen. The results suggest that Met-Enk exerts an immunorestorative activity in aged animals, and that changes in the opioid system may play an important role in the maintenance of immune functions during senescence.

REFERENCES

1. LEWIS, V. M., J. J. TWOMEY, P. BEALMER, G. GOLDSTEIN & R. A. GOOD. 1978. Age, thymic involution, and circulating thymic hormone activity. J. Clin. Endocrinol. Metab. **47:** 145–150.
2. GOLDSTEIN, A. L., G. B. THURMAN, L. K. LOW, G. E. TRIVERS & J. L. ROSSIO. 1979. Thymosin: the endocrine thymus and its role in the aging process. In Aging, Physiology and Cell Biology of Aging. A. Cherkin, N. Kharasch, F. L. Scott, C. E. Finch, T. Makinodan & B. Strehler, Eds. Vol. 8: 51–60. Raven Press. New York, NY.
3. MAKINODAN, T. & M. M. B. KAY. 1980. Age influence on the immune system. Adv. Immunol. **29:** 287–330.
4. ROTH, G. S. & G. D. HESS. 1982. Changes in the mechanisms of hormone and neurotransmitter action during aging: current status of the role of receptor and post-receptor alterations. A review. Mech. Ageing Dev. **20:** 175–194.
5. BURCHINSKY, S. G. 1984. Neurotransmitter receptors in the central nervous system and aging: pharmacological aspect (a review). Exp. Gerontol. **19:** 227–239.
6. KALIMI, M. 1984. Glucocorticoid receptors: from development to aging. A review. Mech. Ageing Dev. **24:** 129–138.
7. BLOOM, E. T., W. J. PETERSON, M. TAKASUGI & T. MAKINODAN. 1985. Immunity and ageing. In Principles and Practice of Geriatric Medicine. M. S. J. Pathy, Ed. 57–65. John Wiley and Sons, Ltd. Chichester, England.
8. JOHNSON, H. M. & B. A. TORRES. 1985. Regulation of lymphokine production by arginine vasopressin and oxytocin-modulation. J. Immunol. **135:** 773s–775s.
9. SNOW, E. C. 1985. Insulin and growth hormone function as minor growth factors that potentiate lymphocyte activation. J. Immunol. **135:** 776s–778s.
10. PAYAN, D. G. & E. J. GOETZL. 1985. Modulation of lymphocyte function by sensory neuropeptides. J. Immunol. **135:** 783s–786s.
11. MOORE, T. C. 1984. Modification of lymphocyte traffic by vasoactive neurotransmitter substances. Immunology **52:** 511–518.
12. MISSALE, C., S. GOVONI, L. CROCE, A. BOSIO, P. F. SPANO & M. TRABUCCHI. 1983. Changes of beta-endorphin and met-enkephalin content in the hypothalamus-pituitary axis induced by aging. J. Neurochem. **40:** 20–24.
13. WYBRAN, J., T. APELBOOM, J. P. FAMAEY & A. GOVAERTS. 1979. Suggestive evidence for receptors for morphine and methionine-enkephalin on normal human blood T lymphocytes. J. Immunol. **123:** 1068–1070.
14. MATHEWS, P. M., C. J. FROELICH, W. L. SIBBITT & A. D. BANKHURST. 1983. Enhancement of natural cytotoxicity by beta-endorphins. J. Immunol. **130:** 1658–1662.
15. SHAVIT, Y., J. W. LEWIS, G. W. TERMAN, R. P. GALE & J. C. LIEBESKIND. 1984. Opioid peptides mediate the suppressive effect of stress on natural killer cell cytotoxicity. Science **223:** 188–190.

16. CARR, D. J. J. & G. R. KLIMPEL. 1986. Enhancement of the generation of cytotoxic T cells by endogenous opiates. J. Neuroimmunol. **12:** 75–87.
17. RUFF, M., S. M. WAHL, S. MERGENHAGEN & C. B. PERT. 1985. Opiate receptor-mediated chemotaxis of human monocytes. Neuropeptides **5:** 363–366.
18. FALKE, N. E. & E. G. FISHER. 1985. Cell shape of polymorphonuclear leukocytes is influenced by opioids. Immunobiology. **169:** 532–539.
19. JOHNSON, H. M., E. M. SMITH, B. A. TORRES & J. E. BLALOCK. 1982. Regulation of the *in vitro* antibody responses by neuroendocrine hormones. Proc. Natl. Acad. Sci. USA **79:** 4171–4174.
20. FARRAR, W. L. 1984. Endorphin modulation of lymphokine activity. *In* Opioid Peptides in the Periphery. F. Faioli, A. Isidora & A. Mazzetti, Eds. 159. Elsevier Sci. Amsterdam.
21. JANKOVIĆ, B. D. & D. MARIĆ. 1986. Modulation of *in vivo* immune responses by enkephalins. Clin. Neuropharmacol. **9**(Suppl. 4): 476–478.
22. JANKOVIĆ, B. D. & D. MARIĆ. 1987. Enkephalins and immunity. I. *In vivo* suppression and potentiation of humoral immune response. Ann. N.Y. Acad. Sci. **496:** 115–125.
23. JANKOVIĆ, B. D. & D. MARIĆ. 1987. Enkephalins and autoimmunity: differential effect of methionine-enkephalin on experimental allergic encephalomyelitis in Wistar and Lewis rats. J. Neurosci. Res. **18:** 88–94.
24. JANKOVIĆ, B. D. & D. MARIĆ. 1987. Enkephalins and anaphylactic shock: modulation and prevention of shock in the rat. Immunol. Lett. **15:** 153–160.
25. MARIĆ, D. & B. D. JANKOVIĆ. 1987. Enkephalins and immunity. II. *In vivo* modulation of cell mediated immunity. Ann. N.Y. Acad. Sci. **496:** 126–136.
26. PAZMINO, N. H. & J. M. JUHAS. 1973. Senescent loss of resistance to murine sarcoma virus (Moloney) in the mouse. Cancer Res. **33:** 2668–2672.
27. GARDNER, I. D. & J. S. REMINGTON. 1978. Aging and immune response. I. Antibody formation and chronic infection in toxoplasma gondii-infected mice. J. Immunol. **120:** 939–943.
28. MAKINODAN, T., S. J. JAMES, T. INAMIZU & M.-P. CHANG. 1984. Immunologic basis for susceptibility to infection in the aged. Gerontology **30:** 279–289.
29. CORBERAND, J. X., P. F. LAHARRAGUE & G. FILLOLA. 1986. Neutrophils of healthy aged humans are normal. Mech. Ageing Dev. **36:** 57–63.
30. SPARROW, P., J. E. SILBERT & J. W. ROWE. 1980. The influence of age on peripheral lymphocyte count in men: a cross-sectional and longitudinal study. J. Gerontol. **35:** 163–166.
31. NAGAKI, K., S. HIRAMATSU, S. INAI & A. SASAKI. 1980. The effect of aging on complement activity (CH 50) and complement protein levels. J. Clin. Lab. Immunol. **3:** 45–50.
32. DWORSKY, R., A. PAGANINI-HILL, A. ARTHUR & J. PARKER. 1983. Immune responses of healthy humans 83–104 years of age. J. Natl. Cancer Inst. **71:** 265–268.
33. LIPSCHITZ, D. A., S. GOLDSTEIN, R. REIS, M. E. WEKSLER, R. BRESSLER & B. A. WEILAN. 1985. Cancer in the elderly: basic science and clinical aspects. Ann. Intern. Med. **102:** 218–228.
34. BLOOM, F. E. 1985. Neuropeptides and other mediators in the central nervous system. J. Immunol. **135:** 743s–745s.
35. CAMMARATA, R. J., G. P. RODNAN & R. H. FENNEL. 1967. Serum antigamma globulin and antinuclear factors in the aged. J. Am. Med. Assoc. **199:** 456–458.
36. AXELSSON, U., R. BACHMAN & J. HALLEN. 1966. Frequency of pathological proteins (M proteins) on 6,995 sera from adult population. Acta Med. Scand. **179:** 235–247.
37. DYBKAER, R., M. LAURITZEN & R. KRAKAUER. 1981. Relative reference values for clinical, chemical and haematological quantities for healthy elderly people. Acta Med. Scand. **209:** 1–9.
38. BESEDOVSKY, H. O., A. DEL REY & E. SORKIN. 1985. Immunoneuroendocrine interactions. J. Immunol. **135:** 750s–754s.
39. ROTH, J., D. LEROITH, E. S. COLLIER, N. R. WEAVER, A. WATKINSON, C. F. CLELAND & S. M. GLICK. 1985. Evolutionary origins of neuropeptides, hormones and receptors: possible application to immunology. J. Immunol. **135:** 816s–819s.

40. JOHNSON, H. M., B. A. TORRES, E. M. SMITH, L. D. DION & J. E. BLALOCK. 1984. Regulation of lymphokine (gamma-interferon) production by corticotropin. J. Immunol. **132:** 246–259.
41. GOLDMAN, R., Z. BAR-SHAVIT & D. ROMEO. 1983. Neuortensin modulates human neutrophil locomotion and phagocytic capability. FEBS Lett. **159:** 63–67.
42. SAGI-EISENBERG, R., Z. BEN-NERIAH, I. PECHT, S. TERRY & S. BLUMBERG. 1983. Structure-activity relationship in the mast cell degranulating capacity of neurotensin fragments. Neuropharmacology **22:** 197–201.
43. BHATHENA, S. J., J. LOUIE, G. P. P. SCHECTER, R. S. REDMAN, L. WAHL & L. RECANT. 1981. Identification of human mononuclear leucocytes bearing receptors for somatostatin and glucagon. Diabetes **30:** 127–131.
44. PAYAN, D. G., D. R. BREWSTER & E. J. GOETZL. 1983. Specific stimulation of human T lymphocytes by substance P. J. Immunol. **131:** 1613–1615.
45. LEVINE, J. D., R. CLARK, M. DEVOR, C. HELMS, M. A. MOSKOWITZ & A. I. BASBAUM. 1984. Intraneuronal substance P contributes to the severity of experimental arthritis. Science **226:** 547–549.
46. CUTZ, E., W. CHAN, N. S. TRACK, A. GOTH & S. SAID. 1978. Release of vasoactive intestinal peptide in mast cells by histamine liberators. Nature **275:** 661–662.
47. BARDEN, N., A. DUPONT, F. LABRIE, Y. MERANDI, D. ROULEAU, H. VAUNDRY & J. R. BOISSER. 1981. Age-dependent changes in the beta-endorphin content of discrete rat brain nuclei. Brain Res. **208:** 209–212.
48. OGAWA, N. 1985. Neuropeptides and their receptors in aged rat brain. Acta Med. Okayama **39:** 315–319.
49. PETKOV, V. V., V. D. PETKOV, T. GRAHORSKA & E. KOUNSTANTINOVA. 1984. Enkephalin-receptor changes in rat brain during aging. Gen. Pharmacol. **15:** 491–495.
50. DUPONT, A., P. SAVARD, Y. MERAND, F. LABRIE & J. R. BOISSIER. 1981. Age-related changes in central nervous system enkephalins and substance P. Life Sci. **29:** 2317–2322.
51. JENSEN, R. A., R. B. MESSING, V. R. SPIEHLER, J. L. MARTINEZ, B. J. VASQEZ & J. L. MCGAUGH. 1980. Memory, opiate receptors, and aging. Peptides **1:** 197–201.
52. WILKINSON, C. W. & D. M. DORSA. 1986. The effect of aging on molecular forms of beta- and gamma-endorphin in rat hypothalamus. Neuroendocrinology **43:** 124–131.
53. PLOTNIKOFF, N. P. 1988. Opioids: immunomodulation. A proposed role in cancer in aging. *In* Neuroimmunomodulation: Interventions in Aging and Cancer. W. Pierpaoli & N. H. Spector, Eds. 312–322. N.Y. Acad. Sci. New York.
54. ZURAWSKI, G., M. BENEDIK, J. B. KAMB, J. S. ABRAMS, S. M. ZURAWSKI & F. D. LEE. 1986. Activation of mouse T-helper cells induces abundant preproenkephalin mRNA synthesis. Science **232:** 772–775.
55. MONSTEIN, H.-J., R. FOLKESSON & L. TERENIUS. 1986. Proenkephalin-A-like mRNA in human leukemia leukocytes and CNS-tissues. Life Sci. **39:** 2237–2241.
56. ZOZULYA, A. A., S. P. PSCHENICHKIN, M. R. SHCHURIN, J. N. KHOMJAKOV & I. A. BESVERSHENKO. 1985. Thymus peptides interacting with opiate receptors. Acta Endocrinol. **110:** 284–288.
57. JANKOVIĆ, B. D., K. ISAKOVIĆ & J. HORVAT. 1965. Effect of lipid fraction from rat thymus on delayed hypersensitivity reactions of neonatally thymectomized rats. Nature **208:** 356–357.
58. TRAININ, N. 1974. Thymic hormones and immune response. Physiol. Rev. **54:** 272–315.
59. WHITE, A. & A. L. GOLDSTEIN. 1970. The role of the thymus gland in the hormonal regulation of host resistance. *In* Control Processes in Multicellular Organisms. G. E. Wolstenholme & J. Knight, Eds. 210–237. Churchill. London.
60. STUTMAN, O. 1977. Two main features of T-cell development: thymus traffic and post thymic maturation. Contemp. Top. Immunobiol. **7:** 1–10.
61. NATIONAL CANCER INSTITUTE MONOGRAPH No. 63. 1983. Biological Response Modifiers: Subcommittee Report. Section IV. Thymic Factors and Hormones 107–137. U.S. Department of Health and Human Services. NIH. Bethesda, MD.

Immunostimulatory Activity of Prothymosin-Alpha in Senescence[a]

DRAGAN MARIĆ, BRANISLAV D. JANKOVIĆ, AND
JELENA VELJIĆ

Immunology Research Center
Vojvode Stepe 458
11221 Belgrade, Yugoslavia

INTRODUCTION

Although the theories of aging postulated by Burnet (1970),[1] Walford (1974),[2] and Makinodan and Kay (1980)[3] consider immunosenescence as the underlying basis of aging, the exact mechanisms of the decline of immunocompetence with age are not clearly understood. Nevertheless, it is generally accepted that the decrease of immune function with age may be directly or indirectly related to thymic involution and depressed thymic hormone production.[4-8] Therefore, numerous efforts have been made to enhance immune function during senescence by means of protein and peptide fractions isolated from the thymus.[9] Thymic hormones, and thymosin-alpha$_1$ in particular, have been widely used for treatment of primary[10,11] and secondary[12] T lymphocyte deficiencies, herpes simplex,[13] and other viral infections,[14] sarcoidosis,[15] melanoma,[16] etc. in young adult and aged animals and humans. Thymosin-alpha$_1$ has been shown to be an effective modulator of helper T cell activity, T cell differentiation, terminal deoxynucleotidyl transferase activity of bone marrow cells, thymocytes and splenocytes, interferon-alpha and -gamma production, T cell dependent IgG, IgA and IgM secondary antibody responses and E-rosette formation.[17-19]

In its native environment, thymosin-alpha$_1$ exists as a 28-amino acid N-terminal part of a 109-amino acid polypeptide molecule named prothymosin-alpha.[20] Since our preliminary experiments have shown that prothymosin-alpha exerts a potent *in vivo* immunoenhancing activity on humoral and cellular immune responses in young adult rats, we attempted in this study to demonstrate the immunorestorative effect of prothymosin-alpha in senescent rats.

MATERIALS AND METHODS

Animals

Experiments were carried out on 8-week-old (180–200 g) and 17-month-old (450–550 g) female Wistar rats. Animals were fed food pellets and had access to tap water *ad libitum*.

[a] This study was supported by the Republic of Serbia Research Fund, Belgrade, and Thymoorgan-Pharmazie, Vienenburg, F.R.G.

Antigens

Antigens used in the experiments were sheep red blood cells (SRBC) and five times crystalized bovine serum albumin (BSA, lot no. 9218) purchased from ICN Pharmaceuticals (Cleveland, Ohio).

Immunization

Animals were immunized with (a) 5×10^9 SRBC in 1 ml of saline, injected intraperitoneally, and (b) 0.5 mg BSA in 0.1 ml of complete Freund's adjuvant (CFA) inoculated into the left hind foot pad.

Prothymosin-Alpha (ProT-Alpha)

This polypeptide (Thymoorgan Pharmazie, Vienenburg, F.R.G.) isolated from the calf thymus was stored at $-20°C$, and dissolved in sterile apyrogenic saline before use.

Treatment Schedules

Rats were intraperitoneally treated with 20 μg of ProT-alpha/kg, a dose shown in our preliminary assays to enhance humoral and cell mediated immune responses in young adult rats. Two schedules were employed: (a) 1 injection every 48 hours, 10 days before and 4 days after immunization with SRBC (a total of 8 injections of ProT-alpha/rat); and (b) 1 injection every 48 hours, 8 days before and 14 days after inoculation of BSA-CFA into foot pad (a total of 10 injections of ProT-alpha/rat). Saline-treated senescent rats, and ProT-alpha- and saline-treated 8-week-old rats served as controls.

Plaque-Forming Cell (PFC) Response

Rats immunized with SRBC were sacrificed 4 days after immunization. The spleens were extirpated and minced through a stainless steel mesh in medium 199, pH 7.2. The isolated splenocytes were washed twice and their concentration adjusted to 1×10^7 cells/ml. Spleen cells were then mixed with a 20% suspension of washed SRBC containing 10% normal guinea pig serum, preadsorbed with SRBC, as a source of complement. Suspensions were incubated in Cunningham's chambers at 37°C for 45 min and the number of hemolytic plaques was determined under a light microscope. PFC response was expressed as the number of hemolysin-producing cells per 10^6 splenocytes.

Hemagglutinin Titer Determination

Agglutinating anti-SRBC antibodies were detected by a microhemagglutination reaction. Blood samples were collected by heart puncture on day 4 after immunization. Sera were inactivated at 56°C for 30 min and then serially twofold diluted in a microtiter plate. To each dilution of serum 1% suspension of SRBC was added, the plates were shaken and incubated at 25°C for 3–4 hours. Antibody titer was expressed as $\log_2$ of the highest serum dilution producing positive hemagglutination.

Hypersensitivity Skin Reactions

All rats sensitized with BSA-CFA were skin tested on day 14 after immunization with 30 μg crystalline BSA in 0.1 ml of saline injected intradermally into the depilated flank. Arthus hypersensitivity skin reactions were read at 4 hours and delayed skin hypersensitivity reactions at 24 hours after administration of antigen. The diameters (mm) of reactions were measured, and degree of edema (Arthus reaction) and induration (delayed reaction) were recorded and graded from 0 to $+ + + +$.

Organ and Body Weights and Histology

Experimental and control animals were weighed at irregular intervals on a small animal scale. Animals were autopsied at the end of the experiment, and thymus and spleen dissected out, weighed and processed for staining with hematoxylin and eosin, and methyl green and pyronin.

Statistical Analysis

Statistical evaluation of results was carried out using Student t test. The significant difference was set up at 0.05.

RESULTS

PFC Response and Hemagglutinin Production

As shown in TABLE 1, there was no significant difference in PFC responses and hemagglutinin titers between saline-treated 8-week-old and 17-month-old rats

TABLE 1. Plaque-Forming Cell (PFC) Response and Antibody Production in 8-Week-Old and 17-Month-Old Rats Immunized with Sheep Red Blood Cells and Treated with ProT-Alpha[a]

Group	Dose (mg/kg b.w.)	PFC/10^6 Splenocytes	Antibody Titer ($\log_2$)
8-week-old rats			
Saline		1,153 + 302	6.1 + 1.9
ProT-alpha	0.02	3,408 + 314[b]	9.7 + 1.3[b]
17-month-old rats			
Saline		1,420 + 218	5.9 + 2.3
ProT-alpha	0.02	4,795 + 506[c]	8.1 + 1.3[c]

[a] No. of rats in group: 20. Figures, mean + SD.
[b] $p < 0.001$, 8-week-old rats treated with prothymosin vs 80-week-old rats treated with saline.
[c] $p < 0.001$, 17-month-old rats treated with prothymosin vs 17-month-old rats treated with saline.

TABLE 2. Arthus Skin Reaction in 8-Week-Old and 17-Month-Old Rats Treated with ProT-Alpha[a]

Group	Dose (mg/kg b.w.)	Arthus Skin Reactivity Mean Diameter (mm) and Intensity (0 to +++++) of Reaction							Mean Score + SD	Mean Diameter (mm + SD)
		0–5 0	6–10 +	11–15 ++	16–20 +++	21–25 ++++	25 +++++			
8-week-old rats										
Saline		0	7	9	4	0	0		1.9 + 0.7	12.8 + 2.1
ProT-alpha	0.02	0	0	5	12	3	0		2.9 + 0.6[b]	15.7 + 2.3[b]
17-month-old rats										
Saline		0	6	12	2	0	0		1.8 + 0.6	13.5 + 2.6
ProT-alpha	0.02	0	0	0	5	5	10		4.2 + 0.8[c]	24.0 + 4.4[c]

[a] No. of rats in group: 20. Figures, mean + SD.
[b] $p < 0.001$, 8-week-old rats treated with ProT-alpha vs 8-week-old rats treated with saline.
[c] $p < 0.001$, 17-month-old rats treated with ProT-alpha vs 17-month-old rats treated with saline.

TABLE 3. Delayed Skin Reaction in 8-Week-Old and 17-Month-Old Rats Treated with ProT-Alpha[a]

Group	Dose (mg/kg b.w.)	Delayed Skin Reactivity Mean Diameter (mm) and Intensity (0 to +++++) of Reaction						Mean Score + SD	Mean Diameter (mm + SD)
		0–5 0	6–10 +	11–15 ++	16–20 +++	21–25 ++++	25 +++++		
8-week-old rats									
Saline		0	3	7	10	0	0	2.3 + 0.7	13.9 + 2.5
ProT-alpha	0.02	0	0	2	10	4	4	3.5 + 0.9[b]	18.0 + 1.6[b]
17-month-old rats									
Saline		6	4	9	1	0	0	1.2 + 0.9	12.7 + 2.7
ProT-alpha	0.02	0	0	0	0	9	11	4.6 + 0.5[c]	26.4 + 3.8[c]

[a] No. of rats in group: 20. Figures, mean + SD.
[b] p <0.001, 8-week-old rats treated with ProT-alpha vs 8-week-old rats treated with saline.
[c] p <0.001, 17-month-old rats treated with ProT-alpha vs 17-month-old rats treated with saline.

immunized with SRBC. On the other hand, these humoral immune reactions markedly increased in rats repeatedly injected with ProT-alpha. The immunoenhancing effect of ProT-alpha was greater in senescent rats compared with young adult controls.

Arthus and Delayed Skin Reactions

Treatment with ProT-alpha produced a significant increase of Arthus (TABLE 2) and delayed (TABLE 3) skin hypersensitivity reactions both in young adult and senescent rats compared to their corresponding saline-treated controls. It should be mentioned, however, that this immunopotentiating effect of ProT-alpha was more pronounced in the aged animals.

Organ Weights and Histology

The thymus and spleen significantly decreased in size in 17-month-old saline-treated rats (TABLE 4). Histologically, in aged rats there were profound changes in

TABLE 4. Thymus and Spleen Weight in 8-Week-Old and 17-Month-Old Rats Treated with ProT-Alpha[a]

Group	Dose (mg/kg b.w.)	Thymus Weight (mg/g)	Spleen Weight (mg/g)
8-week-old rats			
Saline		0.82 ± 0.20	2.90 ± 1.49
ProT-alpha	0.02	1.48 ± 0.19^b	3.06 ± 1.37
17-month-old rats			
Saline		0.32 ± 0.13	1.49 ± 0.25
ProT-alpha	0.02	0.72 ± 0.24^c	1.98 ± 0.33^c

[a] No. of rats in group: 20. Figures, mean ± SD.
[b] $p < 0.001$, 8-week-old rats treated with ProT-alpha vs 8-week-old rats treated with saline.
[c] $p < 0.001$, 17-month-old rats treated with ProT-alpha vs 17-month-old rats treated with saline.

the cellular make-up of the thymus, although cortex and medulla were still recognizable. In the spleen, a striking depletion of lymphocytes occurred in the areas surrounding the white pulp arterioles. On the other hand, the size of the thymus and spleen increased in senescent animals treated with ProT-alpha. The thymus was histologically characterized by an increase in the number of thymocytes in cortical and medullary areas, and a decrease of pyronin-positive cells in the subcortical region. Extensive lymphocyte aggregates in the white pulp were observed in the spleen of ProT-alpha-treated aged rats.

DISCUSSION

Aging is accompanied by a decline in immune responsiveness to foreign antigens and an increase in the incidence of autoimmune and neoplastic phenomena.[21,22] In senescence many performances of immunocompetent cells are altered and lead to depression of the delayed hypersensitivity reactions,[21,23] decline in responses to lectins,[24-27] and allogenic cells,[28] reduction in cytotoxic lymphocytes[29] and helper T-cell activity, and increase in suppressor T-cell function,[30-32] and response to autoantigens.[33] While the absolute number of circulating peripheral blood lymphocytes may remain stable with age,[34] some authors have reported a decline.[35] Although the percentage of circulating T cells has been reported to be unchanged,[27,34,35] a decrease in their proliferative activity, and their lymphokine and IL-2 production has been observed.[36-38] The B cells, on the other hand, show no loss in proliferative ability during senescence and their number may be slightly increased or unaltered.[39,40] The functional state of B cells, however, changes with age, so that during senescence autoantibody synthesis might occur, implying a selective increase in number and type of subpopulations of B cells.[41]

It is also generally considered that alterations in the immune system with age are related to structural and functional changes in the thymus.[4-8] In order to restore the impaired immune function due to thymus insufficiency, functional thymus tissue was implanted into thymus defective animals,[42] and different cell-free extracts of the thymus[43,44] or chemically well-defined thymic hormones[3,45,46] were employed. In a previous study we demonstrated the immunorestorative effects of purified lipid (Thymolip) and protein (Thymex-L) fractions of the calf thymus in senescent and thymectomized at birth young rats,[47] and in elderly humans.[48]

The present study shows that prothymosin-alpha, a native precursor of thymosin-alpha$_1$, also exerts a potent immunorestorative influence in aged rats. The improvement of immune potential was higher in aged than in young adult animals. The treatment with prothymosin alpha, in general, had a greater effect on cell-mediated than on humoral-immune reactions both in young adult and senescent rats, thus suggesting that this polypeptide mainly affects T cell lineages. Repeated injections of prothymosin-alpha significantly improved the cellular make-up of the thymus and thymus-dependent areas of the spleen in senescent rats. The mechanisms underlying the restorative function of thymus-endocrine products are not clear. However, if the pluripotent stem cells of bone marrow and the thymus have preserved functional capacity during senescence,[30,49] then immunosenescence may not be completely dependent on intrinsic changes in immature lymphocytes. Consequently, it is possible that the reexposure of these cells to thymic immunopeptides provokes proliferation, differentiation and maturation of lymphocytes in the functionally insufficient thymus of aged animals, and generation of both T and B cell lineages. In substantial agreement with this hypothesis are the findings of Hiramoto and co-workers (1987),[50] who have shown that bone marrow stem cells and pre-T-stem cells from aged animals are not defective in their regenerative capacity but lack the factors that provide their ability to differentiate and proliferate into more mature forms. Some of these factors have been reported as thymosin, ubiquitin and thymopoietin.[46] Functional maturation of B cells is also controlled to some extent by thymic hormones.[51]

It is possible that the thymus with its endocrine function controls the aging of the immune system and that the immune system plays an important role in influencing general processes of aging. The present results imply that "restoring" thymus endocrine function in aged animals by exogenous administration of its native endocrine products may improve immune system homeostasis in senescence and may thus delay aging to some extent. However, it would be presumptuous to believe that the decline in thymus gland function is the only cause of the general aging process and immune deficiency that take place in animals. Indeed, the immunopotentiating activity of a neuropentapeptide, methionine-enkephalin, in aged animals, as reported elsewhere in this book (Janković and Marić) supports this contention.

SUMMARY

In this study we evaluated the immunorestorative activity of prothymosin-alpha (ProT-alpha) in senescence. Aged rats were repeatedly injected with ProT-alpha after antigen challenge. Both humoral and cell-mediated immune reactions were tested. The results show that ProT-alpha exerted a marked immunopotentiating effect in aged rats. Moreover, ProT-alpha induced enhancement of PFC response, and skin hypersensitivity reactions were more pronounced in senescent rats than in young adult controls. ProT-alpha treatment increased thymus and spleen weights in aged rats, and induced qualitative and quantitative improvements of the cellular make-up of the thymus and thymus-dependent areas of the spleen. The results imply that "restoring" thymus endocrine function by exogenous administration of ProT-alpha may improve immune system homeostasis in senescence.

ACKNOWLEDGMENTS

We would like to thank Dr. Milan Č. Pešić, Institute for Immunology and Thymus Research, Bad Harzburg, F.R.G., for a generous gift of prothymosin-alpha.

REFERENCES

1. BURNET, F. M. 1970. An immunological approach to aging. Lancet **2:** 358–360.
2. WALFORD, R. L. 1974. Immunological theory of aging: current status. Fed. Proc. **33:** 2020–2027.
3. MAKINODAN, T. & M. M. B. KAY. 1980. Age influence on the immune system. Adv. Immunol. **29:** 287–330.
4. TRAININ, N. 1974. Thymic hormones and the immune response. Physiol. Rev. **54:** 272–315.
5. BACH, J. F., M. DARDENNE, J. PLEAU & M. BACH. 1975. Isolation and biochemical characteristics, and biological activity of a circulating thymic hormone in the mouse and in the human. Ann. N.Y. Acad. Sci. **249:** 186–210.
6. LEWIS, V. M., J. J. TWOMEY, P. BEALMEAR, G. GOLDSTEIN & R. A. GOOD. 1978. Age, thymic involution, and circulating thymic hormone activity. J. Clin. Endocrinol. Metab. **47:** 145–150.
7. GOLDSTEIN, A. L., G. B. THURMAN, L. K. LOW, G. E. TRIVIERS & J. L. ROSSIO. 1979. Thymosin: the endocrine thymus and its role in the aging process. In Aging, Physiology and Cell Biology of Aging. A. Cherkin, N. Kharasch, F. L. Scott, C. E. Finch, T. Makinodan & B. Strehler, Eds. Vol. 8: 51–60. Raven Press. New York, NY.
8. SINGH, J. & A. K. SINGH. 1979. Age-related changes in human thymus. Clin. Exp. Immunol. **37:** 507–511.
9. NATIONAL CANCER INSTITUTE MONOGRAPH No. 63. 1983. Biological Response Modifiers: Subcommittee Report. Section IV. Thymic Factors and Hormones 107–137. US Department of Health and Human Services. NIH. Bethesda, MD.
10. WARA, D. W., A. L. GOLDSTEIN, N. DOYLE & A. AMMANN. 1975. Thymosin activity in patients with cellular immunodeficiency. N. Engl. J. Med. **292:** 70–74.

11. DAVIES, E. G. & R. J. LEVINSKY. 1984. Experience in the use of thymic hormones for immunodeficiency disorders. *In* Thymic Factor Therapy. N. A. Byrom & J. R. Hobbs, Eds. Serono Symposia Vol. 16: 155–166. Raven Press. New York, NY.

12. HOBBS, J. R., N. BYROM, R. W. NORRIS, J. K. OATES, R. S. STAUGHTON & N. NAGVEKAR. 1985. Thymic factors in secondary T-lymphocyte deficiencies. *In* Immunopharmacology. P. A. Miescher, L. Bolis & M. Glione, Eds. Serono Symposia Vol. 23: 171–181. Raven Press. New York, NY.

13. DE MAUBEUGE, J., E. HANEKE, D. DJAWARI, K. WOLFF, G. STING, L. MOLIN, E. SCHOPF, R. STENGEL, H. DEGREEF, E. PANCONESI, B. WUTHRICH & K. BOLLA. 1985. Thymopentin treatment of Herpex Simplex infections. An open, monitored, multicenter study. Surv. Immunol. Res. **4**: 30–36.

14. TOVO, P. A., P. COLLESCELLI, R. MINIERO, E. PALOMBA, S. MARTINO, M. G. RONCAROLO, G. PASTORE & A. PUGLIESE. 1984. Thymic factor therapy of viral infections in childhood. *In* Thymic Factor Therapy. N. A. Byrom & J. R. Hobbs, Eds. Serono Symposia Vol. 16: 199–204. Raven Press. New York, NY.

15. SESTINI, P., G. AGOSTINI, G. CARRIERO, A. CIPRIANI, G. FESTI, G. GASPAROTO, M. G. PERARI, R. RAIMONDI, L. ROTTOLI, P. ROTTOLI, G. SEMENZATO & L. LENZINI. 1984. Thymic factor therapy of sarcoidosis. *In* Thymic Factor Therapy. N. A. Byrom & J. R. Hobbs, Eds. Serono Symposia Vol 16: 255–266. Raven Press. New York, NY.

16. BERNENGO, M. G., P. FRA, F. LISA, M. MEREGALLI & G. ZINA. 1983. Thymostimulin therapy in melanoma patients: correlation of immunologic effects with clinical course. Clin. Immunol. Immunopathol. **28**: 311–324.

17. SCHULOF, R. S. & A. L. GOLDSTEIN. 1983. Clinical applications of thymosin and other thymic hormones. *In* Recent Advances in Clinical Immunology. R. A. Thompson & N. R. Rose, Eds. 243–286. Churchill Livingstone. New York, NY.

18. ZATZ, M. M., T. L. K. LOW & A. L. GOLDSTEIN. 1982. Role of thymosin and other thymic hormones in T-cell differentiation. *In* Biological Responses in Cancer. E. Minich, Ed. 219–247. Plenum. New York, NY.

19. DORIA, G., D. FRASCA & L. ADORINI. 1984. Thymosin alpha$_1$-induced modulation of immunoregulatory T-lymphocyte activities. Clin. Immunol. Newsl. **5**: 133–135.

20. HARITOS, A. A., G. J. GOODALL & B. L. HORECKER. 1984. Prothymosin alpha: isolation and properties of the major immunoreactive form of thymosin alpha$_1$ in rat thymus. Proc. Natl. Acad. Sci. USA **81**: 1008–1011.

21. ROBERTS-THOMSON, I. C., S. WITTINGHAM, U. YOUNGCHAIYUD & I. R. MACKAY. 1974. Aging, immune response and mortality. Lancet **2**: 368–370.

22. GOLDSTEIN, A. L., T. L. K. LOW, G. B. THURMAN, M. M. ZATZ, N. R. HALL, C.-P. CHEN, S.-K. HU, P. H. NAYLOR & J. E. MCCLURE. 1981. Current status of thymosin and other hormones of the thymus gland. Rec. Prog. Horm. Res. **37**: 369–415.

23. GOODWIN, J. S., R. P. SEARLES & S. K. TUNG. 1982. Immunologic responses of healthy elderly population. Clin. Exp. Immunol. **48**: 403–410.

24. MAKINODAN, T. & W. H. ADLER. 1975. Effects of aging on the differentiation and proliferation potentials of cells of the immune system. Fed. Proc. **34**: 153–158.

25. WALTERS, C. S. & H. N. CLAMAN. 1975. Age-related changes in cell-mediated immunity in BALB/c mice. J. Immunol. **115**: 1438–1443.

26. INKELES, B., J. B. INNES, M. M. KUNTZ, A. D. KADISH & M. E. WEKSLER. 1977. Immunological studies of aging. III. Cytokinetic basis for the impaired response of lymphocytes from aged humans to plant lectins. J. Exp. Med. **145**: 1176–1187.

27. HALLGREN, H. M., J. H. KERSEY, D. P. DUBUEY & E. J. YUNIS. 1978. Lymphocyte subsets and integrated immune function in aging humans. Clin. Immunol. Immunopathol. **10**: 65–78.

28. MERHAV, S. & H. GERSHON. 1977. The mixed lymphocyte response of senescent mice: sensitivity to antigen and cell replication time. Cell Immunol. **34**: 354–366.

29. SHIGEMOTO, S., S. KISHIMOTO & Y. YAMAMURA. 1975. Change of cell-mediated cytotoxity with aging. J. Immunol. **115**: 307–309.

30. GOIDL, E. A., J. B. INNES & M. E. WEKSLER. 1976. Immunological studies of aging. II.

Loss of IgG and high avidity plaque-forming cells and increased suppressor cell activity in aging mice. J. Exp. Med. **144:** 1037–1048.

31. DORIA, G., G. D'AGOSTARO & M. GARAVINI. 1980. Age-dependent changes of B-cell reactivity and T cell–T cell interactions in the *in vitro* antibody response. Cell. Immunol. **53:** 195–206.

32. KISHIMOTO, S., S. TOMINO, H. MITSUYA & H. NISHIMURA. 1982. Age-related disease in frequencies of B-cell precursors and specific helper T cells involved in the IgG anti-tetanus toxoid antibody production in humans. Clin. Immunol. Immunopathology **25:** 1–10.

33. MEREDITH, P. J. & R. L. WALFORD. 1979. Autoimmunity, histocompatibility and aging. Mech. Ageing Dev. **9:** 61–77.

34. MASCART-LEMONE, F., G. DELESPESSE, G. SERVAIS & M. KUNSTLER. 1982. Characterization of immunoregulatory T-lymphocytes during aging by monoclonal antibodies. Clin. Exp. Immunol. **48:** 148–154.

35. KISHIMOTO, S., S. TOMINO, K. INOMATA, S. KOTEGAWA, T. SAITO, M. KUROKI, J. MITSUYA & S. HISAWITSU. 1978. Age-related changes in subsets and functions of human T-lymphocytes. J. Immunol. **121:** 1773–1780.

36. GIRARD, J. P., M. PAYCHERE, M. CUEVES & F. FERNANDEZ. 1977. Cell-mediated immunity in aging population. Clin. Exp. Immunol. **27:** 85–91.

37. SOHNLE, P. G., C. COLLINS-LOCH & K. E. HUHTA. 1983. Kinetics of lymphokine production by lymphocytes from elderly humans. Gerontology **29:** 169–175.

38. GILLIS, S., R. KOZAK, M. DURANTE & M. E. WEKSLER. 1981. Immunological studies of aging. J. Clin. Invest. **67:** 937–942.

39. HICKS, M. J., J. F. JONES, A. C. THIES, K. A. WEIGLE & L. L. MINNICH. 1983. Age-related changes in mitogen-induced lymphocyte function from birth to old age. Am. J. Clin. Pathol. **80:** 159–163.

40. OTTE, R. G., S. WORMSLEY & J. W. HOLLINGSWORTH. 1983. Cytofluorographic analysis of pokeweed mitogen-stimulated human peripheral blood cells in culture: age-related characteristics. J. Am. Geriatr. Soc. **31:** 49–56.

41. DWORSKY, R., A. PAGANINI-HILL, M. ARTHUR & J. PARKER. 1983. Immune responses of healthy humans 83–104 years of age. J. Natl. Cancer Inst. **71:** 265–268.

42. MILLER, J. F. 1962. Part I. The role of the lymphoid system in homotransplantation immunity. Ann. N.Y. Acad. Sci. **99:** 340–354.

43. JANKOVIĆ, B. D., K. ISAKOVIĆ & J. HORVAT. 1965. Effect of lipid fraction from rat thymus on delayed hypersensitivity reactions of neonatally thymectomized rats. Nature **208:** 356–357.

44. WHITE, A. & A. L. GOLDSTEIN. 1970. The role of the thymus gland in the hormonal regulation of host resistance. *In* Control Processes in Multicellular Organisms. G. E. Wolstenholme & J. Knight, Eds. 210–237. Churchill. London.

45. TRAININ, N., M. SMALL & D. ZIPORI. 1975. Characteristics of THF, a thymic hormone. *In* The Biological Activity of Thymic Hormones. D. W. Van Bekkum, Ed. 117–144. Kooyker Sci. Amsterdam.

46. STUTMAN, O. 1977. Two main features of T-cell development: thymus traffic and postthymic maturation. Contemp. Top. Immunobiol. **7:** 1–10.

47. JANKOVIĆ, B. D. & D. MARIĆ. 1988. Restoration of *in vivo* humoral and cell-mediated immune responses in neonatally thymectomized and aged rats by means of lipid and protein fractions from the calf thymus. *In* Neuroimmunomodulation: Interventions in Aging and Cancer. W. Pierpaoli & N. H. Spector, Eds. Vol. 521: 228–246. Ann. N.Y. Acad. Sci. New York, NY.

48. JANKOVIĆ, B. D., P. KOROLIJA, K. ISAKOVIĆ, L. J. POPESKOVIĆ, M. Č. PEŠIĆ, J. HORVAT, D. JEREMIĆ & V. VAJS. 1988. Immunorestorative effects in elderly humans of lipid and protein fractions from the calf thymus: a double blind study. *In* Neuroimmunomodulation: Interventions in Aging and Cancer. W. Pierpaoli & N. H. Spector, Eds. Vol. 521: 247–259. Ann. N.Y. Acad. Sci. New York, NY.

49. GORCZYNSKI, R. M., M. CHANG, M. KENNEDY, S. MACRAE, K. BENZING & G. B. PRICE. 1984. Alterations in lymphocyte recognition repertoire during aging. I. Analy-

sis of changes in immune response potential on B lymphocytes from non-immunized aged mice, and the role of accessory cells in the expression of that potential. Immunopharmacology **7:** 179–194.

50. HIRAMOTO, R. N., V. K. GHANTA & S.-J. SOONG. 1987. Effect of thymic hormones on immunity and life span. *In* Aging and the Immune Response: Cellular and Humoral Aspects. E. A. Goidl, Ed. 177–198. Marcel Dekker, Inc. New York, NY.
51. SISKIND, G. W. 1979. Ontogeny of B-cell function: a role for the thymus in regulating the maturation of the B-cell population. *In* Ageing and Immunity. S. K. Singhal, N. R. Sinclair & C. K. Stiller, Eds. 35–43. Elsevier/North Holland. New York, NY.

Aging of the Reproductive-Neuroimmune Axis

A Crucial Role for the Hypothalamic Neuropeptide Luteinizing Hormone-Releasing Hormone

BIANCA MARCHETTI, MARIA C. MORALE,
NUNZIO BATTICANE,[a] FRANCESCO GALLO,
ZELINDA FARINELLA, AND MATTEO CIONI

Department of Pharmacology
University of Catania Medical School
Viale Andrea Doria, 6
95125 Catania, Italy

and

[a]OASI Institute for Research on Mental
Retardation and Brain Aging
Troina, Italy

INTRODUCTION

The development of an array of specific and nonspecific mechanisms against alien substances, in higher organisms, has made it possible in adult humans to recognize millions of different antigens (specificity) and to react more intensely when repeatedly exposed to the same antigen (memory).[1] One of the major and most important characteristics of the immune system is the functional diversity of its organization through a delicate system of checks and balances, ensuring that the immune response is activated when needed and turned off when its purpose has been achieved.[1]

Similar to the immune system, the nervous system is analogous to an elaborate system of telegraphy, in which there is a wire connection from the source of initiation of the message to the place where reception of the message has its effect. Then, the development of internal communication systems that can transmit messages from one part to another is the starting point: the transfer of messages as molecules which are recognized by discriminators in sensitive cells, and the elaboration of other molecules, for the final transduction into a biological response. Such a concept forms the basis of the interdisciplinary research area termed "neuroendocrine immunology," since a biochemical network, a sharing of neutransmitters and peptides, connects the three major integrative bodily systems: the central nervous system (CNS), the endocrine system, and the immune system.[2-9] One of the most striking features of the expanding literature in this field is the growing body of experimental information supporting their close intercommunication, with the collaboration of these systems providing this "internal milieu" that Claude Bernard described about a century ago.

In this context, the most fundamental observation linking the immune and reproductive systems is that survival of a living organism depends, besides upon environmental conditions and the availability of nutrients, upon 1. The ability to prevent invasion by other organisms, and 2. The presence of a perfectly operative reproductive axis, for species perpetuation.

The primary communication between the immune and neuroendocrine systems is known to involve the thymus and its peptide secretion.[10] The role of the thymus as a neuroendocrine organ and the significance of the neuroendocrine thymus-lymphoid axis is currently receiving much attention. Detection of mRNA for oxytocin and vasopressin in the human thymus,[10] as well as the direct connection of this gland with the CNS by sympathetic and parasympathetic fibers releasing neurotransmitters including catecholamines and acetylcholine[11,12] as well as a variety of neuropeptides (such as substance P, vasoactive intestinal peptide, neuropeptide Y), are reasons to consider this gland as a "frontier" between the endocrine and the immune systems.

On the other hand, the importance of the thymus gland for the control of reproductive function is known from the studies of Calzolari, almost a century ago (1898).[13,14] More recent findings have shown that neonatal thymectomy decreases luteinizing hormone (LH) and follicle-stimulating hormone (FSH) release from the pituitary gland, reduces plasma estradiol and progesterone levels, delays the onset of puberty and vaginal opening.[15–21] Moreover, profound disturbances (*i.e.*, absence of LH and FSH surges, reduced hypothalamic luteinizing hormone-releasing hormone (LHRH) activity) of gonadotrophin secretion is observed in athymic nude (nu/nu) mice.[18] Sex steroid hormones are, in turn, well known to alter the immune response, especially during pregnancy and after gonadectomy, acting either via specific receptors present in the reticular epithelial matrix of the thymus and lymphocytes, and/or modulating thymic hormonal output.[14]

Conversely, protein factors (*i.e.*, interleukin-1), secreted from immune-associated cells have recently been shown to directly alter ovarian function (FIG. 1).[22] Hormonal interactions between the hypothalamus, the pituitary, the thymus and the gonads permit this intersystem crosstalk to occur. Indeed, two thymic hormones, thymosin fraction 5 and one of its peptide constituents, thymosin β_4 stimulate the release of LHRH from the hypothalamus,[17] which in turn stimulates LH release from the pituitary gland. The increasing levels of sex steroids from the gonads are then believed to depress thymosin release from the thymus[14] (FIG. 2).

In support of the concept for a putative bidirectional network carrying information between the immune and reproductive system, is the recognition that the hypothalamic decapeptide LHRH chiefly involved in the control of reproductive processes[23,24] directly influences thymus function[25–30] (FIG. 2).

In the present paper we shall describe some features of reproductive-immune interconnective pathways, with a particular focus on the role of LHRH as paracrine regulator of thymic cell function, in an attempt to localize the possible common triggers of the aging phenomenon.

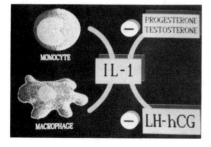

FIGURE 1. Schematic drawing illustrating the direct interaction between the products of activated immune cells (monocyte, macrophage), termed cytokines and the gonadal activity. Interleukin 1 (IL-1) released from monocytes and macrophages after an infection, an antigen challenge or from intra-ovarian stores can directly interfere with gonadal function by decreasing the number of gonadotropin (LH/hCG) receptors and reducing the output of both progesterone and testosterone.

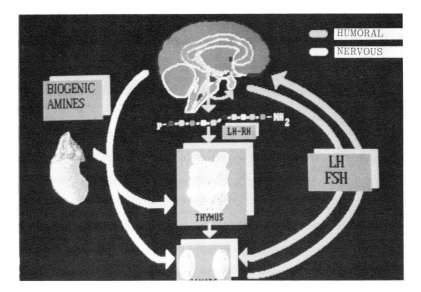

FIGURE 2. The reproductive-neuroimmune axis. The hypothalamic neuropeptide, LHRH, stimulates the secretion of gonadotropins from the anterior pituitary gland. The stimulated levels of circulating sex steroids exert a negative feedback at the hypothalamo-pituitary unit and thymus gland levels. Thymic hormones can then modulate hypothalamic LHRH release. The direct effect of LHRH at the thymus gland level is also illustrated. Moreover, neural inputs coming from the brain directly impinge at the ovarian and thymic gland levels.

LHRH: A MULTIFUNCTIONAL NEUROPEPTIDE ORCHESTRATING REPRODUCTIVE FUNCTION

The hypothalamic peptide, LHRH, directs and coordinates a complex series of biological events occurring in different organs at the appropriate time, to ensure successful reproduction. The menstrual cycle, in primates, like the estrous cycle in other mammals represents, in fact, an extraordinarily complex relationship in time and function among a number of anatomically distant structures. Much of the coordination of these events is achieved by precisely timed fluctuations in the production and secretion rates of hormones.

The presence of LHRH in regions of the CNS as far anteriorly as the olfactory bulbs suggests that this small decapeptide might be involved very early in the initiation of a sexually organized response, from the detection of sexual odors to the induction of mating behavior.[31] While the importance of LHRH functioning in the brain as a neurotransmitter or a neuromodulator has long been recognized,[31-33] only recently has the characterization of specific receptors[34,35] in the CNS provided a morphological substrate for this specific action. On the other hand, in recent years, the importance of the hypophysiotropic signal (LHRH) delivery to the anterior pituitary in order to obtain adequate follicular development and ovulation has been emphasized, while specific LHRH-like proteins have been characterized in rat, ovine and human ovary,[36] underlying a possible paracrine role of this peptide in ovarian physiology.

The complex hormonal regulation of ovarian function is integrated by direct neural pathways coming from the brain,[37-39] which role has been emphasized in recent years. In this context, the development of reproductive acyclicity observed with the process of aging in the female represents one of the most dramatic examples of neuroendocrine changes with age.

We shall summarize some age-dependent changes of the reproductive-immune axis, with the aim of emphasizing the commonality of signals (hormones, peptides, neurotransmitters) and reception mechanisms (receptors) used by the immune and neuroendocrine systems.

LHRH AS A PARACRINE MODULATOR OF CENTRAL AND PERIPHERAL ACTIVITIES

LHRH Receptors in the Brain and the Gonads

The distribution of LHRH outside the regions known to be involved in the control of gonadotropin release suggests that the neuropeptide may have extrahypothalamic nonendocrine functions in the brain. A part its ability to alter the firing rate of neurons within the CNS and to potentiate the effects of centrally acting drugs, such as L-DOPA, LHRH can induce mating behavior in ovariectomized, estrogen-primed rats and anti-LHRH sera or antagonistic analogs of the peptide can inhibit mating.[31–33] Taken collectively these evidences would indicate that LHRH may act as a polypeptide neurotransmitter or neuromodulator of neuronal activity. To perform this function, specific receptors for LHRH should be present in the brain. LHRH receptors in the brain are markedly modulated by changes in the hormonal milieu, since after castration autoradiographic reaction and receptor density are markedly increased, whereas treatment of castrated animals with estrogen in combination with progesterone or androgens (testosterone or dihydrotestosterone) completely counteracts the castration-induced hippocampal LHRH receptor rise.[35] Such findings are in complete agreement with our previous data obtained at the anterior pituitary level and strongly indicate that sex steroids are important modulators of LHRH receptors and action in the brain.

Of interest, developmental changes of LHRH binding sites in the hippocampus follow a pattern strikingly similar to the one observed in the gonads. Following their appearance at 6 days of age, hippocampal LHRH receptors increase to reach maximal density between 20 and 45 days of age. A decline is then observed in adult rats, followed by a progressive increase in receptor density between 11 and 17 months of age. Such findings indicate that changes of hippocampal LHRH binding sites are present during the process of aging, the physiological importance of which as well as their possible involvement in behavioral disturbances observed with the process of aging remain to be determined.

The hypothalamic peptide LHRH has direct antigonadal actions in the rat ovary and specific receptors for the neurohormone have been localized in the ovaries of immature and adult rats.[37–39] The process of aging markedly influences ovarian LHRH receptor activity[38] in a manner similar to the one observed at the CNS level. In fact, in middle-aged animals an important increase of LHRH-R numbers in the afternoon of proestrus indicates that increase of ovarian LHRH-like peptide activity might represent an early signal of reproductive aging. Similarly, animals showing constant vaginal cornification (C.V.C.) or repetitive pseudopregnancies (P.P.) show a significant increase of LHRH-R concentration.[38] The fact that the local injection of a potent LHRH-antagonist completely counteracted the induced LHRH-R levels within the treated ovary[38] clearly indicated that an increase in the production of an LHRH-like protein forms part of the mechanism(s) responsible for ovarian LHRH-R increase observed with aging.[38]

LHRH Receptors in the Thymus and Spleen

The crucial importance of the neuropeptide LHRH in dictating modulatory effects also at the immune system level was revealed by a series of experiments with the aim of assessing 1. the presence of specific LHRH binding sites in the immune organs; 2. the ability of LHRH to influence, *in vitro*, thymic cell function; and 3. the *in vivo* effects of LHRH and its potent agonists (LHRH-A), in situations characterized by a marked decline of immune capacities, such as hypophysectomy and aging.

Characteristics of Thymic LHRH-A Binding

The binding of [125I]buserelin was measured in the 10,000 × g fraction of rat thymic tissue using assay conditions identical to those described for membrane preparations of rat gonadal tissue. [125I]buserelin was specifically bound by membranes prepared from thymus gland obtained from adult (3–4 months) male or female rats at random days of the estrous cycle. The specific binding of the LHRH-A to the rat thymus[26] was saturable (saturability was found at a hormone concentration of 90.5 nM). Binding was dependent on both the temperature and duration of incubation. This pattern of binding was similar to that reported for both pituitary and extra-pituitary tissues.

Specificity of Thymic LHRH-A Binding

The specificity and affinity of the binding site for LHRH in the rat thymus was examined by testing the ability of unlabeled hormones to compete for binding of iodinated buserelin (FIG. 3). For comparison, displacement of [125I]buserelin binding from the rat ovarian LHRH receptor is presented (FIG. 3). To compare the binding of natural sequence of LHRH and the LHRH-A, the binding of [125I]buserelin was measured in the presence of increasing amounts of LHRH or LHRH-A. The binding-inhibition curves obtained with LHRH-A and the natural decapeptide were parallel, consistent with binding of both peptides to the same receptor sites (FIG. 3). However, the affinity of LHRH for these sites was much lower (Ka = 3.8×10^6 M^{-1}) than that of the agonist analog (FIG. 3).

The specificity of the LHRH-A binding was demonstrated by displacement experiments using other hormones. A wide range of peptides (including TRH, arginin vasopressin, angiotensin I, angiotensin II, neurotensin, oxytocin and met-enkephalin, at concentrations up to 2×10^4 M^{-1}) and protein hormones (hCG, oLH, oPRL, up to 10^6 M^{-1}) were unable to displace the specific binding of LHRH-A to rat thymic tissue.[26] Only one peptide tested, somatostatin, was lightly inhibitory at high concentrations (10^6–10^5 M^{-1}), in agreement with what has been reported for hypophyseal LHRH binding sites.

Effect of LHRH and LHRH-A on Blastogenic Transformation of Rat Thymocytes in Vitro

In order to determine the biological function of the thymic LHRH binding site, a culture system was used. In cultures of rat thymocytes, both T-lymphocyte mitosis and DNA synthesis are stimulated by the addition of a mitogenic substance such as concanavalin A (Con-A), and increases in DNA content are then monitored by cellular incorporation of [^{3}H]thymidine. In control cultures, the blastogenic activity increases from 305 ± 38 dpm to 3009 ± 429 78 hrs following stimulation with Con-A (2 μg/ml).[26] On the other hand, when thymocytes were pretreated for 20 hrs with different concentrations of the LHRH-A, D-Trp[6],des-Gly[10]LHRH-N-ethylamide (10^{11}–10^6 M^{-1}), a dose-dependent increase of Con-A-induced stimulation of [^{3}H]thymidine incorporation was observed, reaching a plateau at a concentration of 10^8 M^{-1}.[26]

Effect of LHRH-A on Ornithine Decarboxylase (ODC) Specific Activity

Polyamines are known to be implicated in the process of growth and differentiation in many tissues, including lymphocytes. The increase in ODC activity in gonadotropes of the anterior pituitary gland has been suggested to be part of the mechanism underlying LHRH-induced the LH pro-oestrus surge. We thus thought to determine the effect of LHRH-A on Con-A-induced stimulation of ODC activity in thymocytes. The activity of ornithine decarboxylase rises sharply one day after lectin stimulation, and is maximal 24 hrs later. FIGURE 4 shows ODC activity 24 hrs after addition of the mitogen to the cultures. As observed, incubation of thymocytes with D-Trp[6]-LHRH (10–100 nM) induced a significant ($p < 0.01$) dose-related increase of Con-A-induced stimulation of ODC activity. Superimposable results were obtained using the Ser[6]-LHRH analog.[26]

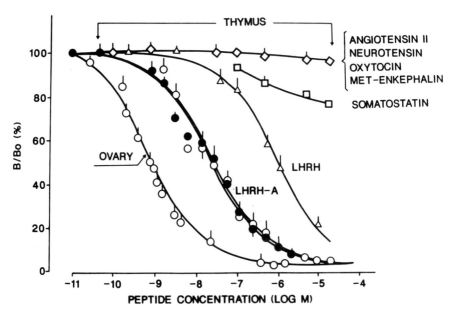

FIGURE 3. Specificity of LHRH agonist binding to rat ovary and thymus gland membrane preparations. Membrane preparations were incubated with ^{125}I-buserelin (150,000–200,000 cpm) and the cold peptides at the indicated concentrations. Only LHRH and its agonist were able to displace LHRH-A binding to both thymus and ovary. As observed, the affinity of the LHRH receptor present in the thymus is lower than that measured in the rat ovary or pituitary.

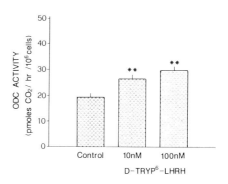

FIGURE 4. Stimulation of ornithine decarboxylase activity (ODC) by the LHRH agonist D-TRYP^6-LHRH. As observed, incubation of thymocyte cultures with the LHRH-A, in the presence of mitogenic substance Con-A, induces a significant potentiation of the enzyme activity, clearly indicating that the rate limiting step in polyamine biosynthesis, ODC, is involved in LHRH action at the thymus gland level.

THE THYMUS

The Clock of Immunological Aging

It is well recognized that the thymus gland is the only clearly individualized primary lymphoid organ believed to play a key role in determining the differentiation of T lymphocytes and involved in the maturation and integrity of the hypothalamo-pituitary unit.[1] An increasing body of evidence points to the thymus as the "clock" of immunological aging, and suggests that involution and atrophy of this gland is one of the keys, if not the principal key, to T-cell aging.[40–44] In fact, available evidence indicates that the decline in immune functions which accompanies aging is due primarily to changes in the T-cell subpopulation. Morphologically, the thymic lymphatic mass decreases with age, primarily as a result of cortical atrophy, in both humans and laboratory animals beginning at the time of sexual maturity.

Furthermore, changes in thymic tissue mass are clearly associated with the loss of T-cell-mediated immune and humoral responses. There is also a direct correlation between the decrease in thymic-dependent immunity and the increase in a variety of diseases associated with aging, including neoplastic and autoimmune diseases.

Neuroendocrine Modulation of the Thymus during the Aging Process: Potential Role of LHRH

While the exact reason for the decline in T-cell function that occurs with aging is unknown, thymic implants, thymic factors and certain anterior pituitary hormones have been shown to partially restore some suppressed T-cell-dependent functions that occur with aging.[40–44] In fact, in addition to the "physiological" regulators, it has been clearly documented that the endocrine system is one of the major systems importantly involved in the regulation of the immune response. Conversely, hormones secreted by lymphocytes and monocytes/macrophages (*i.e.*, lymphokines and monokines) have been shown to alter classical hormone secretion by acting in the brain and/or directly in peripheral endocrine cells.[6–9]

The presence of specific luteinizing hormone-releasing hormone (LHRH) binding sites within the rat thymus gland coupled to the modulatory effects exerted by LHRH and its agonists on thymus function prompted us to determine: 1. The age-dependent changes in LHRH binding sites within the thymus gland; and

2. The ability of a chronic treatment with LHRH agonists (LHRH-A) to influence thymic LHRH binding sites, thymus morphological and functional appearance, as well as thymocyte proliferative capacity during the age-associated decline of immune function.

Effect of Age on Thymus Weight and LHRH Binding Sites

As a first step in studying the LHRH modulation of immune system function during aging, we sought to determine the age-dependent changes in thymic LHRH-A binding sites during the physiological involution of the thymus gland. LHRH binding sites in young adult rats (2–5 months) are measured at 17.8–20.3

TABLE 1. Thymic LHRH Receptor Concentration and Thymus Weights of Aging Male and Female Rats[a]

Groups	Thymus Weight (mg)	LHRH Binding Sites (fmol/mg Protein)
Male		
2 months	300 ± 48	20.35 ± 7.9
5 months	298 ± 36	17.80 ± 6.7
7 months	190 ± 28**	10.50 ± 2.9**
11 months	160 ± 15**	9.30 ± 1.9**
13 months	118 ± 10**	7.30 ± 0.7**
16 months	108 ± 8**	5.10 ± 0.4**
19 months	98 ± 7**	3.10 ± 0.5**
Female		
2 months	270 ± 27	30.10 ± 5.5
5 months	240 ± 20	26.30 ± 4.6
7 months	180 ± 19**	15.80 ± 4.3**
11 months	160 ± 12**	10.90 ± 2.5**
13 months	140 ± 11**	8.10 ± 1.9**
16 months	118 ± 12**	5.00 ± 0.8**
19 months	104 ± 9**	4.00 ± 0.4

[a] LHRH receptor binding assay was carried out in triplicate, in the 10,000 × g fraction of rat thymic tissue, in the presence of ^{125}I-buserelin (150,000 cpm), with or without addition of the unlabelled peptide (10 μg/tube), at 0–4°C for 90 min. Values represent the mean ± SE of 18–20 animals/group. ** p <0.01 compared to 2–5-months rats.

fmol/mg protein in males and 26.3–30.1 fmol/mg protein in females.[27] On the other hand, in 7-month-old rats, a 50% reduction in the number of LHRH-A binding sites (10.5 ± 2.9 fmol/mg protein in males and 15.8 ± 4.3 fmol/mg protein in females) was observed. With increasing age, 11–13-month-old rats showed a 65% decrease in LHRH receptor numbers, and at 16–19 months of age LHRH binding was almost lost, a number of 3.1 fmol/mg protein in males and 4.0 fmol/mg protein in females being measured[27] (TABLE 1).

Thymus weight was reduced 30% in 7-month-old animals, while a 50% reduction in thymic size was reduced at 11 months in male and 13 months in female rats. A further decrease in thymic mass was observed at 16 and 19 months, with weight ranging between 98–110 mg and 104–118 mg in male and female rats, respectively[27] (TABLE 1).

FIGURE 5. Schematic drawing representing the effects of LHRH agonist treatment *in vivo* and *in vitro* in two experimental models characterized by immune deficits, such as aging and hypophysectomy. In both cases treatment *in vivo* with the LHRH-A induces a complete restoration of thymus weight, thymus morphological appearance and thymocyte blastogenic capacity.

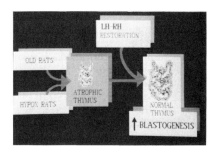

Effect of LHRH-A Treatment of Aging Rats on Thymus Weight and LHRH Binding Sites

In order to study the effect of LHRH on the trophism of the thymus during aging-induced thymus atrophy, 15–16 month-old female and male rats were treated chronically for 45 days with a potent LHRH-A (D-Trp^6-LHRH, 1 μg/day), and the weight of the thymus, its histological appearance, and the number of LHRH binding sites were recorded. In order to compare the effect of surgical removal of the gonads on thymus weight, a group of aging male rats underwent castration. The weight of the thymus at 16–17 months of age was 96 $\pm$ 6 mg in male and 125 $\pm$ 15 mg in female. On the other hand, daily treatment with the super LHRH-A of female rats, produced a 40% increase in thymic size (200 $\pm$ 12 mg), almost counteracting aging-induced decrease of thymus weight (FIG. 5). TABLE 2 shows the effect of both surgical (ORCH) or medical (LHRH-A) castration on thymus weight. It is apparent that ORCH markedly stimulated thymus weight, from 96 $\pm$ 6 mg to 278 $\pm$ 12 mg. On the other hand, LHRH-A treatment produced a 3.5-fold increase in thymic size (380 $\pm$ 18 mg), completely counteracting age-induced thymus atrophy. Similar results were obtained following chronic treatment of aged rats with the D-Ser^6-LHRH analog.[27]

Thymus Histology

The histology of the thymus in 3-month-old rats was characterized by a clear demarcation of cortical and medullary regions, the presence of medullary-epithe-

TABLE 2. Effect of Surgical (ORCH) or Chemical (LHRH-A) Castration on Aging-Induced Decline of Thymic LHRH Binding Sites and Plasma Sex Steroid Levels[a]

Groups	LHRH Binding Sites (fmol/mg Protein)	T (ng/ml)	E_2 (pg/ml)	P (ng/ml)
Male				
Old intact	5.9 $\pm$ 0.5	0.8 $\pm$ 0.05	—	—
Old ORCH	8.9 $\pm$ 0.6**	0.03**	—	—
Old LHRH-A	12.8 $\pm$ 0.7**§	0.3 $\pm$ 0.03**	—	—
Female				
Old intact	7.3 $\pm$ 0.6	—	12 $\pm$ 3	2.4 $\pm$ 0.4
Old LHRH-A	14.8 $\pm$ 2.9**	—	0.5 $\pm$ 0.2**	0.6 $\pm$ 0.1**

[a] Animals' treatment was initiated at 15–16 months of age and rats were sacrificed after 45 days. Results represent mean $\pm$ SEM of 18–20 animals/group. § $p <0.05$ compared to old ORCH; ** $p <0.01$ compared to old intact groups.

lial cells, and rare Hassall's corpuscles.[27] Sixteen–seventeen-month-old rats showed thymus glands lacking a clear demarcation between cortex and medulla, with a marked decrease of T-lymphocyte population, accompanied by a preferential medullary pattern, and a proportionate increase in width of interlobular septa with dilated arterioles.[27] Furthermore, we noticed a sharp increase of perilobular fatty tissue. Both in young and old thymus, plasma cells and mastcells were occasionally observed. Castration of old rats resulted in thymus glands containing lobules with medullary regions surrounded by areas of cortex densely populated with lymphocytes, but not arranged in regular layers, and lobules showing a clear medullary pattern characteristic of the aged rat.

Also observed was a marked hypertrophy and hyperplasia of epithelial cells. Furthermore, broad interlobular septa filled with adipocytes were noted. Treatment of old rats with LHRH-A resulted in thymus glands showing a regularly organized cortex and medulla (with an almost complete restoration of both cortical and medullary compartments towards a young pattern).[27] The cortical region was also markedly increased in width, compared to all the experimental groups studied.[27]

Effect of LHRH-A Treatment of Aging Rats on Blastogenic Transformation of Thymocytes

Since rats undergoing a chronic treatment with LHRH-A had larger thymus glands that appeared to have a normal histological appearance, it was important to determine whether T-cell mitogenesis was enhanced as well. As an index of the suppression in T-cell proliferation induced with aging, thymic cells were prepared from 3-month-old male rats and incubated with Con-A (2 μg/ml). In agreement with earlier studies on mice, rats and humans, the process of aging induces an almost complete loss of the proliferative response of thymocytes to optimal concentrations of Con-A. In fact, while a significative (p <0.01) proliferative response (basal 261 ± 40 vs 3666 ± 335 dpm) was observed in thymocytes cultured from young (3 months) male animals, [^{3}H]thymidine incorporation from control levels of 80 ± 12 dpm, increased to 205 ± 47 dpm after stimulation with Con-A (2 μg/ml) in thymocyte cultures from 17-month-old rats. On the other hand, when equal numbers of thymocytes from 17-month-old rats treated with the LHRH-A for 45 days were cultured with Con-A, cells displayed significantly greater proliferative response (basal: 100 ± 25, stimulated: 2003 ± 235 dpm). It is interesting to notice that while in thymocytes prepared from castrated animals the blastogenic response to the mitogen was similarly increased (from 97 ± 18 to 1740 ± 250 dpm), the combination of both manipulations (ORCH + LHRH-A) resulted in a significant (p <0.01) further increase of the proliferative capacity of thymocytes (from 120 ± 18 to 3970 ± 390 dpm) to respond to Con-A, not distinguishable from that measured in young controls. (FIG. 5).

IMMUNE-REPRODUCTIVE INTERACTIONS

Reproductive Aging

It is recognized that some mammalian aging processes involve effects of steroids on the brain and pituitary. The concept of a critical period during development for the organizing influences of steroids on the sexual differentiation of the rodent nervous system is well established. In fact, estrogens and aromatizable androgens (endogenous or injected) can influence hypothalamic neuronal number and connections during a critical period extending from late fetal development until about 10 days after birth.[46] As a result, males and females have distinct differences in hypothalamic neuroanatomy and in the regulation of LH. It is also becoming clear that the chronic exposure of adult rodents and sheep to estrogens can also have irreversible effects on neuroendocrine functions as manifested by infertility syndromes that are similar in some regards to aging changes.[46]

In a pleiotropic view, aging has been suggested to result from the continuance of developmental processes, which when continued long enough are eventually deleterious to the organism.[46] This pleiotropic view would agree, therefore, with the age-correlated change in the sensitivity of the hypothalamo-pituitary unit to estradiol: a decrease in negative feedback necessary for the regulation of the onset of puberty may continue after puberty and eventually lead to the loss of reproductive capacity.[46]

Major Aspects of Female Reproductive Aging

The processes of female reproductive senescence have attracted the interest of many investigators over the past 20 years. Loss of fertility during midlife occurs in the female of many mammalian species. A major question concerned with aging of the reproductive system is the loss of estrous/menstrual cycles, which is a characteristic in many spontaneous ovulators, including mice, rats and humans.[45,46]

The 28-day cycle of women (or the 4–5-day-cycle of the rodent) is based on multiple and highly precise neurohormonal interactions taking place at the level of the brain, anterior pituitary gland and ovary, responsible for the LH surge that leads to ovulation. The increased secretion of ovarian estrogens from the maturing follicle is thought to trigger LHRH secretion from the hypothalamus and to facilitate the action of the neurohormone at the anterior pituitary level by increasing the LH and FSH responsiveness to LHRH.[31] In the past few years, it has become increasingly clear how the hypothalamic-hypophyseal-gonadal system represents one of the most sophisticated examples of hard-wired circuit, constantly tuned by chemical signals, the efficiency of which is strictly dependent upon the perfect functioning of the "hardware" (hypothalamic neurons, gonadotrophs, gonads) and "software" (neurohumoral factors impinging on hypothalamic LHRH machinery) components of the fertility program. In this context, the development of reproductive acyclicity in the female represents, perhaps, one of the most dramatic examples of neuroendocrine changes with age.

In fact, the secretory response of the gonadotroph to LHRH as well as the concentration of gonadotropic hormones are dependent upon the patterning of the LHRH stimulus, and subtil changes in the frequency of LHRH stimulation have profound effects on the quality of follicular development. The rhythm of hypophysiotropic signal frequency is dictated by the complex integration of aminergic and peptidergic signals acting both at central (hypothalamic) and peripheral (hypophyseal, ovarian) levels and whose integrity ensures a physiological menstrual cycle.

Common Pacemakers for Aging of the Reproductive and Immune Systems? Role of LHRH

The primary cause for the disappearance of ovarian function in women is not completely understood. A point is represented by the fact that the mammalian ovary acquires its fixed stock of oocytes during development and that this stock is irreversibly lost during postnatal development and aging.[46]

A potential neuroendocrine component in menopause concerns the frequency of gonadotropin pulses, which has been shown to have a major influence on follicular development. In fact, experimentally retarding the frequency of LHRH pulses from once/60 min to once/120 min can cause anovulatory cycles with lower peak of estradiol, while slowing to once/180 min, results in the absence of any follicular development, despite the normal circulating FSH levels.[32] It is therefore clear that Knobil's (1980) suggestion that little changes in the frequency and/or amplitude of LHRH secretion which have a major influence on initiation of puberty, could be extended to consider a role of LHRH pulse frequency during aging, responsible for lengthening of cycles.[31] Substantial evidence indicates that LHRH levels in the portal vessel is probably elevated during the postmenopausal stage as well as in hypogonadal conditions, when ovarian steroids are absent. Furthermore, recent studies, reviewed by Finch and co-workers,[46] have shown that the amount of LHRH in the hypothalamus of women varied as a function of age and reproductive status. In premenopausal women (16–49 years of age), the mean hypothalamic content of LHRH was twice that in postmenopausal women who were 50–78 years old.[46] Of interest, in this study, was the observation that the amount of LHRH in the hypothalami of castrated premenopausal women was as low as that in the postmenopausal women, suggesting that the reduction in the hypothalamic LHRH content in postmenopausal women was not the result of aging per se, but rather a consequence of diminished ovarian function occurring at the time of menopause.[46]

Because of the crucial importance of ovarian steroids in triggering the phasic LHRH discharge, exerted possibly via a critical combination of threshold doses (adequate estradiol and progesterone concentrations) of sex steroids, sensitivity of the hypothalamic norepinephrinergic system and decrease of opiatergic tone, it seems likely that alterations in the rate and/or ratio of ovarian steroid secretion and/or metabolism during the approach of menopause could influence the frequency of LHRH pulses, thereby influencing folliculogenesis.

CONCLUSION

As observed from the information presented in this paper, the process of aging is a complex phenomenon involving changes in neural, endocrine and immune activities. The subtle alterations in the degree of sensitivity of the different target cells to the hypophysiotropic hormones, trophic factors and neuroactive substances, has now to face possible compensatory homeostatic mechanism(s), for instance, involving production of neuropeptides and endocrine hormone from the immune cells, in an attempt to restore and/or to balance the neuroendocrine axes dysfunctions.

In terms of reproductive decline induced by the process of aging, the available information points to LHRH as the major factor involved in reproductive senescence. The significant role played by the hypothalamic neuropeptide in the modulation of immune responsiveness would indicate LHRH as the signal conveying information to both the neuroendocrine and immune cells, with the role of informing and then transducing the messages into appropriate biological responses. The widespread therapeutical application of LHRH agonists in a large number of pathologies, such as pediatric, gynecologic, urologic and oncologic medicine, would perhaps include this class of compounds as possible immunomodulators.

Conversely, thymic peptides could found important applications in endocrinological gynecology. A clear example of such a situation is given by the important positive effects of the LHRH-A therapy in postmenopausal breast cancer patients, where the desensitization of the pituitary-gonadal axis cannot be invoked to explain the regression of metastases in these patients, and a possible immunorestorative effect could be postulated.

Further studies on the molecular mechanisms which form the bases for the crosstalk communication between the reproductive and immune systems will not only give us new insights into the problems of fertility regulation and in more general issues of aging and aging-related diseases, but will also provide us with a variety (neural, endocrine, immune) of tools that can be used to reverse, minimize or postpone some age-dependent events, with positive implications for the elderly population.

REFERENCES

1. PATRICK, C. C., J-M. GOUST & G. VIRELLA. 1986. Tissues and cells of the immune system. *In* Introduction to Medical Immunology. C. C. Patrick, J-M. Goust, H. H. Fudenberg & G. Virella, Eds. 7. Marcel Dekker. New York and Basel.
2. PIERPAOLI, W. & E. SORKIN. 1967. Relationship between thymus and hypophysis. Nature **215:** 834.
3. PIERPAOLI, W. & H. O. BESEDOVSKY. 1975. Role of the thymus in programming of neuroendocrine functions. Clin. Exp. Immunol. **20:** 323.
4. PIERPAOLI, W., H. G. KOPP, J. MULLER & M. KELLER. 1977. Interdependence between neuroendocrine programming and the generation of immune recognition in ontogeny. Cell. Immunol. **29:** 16.
5. PIERPAOLI, W. 1981. Integrated phylogenetic and ontogenetic evolution of neuroendocrine and identity-defense immune functions. *In* Psychoneuroimmunology. R. Ader, Ed. 575. Academic Press. New York.
6. BLALOCK, J. E. 1984a. Relationships between neuroendocrine hormones and lymphokines. Lymphokines **9:** 1.
7. BLALOCK, J. E. 1984b. The immune system as a sensory organ. J. Immunol. **132:** 1067.
8. BLALOCK, J. E., K. L. BOST & E. M. SMITH. 1985. Neuroendocrine peptide hormones and their receptors in the immune system: production, processing and action. J. Neuroimmunol. **10:** 31.
9. WEIGENT, D. A. & J. E. BLALOCK. 1987. Interactions between the neuroendocrine and immune systems: common hormones and receptors. Immunol. Rev. **100:** 79.
10. GEENEN, V., J. J. LEGROS, P. FRANCHIMONT, M. BAUDRIHAYE, M. P. DEFRESNE & J. BONIVER. 1986a. The neuroendocrine thymus: coexistence of oxytocin and neurophysin in the human thymus. Science **232:** 508.
11. LIVNAT, S., S. Y. FELTEN, S. L. CARLSON, D. L. BELLINGER & D. L. FELTEN. 1985. Involvement of peripheral and central catecholamine systems in neural-immune interactions. Neuroimmunology **10:** 5.
12. ROSZMAN, T. L. & W. H. BROOKS. 1985. Neural modulation of immune function. J. Neuroimmunol. **10:** 59.
13. CALZOLARI, A. 1898. Recherches experimentales sur un rapport probable entre la fonction du thymus et celle des testicules. Arch. Ital. Biol. Torino **307:** 71.
14. GROSSMAN, C. J. 1985. Interactions between the gonadal steroids and the immune system. Science **227:** 257.
15. BESEDOVSKY, H. O. & E. SORKIN. 1974. Thymus involvement in female sexual maturation. Nature **249:** 356.
16. HALL, N. R., J. P. McGILLIS & A. L. GOLDSTEIN. 1984. Activation of neuroendocrine pathways by thymosin peptides. *In* Stress, Immunity and Aging. E. L. Cooper, Ed. 209. Dekker. New York.
17. REBAR, R. W., A. MIYAKE, T. K. L. LOW & A. L. GOLDSTEIN. 1981a. Thymosin stimulates secretion of luteinizing hormone-releasing factor. Science **214:** 669.

18. REBAR, R. W., I. C. MORANDINI, G. F. ERICKSON & J. E. PETZE. 1981b. The hormonal basis of reproductive defect in athymic mice. I. Diminished gonadotrophic concentrations in prepuberal females. Endocrinology **108:** 120.
19. MICHAEL, S. D., O. TAGUCHI & Y. NASHIZUKA. 1980. Effect of neonatal thymectomy on ovarian development and plasma LH, FSH, GH, and PRL in the mouse. Biol. Reprod. **22:** 343.
20. REBAR, R. W., A. MIYAKE, G. F. ERICKSON, T. L. K. LOW & A. L. GOLDSTEIN. 1983. *In* Factors Regulating Ovarian Function. G. S. Greenwald & P. F. Terranova, Eds. 465. Raven Press. New York.
21. REBAR, R. W., I. C. MORANDINI, S. A. DESILVA, G. F. ERICKSON & J. E. PETZE. 1981c. The importance of the thymus gland for normal reproductive function in mice. *In* Dynamics of Ovarian Function. N. Schwartz & M. Hunzicker-Dunn, Eds. 285. Raven Press. New York.
22. GOTTSCHALL, P. E., A. UEHARA, S. TALBOT HOFFMANN & A. ARIMURA. 1987. Interleukin-1 inhibits follicle stimulating hormone-induced differention in rat granulosa cells *in vitro*. Biochem. Biophys. Res. Commun. **149:** 502.
23. MARCHETTI, B., G. PELLETIER, M. CIONI, M. BADR, G. PALUMBO & U. SCAPAGNINI. 1988. Age-dependent changes in luteinizing hormone releasing hormone (LHRH) receptor systems: role of central and peripheral LHRH in the decline of reproductive function. *In* The Brain and Female Reproductive Function. A. R. Genazzani, U. Montemagno, C. Nappi & F. Petraglia, Eds. 207. Parthenon Press.
24. MARCHETTI, B., F. LABRIE, G. PELLETIER, L. PROULX-FERLAND & J. J. REEVES. 1983. Hormonal control of pituitary luteinizing hormone-releasing hormone receptors. *In* Recent Advances in Male Reproduction. Molecular Basis and Clinical Implications. R. D'Agata, M. B. Lipsett & H. J. van der Molen, Eds. Raven Press. New York.
25. MARCHETTI, B., V. GUARCELLO & U. SCAPAGNINI. 1988. Luteinizing hormone-releasing hormone (LHRH-A) binds to lymphocytes and modulates the immune response. *In* Biology and Biochemistry of Normal and Cancer Cell Growth. L. Castagnetta & I. Nenci, Eds. 149. Harwood Academic Press. London.
26. MARCHETTI, B., V. GUARCELLO, M. C. MORALE, G. BARTOLONI, Z. FARINELLA & U. SCAPAGNINI. 1989. Luteinizing hormone-releasing hormone binding sites in the rat thymus: characteristics and biological function. Endocrinology **125:** 1025.
27. MARCHETTI, B., V. GUARCELLO, M. C. MORALE, G. BARTOLONI, F. RAITI, G. PALUMBO, JR., Z. FARINELLA, S. CORDARO & U. SCAPAGNINI. 1989. Endocrinology **125:** 1037.
28. MARCHETTI, B., V. GUARCELLO, G. TRIOLO, M. C. MORALE, Z. FARINELLA & U. SCAPAGNINI. 1989. Luteinizing hormone-releasing hormone (LHRH) as natural messenger in neuroendocrine-immune communications. *In* Interactions among CNS, Neuroendocrine and Immune Systems. W. Hadden, K. Masek & G. Nisticò, Eds. 127. Pythagora Press. Rome and Milan.
29. MARCHETTI, B., M. C. MORALE, V. GUARCELLO, N. CUTULI, F. RAITI, N. BATTICANE, G. PALUMBO, JR., Z. FARINELLA & U. SCAPAGNINI. 1990. Crosstalk communication in the neuroendocrine-reproductive-immune axis: age-dependent changes in the common communication networks. *In* Neuropeptides and Immunopeptides: Messengers in a Neuroimmune Axis. M. S. O'Dorisio & A. Panerai, Eds. Vol. 594: 309. New York Academy of Sciences. New York.
30. MARCHETTI, B., C. C. MAIER, R. D. LEBOEUF & J. E. BLALOCK. 1990. Luteinizing hormone-releasing hormone gene expression in the thymus. 20th Ann. Meet. Soc. Neurosci. Abst. 1895.
31. KNOBIL, E. & J. D. NEILL. 1988. The Physiology of Reproduction. Vol. 2. L. L. Ewing, G. S. Greewald, C. L. Markert & D. W. Pfaff, Associate Eds. Raven Press. New York.
32. CONN, P. M., A. J. W. HSUEH & W. F. CROWLEY, JR. 1983. Gonadotropin-releasing hormone: molecular and cell biology, physiology, and clinical applications. *In* GnRH Regulation of the Gonadotropins. Symposium Summary. 67th Ann. Meet. Fed. Am. Soc. Exp. Biol. Chicago. 2351.

33. HSUEH, A. J. & J. M. SCHAEFFER. 1985. Gonadotropin-releasing hormone as a paracrine hormone and neurotransmitter in extra-pituitary sites. J. Steroid Biochem. **23(5B):** 757.
34. BADR, M. & G. PELLETIER. 1987. Characterization and autoradiographic localization of LHRH receptors in the rat brain. Synapse **1:** 567.
35. BADR, M., B. MARCHETTI & G. PELLETIER. 1988. Modulation of hippocampal LHRH receptors by sex steroids in the rat. Peptides **9:** 441–442.
36. MARCHETTI, B., G. PALUMBO, E. CITTADINI, A. CIANCI, R. PALERMO, L. LOMEO, S. CIANCI & U. SCAPAGNINI. 1987b. LHRH receptors in human ovary and corpus luteum: possible role in the intragonadal regulation of human reproductive function. *In* Proc. 12th Congress on Fertility and Sterility. 225. Parthenon. Carnforth.
37. MARCHETTI, B., M. CIONI & U. SCAPAGNINI. 1985. Ovarian LHRH receptors increase following lesions of the major LHRH structures in the rat brain: involvement of a direct neural pathway. Neuroendocrinology **41:** 321.
38. MARCHETTI, B. & M. CIONI. 1988. Opposite changes of ovarian and pituitary receptors for LHRH in ageing rats: further evidence for a direct neural control of ovarian LHRH receptor activity. Neuroendocrinology **48:** 242.
39. MARCHETTI, B., M. CIONI & U. SCAPAGNINI. 1986b. Ovarian receptors for luteinizing hormone-releasing hormone (LHRH) are finely modulated by direct neural influences: role of central and peripheral LHRH systems. *In* Endocrinology 85. G. M. Molinatti & L. Martini, Eds. 349. Excerpta Medica. Amsterdam.
40. FABRIS, N. 1981. In handbook of Immunology of Aging. M. Kay & T. Makinodan, Eds. 61. CRC Press, Inc. Boca Raton, FL.
41. MAKINODAN, T. 1978. The thymus in aging. *In* Geriatric Endocrinology. (Aging: Vol. 5.) R. B. Greenblatt, Ed. 217. Raven Press. New York.
42. FABRIS, N., W. PIERPAOLI & E. SORKIN. 1972. Lymphocytes, hormones and aging. Nature **240:** 557.
43. KELLEY, K. W., S. BRIEF, H. J. WESTLY, J. NOVAKOFSKI, P. J. BECHTEL, J. SIMON & E. R. WALKER. 1986. GH₃ pituitary adenoma cells can reverse thymic aging in rats. Proc. Natl. Acad. Sci. USA **83:** 5663.
44. PIERPAOLI, W. & N. H. SPECTOR, EDS. 1988. Neuroimmunodulation: Interventions in Aging and Cancer. Vol. 521. New York Academy of Sciences. New York.
45. SCAPAGNINI, U., M. CIONI & B. MARCHETTI. 1986. The ageing brain as a major pacemaker in the decline of reproductive function: evidence for a direct neural involvement in ovarian failure. *In* Gynecological Endocrinology. A. R. Genazzani, A. Volpe & F. Facchinetti, Eds. 75. Parthenon. Carnforth.
46. FINCH, C. E., L. S. FELICIO, C. V. MOBBS & J. F. NELSON. 1984. Endocrinol. Rev. **5:** 476.

Age-Related Changes of Beta-Endorphin and Cholecystokinin in Peripheral Blood Mononuclear Cells

ALBERTO E. PANERAI, BARBARA MANFREDI,
LUISA LOCATELLI, FRANCESCA RUBBOLI,
AND PAOLA SACERDOTE

Department of Pharmacology
University of Milan
School of Medicine
Via Vanvitelli, 32
20100 Milan, Italy

Aging is well known for being associated with a decline in cognitive[1] a well as in immune functions.[2] For this reason, it looked worthwhile to investigate whether the decline of immune responses could be associated with changes of neuropeptide content in immune cells. Therefore, we studied the concentrations of beta-endorphin (BE) and cholecystokinin (CCK) in peripheral blood mononuclear cells (PBMC) from subjects of different age groups, both immediately after sampling and after culture as well as in the presence or absence of appropriate stimuli.

Moreover, we looked at the same parameters in patients affected by Alzheimer's disease or Down's syndrome, two pathologies thought of as being characterized by precocious aging.

MATERIALS AND METHODS

Subjects

For the studies in normal subjects, samples were obtained from over fifty 20–99-year-old volunteers, healthy in relation to their respective age. In order to evaluate peptide concentrations at different ages, samples were grouped according to the age of the donors into ages 20–30 (mean + SD = 23 + 2.4; 20 women and 20 men), 31–50 (39 + 4.0; 16 women and 18 men), 51–70 (59 + 6.0; 18 women and 18 men), 71–99 (88 + 7.8; 12 women and 10 men). For the study in Down patients, samples were obtained from 20 patients (19 men and 1 woman) in the age groups 10–20 (young) and 40–50 (old). Samples were also obtained from 6 Alzheimer male patients, age 65–80.

Separation of Peripheral Blood Mononuclear Cells

Peripheral blood was obtained between 0900 and 1100 in the morning, and collected into tubes containing 1000 U/ml heparine. PBMC were separated by gradient sedimentation over Ficoll-Paque (Pharmacia),[3] and the cells pelleted to 20×10^6 PBMC. Aprotinine 1,000 K.I.U./ml was added to all samples before storage at $-20°C$ till further processing, in order to inhibit enzymatic degradation of the peptides.[4]

Pelletted cells were resuspended in 1.0 ml 0.1 N acetic acid, homogenized in a blade homogenizer and sonicated. Samples were centrifuged at 20.000 × g for 10 minutes and the pellets were used for protein determination,[5] while the supernatants were frozen till further processing by radioimmunoassay.

PBMC Cultures

Macrocultures of PBMC obtained from subjects of the different age groups were set up with 2×10^6 cells/ml in RPMI 1640, 10% fetal calf serum, 1% glutamine, penicillin 100 U/ml, streptomycin 100 μg/ml, containing or not containing phytohemagglutinin (PHA) 4 μg/ml (GIBCO, Grand Island, NY), and incubated at 37°C, 5% CO_2 for 48 hr. After incubation, cells were collected, and Aprotinine 1,000 K.I.U./ml was added to the pellets, which were then treated as previously described. Concomitantly, PHA-stimulated microcultures from the same subjects were carried out in order to evaluate cell proliferation.[6,7] After 48 hr incubation at 37°C all cultures received 0.5 mCi of ^{3}H-thymidine (specific activity 2 Ci/mmol, Amersham, UK). Four hr later, cells were harvested by an automated cell harvester (Skatron) and radioactivity was measured in a liquid scintillation counter (Packard, Downers Grove, IL).

Measurement of BE and CCK in PBMC

Peptides were measured by radioimmunoassay with C-terminal directed antibodies specific for BE or the sulphated fragment 26–33 of CCK. The antisera and whole radioimmunoassays procedures were previously described and validated.[4,8,9]

Statistical Analysis of Results

Student *t* test and analysis of variance followed by Dunnett's test for multiple comparisons were used.

RESULTS

BE and CCK in PBMC from Subjects at Different Ages

FIGURE 1 shows that BE concentrations in fresh resting lymphocytes increase significantly with age. BE and CCK concentrations increase significantly after 30

FIGURE 1. Beta-endorphin concentrations in peripheral blood mononuclear cells from healthy subjects of different age.

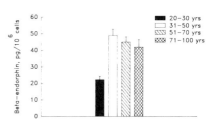

years of age vs younger subjects ($p < 0.01$), and remain constantly higher in the 51–70- and 71–99-year-old subjects ($p < 0.01$). In Down and Alzheimer patients, BE concentrations in PBMC are comparable to those present in healthy subjects.

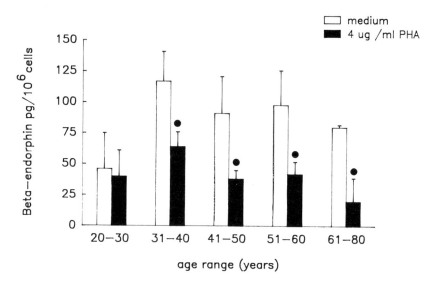

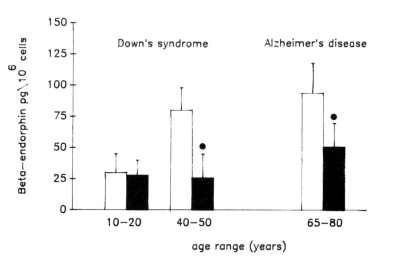

FIGURE 2. Beta-endorphin concentrations in cultured peripheral blood mononuclear cells obtained from healthy subjects of different age (*upper panel*) or Down and Alzheimer patients (*lower panel*) before and after stimulation with PHA. ● = $p < 0.001$ vs medium alone.

TABLE 1. PHA-Induced Proliferation of Lymphocytes Obtained from Healthy Subjects of Different Age Groups, and Down or Alzheimer Patients

Subjects	Age (n)	Proliferation (c.p.m.)
Healthy	20–30 (18)	98561 + 25717*
Healthy	31–50 (16)	89775 + 29741
Healthy	51–70 (17)	74388 + 21544
Healthy	71–99 (16)	65554 + 21482
Down	10–20 (12)	47799 + 13825
Down	40–50 (12)	17340 + 11909
Alzheimer	65–80 (6)	44500 + 16520

* = mean + SD.

BE and CCK in Cultured PBMC

FIGURE 2 shows that BE concentrations are higher after 48 hr culture in the absence of stimuli in PBMC obtained from subjects over 30 years of age, when compared to PBMC obtained from young subjects. PHA stimulation does not induce any change in BE concentrations of PBMC obtained from healthy subjects in the 20–30 age group and in young Down, while it significantly decreases the concentrations of the opioid peptide in PBMC obtained from subjects of the 31–50, 51–70, and 71–99 age group, in old Down and Alzheimer patients. The BE decrease can be evidentiated whatever the parameters used for calculation are, *i.e.*, pg/mg of protein, pg/10^6 cells, or total content of BE/total number of cells. CCK concentrations in PBMC were not affected by stimulation by PHA in any of the age groups studied.

TABLE 1 shows PHA-induced PBMC proliferation from normal subjects of the different age groups, young and old Down, and Alzheimer patients. Neither for young nor for old cells was a correlation between the degree of proliferations and concentrations of the opioid found.

DISCUSSION

While data are rapidly accumulating on the effects of neuropeptides on immune functions,[10,11] less is known on neuropeptides in immune cells. In this study we attempt to correlate the concentrations of BE and CCK in resting and mitogen-stimulated PBMC to the age of donors.

BE and CCK are present in fresh PBMC obtained from healthy subjects of different age and Down or Alzheimer patients. The previous identification in PBMC of the BE precursor POMC and of lipotropin confirms that BE is synthesized in PBMC and not taken up from plasma or culture media.[8]

According to our results, aging seems to be associated with an increase in BE and CCK concentrations either in fresh resting cells and in PBMC cultured without the mitogen. On the other hand, PHA stimulation induced a decrease in BE, but not in CCK, showing an age-related pattern comparable to that of the increase in absolute concentrations of this peptide in fresh unstimulated PBMC. At present we cannot find any consistent hypothesis for the PHA-induced decrease in BE contents nor can we find any correlation with the immune functions studied. Moreover, since BE concentrations in cell culture supernatants did not change after PHA stimulation (data not shown), it looks like that observed into cells did not simply reflect the release of BE from PBMC. The behavior of PBMC from Down patients deserves special attention. As previously shown, PBMC obtained from young or old Down patients showed a decreased proliferation in response to PHA more pronounced than that observed in old healthy subjects and Alzheimer patients. However, the content of BE in resting and PHA-stimulated PBMC of young Down patients was similar to that of 20–30-year-old healthy subjects. These data further point out that proliferative responses and neuropeptide contents dissociate. Moreover, the time course of changes in BE and CCK concentrations observed in fresh and cultured cells from subjects of different ages does not directly correlate to the time course of immune defects found during aging. In fact, the changes we observe are already present in the 31–50 age group, while immunological signs of aging, *e.g.,* impaired mitogen-induced proliferation or IL-2 production, appear at older age (>60).[7]

The only correlation that can be envisaged between the time course of PBMC CCK and BE changes and the age-associated immune defects is in the atrophy of the cellular matrix of the thymus and the initial decline of thymic hormone plasma levels that seems to take place with the same age pattern.[12] This observation might induce to speculate on a possible inhibitory effect of thymic factors on PBMC BE and CCK or, alternatively, on an inhibitory effect of BE and/or CCK on the thymus.

REFERENCES

1. Rowe, J. W. & R. L. Kahn. 1987. Human aging: usual and successful. Science 237: 143–149.
2. Weskler, M. E. & G. W. Siskind. 1984. The cellular basis of immune senescence. Monogr. Dev. Biol. 17: 110–121.
3. Sacerdote, P. & A. E. Panerai. 1989. Analysis of the beta-endorphin structure-related activity on human monocyte chemotaxis: importance of the N- and C-terminal. Peptides 10: 565–569.
4. Panerai, A. E., A. Martini, A. M. Di Giulio, F. Fraioli, C. Vegni, G. Pardi, A. Marini & P. Mantegazza. 1983. Plasma β-endorphin, β-lipotropin, and met-enkephalin concentrations during pregnancy in normal and drug-addicted women and their newborn. J. Clin. Endocrinol. Metab. 57: 537–543.
5. Lowry, O. H., N. J. Rosebrough, A. L. Farr & R. J. Randall. 1951. Protein measurement with the Folin phenol reagent. J. Biol. Chem. 193: 265–275.
6. Alvarez-Mon, A., J. H. Kehrl & A. S. Fauci. 1985. A potential role for adrenocorticotropin in regulating human B lymphocyte functions. J. Immunol. 135: 3823–3826.
7. Barcellini, W., M. O. Borghi, C. Sguotti, R. Palmieri, D. Frasca, P. L. Meroni & C. Zanussi. 1988. Heterogeneity of immune responsiveness in healthy elderly subjects. Clin. Immunol. Immunopathol. 47: 142–151.
8. Ogawa, N., A. E. Panerai, S. Lee, G. Fosbach, V. Havliceck & H. G. Friesen. 1979. Beta-endorphin concentrations in the brain of intact and hypophysectomized rats. Life Sci. 25: 317–326.
9. Salerno, F., C. Bonato, A. E. Panerai, A. Martini & A. Malesci. 1983. Brain cholecystokinin-8 immunoreactivity in rats with experimental liver cirrhosis. Life Sci. 33: 377–381.
10. Blalock, J. E. 1989. A molecular basis for bidirectional communication between the immune and neuroendocrine system. Physiol. Rev. 69: 1–32.
11. Morley, J. E., N. E. Kay, G. F. Solomon & N. P. Plotnikoff. 1987. Neuropeptides: conductors of the immune orchestra. Life Sci. 41: 527–544.
12. Goldstein, G. & T. K. Audhya. 1985. Thymopoietin to thymopentin: experimental studies. Surv. Immunol. Res. 4(Suppl. 1): 1–10.

Band 3 in Aging and Neurological Disease[a]

MARGUERITE M. B. KAY[b]

*Departments of Medicine, Medical Microbiology and
Immunology, and Biochemistry and Genetics
Texas A & M University
Olin E. Teague Veterans Center
Temple, Texas 76504*

INTRODUCTION

Senescent cell antigen (SCA), an aging antigen, was discovered in 1975.[1] It is a protein that appears on old cells and acts as a specific signal for the termination of that cell by initiating the binding of IgG autoantibody and subsequent removal by phagocytes.[1-29] This appears to be a general physiologic process for removing senescent and damaged cells in mammals and other vertebrates.[4] Although the initial studies were done using human erythrocytes as a model, senescent cell antigen was discovered on cells besides erythrocytes in 1981.[4] It occurred on all cells examined.[4] The aging antigen itself is generated by the degradation of an important structural and transport membrane molecule, protein band 3.[5] Besides its role in the removal of senescent and damaged cells, senescent cell antigen also appears to be involved in the removal of erythrocytes in clinical hemolytic anemias and the removal of malaria-infected erythrocytes.[7,18] Oxidation generates senescent cell antigen *in situ*.[6]

The presence of band 3-related molecules in nonerythroid tissues was first demonstrated in 1983.[30] A protein immunologically related to band 3 was demonstrated in such diverse cell types as isolated neurons, hepatocytes, squamous epithelial cells, alveolar (lung) cells, lymphocytes, neurons, and fibroblasts using an antibody to band 3 that reacts with the transmembrane, anion transport domain of band 3.[30] The band 3-like protein in many of these cell types appeared to be a truncated version of the erythroid protein based on its molecular weight of ~60,000 estimated from its migration in polyacrylamide gels. We suggested that part of the cytoplasmic amino terminus segment was missing from the band 3-like protein in these cell types, and that band 3 protein was modified to perform functions in different environments.[30] Since then, band 3 has been described in numerous cell types and tissues including fibroblasts, hepatoma cells, and lymphoid cells. Band 3 is also present in nuclear,[30] Golgi,[31] and mitochondrial membranes[32] as well as in cell membranes. Band 3-like proteins in nucleated cells participate in band 3 antibody-induced cell surface patching and capping.[30] A truncated version of band 3 which lacks the amino terminus has also been described in kidney.[33] Band 3 is present in the central nervous system, and differ-

[a] This work was supported by a Veterans Administration Merit Review, the International Foundation for Biomedical Aging Research, and National Institutes of Health Grants AG08444, AG08574.

[b] Address for correspondence: Marguerite M. B. Kay, Regents' Professor, University of Arizona Health Sciences Center, Room 644 LSN, 1501 North Campbell Avenue, Tucson, AZ 85724.

ences described in band 3 between young and aging brain tissue.[34] One autosomal recessive neurological disease, choreoacanthocytosis, is associated with band 3 abnormalities.[17,19] The 150 residues of the carboxyl terminus segment of band 3 appear to be altered.[19] In brains from Alzheimer's disease patients, antibodies to aged band 3 label the amyloid core of classical plaques and the microglial cells located in the middle of the plaque in tissue sections and an abnormal band 3 in immunoblots. However, our knowledge of band 3 in nonerythroid cells is limited to the observation that it is present. The question of whether band 3 in nonerythroid tissues performs the same functions as it does in erythrocytes is addressed in the last section of this article.

MATERIALS AND METHODS

IgG Binding and Inhibition Assay

Details of the methods are given in the articles referred to in the text. IgG was isolated from senescent RBC from 50 liters of blood and purified as previously described.[2,4] IgG eluted from senescent cells, rather than serum IgG, was used because normal serum contains antibodies to spectrin, actin, 2.1, etc.[8,9,11] Competitive inhibition studies were performed using synthetic peptides to absorb the IgG isolated from senescent erythrocytes. SCIgG (3^* μg) was absorbed with synthetic peptides at the concentrations indicated or purified SCA, as a control, for 60 min at room temperature, and incubated with stored red cells for 60 min at room temperature.[1,2,4,18] The number of red cell-bound IgG molecules were quantitated before and after absorption using equilibrium binding kinetics.[7,18] Scatchard analysis was performed.[7,18] Percent inhibition was calculated from the following formula: $100 [1 - (x - b/T - b)]$ where x = molecules of IgG autoantibody bound per cell; T = total number of IgG antibody molecules bound in the absence of inhibitor; b = background Protein A binding.

Peptides

Peptides were prepared by solid phase synthesis using an Applied Biosystems 430A automatic peptide synthesizer. They were analyzed by amino acid analysis, HPLC, sequencing, and/or FABS to determine purity. Amino acids are referred to by the standard single letter code.

Brain Tissue Preparation

Perfused brains were obtained from young Sprague-Dawley rats (Charles River Laboratories, Wilmington, MA). Rats were anesthetized with Nembutal and perfused intracardially with phosphate buffered saline (PBS). They were immediately decapitated, the entire brain was rapidly removed, and tissues were frozen in isopentane cooled on dry ice. Brains were stored at $-70°C$ for biochemical analysis.[15,16]

Brain Anion Transport

Influx of sulfate was performed essentially according to the method of Elgavish et al.[35]

Immunohistochemical Analysis

Perfused brains were obtained from adult male C57Bl mice (Jackson Laboratories, Bar Harbor, ME) as described above. Human cerebellar tissue was obtained from normal individuals at autopsy and frozen immediately in isopentane.

RESULTS AND DISCUSSION

Mechanism of Removal of Senescent Cells: Early Studies

The first hint that a "neo-antigen" appeared on senescent cells came from studies showing that IgG autoantibodies selectively bind to old human red blood cells (RBC) aged *in situ*[1,2] during investigations of the mechanism by which macrophages distinguish between senescent and other "self" cells.

RBC as a Model

Human RBC were used as a model for these studies because of the ready availability of these cells and the ease with which populations of different ages can be separated. In addition, RBC do not synthesize proteins. Therefore, they provide information on cumulative protein aging and damage.

Hypothesis

It was hypothesized that Ig in normal human serum attaches to the surface of senescent RBC until a critical level is reached which results in phagocytosis.

IgG Binds to Old but Not Young Cells

To test this hypothesis, RBC separated by density centrifugation from freshly drawn blood was incubated with specific antibodies to human immunoglobulins (Ig) conjugated to scanning immunoelectron microscopy markers. Old RBC had IgG but no IgA or IgM or their surface as determined by scanning immunoelectron microscopy.[1] Young RBC did not have immunoglobulin on their surface. Incubation of old RBC with autologous macrophages resulted in their phagocytosis regardless of whether incubations were performed in medium with serum, autologous Ig-depleted serum or whole serum.[1] Young RBC were not phagocytized under any of these conditions. Thus, it appeared that the IgG attached *in situ* to senescent human RBC and rendered them vulnerable to phagocytosis by macrophages. The presence of IgG autoantibodies on the surface of old cells indicates that a new antigen had appeared that was not present on other cells. This was the first indication that a "neo-antigen" appears on senescent cells.

Senescent Cell IgG Is an Autoantibody

IgG attached to senescent cells *in situ* was shown to be an autoantibody.[2] The antibodies could be dissociated from senescent cells. The dissociated antibodies specifically reattached via the antigen binding (Fab) portion of the IgG molecule to homologous senescent, but not to autologous or allogeneic mature or young cells.[3] Fab binding was demonstrated by antigen blockade studies, scanning immunoelectron microscopy, and ^{125}I labeled Protein A binding to the Fc region of IgG bound to senescent cells and vesicles.[2,8,9,11] Thus, the antibody to the senescent cell antigen is an autoantibody and not a nonspecific or a cytophilic antibody.[2] It exhibited specific immunologic binding via the Fab region.

Other investigators have confirmed the presence of IgG on senescent, damaged, and stored red cells[1–13,22–29] (for review see REFS. 9, 11). The amount of IgG on the surface of cells increases with storage.

Glass et al.[23] have found a 44% reduction in the mean life span of RBC in old, specific pathogen-free rats, as compared to the life span in young rats, as determined by ^{59}Fe pulse-labeling in vivo. The proportion of young cells circulating in the blood of old animals was increased. In old rats, young as well as old RBC were heavily labeled with IgG; whereas predominantly old cells carried IgG in young rats. Extending their studies to humans, Glass et al.[24] found a significant increase in reticulocytes in healthy elderly humans even though their hematocrits were the same as those of younger individuals. A significant increase in autologous IgG on lower middle aged cells was consistently demonstrated in these elderly individuals. These findings suggest that young cells age prematurely in old individuals. Bartosz et al.[25] have found increased amounts of cell-membrane bound IgG on RBC from patients with Down's syndrome and suggest that accelerated red cell aging occurs in these individuals. Accelerated aging of other cells and systems, including the immune system, has been reported in patients with Down's syndrome. Bosman et al.[36] have found that erythrocytes from patients with Alzheimer's disease but not multiinfarct dementia show characteristics of accelerated aging.

The results of studies described above demonstrate that Ig was required to initiate phagocytosis of senescent and stored cells and that IgG attaches in situ to senescent human RBC.[1,2]

Red Cell Life Span Studies

These results were confirmed in vivo using mice which were bred and maintained in a Maximum Security Barrier devoid of viruses, mycoplasma, and pathogenic bacteria; thus, excluding an exogenous source for the senescent cell antigen.[3] RBC were labeled in situ with ^{59}Fe which labeled the newly synthesized hemoglobin in young cells. Red cells were separated on Percoll gradients, 1 or 40 days after radioactive iron injection, into young and old populations, and injected into separate groups of syngeneic mice. Kinetic studies revealed that <90% of the ^{59}Fe-labeled young RBC were removed from the circulation within 45 days. In contrast, >90% of the ^{59}Fe-labeled old RBC were removed within 20 days. The difference in the rate of removal of young and old RBC was statistically significant ($p \leq 0.001$). Kinetic studies on density-separated spleen cell populations revealed that the radioactivity decreased in the RBC fraction concomitantly with an increase in radioactivity in the splenic macrophage fraction. The radioactivity was found to be inside macrophages.[3]

Studies performed in vitro with mouse splenic macrophages and autologous young and old RBC revealed that mouse macrophages phagocytized senescent but not young RBC ($p \leq 0.001$). The phagocytosis of middle-aged RBC (~23%) was intermediate between that of young RBC (5%) and old RBC (~50%). This suggested that the appearance of the senescent cell antigen, and, thus, molecular aging of membranes, was a cumulative process.

Cellular Removal in Other Vertebrates

Numerous investigators have confirmed the presence of IgG on old human cells using different methods. In addition, IgG binding to erythrocytes has been shown to be a mechanism of removal of old red cells in SPF mice,[3] conventionally housed mice,[22] germ-free rats,[23] cows,[25] rabbits,[28] and chickens (Bosman, Harris, and Kay, in preparation). Anion transport by old erythrocytes from chickens was consistent with band 3 aging (Bosman, Harris, and Kay, in preparation).

Role of Sialic Acid and Carbohydrate in Recognition and/or Removal of Senescent Cells

Other groups, extrapolating from the classical experiments of Ashwell and co-workers who showed that the lifetime of serum glycoproteins could be drastically shortened by removal of external carbohydrates, have suggested that binding and phagocytosis of old erythrocytes requires disappearance of terminal sialic acid residues and subsequent exposure of penultimate galactose residues.

In order to determine what role, if any, galactose has in the physiological removal of old erythrocytes, we tried to elute IgG from intact senescent erythrocytes, as well as from their membranes, with buffer containing galactose.[37] Incubation of senescent RBC with galactose did not inhibit their phagocytosis by macrophages indicating that galactose did not displace senescent cell IgG. Incubation with galactose did not elute senescent cell IgG from the membranes of red cells. In addition, absorption of senescent cell IgG with the carbohydrate portion of band 3 did not alter binding to band 3 in immunoblots. The fraction specifically eluted from affinity columns containing the carbohydrate portion of band 3 did not bind to erythrocyte membranes in immunoblots. These results suggest that the IgG binding specifically to senescent erythrocytes was not directed against galactose residues. In addition, our synthetic peptide studies described below show that carbohydrate is not required for senescent cell IgG binding because it binds to synthetic peptides which have no carbohydrate attached.

In summary, macrophages recognize old and damaged RBC on the basis of binding of a specific IgG autoantibody to old cells. IgG is required for phagocytosis of old RBC.

Neoantigen Appears on Old Cells

Binding of an IgG autoantibody to senescent RBC through immunologic mechanisms indicated that antigenic determinants recognized by these IgG autoantibodies appeared on the membrane surface as RBC aged.

Isolation of Senescent Cell Antigen

As an approach to isolating and identifying this neoantigen, affinity columns were prepared with IgG isolated from old cells. Senescent cell antigen was isolated from sialoglycoprotein mixtures with affinity columns prepared with IgG eluted from senescent cells.[4] Material specifically bound by the column was eluted with glycine-HCl buffer, pH 2.3. Both glycoprotein and protein stains of gels of the eluted material revealed a band migrating at a relative molecular weight of

62,000 in the component 4.5 region. These experiments suggested that the 62,000 M_r glycopeptide carried the antigenic determinants recognized by IgG obtained from freshly isolated senescent cells. The 62,000 M_r peptide, but not the remaining sialoglycoprotein mixture from which it is isolated, abolished the phagocytosis-inducing ability of IgG eluted from senescent RBC in the erythrophagocytosis assay.[4] This indicated that the 62,000 M_r peptide is the antigen which appeared on the membrane of cells as they aged.

Senescent Cell Antigen is Present on Nucleated Cells

Examination of other somatic cells for the antigen which appears on senescent RBC revealed its presence on lymphocytes, platelets, neutrophils, and cultured human adult liver cells and primary cultures of human embryonic kidney cells as determined by a phagocytosis inhibition assay[4] (TABLE 1). The senescent cell antigen was isolated from lymphocytes[4,38] with the senescent RBC IgG affinity column. Gel electrophoresis of the material obtained from the column revealed a band migrating at a M_r of 62,000 at the same position as the antigen isolated from senescent RBC.[4] This finding confirmed the results obtained with the phagocytosis inhibition assay, indicating that the antigen which appeared on senescent RBC also appeared on other somatic cells.

Appearance of the 62,000 M_r antigen on RBC initiated binding of IgG autoantibodies *in situ* and phagocytosis of senescent cells by macrophages.[1-4] The antigen was present on stored human lymphocytes, platelets, and neutrophils, and on cultured liver and kidney cells. In addition, IgG autoantibodies in normal serum have been shown to bind to senescent RBC *in situ* in humans,[1,2] mice,[3] rats,[35] cows,[31] rabbits,[32] and chickens (Bosman, Harris, Kay, in preparation). Thus, the immunological mechanism for removing senescent and damaged red cells appears to be a general physiological process for removing cells programmed for death in mammals and, possibly, other vertebrates.[1,2,4]

Identification of Senescent Cell Antigen as a Band 3 Product

Since mature erythrocytes cannot synthesize proteins, senescent cell antigen is probably generated by modification of a preexisting protein of higher molecular weight.[8,10,11] It is postulated that senescent cell antigen is a component of the 4.5 region that is derived from band 3[8,10,11] based on both extraction and isolation conditions, relative molecular weight, and its characterization as a glycosylated peptide.[4]

Experiments designed to test this hypothesis revealed that senescent cell antigen is immunologically related to band 3 and may represent a physiologically significant breakdown product of the parent molecule.[8,10,11] Both band 3 and senescent cell antigen abolished the phagocytosis inducing ability of IgG eluted from senescent cells; whereas, spectrin, bands 2.1 and 4.1, actin, glycophorin A, PAS staining band 1–4, and desialylated PAS staining bands 1–4 did not. In addition, rabbit antibodies to both purified band 3 and senescent cell antigen, and IgG eluted from senescent cells reacted with band 3 and its breakdown products as determined by immunoautoradiography of RBC membranes indicating that these molecules share common antigenic determinants not possessed by other red cell membrane components.[8,10,11]

These results confirmed those obtained with the erythrophagocytosis assay by indicating that band 3 carries the antigenic determinants of senescent cell antigen. Thus, senescent cell antigen is immunologically related to band 3 and may be derived from it.

Senescent cell antigen was mapped along the band 3 molecule using topographically defined fragments of band 3. Both binding of IgG eluted from senescent red blood cells ("senescent cell IgG") to defined proteolytic fragments of band 3 in immunoblots, and two-dimensional peptide mapping of senescent cell antigen, band 3, and defined proteolytic fragments of band 3 was used to localize senescent cell antigen along the band 3 molecule.[10] The data suggested that the antigenic determinants of senescent cell antigen that was recognized by physiologic IgG autoantibodies resided on an external portion of a naturally occurring transmembrane fragment of band 3 that had lost an M_r 40,000 cytoplasmic (NH_2-terminal) segment and part of the anion transport region. A critical cell age specific cleavage of a band 3 appeared to occur in the transmembrane, anion transport region of band 3.

TABLE 1. Inhibition of the Phagocytosis-Inducing Ability of IgG Autoantibody Eluted from Senescent RBC by Previous Absorption with (A) Stored Platelets, Lymphocytes, or Neutrophils, and (B) Human Adult Liver Cells or Embryonic Kidney Cells[a]

		Cell Type Used for Absorption	Phagocytosis (%) (Mean ± s.d.)
A		none	37 ± 4
		platelets	2 ± 2
		lymphocytes	0
		neutrophils	0
B		none	38 ± 6
		liver	0
		kidney	7 ± 7

[a] From Kay.[4] Reprinted by permission from *Nature*.

Band 3 Aging

The demise of band 3, which is synonymous with generation of senescent cell antigen, occurred in two distinct steps. Structurally, band 3 underwent an as yet uncharacterized initial change during cellular aging that triggered a series of events terminating the life of the cell. We recently developed antibodies against aged band 3 that recognized this change because they bound to a distinct region of band 3 in old but not middle-age or young cells.[7] Following the change in intact band 3 with aging, band 3 underwent degradation, presumably catalyzed by an enzyme.[38] Preliminary experiments indicated that it was a calcium-dependent membrane-bound protease and suggested that the protease may be calpain. Cleavage of band 3 occurred in the transmembrane, anion transport region.[5-7,8,10,11,38] Fragments of band 3 were detected in membranes of old but not young cells by immunoblotting with antibodies to normal band 3. Following degradation, band 3 underwent a change in tertiary structure[38] becoming senescent cell antigen. A physiologic IgG autoantibody bound to senescent cell antigen and initiated cellular removal.

Since our previous studies had indicated that senescent-cell antigen is derived from band 3 by cleavage in the transmembrane anion transport region,[5,8,9,38] we suspected that anion transport might be altered with cellular aging.[6] If this suspicion proved to be correct, then we would have a functional assay for aging of band 3, the major anion transport protein of the erythrocyte membrane.

Transport studies on age-separated rat erythrocytes indicated that anion transport decreased with age.[6] The Michaelis constant (K_m) increased, and the maximal velocity (V_{max}) decreased in old erythrocytes as compared to middle-aged erythrocytes. These data provided us with another assay of cellular function to use to determine whether erythrocytes are "senescent." However, it is doubtful that the number of molecules of band 3 to which IgG was bound (100 per cell) was adequate to account for the magnitude of change in anion transport. Therefore, we suspect that another as yet unidentified change preceded events initiating IgG binding and was responsible for the observed changes in anion transport.

The following functional changes in band 3 occurred as red cells aged. These changes were: decreased anion transport activity (increased K_m; decreased V_{max}), decreased number of high affinity ankyrin binding sites, and binding of physiologic IgG autoantibodies *in situ*.[39] In addition, band 3 underwent an as yet undefined change that resulted in binding of 980 antibodies to aged band 3.[7] These 980 antibodies recognized band 3 that had aged prior to its formation of senescent cell antigen. Degradation of band 3 generated senescent cell antigen.

Models for Cellular Aging

Oxidation and Vitamin E

We postulated that generation of senescent cell antigen may result from oxidation-induced cross-linking followed by proteolysis.[6] As an approach to evaluating oxidation as a possible mechanism responsible for generation of senescent-cell antigen, we studied erythrocytes from vitamin E-deficient rats.[6] The importance of vitamin E as an antioxidant, providing protection against free radical-induced membrane damage, has been well documented (see REF. 6). Vitamin E is primarily localized in cellular membranes, and a major role of vitamin E is the termination of free-radical chain reactions propagated by the polyunsaturated fatty acids of membrane phospholipids. Vitamin E-deficient erythrocytes are defective in their ability to scavenge free radicals. It is interesting that there is a correlation between life span and natural antioxidant levels in a variety of species and that the level of such antioxidants appears to correlate with metabolic activity of individual species. Specific biochemical alterations in the membrane of erythrocytes from vitamin E-deficient rhesus monkeys have been described (see REF. 6). Furthermore, vitamin E deficiency represents a "physiological" method for rendering cells susceptible to free-radical damage and may simulate conditions encountered *in situ*. We used vitamin E deficiency as a model for studying oxidation because studies show that, in mammals, vitamin E functions as an antioxidant, and because vitamin E deficiency simulates conditions encountered *in situ* more closely than does chemical treatment of cells *in vitro*. Red cells from vitamin E-deficient rats behaved like old erythrocytes in the phagocytosis assay, and in anion transport and glyceraldehyde-3-phosphate dehydrogenase activity. In addition, increased breakdown products of band 3 was observed in erythrocyte membranes from vitamin E-deficient rats. Vitamin E-deficient rats developed a compensated hemolytic anemia as is observed in vitamin E-deficient humans.

Middle-aged erythrocytes from vitamin E-deficient rats behaved like old cells based on the phagocytosis assay, anion transport studies, and immunoblotting studies[6] (see tables in REF. 9).

Immunoblotting studies revealed increased breakdown products of band 3 in cells from vitamin E-deficient rats as is observed in old cells.[6] Thus, vitamin E deficiency leads to accelerated red cell aging, presumably through oxidation.

We have not observed high molecular weight complexes containing band 3 in membranes from vitamin E-deficient rats or old cells aged *in situ,* except under conditions that precipitate IgG (unpublished observations).

Results of the experiments on vitamin E deficiency suggest that oxidation can cause aging of band 3. We suspect that this may be one of the mechanisms of cellular aging *in situ.* At this time, it appears that general cellular damage such as lysis (Kay, unpublished) and oxidation can result in the generation of senescent cell antigen. We suspect that many different cellular insults have a final common pathway that results in generation of senescent cell antigen.

Chemical Models

As part of our systematic ongoing studies of mechanisms of cellular and molecular aging, we developed a "biochemical profile" of senescent human red cells.[39] This "red cell aging" panel allows us to assess functional red cell age independent of chronological age. The panel used to obtain this profile includes IgG binding, phagocytosis, enzyme activity, anion transport, ankyrin binding and immunoblotting with antibodies to band 3. We also searched for models of accelerated and decelerated cellular aging, anticipating that such models would allow us to dissect molecular aging and provide insight into mechanisms. Initially, we investigated models for aging *in vitro.*[39]

Free Radical Generating Systems

We subjected intact human erythrocytes to treatments that have been reported to result in changes in band 3 and/or to mimic aging *in vitro.* The validity of these treatments as model systems for erythrocyte aging was evaluated using a "red cell aging panel" which provided a biochemical profile of a senescent red cell.[6,7,39] Treatments were assessed for their ability to induce the following changes *in vitro* that were observed in normal erythrocytes aged *in vivo:* 1, increased breakdown of band 3 as detected by immunoblotting; 2, decrease in anion transport efficiency as detected with a sulfate self-exchange assay; 3, decrease in total glyceraldehyde 3-phosphate dehydrogenase (G3PDH) activity with an increase in membrane-bound activity; and 4, increase in the binding of autologous IgG as detected with a protein A-binding assay. Neither incubation with the free radical-generating xanthine oxidase/xanthine system, nor treatment with malondialdehyde, an end product of free radical-initiated lipid (per) oxidation, resulted in age-specific changes.[39] Loading of the cells with calcium, and oxidation with iodate resulted in increased breakdown of band 3, but did not lead to increased binding of autologous IgG. Only erythrocytes that had been stored for 3–4 weeks showed the same structural and functional changes as observed during aging *in vivo.*[39]

Hemoglobin Cross-Linking

Cross-linking of band 3 by hemoglobin has been suggested as a mechanism for generating senescent cell antigen. Results of experiments in which cells are treated with phenylhydrazine in order to cross-link band 3 revealed increased binding of autologous IgG. However, phenylhydrazine in the amounts used caused red cell lysis. Lysis by itself initiates IgG binding. For example, IgG binding by control red cells that was not exposed to phenylhydrazine and had 0% lysis as determined by the loss of red cells after incubation in PBS +10 mM glucose pH 7.4 for 1 hour at 37°C (5% hematocrit) was 18 ± 2 molecules IgG/cell (mean ± 1 standard deviation). When the incubation was performed with 5 mM phenylhydrazine in the solution, 20% hemolysis was observed and IgG binding increased to 115 ± 7. At 10 mM phenylhydrazine, hemolysis increased to 50% and IgG binding is 129 ± 7. At 15 mM phenylhydrazine, hemolysis was 60% and IgG binding was 200 ± 34. Similar results were obtained with acridine orange at the concentrations employed to induce "cross-linking" of band 3. This supports our early finding that lysis can initiate IgG binding but does not provide any insight into the role of cross-linking in the generation of senescent cell antigen. Drs. Linss, Simon, Halbhuber and Neyer have shown independently that IgG binding in the induced Heinz body system is an artifact (presented at the XIIth International Symposium on the Structure and Function of Erythroid Cells, Berlin, GDR, 1989). Thus, it appears that hemichrome formation generates artifacts. The other problem with this suggested hypothesis for the generation of senescent cell antigen is that it is limited to RBC and cannot explain the formation of senescent cell antigen in cells besides RBC.

Cell Mutations/Alterations

Hemoglobin Koln and G6PD Deficiency

We then began a search for "experiments of nature" that might provide insights into the process of normal cellular aging.[39] Initially, we studied glucose 6-phosphate dehydrogenase deficiency (G6PD) and hemoglobin Kln as potential models.[12,39] Membranes from both the G6PD-deficient and hemoglobin Kln cells which we studied have been reported to contain high molecular weight polymers.[12] In addition, hemoglobin Kln cells contain hemoglobin precipitates. We used the red cell aging panel to compare the biochemical profile of glucose 6-phosphate dehydrogenase-deficient and hemoglobin Kln cells containing high molecular weight protein polymers or hemoglobin precipitates with that of normal senescent cells. However, accelerated cellular aging is not present as determined by a "red cell aging panel" including lack of phagocytosis and IgG binding to young and middle-aged erythrocytes, normal ankyrin binding, normal anion transport, normal G3PDH activity, and no increase in band 3 breakdown products.[12] We found no evidence in support of the concept that aggregation of band 3 plays a role in the mechanism for generating senescent cell antigen. Observations like these support the hypothesis that degradation of band 3, not aggregation, is a critical event in IgG binding and normal erythrocyte aging.

Band 3 Mutations/Alterations

We began a search for mutations and/or clinical alterations of erythrocyte band 3. Our search for band 3 protein alterations resulted in the discovery of the first band 3 alterations/mutations in any species. All three different alterations were discovered in humans.[7,14,17,19] Anion and glucose transport of all three is summarized in TABLE 2. One mutation, high molecular weight band 3, results from an addition of tyrosine containing peptides in the transmembrane, anion transport region of band 3.[14] It appears to be an autosomal recessive. This mutation is associated with acanthocyte ("thorny" cell) formation. However, erythrocyte survival is normal *in situ* as determined by the reticulocyte count, and the erythrocytes do not exhibit accelerated aging as determined by the "red cell aging panel."[39]

A second band 3 alteration also exhibits acanthocytosis.[17,19] This alteration is associated with ion and glucose transport abnormalities and neurologic disease. The neurological disease is an autosomal recessive.

TABLE 2. Anion and Glucose Transport by Middle-Aged and Old Erythrocytes from Normal Individuals and Erythrocytes from Individuals with Band 3 Alterations[a]

| | | Anion | | K_m | Glucose V_{max}[d] | |
Cells	Km[b]	V_{max}[c]			Efflux	Influx
Middle-aged	0.9 ± 0.1	13.2 ± 1.4		8.9 ± 1.2	19.0 ± 2.9	12.8 ± 1.9
Old	1.6 ± 0.1[+]	7.7 ± 1.1[+]		22.1 ± 3.8	33.4 ± 5.3	6.7 ± 1.7
HMW						
Control	0.6 ± 0.1	11.1 ± 0.6		18.5 ± 2.5	9.2 ± 2.8	13.9 ± 3.4
Propositus	0.5 ± 0.1	22.3 ± 1.0*		11.5 ± 2.6+	10.1 ± 0.3[+]	12.9 ± 1.0
Neuro						
Control	0.7 ± 0.1	13.5 ± 0.7		ND	16.5 ± 0.6	10.1 ± 0.9
Proposita	0.9 ± 0.1	29.0 ± 1.0+		ND	8.2 ± 0.3	9.8 ± 1.2
Fast aging						
Control	1.0 ± 0.1	12.4 ± 0.7			8.1 ± 1.1	13.2 ± 1.0
Propositus	1.7 ± 0.2+	9.9 ± 1.0+		16.4 ± 0.4[+]	21.2 ± 0.7+	8.1 ± 1.1+

[a] Results are presented as the mean ± one standard deviation; *$p \leq 0.001$ compared to control; +$p \leq 0.01$ compared to control.

[b] K_m, exchange constant, *i.e.*, the sulfate concentration (in mM) at which the transport rate is half the maximal value, as determined from a Lineweaver-Burk plot of the ascending branch of the rate curve.

[c] V_{max}, the maximal velocity in moles $\times 10^{-8}/10^8$ cells/min.

[d] μmoles/ml cells/min; efflux, zero-trans-efflux.

The third alteration of band 3 alteration is characterized by accelerated cellular aging as determined by a "red cell aging panel," and cellular removal. The propositus' reticulocyte count is ~20%, indicating the destruction and replacement *in situ* of 20% of circulating erythrocytes daily, and there is increased IgG binding to middle-aged cells (TABLE 3). Both peripheral blood findings (*e.g.*, the presence of nucleated erythrocytes and precursors of monocytes and lymphocytes) and bone marrow biopsy are consistent with a hemolytic anemia.[7] We gave this band 3 alteration the descriptive name "fast aging" band 3 because the propositus' young and middle-aged cells exhibit all the characteristics of old erythrocytes (*e.g.*, increased IgG binding and decreased anion and altered glucose transport, and increased breakdown products of band 3 is observed on immunoblots). Aged band 3 antibodies, which do not bind to young or middle-aged cells, bind to a distinct region of band 3 in immunoblots of membranes of middle-aged red cells, and to intact middle-aged red cells as determined by immunoelectronmicroscopy. We suspect that "fast aging" band 3 is more susceptible to proteolysis than is normal band 3.

The data indicate that the band 3 alteration that results from an addition to band 3 does not alter red cell life span or produce clinical disease. In contrast, band 3 alterations that are associated with band 3 aging and/or degradation are characterized by shortened red cell life span and clinical diseases. We suspect that these latter alterations result from deletions or substitution in the band 3 gene.

The three band 3 mutations/alterations provide support for the hypothesis that the membrane spanning domain of the anion transporter and glucose transporter(s) is functionally and structurally related. For example, high molecular weight band 3 containing cells exhibit changes in band 3 structure and function that is probably caused by a redundant segment in the anion transport region.

TABLE 3. IgG Binding to RBC from Individuals with Normal or "Fast Aging" Band 3 as Determined by an ^{125}I-Protein A Binding Assay[a]

Individual	Cell Age[b]	IgG Molecules/Cell[c]
Control	unsep	8 ± 2
Propositus	unsep	106 ± 10*+
Control	MA	9 ± 2
Propositus	MA	99 ± 4*
Control	old	102 ± 11*
Propositus	old	119 ± 12*

[a] Data are presented as the mean ± one standard deviation of the mean from different experiments; n = 8–12.

[b] Unsep, unseparated; MA, middle-aged; old, second band of 4 bands of old cells.

[c] +$p \leq 0.001$ compared to control; *$p \leq 0.001$ compared to control middle-aged cells.

Changes in other membrane proteins or lipids were not detected. The other parameter that is altered is the V_{max} of glucose efflux. External modifications of band 3, probably at its cytoplasmic domain, that occurred in G6PD-deficient cells or in cells containing unstable hemoglobin Koln had no effect on anion transport and did not affect glucose transport. At the present time, we cannot reconcile the sequence data of the available glucose transport proteins with the genetic, functional, cell biological, and immunological data which indicate a relationship between band 3 and glucose transport.

The results of the studies on aging *in vivo* indicate that IgG binding and anion transport are the two most sensitive screening assays for determining cellular age.

Molecular Mapping of Senescent Cell Antigen

We concluded from previous studies that senescent cell antigen is a degradation product of band 3 that includes most of the ~38,000 Da carboxyl terminal segment and ~30% of the ~17,000 Da anion transport region.[5] Both immunoblotting studies with IgG isolated from senescent cells and two dimensional peptide mapping studies of senescent cell antigen indicated that senescent cell antigen lacks a ~40,000 molecular weight cytoplasmic segment which contains the amino terminus and, possibly, additional peptides of band 3.[5] Peptide mapping studies and anion transport studies suggested that a cleavage of band 3 occurred in the anion transport region.[5] Furthermore, breakdown products of band 3 were observed in the oldest cell fractions but not in young or middle-aged cell fractions, and anion transport was impaired in old cells.[5-7,39] The following changes are characteristic of old erythrocytes: increased IgG binding to senescent cell antigen, decreased anion transport (decreased V_{max} and increased K_m), and increased breakdown products of band 3.[6,39]

Based on this structural, biochemical, immunological and physiological data,[1-7] we selected four peptides of band 3 for testing.[18,20] We synthesized peptides of erythrocyte band 3 from the anion transport region or with suspected anion transport activity. We selected one band 3 segment which appears to be exposed to the outside of the cell and one that is further along the molecule towards the amino terminus and outside the region that we speculated was included in senescent cell antigen.[5] The first peptide, pep-ANION 1, contains a covalent binding site for the anion transport inhibitor, diisothiocyano dihydrostilbene disulphonate (DIDS), and a tyrosine that is exposed to the outside.[40] Thus, we know that this peptide is located on the cell surface. The second peptide, pep-ANION 2, is situated toward the end of the region and is probably intracellular.[18,20,21] It has anion transport capability.[21] This peptide would be predicted to lack inhibitory activity because it would not be presented as an antigen on native band 3. The last peptide, pep-COOH, is from the carboxyl terminus region and contains an anion transport region.[18,20,21] The lysines found in this region comprise another binding site for DIDS.[41,42] As a control, we used a peptide, pep-CYTO, from the cytoplasmic segment of band 3 within the region of the putative ankyrin binding site.[40]

Competitive inhibition studies are performed using the synthetic peptides to absorb the IgG isolated from senescent erythrocytes. This is the same IgG that initiates phagocytosis *in situ*. The Fab region binds to the aging antigen, and the Fc portion of IgG is available for binding by macrophages as is the case *in situ*.[2,8,9,11] IgG binding and inhibition was determined with a protein A binding assay.[7] This biological assay measures the fate of erythrocytes *in vitro* and *in vivo*.[7,9,11,27]

Results of these studies suggest that the regions pep-ANION 1 (538–554) and pep-COOH (812–827) contain antigenic determinants recognized by senescent cell IgG (FIG. 1A,B). pep-ANION 2 is only weakly inhibitory and pep-CYTO does not inhibit. Immunoblotting studies demonstrate binding of senescent cell IgG to peptides pep-ANION 1 and 2 and pep-COOH but not to pep-CYTO.[18,20] Immunoblotting studies showed binding of IgG from senescent cells to peptides pep-ANION 1, pep-ANION 2, pep-COOH, but not to pep-CYTO (not shown here, see REF. 20) or to pep-GLYCOS (FIG. 2), an external peptide that provides an anchorage for carbohydrate chains attached to band 3. This peptide was included as an additional control.

The results of these experiments indicate that pep-ANION 1 and pep-COOH carry active aging antigenic determinants, and synthetic peptides alone, without carbohydrate attached, abolish binding of senescent cell IgG to red cells. Therefore, carbohydrate moieties are not required for the antigenicity or recognition of senescent cell antigen. The peptide to which band 3 carbohydrate attaches (pep-GLYCOS) does not significantly inhibit IgG binding to old cells. A cytoplasmic peptide is not involved in senescent cell antigen activity.

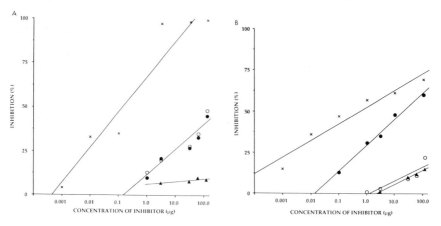

FIGURE 1. Inhibition of senescent cell IgG binding to erythrocytes by synthetic peptides or synthetic peptide mixtures. Competitive inhibition studies were performed as described in materials and methods at the concentrations indicated on the graph. For peptide mixtures, the total peptide used was the amount indicated with each peptide constituting half of that amount. **(A)** (▲) pep-CYTO (R139–159); (●) pep-ANION 1 (R538–554); (○) pep-COOH (R812–827); (X) pep-ANION 1 and pep-COOH mixture. **(B)** (●) pep-COOH hexamer (N6) consisting of 6 amino acids on the amino side of pep-COOH; (x) pep-COOH hexamer (N6) and pep-ANION 1 mixture; (○) pep-GLYCOS (R630–648); (▲) pep-ANION 2 (R588–602). The data for peptides pep-ANION 1, pep-COOH, and their admixtures are the averages of three separate inhibition experiments, each of which consisted of replicative determinations. Lines are fitted by the method of least squares. The data of pep-ANION 1 and pep-COOH could be fitted by a single line in (A). Other pep-COOH subpeptides gave the following percent inhibition: R818–827 (17 μM, 12.2 μg), 54 ± 7; R818–823 (17 μM, 6.9 μg), 27 ± 4; R822–827 (70.6 μM, 30 μg), 30 ± 2.

Red blood cells were separated into populations of different ages on Percoll gradients as previously described.[3] Middle-aged cells were stored at 4°C for 3 weeks in Alsever's solution. Storage mimics normal aging *in situ* immunologically and biochemically.[1-8,11,39] Senescent cell IgG was isolated from senescent erythrocytes as described[2,4] and 0.71 μg incubated with peptides or buffer in 0.5 ml for 90 min at room temperature. Intact erythrocytes[2,4] were added to the IgG, and samples were incubated for 90 min at room temperature. Cells were washed and the amount of IgG on cells was quantitated using ^{125}I-labeled Protein A.[7] Percent inhibition was calculated from the formula: $100 - [1 - (x - b/T - b)]$ where x = molecules of senescent cell IgG autoantibody bound in the absence of inhibitor and b = background protein A binding. T is the total number of molecules of IgG autoantibody bound in the absence of inhibitor.

Peptides were prepared by solid phase synthesis using an Applied Biosystems 430A automatic peptide synthesizer. Purity of peptides as determined by amino acid composition was as follows: pep-CYTO: 98%; pep-ANION 1, 97%; pep-ANION 2, 95%; pep-COOH, 97%. The peptide sequence was as follows: pep-ANION 1, position 538–554; SER-LYS-LEU-ILE-LYS-ILE-PHE-GLN-ASP-HIS-PRO-LEU-GLN-LYS-THR-TYR-ASN; pep-ANION 2, 588–602; LEU-ARG-LYS-PHE-LYS-ASN-SER-SER-TYR-PHE-PRO-GLY-LYS-LEU-ARG; pep-COOH, 812–827: LEU-PHE-LYS-PRO-PRO-LYS-TYR-HIS-PRO-ASP-VAL-PRO-TYR-VAL-LYS-ARG; pep-CYTO, 139–159: ALA-GLY-VAL-ALA-ASN-GLN-LEU-LEU-ASP-ARG-PHE-ILE-PHE-GLU-ASP-GLN. (From Kay and Lin.[21] Reprinted by permission from *Gerontology*.)

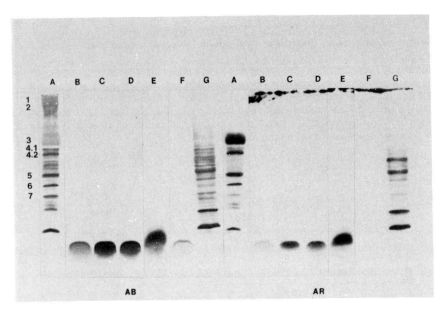

FIGURE 2. Binding of senescent cell IgG to erythrocyte and brain membranes and synthetic peptides in immunoblots. AB, amido black stain for proteins; AR, autoradiograph of senescent cell IgG binding. *Lanes:* A, erythrocyte membrane; B, pep-ANION 1; C, pep-ANION 2; D, pep-COOH; E, pep-COOH hexamer; F, pep-GLYCOS; F, brain membranes prepared from perfused rat brain cerebral cortex.

Synthetic Senescent Cell Antigen

We decided to mix the two inhibitory peptides, pep-ANION 1 and pep-COOH, to determine whether they acted synergistically for two reasons. First, both are inhibitory, but the inhibition is not complete. Second, the results of our earlier peptide mapping studies with topographically defined segments of band 3 suggested that senescent cell antigen was composed of peptides from both the anion transport transmembrane region and the 35,000–38,000 Da carboxyl terminal segment.[5] Mixing of these two regions produced a peptide map that closely resembled senescent cell antigen even though it contained more peptides. Although 3 μg of pep-ANION 1 alone only produced 16% inhibition, and pep-COOH alone produced 22% inhibition, the mixture containing 1.5 μg of each produced 97% inhibition (FIG. 1A). This suggests that the two peptides interact together to form a three-dimensional aging antigen. In other words, both peptides contribute amino acids to the configuration recognized by the antigen binding site on the IgG molecule. A mixture of 30 μg pep-ANION 2 and pep-COOH did not produce synergy (18 ± 4% inhibition).

Synthetic peptides are usually not as effective as the native molecule from which they are derived in physiologic studies because short peptide segments do not assume the same tertiary configuration as that of the whole molecule. The synergism of peptides pep-ANION 1 and pep-COOH suggests that the conformation of the determinants of these two peptides interacting with each other is similar to that of the intact aging antigen and that these two determinants must be spatially close in the native molecule. Therefore, we refer to the synergistic mixture of pep-ANION 1 and pep-COOH as "synthetic senescent cell antigen." These results suggest that these peptides lie in close spatial proximity in the folded, tertiary structure of native band 3 even though they are separated by ~300 amino acids in the primary structure of the 911 amino acid band 3 molecule (FIG. 3). An alternative explanation is that a change in aged band 3 alters its configuration and results in the three-dimensional alignment of these two sites. We suspect that the three-dimensional structure of band 3 is a ring in which the two external loops on which pep-ANION 1 and pep-COOH reside are in close spacial proximity forming senescent cell antigen as cells age.

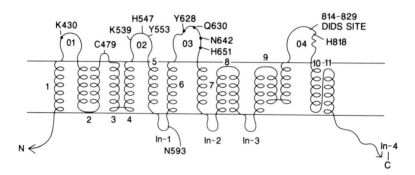

FIGURE 3. Model of membrane associated and external regions of anion transport protein band 3, approximate residues (R) 400–870. K, lysine; C, cysteine; H, histidine; Y, tyrosine; N, asparagine; the *number following a letter* indicates residue number; In, inside the cell; O, outside of the cell; *arrow* C, carboxyl terminus; *arrow* N, amino terminus. The model was constructed using the program PEPPLOT of the GCG package to identify membrane spanning nonpolar helices and intervening hydrophilic loops. The location of the hydrophilic loops as extracellular or intracellular was predicted on the basis of established chemical or biological markers, *e.g.*, the demonstration that residues 814–829 contain a DIDS binding site accessible from the outside[41,42,44] or external radioiodination of the tyrosine (Y) at position 553.[40] Key residues are identified to facilitate their identification within the sequence. This is a two-dimensional representation that does not reflect three-dimensional associations of residues that are separated by long stretches of sequence. Our present results show, however, that close steric association must be maintained by external loops 02 and 04. If these regions are associated on the same band 3 monomer, then band 3 loops back upon itself so that these regions are contiguous. Alternatively, the functional assembly may be dimers in which close associations of 02 and 04 form between separate molecules. (From Kay *et al.*[20] Reprinted by permission from the National Academy of Sciences.)

Active Aging Antigenic Amino Acids

In order to define the aging antigenic site along the band 3 molecule and to determine the active antigenic residues, we tried substituting a neutral or positively charged amino acid for the positively charged lysine in pep-COOH peptide (LFKPPKYHPDVPYVKR) during synthesis. Substitution of either neutral glycines (pep-COOH-G: LFGPPGYHPDVPYVGR) or positively charged arginines (pep-COOH-R: LFRPPRYHPDVPYVRR) for lysine in pep-COOH reduced but did not abolish its activity in the competitive inhibition assay with senescent cell

IgG.[21] This suggests that (a) charge alone is not the critical determinant of antigenicity, and (b) lysines contribute to the antigenicity of the aging antigen. Since we changed all three of the lysines in the synthetic peptide pep-COOH, we cannot determine at this time whether all lysines are critical or whether antigenicity depends on a specific lysine.

We have used synthetic peptides to locate a crucial aging antigen on band 3 and to create a synthetic senescent cell antigen. Results indicate that pep-ANION 1 (residues 538–554) and pep-COOH residues (812–827) may be the aging antigenic sites of the band 3 molecule, and that lysine(s) is required for antigenicity. Generation of senescent cell antigen initiates IgG binding and removal of cells *in situ*. These results are consistent with the physiological data demonstrating that old erythrocytes have impaired anion transport,[6,7,11,39] and the biochemical and immunological data indicating that band 3 undergoes degradation with loss of a cytoplasmic segment during the aging process.[4–8,9,11,39]

Band 3 and Senescent Cell Antigen in Neural Tissue

Since band 3 is such a crucial structural and functional protein and is intimately involved in cellular aging, we investigated its location, structure, and function in mammalian brain. We then determined whether senescent cell antigen, a terminal differentiation antigen, is generated in brain. The presence of band 3 related molecules in nonerythroid tissues was first demonstrated in 1983.[30]

Detection of Polypeptides Immunologically Related to Erythroid Band 3 and Senescent Cell Antigen in Immunoblots with Antibodies to Human Erythroid Band 3 and Synthetic Peptides of Band 3

Multiple polypeptides immunologically related to erythrocyte band 3 were detected with both antibodies to the whole human erythrocyte band 3 molecule and antibodies to synthetic peptides synthesized from the sequence data of human erythroid[40] or K562[43] band 3.[43] Thus, these antibodies were binding to a band 3 protein. Staining of these bands was blocked by absorption of antisera with whole human erythroid band 3. Since multiple band 3 polypeptides were observed in membranes from snap-frozen, saline perfused rat brains prepared with potent protease inhibitors, it is unlikely that these bands represented degradation products of band 3. The finding that antibodies to different synthetic peptides from human erythroid and K562 band 3 recognized bands migrating at different molecular weights suggests that there are different forms of band 3 in brain membranes. Because there are many cell types in the brain, we cannot tell whether there is more than one type of band 3 in a cell type or whether different cell types have different band 3 molecules. This requires further study. We suspect that there are multiple forms of band 3 protein that are adapted to various functions in neural and other tissue.

Binding of antibodies to synthetic peptides of erythroid band 3 to brain membranes suggests that the primary structure of these segments that are recognized by the antibodies are similar in brain and erythrocytes. Senescent cell antigen has been mapped to erythroid band 3 residues 538–554 and 788–827.[18,20]

IgG eluted from senescent erythrocytes binds to band 3 in erythrocytes and band 3 related polypeptides in membranes of saline perfused rat brains as determined by immunoblotting. Absorption of senescent cell IgG with brain membranes resulted in inhibition of binding in the IgG binding/inhibition assay (80 ± 2%). For comparison, absorption with purified erythroid senescent cell antigen itself resulted in a 74 ± 6% inhibition of binding. Absorption with pep-CYTO and pep-GLYCOS resulted in 0 and 24 ± 2% inhibition, respectively. This suggests that senescent cell antigen, an aging antigen that terminates the life of cells, is generated on brain band 3.

Immunohistochemical Localization of Band 3-Like Proteins in Brain Using Antibodies to Erythroid Band 3 and Synthetic Peptides of Human Erythroid Band 3

Antibodies to the whole band 3 molecule and to synthetic peptides bound to Purkinje cell soma, axons, glomeruli (areas of synaptic contact) in the internal granule layer (IGL), pia, internal granule layer, neural cells, ependymal cells lining the ventricles, and the choroid plexus as determined by rhodamine and peroxidase staining (FIGS. 4 and 5). Some axonal staining occurred in the medullary layer (MED), but distinct axons were not observed. The presence of band 3 in the choroid plexus was not surprising in view of its role as the "kidney" for the brain. The choroid plexus maintained the chemical stability of the cerebral spinal fluid.

Ankyrin Binding

Erythrocyte band 3 binds to ankyrin which anchors it to spectrin. Therefore, we examined the interaction between brain band 3 and erythrocyte ankyrin. Ankyrin binding studies gave the following results: $N = 16 ± 3$ μg ankyrin/mg protein after removal of cytoskeletal proteins; $K_D = 33 ± 5$ nM. Incubation of ankyrin with whole human erythroid band 3 conjugated to Sepharose 4B prior to incubation with brain membranes abolished ankyrin binding. Addition of the M_r 40,000 cytoplasmic fragment of human erythroid band 3 with ankyrin to brain vesicles abolished binding. Thus, brain band 3 appears to perform the same structural function of stabilizing the plasma membrane and linking it to the internal cytoskeleton as does erythrocyte band 3.

Anion Transport Studies

Anion transport studies were performed on cerebral cortex using both the tube and the chamber techniques.[15,16] The presence of 4,4'-diisothiocyano-2,2' disulfonic acid (DIDS) inhibitable anion transport systems in brain was detected with both methods.

We compared the effect of the anion transport inhibitors DIDS, phenylglyoxal, and furosemide on brain and erythrocyte anion transport (FIG. 6). Sulfate exchange was inhibited in erythrocytes by (DIDS), phenylglyoxal, and furosemide. Stilbenedisulfonate derivatives such as DIDS inhibited anion transport by binding to at least two lysine residues in the membrane-spanning region of band 3.[18,21,42,44] DIDS is a specific, irreversible, inhibitor of anion transport. It binds covalently. Phenylglyoxal modifies an arginine involved in anion transport that is located on the 35,000 carboxyl segment of band 3.[45] The diuretic furosemide inhibits NaCl cotransport by acting at a chloride transport site. The compounds that inhibit anion transport in erythrocytes also inhibit transport in brain. Transport by brain vesicles was reduced to a level ~74% of normal by DIDS, ~65% by furosemide, and ~45% by phenylglyoxal. In contrast, transport in erythocytes was reduced by 100% by DIDS, and ~95% by furosemide. Inhibition by phenylgloxal was the

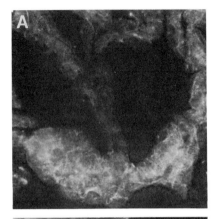

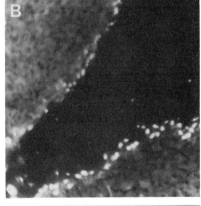

FIGURE 4. Antibodies to human erythroid band 3 synthetic peptide pep-ANION 1 (residues 538–554 SKLIKIFQDHPLQKTYN) included in senescent cell antigen react with frozen sections of mouse brain as detected with rhodamine staining. Mouse cerebellum: **(A)** choroid plexus of the fourth ventricle stained; **(B)** ependyma of the fourth ventricle; **(C)** control consisting of antisera absorbed with pep-ANION 1.

same for brain and erythrocytes. Since brain anion transport was significantly inhibited but not abolished by DIDS, the data suggest the presence in brain of more than one anion transport system (*i.e.,* a transport system[s] that is DIDS inhibitable and another (or others) that is not) and/or ~20% of the sulfate influx is

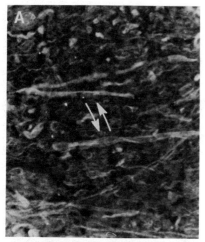

FIGURE 5. Mouse frozen brain sections stained with antibodies to human erythroid band 3 synthetic peptide pep-ANION 1 (residues 538–554 SKLIKIFQDHPLQKTYN) included in senescent cell antigen. **(A)** Axons; **(B)** control consisting of antisera absorbed with the peptide.

due to leakage. There may be many transporters in each cell type present in the brain or there may be different transporters in different cell types. We suspect that the former is the case. However, the next obvious step is to examine pure cell types from brain tissue.

Peptide Inhibition of Anion Transport

Peptides from putative human erythroid transport region were used to inhibit sulfate transport into erythrocytes and brain vesicles (FIG. 7). Peptides used were pep-ANION 1, pep-ANION 2, pep-COOH, and pep-COOH-N6. pep-COOH-6 is on the amino end of pep-COOH and contributes a significant amount of the antigenicity of senescent cell antigen.[20] In previous experiments, we showed that pep-ANION 1, a putative transport region, does not inhibit anion transport in erythrocytes.[26,57] Thus, it serves as a negative control for these experiments. Results of these experiments showed that the same peptides that inhibited anion transport in erythrocytes inhibit transport in brain. This suggests that the transport site(s) in erythroid and neural tissue is similar.

The results of these studies indicate that one or more band 3 proteins are present in mammalian brain that perform the same functions as that of erythroid band 3. These functions are anion transport, ankyrin binding, and generation of senescent cell antigen, an aging antigen that terminates the life of cells. Proteins with which and 3 interacts in erythrocytes to provide structural stability to the membrane are present in neural tissue (see REF. 18). The anion transport segments of erythoid and brain band 3 must be similar since synthetic peptides from transport regions of erythroid band 3 inhibit anion transport by brain vesicles as well as erythrocytes. In addition the inhibitors of anion transport in erythrocytes (DIDS, phenylgloxal, and furosemide) also inhibit anion transport by brain membranes. Since senescent cell antigen is derived from band 3 and (a) IgG specific for this antigen binds to brain membranes in immunoblots and a senescent cell IgG binding-inhibition assay, and (b) antibodies to the segments of band 3 on which senescent cell antigen resides react with brain in immunoblots and tissue sections, the data suggest that senescent cell antigen may be involved in the removal of neurons in aging and disease. This supports the hypothesis that the immunological mechanism of maintaining homeostasis is a general physiologic process for removing senescent and damaged cells in mammals and other vertebrates.[4]

Band 3 in Neurological Aging and Disease

That band 3 may play a role in neurological health and disease is suggested by several lines of indirect evidence. First, preliminary studies indicate that antibodies to aged band 3 labeled the core of classical plaques and microglial cells located in the middle of the plaque. Second, an autosomal recessive neurologic disorder (choreoacanthocytosis) that has both red cell and neurologic abnormalities,[17,19] has band 3 defects.

Because senescent cell antigen is derived from band 3 and defects in band 3 are associated with neurological disease,[16] we performed pilot studies to determine whether senescent cell antigen might play a role in band aging and disease. Exam-

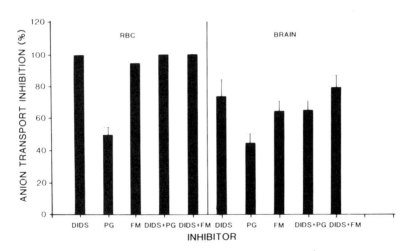

FIGURE 6. Anion transport inhibition of erythrocyte or brain anion transport by the anion transport inhibitors 4,4'-diisothiocyano-2,2' disulfonic acid (DIDS), phenylglyoxal (PG), furosemide (FM), DIDS + PG, OR DIDS + FM. Results are plotted as the mean ± standard deviation. (From Kay et al.[15] Reprinted by permission from the National Academy of Sciences.)

ination of frozen brain sections from 10-year-old and 96-year-old individuals revealed labeling of fibrillary structures and processes with senescent cell antigen-band 3 antibodies in sections from old but not young brains.[34]

Preliminary studies performed with Dr. Robert Terry, University of California, San Diego, show selective binding of band 3 antibodies to human cerebellum and cerebral cortex. Controls which consisted of preimmune serum incubated with brain tissue, liver and myocardium are negative. In normal brains from elderly individuals, band 3 antibodies react with cortex neurons in layers III and IV, Purkinje cells and their dendrites extending into the molecular layer, and cerebellar dentate nucleus neurons. Aged band 3 (presenescent cell antigen) antibodies 980 reacted with astrocytes in the white matter, a "mossy fiber" distribution in the cerebellum, and select Purkinje cells. Dentate neurons are strongly reactive, especially those containing lipofuscin, but the staining did not resemble that of lipofuscin. There was a moderately strong reaction with many, but not all, large neurons in the cerebrum. Aged band 3 antibodies 980 recognize old band 3 before senescent cell antigen is formed.

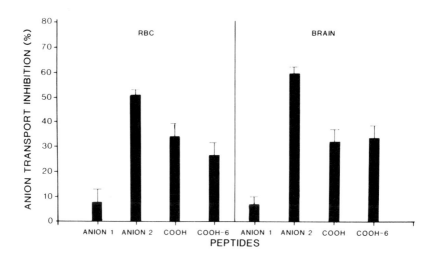

FIGURE 7. Inhibition of erythrocyte or brain anion transport by synthetic peptides of human erythroid band 3. Peptides and sulfate were used in equimolar amounts. Peptides used were ANION 1 (residues 538–554: SKLIKIFQDHPLQKTYN), ANION 2 (residues 588–602: LRKFKNSSYFPGKLR), COOH (residues 812–827: LFKPPKYHPDVPYVKR), and COOH-6 (residues 813–818: FKPPKY). (From Kay et al.[15] Reprinted by permission from the National Academy of Sciences.)

In brains from Alzheimer's disease patients, aged band 3 antibodies labeled the amyloid core of classical plaques and the microglial cells located in the middle of the plaque. Adjacent neurons displayed a stronger and more widespread reaction than normals. In contrast, band 3 antibodies labeled the neuritic components of plaques with some reaction noted in microglial cells, adjacent astrocytes, and neurons. While these results are preliminary, they suggest that band 3 may be altered in Alzheimer's disease. Bosman and colleagues found that red cell band 3 undergoes accelerated aging in Alzheimer's disease.[36] Thus, band 3 appears to be involved in brain aging and disease.

By determining primary structure(s) and amino acids recognized by physiologic autoantibodies involved in the removal of aged cells, we have prepared the foundation for manipulation of these aging sites. Synthetic senescent cell antigen blocks the biological activity of physiologic autoantibodies that initiate removal of senescent cells *in vitro*. We postulate that it can be used to manipulate the life span of cells *in vivo*. Alteration of the antigen itself on living cells could block their removal *in situ*.

SUMMARY

Senescent cell antigen appears on old cells and marks them for death by initiating the binding of IgG autoantibody and subsequent removal by phagocytes in mammals and other vertebrates. We have created a synthetic aging antigen that blocks binding of IgG to senescent cells *in vitro*. Synthetic senescent cell antigen might be effective in preventing cellular destruction *in vivo* in certain diseases, and can be used to manipulate cellular life span *in situ*.

Senescent cell antigen is generated by the modification of an important structural and transport membrane molecule, protein band 3. Band 3 is present in cellular, nuclear, Golgi, and mitochondrial membranes as well as in cell membranes. Band 3 proteins in nucleated cells participate in cell surface patching and capping. Band 3 maintains acid-base balance by mediating the exchange of anions (*e.g.*, chloride, bicarbonate), and is the binding site for glycolytic enzymes. It is responsible for CO_2 exchange in all tissues and organs. Thus, it is the most heavily used anion transport system in the body. Band 3 is a major transmembrane structural protein which attaches the plasma membrane to the internal cell cytoskeleton by binding to band 2.1 (ankyrin). Oxidation generates senescent cell antigen *in situ*.

Band 3 is present in the central nervous system, and differences have been described in band 3 between young and aging brain tissue. One autosomal recessive neurological disease, choreoacanthocytosis, is associated with band 3 abnormalities. The 150 residues of the carboxyl terminus segment of band 3 appear to be altered. In brains from Alzheimer's disease patients, antibodies to aged band 3 label the amyloid core of classical plaques and the microglial cells located in the middle of the plaque in tissue sections, and an abnormal band 3 in immunoblots.

Band 3 protein(s) in mammalian brain performs the same functions as that of erythroid band 3. These functions is anion transport, ankyrin binding, and generation of senescent cell antigen, an aging antigen that terminates the life of cells. Structural similarity of brain and erythroid band 3 is suggested by the reaction of antibodies to synthetic peptides of erythroid band 3 with brain band 3, the inhibition of anion transport by the same inhibitors, and an equal degree of inhibition of brain and erythrocyte anion transport by synthetic peptides of erythroid band 3. One of these segments, pep-COOH, contains antigenic determinants of senescent cell antigen. These findings suggest that the transport domain of erythroid and neural band 3 is similar functionally and structurally, and support the hypothesis that the immunological mechanism of maintaining homeostasis is a general physiologic process for removing senescent and damaged cells in mammals and other vertebrates.

ACKNOWLEDGMENTS

We are grateful to Bobby Poff and Gordon Purser for assistance with the figures.

REFERENCES

1. KAY, M. M. B. 1975. Mechanism of removal of senescent cells by human macrophages *in situ*. Proc. Natl. Acad. Sci. USA **72**: 3521–3525.
2. KAY, M. M. B. 1978. Role of physiologic autoantibody in the removal of senescent human red cells. J. Supramol. Struct. **9**: 555–567.
3. BENNETT, G. D. & M. M. B. KAY. 1981. Homeostatic removal of senescent murine erythrocytes by splenic macrophages. Exp. Hematol. **9**: 297–307.
4. KAY, M. M. B. 1981. Isolation of the phagocytosis inducing IgG-binding antigen on senescent somatic cells. Nature (London) **289**: 491–494.
5. KAY, M. M. B. 1984. Localization of senescent cell antigen on band 3. Proc. Natl. Acad. Sci. **81**: 5753–5757.
6. KAY, M. M. B., G. J. C. G. M. BOSMAN, S. S. SHAPIRO, A. BENDICH & P. S. BASSEL. 1986. Oxidation as a possible mechanism of cellular aging: vitamin E deficiency causes premature aging and IgG binding to erythrocytes. Proc. Natl. Acad. Sci. USA **83**: 2463–2467.
7. KAY, M. M. B., N. FLOWERS, J. GOODMAN & G. J. C. G. M. BOSMAN. 1989. Alteration in membrane protein band 3 associated with accelerated erythrocyte aging. Proc. Natl. Acad. Sci. USA **86**: 5834–5838.
8. KAY, M. M. B., K. SORENSEN, P. WONG & P. BOLTON. 1982. Antigenicity, storage & aging: physiologic autoantibodies to cell membrane and serum proteins and the senescent cell antigen. Mol. Cell. Biochem. **49**: 65–85.
9. KAY, M. M. B. 1983. Appearance of a terminal differentiation antigen on senescent and damaged cells and its implications for physiologic autoantibodies. Biomembranes **11**:119–150.
10. KAY, M. M. B., S. GOODMAN, K. SORENSEN, C. WHITFIELD, P. WONG, L. ZAKI & V. RUDOLOFF. 1983. The senescent cell antigen is immunologically related to band 3. Proc. Natl. Acad. Sci. **80**: 1631–1635.
11. KAY, M. M. B. 1986. Senescent cell antigen: a red cell aging antigen. *In* Red Cell Antigens and Antibodies. G. Garratty, Ed. 35–82. American Association of Blood Banks. Arlington, VA.
12. KAY, M. M. B., G. J. C. G. M. BOSMAN, G. JOHNSON & A. BETH. 1988. Band 3 polymers and aggregates, and hemoglobin precipitates in red cell aging. Blood Cells **14**: 275–289.
13. KAY, M. M. B. 1988. Immunologic techniques for analyzing red cell membrane proteins. *In* Methods in Hematology: Red Cell Membranes. S. Shohet & N. Mohandas, Eds. 135–170. Churchill Livingston, Inc. New York.
14. KAY, M. M. B., G. J. C. G. M. BOSMAN & C. LAWRENCE. 1988. Functional topography of band 3: a specific structural alteration linked to functional aberrations in human erythrocytes. Proc. Natl. Acad. Sci. USA **85**: 492–496.
15. KAY, M. M. B., J. HUGHES, I. ZAGON & F. LIN. 1990. Brain membrane protein band 3 performs the same functions as erythrocyte band 3. Proc. Natl. Acad. Sci. USA. In press.
16. KAY, M. M. B., J. EARLE-HUGHES & I. ZAGON. 1990. Aging of cell membrane molecules: Band 3 and senescent cell antigen in neural tissue. Proc. Heidelberg Acad. Sci. In press.
17. KAY, M. M. B., J. GOODMAN, S. GOODMAN & C. LAWRENCE. 1990. Membrane protein band 3 alteration associated with neurologic disease and tissue reactive antibodies. Clin. Exp. Immunogenet. In press.
18. KAY, M. M. B., F. LIN, G. BOSMAN, J. J. MARCHALONIS & S. F. SCHLUTER. 1990. Human erythrocyte aging: cellular and molecular biology. Trans. Med. Revs. In press.

19. KAY, M. M. B., J. GOODMAN, C. LAWRENCE & G. BOSMAN. 1990. Membrane channel protein abnormalities and autoantibodies in neurological disease. Brain Res. Bull. **24:** 105–111.

20. KAY, M. M. B., J. J. MARCHALONIS, J. HUGHES, K. WATANABE & S. F. SCHLUTER. 1990. Definition of a physiologic aging autoantigen using synthetic peptides of membrane protein band 3: localization of the active antigenic sites. Proc. Natl. Acad. Sci. USA. In press.

21. KAY, M. M. B. & F. LIN. 1990. Molecular mapping of the active site of an aging antigen: senescent cell antigen requires lysines for antigenicity and is located on an anion binding segment of band 3 membrane transport protein. Gerontology. In press.

22. SINGER, J. A., L. K. JENNINGS, C. JACKSON, M. E. DOCTKER, M. MORRISON & W. S. WALKER. 1986. Erythrocyte homeostasis: antibody-mediated recognition of the senescent state by macrophages. Proc. Natl. Acad. Sci. USA **83:** 5498–5501.

23. GLASS, G. A., H. GERSHON & D. GERSHON. 1983. The effect of donor and cell age on several characteristics of rat erythrocytes. Exp. Hematol. **11:** 987–995.

24. GLASS, G. A., D. GERSHON & H. GERSHON. 1985. Some characteristics of the human erythrocyte as a function of donor and cell age. Exp. Hematol. **13:** 1122–1126.

25. BARTOSZ, G., M. SOSYNSKI & A. WASILEWSKI. 1982. Aging of the erythrocyte XVII. Binding of autologous immunoglobin. Mech. Ageing Dev. **20:** 223–232.

26. BARTOSZ, G., M. SOSYNSKI & J. KREDZIONA. 1982. Aging of the erythrocyte. VI. Accelerated red cell membrane aging in Down's syndrome. Cell Biol. Int. Rep. **6:** 73–77.

27. KHANSARI, N., G. F. SPRINGER, E. MERLER & H. H. FUDENBERG. 1983. Mechanisms for the removal of senescent human erythrocytes from circulation: specificity of the membrane-bound immunoglobulin G. J. Mech. Aging Dev. **21:** 49–58.

28. KHANSARI, N. & H. H. FUDENBERG. 1983. Immune elimination of autologous senescent erythrocytes by Kupffer cells *in vivo*. Cell. Immunol. **80:** 426–430.

29. WALKER, W. S., J. A. SINGER, M. MORRISON & C. W. JACKSON. 1984. Preferential phagocytosis of *in vivo* aged murine red blood cells by a macrophage-like cell line. Br. J. Haematol. **58:** 259–266.

30. KAY, M. M. B., C. M. TRACEY, J. R. GOODMAN, J. C. CONE & P. S. BASSEL. 1983. Polypeptides immunologically related to erythrocyte band 3 are present in nucleated somatic cells. Proc. Natl. Acad. Sci. USA **80:** 6882–6886.

31. KELLOKUMPU, S., L. NEFF, S. JAMSA-KELLOKUMPU, R. KOPITO & R. BARON. 1988. A 115-kD polypeptide immunologically related to erythrocyte band 3 is present in Golgi membranes. Science **242:** 1308–1311.

32. SCHUSTER, V. L., S. M. BONSIB & M. L. JENNINGS. 1986. Two types of collecting duct mitochondria-rich (intercalated) cells: lectin and band 3 cytochemistry. Am. J. Physiol. **251:** C347–C355.

33. KUDRYCKI, K. E. & G. E. SHULL. 1989. Primary structure of the rat kidney band 3 anion exchange protein deduced from a cDNA. J. Biol. Chem. **264:** 8185–8192.

34. KAY, M. M. B., G. BOSMAN, M. NOTTER & P. COLEMAN. 1988. Life and death of neurons: the role of senescent cell antigen. Ann. N.Y. Acad. Sci. **521:** 155–169.

35. ELGAVISH, A., J. B. SMITH, D. J. PILLION & E. MEEZAN. 1985. Sulfate transport in human lung fibroblasts (IMR-90). J. Cell. Physiol. **125:** 243–250.

36. BOSMAN, G., I. BARTHOLOMEUS & W. DEGRIP. 1990. Alzheimer's disease and cellular aging: membrane-related events as clues to primary mechanisms. Gerontology. In press.

37. KAY, M. M. B. & G. J. C. G. M. BOSMAN. 1985. Naturally occurring human "antiga-lactosyl" IgG antibodies are heterophile antibodies recognizing blood group related substances. Exp. Hematol. **13:** 1103–1112.

38. KAY, M. M. B. 1985. Aging of cell membrane molecules leads to appearance an aging antigen and removal of senescent cells. Gerontology **31:** 215–235.

39. BOSMAN, G. J. C. G. M. & M. M. B. KAY. 1988. Erythrocyte aging: a comparison of model systems for simulating cellular aging *in vitro*. Blood Cells **14:** 19–35.

40. TANNER, M. J. A., P. G. MARTIN & S. HIGH. 1988. The complete amino acid sequence of the human erythrocyte membrane anion-transport protein deduced from the cDNA sequence. Biochem. J. **256:** 703–712.

41. KAY, M. M. B. 1990. Molecular mapping of human band 3 anion transport regions and stilbene disuphonate binding site using synthetic peptides. Proc. Natl. Acad. Sci. USA. Submitted.
42. JENNINGS, M. L., M. P. ANDERSON & R. MONAGHAN. 1986. Monoclonal antibodies against human erythrocyte band 3 protein. Localization of proteolytic cleavage sites and stilbenedisulfonate-binding lysine residues. J. Biol. Chem. **261:** 9002–9010.
43. DEMUTH, D. R., L. C. SHOWE, M. BALLANTINE, A. PALUMBO, P. J. FRASER, L. CIOE, G. ROVERA & P. J. CURTIS. 1986. Cloning and structural characterization of a human non-erythroid band 3-like protein. EMBO J. **5:** 1205–1214.
44. JENNINGS, M. L. 1989. Structure and function of the red blood cell anion transport protein. Annu. Rev. Biophys. Biophys. Chem. **18:** 397–430.
45. BJERRUM, P. J., J. O. WIETH & S. MINAKAMI. 1983. Selective phenylglyoxalation of functionally essential arginyl residues in the erythrocyte anion transport protein. J. Gen. Physiol. **81:** 453–484.

Platelet Autoantibodies in Dementia and Schizophrenia

Possible Implication for Mental Disorders[a]

MEIR SHINITZKY,[b,c] MICHAEL DECKMANN,[c]
ABRAHAM KESSLER,[c] PINCHAS SIROTA,[d]
ABRAHAM RABBS,[d] AND AVNER ELIZUR[d]

[c]Department of Membrane Research
The Weizmann Institute of Science
76100 Rehovot, Israel

and

[d]Abarbanel Mental Hospital
Bat Yam, Israel

Several studies have demonstrated significant changes in lymphocyte subpopulation distribution and activity in blood of schizophrenic[1,2] and demented[3–5] patients. It has also been reported that platelets from schizophrenic patients exhibit some abnormal activities.[6,7] In view of the apparent resemblance between neurological tissues and platelets[8,9] and their apparent involvement in leukocyte activities,[10] we have investigated in this study the possibility that in mental disorders platelet antigens may serve as triggering sites for autoimmune reaction that eventually propagates into the central nervous system.

SUBJECTS AND METHODS

All tests and analytical procedures were carried out simultaneously with blood samples of patients and normal donors drawn on the same day (see below). Most subjects were tested more than once during this 6-month study.

Patients

The participating patients were either hospitalized in the Abarbanel Mental Hospital or were outpatients who were closely inspected and supervised. In line with the aim of this study, patients were only grossly categorized into 4 major groups: schizophrenia, affective disorders (bipolar, depression and personality disorder), dementia (mild Alzheimer, severe Alzheimer and multi infarct) and dementia treated with neuroleptics. Schizophrenic and affective disordered patients were diagnosed and rated according to the DSM-III criteria of the American

[a] This work was supported in part by a grant from the Belle S. and Irving E. Meller Center for the Biology of Aging, the Weizmann Institute of Science.
[b] To whom correspondence should be addressed.

Psychiatric Association 1987 and further verified by the BPRS test.[11] All schizo-phrenic patients reported here were either newly diagnosed or free from neurolep-tic treatment for at least one month.

Demented patients were classified by a series of conventional psychometric tests.[12-14] They were divided into 2 separate groups—untreated and treated with neuroleptics.

A detailed outline of the groups participating in this study is given in TABLE 1.

Normals

Young healthy volunteers, most of them belonging to the hospital staff, consti-tuted the young control group. Subjects of the old-age control group were patients from a local hospital who suffered from nonorganic problems and were all men-tally sound and clear.

TABLE 1. Category of Subjects Participating in This Study

Group	Number of Subjects	Age Range (Years)	Average Age ± S.D. (Years)
I. Schizophrenia (untreated)	23	20–62	34 ± 11.6
II. Affective disorders			
Bipolar	13	25–40	31 ± 4.0
Depression	10	22–66	38 ± 10.0
Personality disorder	7	28–39	32 ± 4.2
III. Dementia (untreated)			
Mild Alzheimer	22	60–83	71 ± 6.3
Severe Alzheimer	17	62–85	80 ± 7.4
Multi infarct	9	55–84	74 ± 8.1
IV. Dementia (treated with neuroleptics)	27	51–79	65 ± 6.2
V. Normal (control subjects)			
Young	12	27–44	34 ± 6.0
Old	28	61–87	76 ± 8.2

Platelets

Venous blood (10 ml) was drawn with heparin as anticoagulant in the morning. Within 2 hours after drawing, platelet-rich plasma (PRP) was separated by centrif-ugation (100 g, 15 min, 22°C) and the number of platelets per ml PRP was scored microscopically.

Platelet Associated Antibodies (PAA)

The presence of antibodies on platelets was determined by an enzyme linked immunoassay based on color development after reaction with anti-human im-munoglobulin bund to horseradish peroxidase.[15] Aliquots of 0.3 ml PRP were mixed with 1 ml phosphate buffered saline (PBS) and platelets were spun down by centrifugation in an Eppendorf centrifuge (1 min, 4°C). After an additional washing with 1 ml PBS, platelets were resuspended in 0.15 ml PBS containing a mixture of anti-human antibodies against IgA, IgE, IgG, and IgM linked to horse-radish peroxidase (Bio-Yeda, Cat. No. 3634-1) at a final dilution of 1 : 1000 and incubated for 30 min at 36°C. The same batch of anti-human antibodies was used throughout this study. After 4 washings with 1 ml PBS at 4°C, platelets were incubated with 1 ml freshly prepared color reagent (99 ml PBS + 10 mg ortho-phenylenediamine in 1 ml methanol + 0.015 ml 30% H_2O_2) for 1 h at 36°C. The enzymic reaction was stopped by adding 0.1 ml 6N sulfuric acid and optical density (O.D.) was measured spectrophotometrically at 480 nm in a 1 cm cuvette. After background subtraction (approx. 0.3 O.D.), the O.D. was normalized for 10^8 platelets in 1 ml. This procedure gave reproducible results with standard deviation better than 5% and was, therefore, routinely applied throughout this study.

Isolation of Antigens

Antibodies were removed from pelleted platelets by lowering the pH (0.1 M glycine-HCl buffer, pH 3.0) and then purified by protein A-affinity chromatography[16] on protein A-agarose column (Sigma). The isolated antibodies were coupled to N-hydroxysuccinimide-agarose column (Sigma) as described.[17] Coupled IgG amounted to 3–4 mg IgG/ml agarose. Human platelets or P_2m-membranes[18] from rat frontal cortex, striatum or cerebellum were solubilized with 1% Triton X-100 in PBS and ultracentrifuged (100000 g, 1 h, 4°C). Supernatants (about 5 mg protein in 5 ml) were then applied to the affinity IgG-agarose column. After washing with 1% Triton X-100/PBS bound antigens were eluted with 0.1% Triton X-100 in glycine-HCl buffer, pH 3.0, radioiodinated with ^{125}I by the chloramine T method,[19] separated from free ^{125}I by exclusion chromatography (Sephadex G25 medium; Pharmacia) and visualized by autoradiography after SDS-polyacryl-amide gradient (7.5–15%) gel electrophoresis.

Data Analysis

Curve fitting, statistical evaluation and graphics were carried out with a Mac-intosh II computer (Apple, Inc.).

RESULTS

Platelet count and level of platelet associated antibodies (PAA) were deter-mined in triplicate within 4 hours after blood drawing. The results obtained for the level of PAA in the various groups (TABLE 1) are summarized in FIGURE 1. As shown, the mean levels of PAA on platelets from schizophrenic and demented patients (0.86 and 1.02 O.D. units, respectively) are significantly higher ($p < 0.01$) than those obtained for the age-matched control groups (0.37 and 0.65 O.D. units, respectively). In the demented patients some variations between the subgroups was noticed (FIG. 1) but were assumed to be insignificant due to small sample numbers. The difference in PAA levels of normals and patients with affective disorders (mean value of 0.29 O.D. units) was of lower significance ($p < 0.05$). For the cases of schizophrenia and dementia PAA values corresponding to O.D. = 1.1 and O.D. = 1.3, respectively, could be assigned as cut-off values for the normal range.

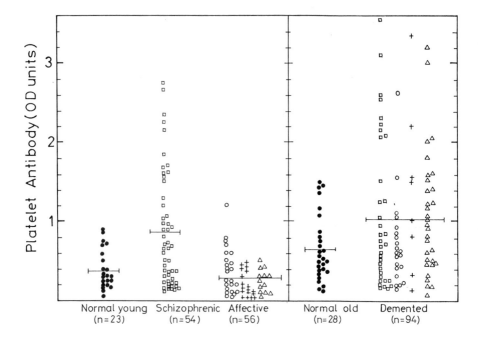

FIGURE 1. Level of platelet associated antibodies (PAA) expressed in O.D. units of radioimmunoassay with 10^8 platelets. Groups from left to right (n = number of samples): Normal young, n = 23; Schizophrenia, n = 54; Affective disorders, n = 56 (O = bipolar, + = depression, △ = personality disorder); Normal old, n = 28; Demented, n = 94 (□ = mild Alzheimer, O = severe Alzheimer, + = multi infarct, △ = Demented treated with neuroleptics). The *horizontal bars* represent the mean values.

FIGURES 2–4 present the results obtained for schizophrenia and the various groups of dementia as platelet number versus level of PAA. In the normal group no significant correlation between platelet number and PAA could be resolved in either the young or the old group, separately, or in combination (not shown). In the group of schizophrenic patients (FIG. 2) a significant inverse correlation ($R^2 = 0.741$; $R = 0.87$) between platelet number and PAA was observed. The results obtained for PRP samples from untreated mild and severe Alzheimer patients and untreated multi infarct demented patients are shown in FIGURE 3. An inverse correlation between platelet number and PAA level of moderate significance ($R^2 = 0.529$; $R = 0.73$) was observed in the combined presentation. An inverse correlation, similar to that displayed in FIGURE 3, was also observed in PRP samples from Alzheimer and demented patients who were under treatment with neuroleptics (FIG. 4).

In our study, most of the subjects were tested more than once over a period of 6 months. Twelve of the schizophrenic patients and 9 of the severe Alzheimer patients were tested 3 times. The results for these patients are presented on an individual basis in FIGURES 5 and 6. As shown, the trend of an inverse correlation between platelet number and PAA is also displayed for most patients. The combined presentation of the individual results is similar to that presented in FIGURES 2 and 3, respectively. The large variations in platelet number and PAA in one individual comply with the possibility that the level of PAA in these patients changes, or even oscillates, with time and the platelet count is modulated with respect to these changes.

In an attempt to resolve the mechanism underlying the inverse correlation between platelet number and level of PAA described above, the results presented in FIGURES 2–4 were analyzed according to a plausible mechanism outlined in the following. Under normal circumstances the steady-state level of platelets in the blood can be ascribed to an equilibrium between a constant rate of platelet (P) production, $dp/dt = k_1$, and a first order rate of platelet clearance, $-dp/dt = k_2P$, which at steady-state yields $P = k_1/k_2$.[20,21] Under ordinary physiological conditions k_2 combines all rate constants of natural routes of platelet clearance. When antibodies are associated with the platelets, they may add an additional route of platelet clearance,[22,23] which may act either independently of platelet concentration (*e.g.,* by association with macrophages via the Fc part of the antibody or by complement fixation) or in association with platelet aggregation caused by random crosslinking of adjacent platelets by PAA. In both mechanisms the idiopathic release of PAA into the blood stream is assumed to oscillate with time as in other cases of autoimmune response.[23] The rate of platelet elimination can be then presented as:

$$-\frac{dp}{dt} = k_2P + k_3A^nP \tag{1}$$

where A is the average level of PAA on a fixed number of platelets and n is the cooperativity factor of PAA in the process of platelet clearance. In a steady-state

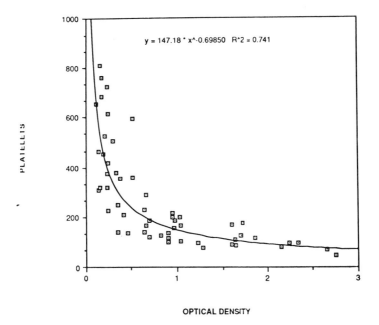

FIGURE 2. Platelet count (per n·liter) versus level of PAA (in units of O.D. per 10^8 platelet/ml) in plasma of schizophrenic patients.

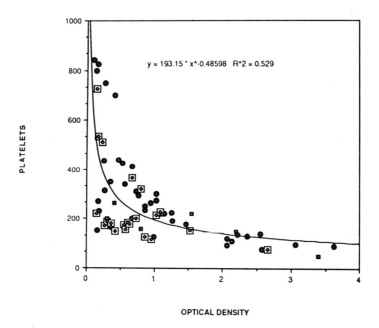

FIGURE 3. Platelet count (per n·liter) versus level of PAA (in units of O.D. per 10^8 platelet/ml) in plasma of untreated patients with dementia (○ = mild Alzheimer; ⊘ = severe Alzheimer; □ = multi infract).

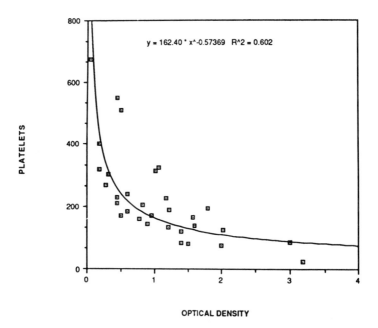

FIGURE 4. Platelet count (per n·liter) versus level of PAA (in units of O.D. per 10^8 platelet/ml) in plasma of dementia patients under treatment with neuroleptics.

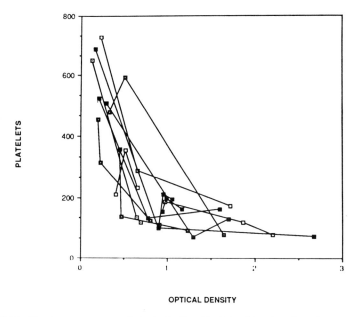

FIGURE 5. Platelet count versus O.D. (as in FIG. 2) of 12 schizophrenic patients. Each line represents the results of 3 consecutive monthly tests, of a specific patient.

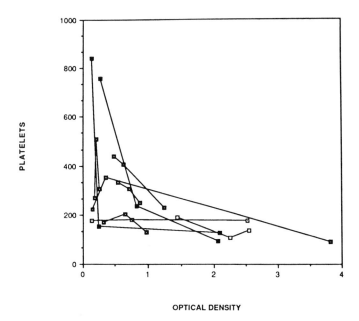

FIGURE 6. Platelet count versus O.D. (as in FIG. 3) of 9 patients with severe Alzheimer dementia. Each line represents the results of 3 consecutive monthly tests, of a specific patient.

under such a mechanism: $k_1 = k_2P + k_3A^nP$ (rate of platelet production is equal to the sum of the rates of platelet clearance). Accordingly

$$\frac{1}{P} = \frac{k_2}{k_1} + \frac{k_3}{k_1} A^n \tag{2}$$

This reciprocal relation may, in principle, agree with the experimental correspondence between P and A which is displayed in FIGURES 2–4. Transformation of the data in these figures according to EQ. 2 revealed best fitting when n = 1. The corresponding replots of the data presented in FIGURES 2–4 are presented in FIGURES 7–9. As shown, for the cases of schizophrenia (FIG. 7), untreated dementia (FIG. 8) and treated dementia (FIG. 9), the linear dependence between 1/P and A is significant and with a correlation factor of around $R = 0.8$. It is interesting to note that in schizophrenia the presumed rate constant of platelet clearance mediated by PAA, k_3, is significantly greater than the basal rate constant of platelet

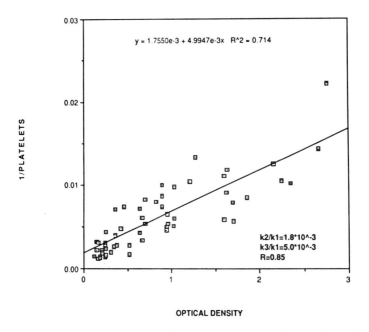

FIGURE 7. Replot of the data presented in FIGURE 2 as the reciprocal of platelet count (1/platelet) versus O.D.

clearance, k_2 ($k_3/k_2 = 2.6$, see FIG. 7). In Alzheimer patients (FIG. 8) and treated demented patients (FIG. 9) the ratio of these rate constants is approximately 1 and 1.6, respectively. This analysis therefore predicts that the average life span of platelets in schizophrenia and dementia, especially in cases of high level of PAA, is significantly shorter than the average normal life span.

Preliminary experiments indicated that the majority of the PAA in the mentally disordered patients belong to the IgG class and that they cross-react with

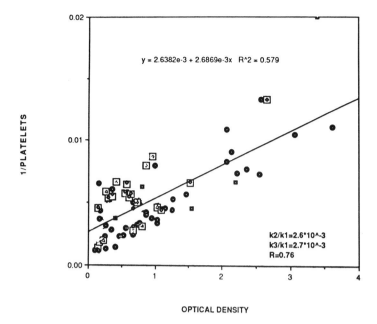

FIGURE 8. Replot of the data presented in FIGURE 3 as the reciprocal of platelet count (1/platelet) versus O.D.

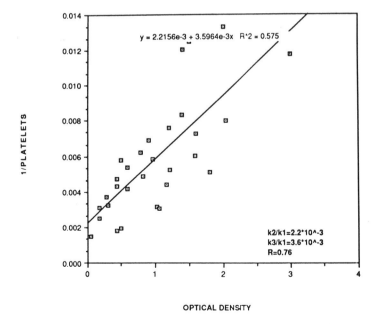

FIGURE 9. Replot of the data presented in FIGURE 4 as the reciprocal of platelet count (1/platelet) versus O.D.

platelets from normal donors irrespective of blood group (see TABLE 2). PAA isolated from platelets of demented patients were also found to cross-react with specific regions of the rat brain, and only insignificantly with other rat tissues (TABLE 2). We have also observed that PAA from schizophrenic patients inhibit dopamine transport and block dopamine binding to P_2m membranes from rat brain (A. Kessler et al., to be published). On the other hand, PAA isolated from normal subjects reacted only weakly with human platelets and did not react with sections of the rat brain. Affinity purification of the antigens from rat brain indicated that antigens with similar molecular weight were recognized by the PAA from Alzheimer dementia. However, different antigenic proteins were found to exist in different brain regions (TABLE 3). Further investigation on the nature of the platelet antigens relevant to mental disorders is currently underway.

DISCUSSION

Circulating platelets from both normal subjects and mentally disordered patients were found to bear platelet associated antibodies (PAA). The level of PAA detected in schizophrenia and the various cases of dementia was considerably higher than that detected in the age-matched normal cases (see FIG. 1). It is reasonable to assume that the PAA detected on platelets from normals are actually heterogeneous plasma immunoglobulins which are associated with the platelet surface either by nonspecific adherence or by binding to the platelet Fc receptor.[25]

The observed inverse correlation between platelet associated antibodies and platelet number in schizophrenic (FIG. 2), and demented subjects (FIGS. 3 and 4) strongly suggests that these antibodies include a distinct population of autoimmune antibodies, reacting against specific platelet antigens. This possibility is supported by the finding that these antibodies cross-react with platelets from normal subjects (TABLE 2), and unlike antibodies isolated from platelets of normals, these antibodies exhibit cross-reactivity with a distinct group of antigens in various regions of the rat central nervous system (TABLE 3). This intriguing cross-reactivity might hint of a basic autoimmune implication for the etiology of mental disorders as was suggested previously.[26,27]

TABLE 2. Cross-Reactivity of Platelet Associated Antibodies from Alzheimer and Multi Infarct Dementia with Other Tissues

Tissue	Cross Reactivity[a]
Platelets (normal human)	+++
Erythrocytes (normal human)	0
Muscle (rat)	+
Heart (rat)	+
Liver (rat)	0
Kidney (rat)	+
Spleen (rat)	+
Cerebellum (rat)	+++
Cortex (rat)	+++
Striatum (rat)	+++

[a] +: weak; ++: mild; +++: strong.

TABLE 3. Antigens Present on Rat Brain Plasma Membranes (P_2m) Recognized by Antibodies Removed from Platelets of Untreated Alzheimer Patients, Drug-Treated Dementia Patients, and Control Subjects[a]

	Alzheimer	Treated Dementia	Control
Cerebellum	29,53(K)	29,53(K)	none
Frontal cortex	53(K)	53(K)	none
Striatum	47,53(K)	47,53(K)	none
Whole brain	21,22,25,29,47,53,68(K)	21,22,25,29,47,53,68(K)	none

[a] Molecular weights are given in Kilo-Dalton and were determined under reducing conditions, *i.e.*, when subunits are dissociated.

Kinetic considerations of the dependence of platelet number on level of PAA in schizophrenia (FIG. 7), Alzheimer dementia (FIG. 8), and drug-treated dementia (FIG. 9) could comply with a mechanism involving complement fixation or ingestion by macrophages after association via the Fc receptor.[22,23] Another plausible mechanism involves cross-linking by PAA leading to platelet microaggregation which is then cleared out by the reticuloendothelial system, liver, or spleen. The latter mechanism raises the intriguing possibility that a burst of release of serotonin and its derivatives, ensuing from such platelet aggregation, may affect directly or indirectly mental dysfunction in schizophrenia or dementia.

Significant reduction in platelet life span in schizophrenia, and to a lesser extent in dementia, is implied from the ratios of the platelet clearance rate mediated by PAA, k_3, and the basal clearance rate, k_2, (FIGS. 7–9). A direct experimental verification of this prediction will lend further support to the possible involvement of PAA and platelet antigens in mental disorders.

SUMMARY

Platelets isolated from blood of demented and schizophrenic patients were found to bear surface antibodies at a considerably higher titer than those found on platelets from normal age-matched groups or patients with affective disorders. The platelet count in demented and schizophrenic patients correlated inversely with the level of the platelet associated antibodies (PAA) which suggested an autoimmune route of opsonization. In most individual cases of dementia or schizophrenia PAA and platelet count were found to oscillate with time between high PAA–low platelet number and low PAA–high platelet number in approximately inverse correlation. PAA isolated from demented patients were found to cross-react with platelets from normals and with brain tissue from rats. Furthermore, molecular weights of specific brain antigens were identified by binding to PAA. These observations support the possibility that PAA might be implicated in the etiology of some mental dysfunctions associated with dementia and schizophrenia.

REFERENCES

1. BALDWIN, J. A. 1979. Schizophrenic and physical disease. Psychol. Med. **9:** 611–618.
2. BESSLER, H., J. EVIATAR, M. MESHULAN, S. TYANO, M. DJALDETTI & P. SIROTA. 1987. Theophylline-sensitive T-lymphocyte subpopulation in schizophrenic patients. Biol. Psychiatr. **22:** 1025–1029.

3. TAVOLATO, B. & V. ARGENTINO. 1980. Immunological indices in presenile Alzheimer disease. J. Neural. Sci. **46:** 325–331.
4. WALFORD, R. L. 1982. Immunological studies of Down's syndrome and Alzheimers disease. Ann. N.Y. Acad. Sci. **396:** 95–106.
5. KHANSARI, N., H. D. WHITTEN, Y. K. CHOU & H. H. FUDENBERG. 1985. Immunological dysfunction in Alzheimer disease. J. Neuroimmunol. **7:** 279–286.
6. BOULLIN, D. J., M. W. ORR & J. R. PETERS. 1978. The platelet as a model for investigating the clinical efficacy of centrally acting drugs in schizophrenics. *In* Platelets: A Multodiciplinary Approach. G. de Gaetano & S. Garatini, Eds. 389–410. Raven Press. New York.
7. ROTMAN, A., A. SHATZ & J. SZEKELY. 1983. Correlation between serotonin uptake and imipramine binding in platelets of schizophrenic patients. Prog. Neuropsychopharmacol. Biol. Psychiatr. **6:** 57–61.
8. PLETSCHER, A. & E. LAUBSCHER. 1980. Use and limitations of platelets as models for neurons. Amine release and shape change reaction. *In:* Platelets: Cellular Response Mechanisms and Their Biological Significance. A. Rotman *et al.,* Eds. 267–276. Wiley Interscience. Chichester, UK.
9. ROTMAN, A. 1983. Blood platelets in psychopharmacological research. Prog. Neuropsychopharmacol. Biol. Psychiatr. **6:** 135–151.
10. MARCUS, A. J., L. B. SALIER, H. L. ULLMAN, T. ISLAMA, M. J. BROEKMAN, J. R. FALCK, S. FISCHER & C. VON SCHACKY. 1988. Platelet-neutrophil interactions. J. Biol. Chem. **263:** 2223–2229.
11. OVERALL, J. E. & D. R. GORMAN. 1962. The brief psychiatric rating scale. Psychol. Rep. **10:** 799–812.
12. WECHSLER, D. 1945. A standardized memory scale for clinical use. J. Psychol. **19:** 87–95.
13. PFEIFFER, E. 1975. A short partable mental status questionnaire for the assessment of organic brain deficit in elderly patients. J. Am. Geriatr. Soc. **23:** 433–441.
14. FOLSTEIN, M. F., S. E. FOLSTEIN & P. R. McHUGH. 1975. "Mini-Mental State": a practical method for grading the cognitive state of patients for the clinician. J. Psychiatr. Res. **12:** 189–198.
15. LEPORRIER, M., G. DIGHIERO, M. AUZEMERY & J. L. BINET. 1979. Detection and quantification of platelet bound antibodies with immunoperoxidase. Br. J. Haematol. **42:** 605–611.
16. TUCKER, D. F., R. H. J. BEGENT & N. M. HOGG. 1978. Characterization of immune complexes in serum by adsorption staphylococcal protein A. J. Immunol. **121:** 1644–1653.
17. WILCHEK, M. & T. MIRON. 1982. Immobilization of enzymes and affinity ligands onto agarose via stable and uncharged carbamate linkages. Biochem. Int. **4:** 629–635.
18. MORGAN, J. G., L. S. WOLFE, P. MANDEL & G. GOMBES. 1971. Isolation of plasma membranes from rat brain. Biochim. Biophys. Acta **241:** 737–751.
19. GREENWOOD, F. C., W. M. HUNTER & J. S. GLOVER. 1963. Radioiodination of proteins with chloramine T. Biochem. J. **89:** 114–123.
20. MURPHY, E. A., G. A. ROBINSON, H. C. ROWSELL & J. F. MUSTARD. 1967. The pattern of platelet disappearance. Blood **30:** 26–29.
21. KOTILAINEN, M. 1969. Platelet kinetics in normal subjects and haematological disorders with special reference to thrombocytopenia and to the role of the spleen. Scand. J. Haematol. (Suppl.) **5:** 9–11.
22. MUELLER-ECKHARDT, C., W. KAYSER & K. MERSCH-BAUMERT. 1980. Clinical significance of platelet-associated IgG: a study on 298 patients with various disorders. Br. J. Haematol. **46:** 123–131.
23. KELTON, J. G. & S. GIBBONS. 1982. Autoimmune platelet destruction: idiopathic thrombocytopenic purpura. Semin. Thromb. Hemostasis **8:** 83–104.
24. CARNEGIE, P. R. & I. R. MacKAY. 1975. Vulnerability of cell surface receptors to autoimmune reactions. Lancet II: 684–687.
25. PFUELLER, S. L., S. WEBER & E. F. LUESCHER. 1977. Studies of the mechanism of the human platelet reaction induced by immunologic stimuli. J. Immunol. **118:** 514–524.

26. ABRAMSKY, O. & Y. LITVIN. 1978. Autoimmune response to dopamine-receptor as a possible mechanism in the pathogenesis of Parkinson disease and schizophrenia. Perspect. Biol. Med. **22:** 104–114.
27. DeLISI, L. E. & T. J. CROW. 1986. Is schizophrenia a viral or immunological disorder? Psychiatr. Clin. North Am. **9:** 115–132.

Calcitonin Gene-Related Peptide in the Developing and Aging Thymus

An Immunocytochemical Study

K. BULLOCH, J. HAUSMAN, T. RADOJCIC,
AND S. SHORT[a]

Departments of Psychiatry and [a]Pediatrics
School of Medicine, 0603
University of California, San Diego
La Jolla, California 92093-0603

INTRODUCTION

The neuropeptide calcitonin gene-related peptide (CGRP) has been identified in both the central and the peripheral nervous system and in peripheral tissues. CGRP-like immunoreactivity (CGRP-IR) is evident in many afferent sensory neurons which supply the ear, eye, nose, taste buds, and skin,[1–3] and in sensory and parasympathetic ganglia.[4] CGRP-IR fibers have also been found in the lymph nodes and thymus of several mammalian species,[5,6] and receptor sites specific for CGRP have been reported in lymph nodes, spleen, and bone marrow.[7–9] The source of thymic CGRP is unclear, but it is well known that the thymus is innervated by the autonomic nervous system and that the nucleus ambiguus and retrofacial nucleus send efferent fibers to the thymus.[10–13] Both CGRP mRNA[14] and CGRP-IR[15,16] have been demonstrated in these brainstem vagal nuclei.

During embryogenesis vagal fibers penetrate the thymic primordium prior to the entry of lymphocytes.[17–19] The thymus also undergoes a characteristic involution with aging. Although CGRP-IR has been found in the thymus, little is known about its developmental distribution or its role in T cell differentiation. However, CGRP is able to indirectly influence T cells *in vitro*. Murine splenic and lymph node lymphocyte proliferation in response to the mitogens Con A and PHA, but not LPS, is inhibited by 10^{-10} M to 10^{-7} M CGRP. It has been suggested that this effect is mediated by cAMP.[20]

In the following study we have mapped the distribution of CGRP within the mouse thymus during different stages of development and aging in order to gain a better understanding of the role of this peptide in thymic function.

METHODS

Animals

Sixty BALB/c (male and female) mice ranging in age from embryonic day 17 to 18 months were used in this study. The adult animals were housed 4 to 5 per cage, had free access to food and water and were kept on a diurnal lighting schedule.

Chemicals

Rabbit anti-CGRP was obtained from Cambridge Research Biochemicals. Antibody specificity was determined by absorption of the activity with 1×10^{-5} M CGRP. Normal rabbit serum was kindly donated by Dr. Steven Baird of the VA Medical Center in La Jolla. ABC rabbit stain kits were purchased from Vector Laboratories.

Immunocytochemical Techniques

Mice were lethally anesthetized with sodium pentobarbital and perfused with dextrose and saline followed by Zamboni's fixative.[21] A 2-hour postfixation of excised thymus tissue was also carried out in Zamboni's fixative. The tissue was cryoprotected in 30% sucrose and sectioned at 24 μ in a cryostat. The slides were passed through three 10-minute rinses in 50 mM PBS followed by 15 minutes in 0.3% H_2O_2. In order to eliminate background binding, all sections were preincubated for 30 minutes at room temperature with normal goat serum (in 50 mM PBS,

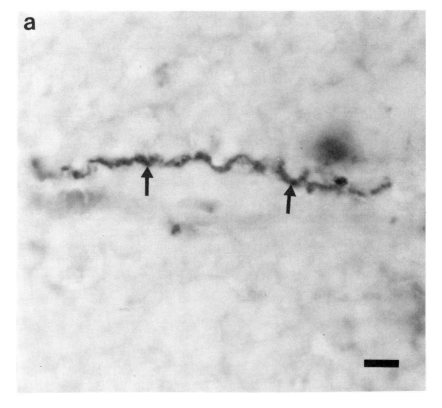

FIGURE 1. Thymus from a seventeen-day-old mouse embryo. (a) Large nerve bundle (*arrows*) running along a blood vessel (marker bar = 15 μ).

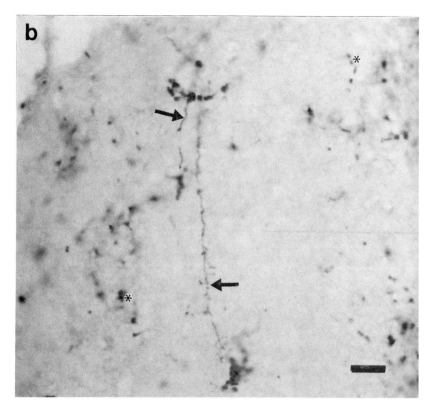

FIGURE 1. (b) A few delicate nerve fibers (*arrows*) extend into the parenchyma of the gland. Scattered, darkly staining small cells (*asterisks*) are also seen near the cortico-medullary junction (marker bar = 100 μ).

0.4% Triton X-100, 1.0% BSA). They were then washed in 50 mM PBS, 0.02% Triton X-100 buffer and transferred to the primary antibody solution for overnight incubation. The following day, the slides were washed ten times in buffer (10 minutes each) and incubated at room temperature for 1 hour in biotinylated goat antirabbit gamma globulins. They were then rinsed four times in buffer, reacted in ABC reagent at room temperature for 1 hour, rinsed again and transferred to DAB solution at pH 7.2 for 7 minutes. Finally, the slides were passed through a wash of buffer and water, dehydrated and mounted in Permount.

RESULTS

In order to determine optimal experimental conditions serial dilutions of the anti-CGRP, ranging from 1 : 100 to 1 : 3200, were tested. A final concentration of 1 : 400 gave excellent staining for CGRP with the lowest background.

In the 17-day-old embryo several large CGRP-IR nerves penetrated the dorsal aspect of the gland. From these nerves, smaller CGRP-IR fibers followed the blood vessels into the body of the thymus. Small intensely stained cells were also observed in the medulla near the cortico-medullary junction (FIG. 1).

The thymus of the postembryonic three-week-old mouse displayed a dense matrix of the small CGRP-IR cells at the cortico-medullary boundary (FIG. 2). Subcapsular and trabecular mast cells, most of which contained CGRP-IR, were also evident. Many nerve fibers located within the three- to eight-week-old thymus also stained positively for CGRP. Major nerve bundles entered at the mid-dorsum of the gland and ran through connective tissue in the capsule and inter-lobular regions; however, other fibers in the nerve bundles were unstained (FIG. 3). Generally, large CGRP-IR nerve trunks could be found coursing near the larger blood vessels. Deeper in the gland, some of the smaller CGRP-IR fibers formed perivascular plexuses, but many fine fibers branched off the trunk, traversed great spans of thymic tissue, and developed varicosities near both types of CGRP-IR cells (FIG. 4).

Similar patterns of CGRP-IR cells and nerves were observed in the six-month-old mouse thymus. The small cortico-medullary cells were still observed within the gland, but by six months there was a slight decrease in their overall number.

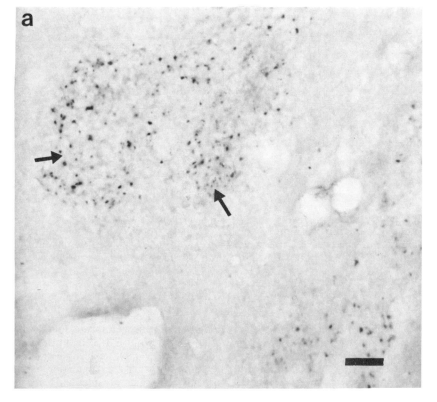

FIGURE 2. Adjacent thymus sections from a three-week-old mouse. (a) Many small CGRP-IR cells (*arrows*) are seen near the cortico-medullary boundary (marker bar = 200 μ).

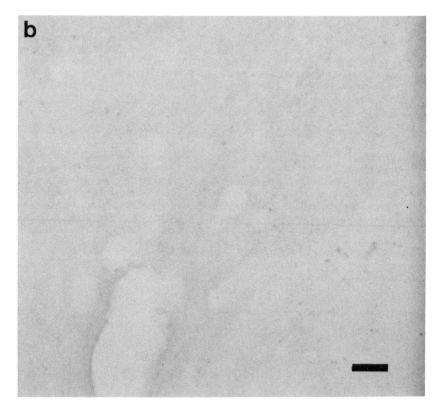

FIGURE 2. (b) Negative control from an adjacent section incubated with buffer (marker bar = 200 μ).

Conversely, beyond six weeks there was a steady increase in the number of mast cells (FIG. 5).

These trends were even more striking in the thymus from the 18-month-old mouse. Mast cells were predominant, and there were very few small CGRP-IR cells. At this age nerves were in very close association with the vasculature with little branching into the parenchyma of the gland (FIG. 6).

DISCUSSION

Evidence that the neuropeptide CGRP and its receptors are found in the immune system led us to investigate the distribution of CGRP-IR in the mouse thymus during different stages of development.[6,15] Our studies demonstrated extensive CGRP-IR within intrathymic nerves. Surprisingly, a population of small cells at the cortico-medullary junction as well as most subcapsular and trabecular mast cells were also immunoreactive for CGRP.

The pattern of nerves and cells demonstrating CGRP-IR changed throughout development and may be important for T cell differentiation. In the 17-day-old mouse embryo, CGRP-IR intrathymic nerves were largely confined to the connective tissue and ran along the vasculature with little branching into the parenchyma. Small CGRP-IR cells, which may be lymphocytes, were scattered near the cortico-medullary junction.

The 3- to 8-week-old mouse thymus contained many CGRP-IR cortico-medullary cells as well as CGRP-IR and negative mast cells. At this stage of development CGRP-IR nerves paralleled the vasculature but the majority of fibers were not invested in the arteries. The nerves branched extensively and formed varicosities among the CGRP positive and negative cells.

As the mouse ages, there was a steady decrease in the number of small CGRP-IR cortico-medullary cells and an increase in the number of mast cells. The general pattern of CGRP-IR nerves remained the same though there appeared to be less branching of the nerves in the 18-month-old mouse.

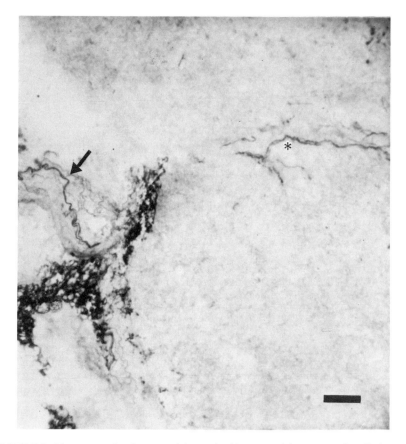

FIGURE 3. Thymus section from an eight-week-old mouse. A large nerve bundle (*arrow*) containing both CGRP-IR and negative fibers penetrates the dorsal aspect of the gland. A major branch (*asterisk*) runs along a blood vessel (marker bar = 200 μ).

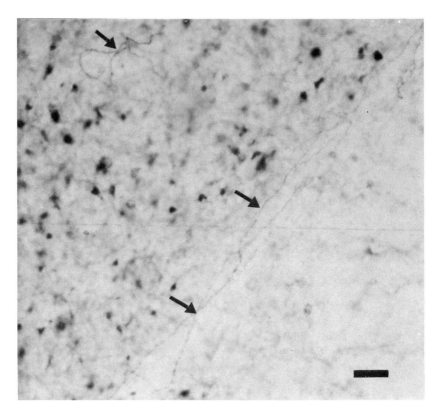

FIGURE 4. Same thymus as in FIGURE 3. Fine fibers containing varicosities (*arrows*) run along the vasculature at the cortico-medullary junction among the small CGRP-IR cells (marker bar = 50 μ).

In mammals, the thymus primordium is first innervated by fibers of the vagus nerve while the gland is still in its cervical location.[18–20] Retrograde transport studies show that the ambiguus and retrofacial nuclei of the brainstem vagal complex project to the thymus.[10–13] Both immunohistochemical staining[15,16] and *in situ* hybridization[14] reveal that these nuclei contain CGRP. Taken collectively these two studies suggest that the CGRP nerves of the thymus are derived from the brain stem vagal nuclei. Furthermore, Al-Shawaf *et al.*[22] have shown that after chemical sympathectomy with 6-hydroxydopamine, nerves containing VIP, CGRP, and AChE are unaffected in the thymus. Further studies combining CGRP immunocytochemistry of the brain stem vagal nucleus with thymic retrograde transport techniques are needed to verify this hypothesis.

Some of the CGRP-IR fibers appeared to terminate near both types of CGRP-IR cells. Primary sensory afferents (C fibers) containing CGRP and substance P are known to have neuroeffector junctions with mast cells. These neuropeptides are present in the nodose ganglion and in the dorsal root ganglia (C1–C7),[4] which are known to contain cell bodies of thymic afferent nerves.[13,23] It has been postulated that mast cells are target cells for these neuropeptides. Both substance P and

CGRP release histamine, which induces a wheal and flare reaction when injected into the skin. CGRP also causes prolonged and delayed vasodilatation,[24–26] which may be mediated through ATP-sensitive potassium channels in arterial smooth muscle.[27]

Although intrathymic nerves containing substance P and CGRP seem to overlap,[6] Geppetti *et al.*[28] have shown that while capsaicin almost completely depletes substance P in the rat thymus it has little effect on the content of CGRP. These authors hypothesized that a significant part of the CGRP in the thymus is extraneuronal and thus insensitive to capsaicin. This hypothesis is supported by our results showing CGRP-IR in the mast and cortico-medullary cells.

SUMMARY

Calcitonin gene-related peptide (CGRP) is known to block Con A and PHA induced T cell proliferation. As a first step in determining the role of this peptide

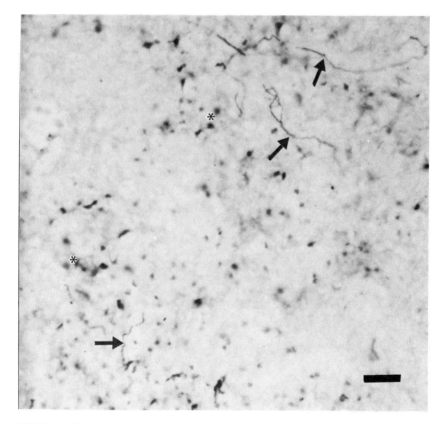

FIGURE 5. Thymus from a six-month-old mouse. There is a slight decrease in the density of the small CGRP-IR cells (*asterisks*). As in FIGURE 4, delicate nerve fibers (*arrows*) can be seen among these cells (marker bar = 100 μ).

in T cell education and function we have studied the distribution of CGRP within the developing mouse thymus using immunocytochemistry. CGRP-like immunoreactivity (CGRP-IR) was found in thymic nerves in close proximity to blood vessels in the 17-day-old embryonic mouse thymus. A discrete population of small

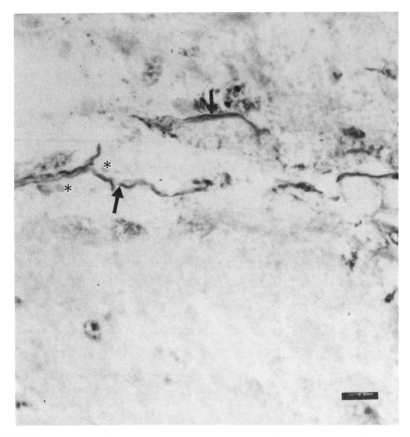

FIGURE 6. Section of thymus from an eighteen-month-old mouse showing dense nerve bundles (*arrows*) along the vasculature, many mast cells (*asterisks*) in the abundant connective tissue, and a paucity of small CGRP-IR cells in the parenchyma (marker = 50 μ).

cells at the cortico-medullary junction also stained intensely for CGRP. As the mouse thymus reached maturity (three to eight weeks) CGRP innervation became more dense, with fibers running along the vasculature at the cortico-medullary boundary, then branching into the cortical and medullary regions. Some fibers were invested in the blood vessels while a large portion formed varicosities among the cells of the thymus. In the mature thymus, the small CGRP-IR cortico-medullary cells were more numerous, and CGRP-IR was also found in subcapsular and trabecular mast cells. The pattern of innervation remained the same in the aging mouse thymus (six months), but there appeared to be somewhat fewer cortico-medullary cells and an increase in mast cell number. In the aged (eighteen months) thymus, the small CGRP-IR cortico-medullary cells were rarely seen, but mast cells were more numerous, most of which stained positively for CGRP, in the connective tissue. Nerves containing CGRP-IR generally had the same distribution as in the younger mice but appeared somewhat truncated. The distribution of CGRP-IR nerves in the mouse thymus at different stages of development was similar to that reported for cholinergic (AChE-positive) nerves. Since the brain-stem vagal nuclei have been shown by retrograde transport studies to project to the thymus as well as to contain CGRP-IR neurons, our findings suggest that CGRP-IR thymic nerves may be derived from the vagus complex.

REFERENCES

1. WALLENGREN, J., R. EKMAN & F. SUNDLER. 1987. Occurrence and distribution of neuropeptides in human skin. Acta Derm. Venereol. (Stockholm). **67:** 185–192.
2. ALVAREZ, F. J., C. CERVANTES, I. BLASCO, R. VILIABLA, R. MARTINEZ-MURILLO, J. M. POLAK & J. RODRIGO. 1988. Presence of calcitonin gene-related peptide (CGRP) and substance P (SP) immunoreactivity in intraepidermal free nerve endings of cat skin. Brain Res. **442:** 391–395.
3. SILVERMAN, J. D. & L. KRUGER. 1989. Calcitonin-gene related peptide-immunoreactive innervation of the rat head with emphasis on specialized sensory structures. J. Comp. Neurol. **280:** 303–330.
4. SPRINGALL, D. R., A. CADIEUX, H. OLIVEIRA, H. SU, D. ROYSTON & J. M. POLAK. 1987. Retrograde tracing shows that CGRP-immunoreactive nerves of rat trachea and lung originate from vagal and dorsal root ganglia. JANS **20:** 155–165.
5. FINK, T. & E. WEIHE. 1988. Multiple neuropeptides in nerves supplying mammalian lymph nodes: messenger candidates for sensory and autonomic neuroimmunomodulation? Neurosci. Lett. **90:** 39–44.
6. WEIHE, E., S. MULLER, T. FINK & H. J. ZENTEL. 1989. Tachykinins, calcitonin gene-related peptide and neuropeptide Y in nerves of the mammalian thymus: interactions with mast cells in autonomic and sensory neuroimmunomodulation? Neurosci. Lett. **100:** 77–82.
7. POPPER, P., C. R. MANTYH, S. R. VIGNA, J. E. MAGGIO & P. W. MANTYH. 1988. The localization of sensory nerve fibers and receptor binding sites for neuropeptides in canine mesenteric lymph nodes. Peptides **9:** 257–267.
8. HENKE, H., S. SIGRIST, W. LANG, J. SCHNEIDER & J. A. FISCHER. 1987. Comparison of binding sites for the calcitonin gene-related peptides I and II in man. Brain Res. **410:** 404–408.
9. NAKAMUTA, H., Y. FUKUDA, M. KOIDA, N. FUJII, A., OTAKA, S. FUNAKOSHI, H. YAJIMA, N. MITSUYASU, AND R. ORLOWSKI. 1986. Binding sites of calcitonin gene-related peptide (CGRP): abundant occurrence in visceral organs. Jpn. J. Pharmacol. **42:** 175–180.
10. BULLOCH, K. 1985. Neuroanatomy of lymphoid tissue: a review. *In* Neural Modulation of Immunity. R. Guillemin *et al.*, Eds. 111–141. Raven Press. New York.
11. BULLOCH, K. & R. Y. MOORE. 1981. Innervation of the thymus gland of brain stem and spinal cord in mouse and rat. Am. J. Anat. **162:** 157–166.
12. TOLLEFSON, L. & K. BULLOCH. 1990. Dual-label retrograde transport: CNS innervation of the mouse thymus distinct from other mediastinum viscera. J. Neurosci. Res. **25**(1): 20–28.
13. MAGNI, F., F. BRUSCHI & M. KASTI. 1987. The afferent innervation of the thymus gland in the rat. Brain Research. **424:** 379–385.
14. AMARA, S. G., J. L. ARRIZA, S. E. LEFF, L. W. SWANSON, R. M. EVANS & M. G. ROSENFELD. 1985, Sept. 13. Expression in brain of a messenger RNA encoding a novel neuropeptide homologous to calcitonin gene-related peptide. Science. **229:** 1094–1097.

15. WIMALAWANSA, S. J., P. EMSON & I. MACINTYRE. 1987. Regional distribution of calcitonin gene-related peptide and its specific binding sites in rats with particular reference to the nervous system. Neuroendocrinology **46:** 131–136.
16. MCWILLIAM, A. V., A. MAQBOOL & T. F. BATTEN. 1989. Distribution of calcitonin gene-related peptide-like immunoreactivity in the nucleus ambiguus of the cat. J. Comp. Neurol. **282**(2): 206–214.
17. HAMMAR, J. A. 1932. Glasrekonstruktionen zur Beleuchtung der frühen embryonalen entwicklung der thymus-innervation. Vers. Verh. Anat. Ges. **41:** 234–235.
18. HAMMAR, J. A. 1935. Konstitutionsanatomische studien uber die neirotisierung des menschenembryos. IV. Uber die innervations-verhaltnisse der inkretorgane un der thymus bis in den 4 fotalmonat. Z. Mikrosk. Anat. **38:** 253–293.
19. BULLOCH, K. 1982. A light and ultrastructural analysis of the innervation of the thymus gland during the prenatal period. Soc. Neurosci. Abstr. **8:** 72.
20. UMEDA, Y., M. TAKAMIYA, H. YOSHIZAKI & M. ARISAWA. 1988. Inhibition of mitogen-stimulated T lymphocyte proliferation by calcitonin gene-related peptide. Biochem. Biophys. Res. Commun. **154**(1): 227–235.
21. ZAMBONI, L. & C. DEMARTINO. 1967. Buffered picric acid-formaldehyde: a new, rapid fixative for electron microscopy. J. Cell Biol. **35:** 148A.
22. AL-SHAWAF, A., T. COWAN, J. ABERDEEN & M. D. KENDALL. 1990. A comparison of VIP, PGP 9.5, NP-Y and CGRP immunofluorescence, SPG catacholamine fluorescence and AChE histochemistry in the rat thymus before and after chemical sypathectomy. ABSTRACTS of 1st Int. Congress ISNIM. Abstr. **216:** 298.
23. BULLOCH, K., E. ROTH & M. R. CULLEN. 1984. Nodose and superior cervical ganglia project into rat thymus. Soc. Neurosci. Abstr. **10**(Part 2): 725.
24. GUNNAR, N., K. ALVING, S. AHLSTEDT, T. HÖKFELT & J. M. LUNDBERG. Peptidergic innervation of rat lymphoid tissue and lung: relation to mast cells and sensitivity to capsaicin and immunization. Submitted for publication (from her book, Modulation of the Immune Response in Rat by Utilizing the Neurotoxin Capsaicin).
25. FOREMEN, J. C. 1987. Substance P and calcitonin gene-related peptide: effects on mast cells and in human skin. Int. Arch. Allergy Appl. Immunol. **82:** 366–371.
26. BRAIN, S. D., T. J. WILLIAMS, J. R. TIPPINS, H. R. MORRIS & I. MACINTYRE. 1984. Calcitonin gene-related peptide is a potent vasodilator. Nature **313:** 54–56.
27. NELSON, M. T., Y. HUANG, J. E. BRAYDEN, J. K. HESCHELER & N. B. STANDEN. 1990. Calcitonin gene-related peptide (CGRP) dilates arteries by activating ATP-sensitive K+ channels (K_{ATP}). Biophys. J. **57:** 315a.
28. GEPPETTI, P., S. FRILLI, D. RENZI, P. SANTICIOLI, C. A. MAGGI, E. THEODORSSON & M. FANCIULLACCI. 1988. Distribution of calcitonin gene-related peptide-like immunoreactivity in various rat tissues: correlation with substance P and other tachykinins and sensitivity to capsaicin. Regul. Pept. **23:** 289–298.

Developmental Changes in Bone Marrow Thymocyte Progenitors and Thy1$^+$ Cells in Aging[a]

AYALA SHARP, SHAI BRILL, TOVA KUKULANSKY, AND AMIELA GLOBERSON[b]

Department of Cell Biology
Weizmann Institute of Science
P.O. Box 26
76 100 Rehovot, Israel

INTRODUCTION

The idea that immunosenescence is based at least in part on developmental failures has gained support from various types of experimental evidence. These have been linked with thymic involution which causes a decrease in thymic hormonal[1-3] and microenvironmental effects.[4,5] The effects of aging on bone marrow T cell progenitors were studied in experiments in which bone marrow from old donors was grafted into young irradiated recipients.[6-10] However, whereas lymphoid reconstitution with cells of the old was achieved within six weeks, just as in the case of transplants from young donors, a decline in T cell functions in the recipients became apparent after 6 months.[9,10] The basis for age-related changes in bone marrow has yet to be elucidated. We employed a variety of *in vitro* experimental models to analyse the potential of bone marrow cells for self renewal and differentiation and to establish whether any quantitative or qualitative age-related changes occur in thymocyte progenitors in the bone marrow, which might contribute to immunosenescence in T cells. In parallel we characterized the Thy1$^+$ cells, found to increase in the bone marrow in aging, to elucidate whether this increase represented a change in hemopoietic progenitors or in mature T cells.

RESULTS AND DISCUSSION

Thymocyte Progenitors in Bone Marrow

The Experimental Model

Mechanisms underlying the age-related decrease in the developmental capacity of thymocyte progenitors from bone marrow were analyzed by seeding the cells onto thymocyte-depleted fetal thymus explants. This strategy was based on

[a] Supported by a grant from the Chief Scientist, Israel Ministry of Health, and by the SANDOZ Foundation for Gerontological Research. A.G. is the incumbent of the Harriet and Harold Brady Chair in Cancer Research.
[b] Corresponding author.

our original findings that a urethane-treated fetal thymus, reconstituted *in vitro* by bone marrow cells, could resume lymphoid development.[11] To achieve maximal thymocyte depletion in the fetal thymus we employed 2-deoxyguanosine as previously described.[12] Reconstitution of the lymphocyte-depleted thymuses was performed by incubation of 14-day fetal thymus explants with the colonizing cells for 72 hrs in hanging drop cultures. The explants were rinsed to remove any cells that did not seed the thymus, and then transferred to organ culture, in which lymphoid differentiation proceeded.[13] Our studies using this system indicated that the patterns of reconstitution of fetal thymuses by bone marrow cells from young (2–3 months) and old (24 months) C57BL/6J (H-2^b, Thy1.2) or C57BL/Ka (H-2^b, Thy1.1) mice were similar, as determined by the levels of Thy1$^+$ cells per explant, including CD4 and CD8 subsets.[14]

We could thus conclude that there is no difference in the developmental potential of bone marrow cells from young and old donors. Accordingly, we predicted that if this is indeed the case, then seeding of a 1 : 1 mixture of cells from the two age groups would lead to development of cells from the two sources in equal proportions.

When mixtures of cells from the young and old Thy1 congenic bone marrow donors were seeded onto the same individual thymic lobe, a developmental advantage of the cells from the young donors was apparent.[14] Hence, this strategy of competitive reconstitution enabled the detection of differences in developmental capacity, and it could serve as an experimental model to analyze the effects of aging on the differentiation of thymocytes from their progenitors in bone marrow.

Quantitative Age-Related Changes in Bone Marrow Thymocyte Progenitors Manifested under Competitive Reconstitution of the Thymus

We considered different possible mechanisms to account for the results described above. The first possibility, that aging is associated with a decline in the frequency of thymocyte progenitors, was examined by seeding the thymus explants with limiting cell doses to achieve clonal colonization and measuring the proportion of thymic lobes that were reconstituted. The results[15] revealed a decline in frequency of colonizing cells in the old mouse bone marrow, as compared with the young.

We next applied limiting doses of mixtures of bone marrow cells from both age groups, at the clonal level, and compared them with the seeding of saturating amounts of cells (500 cells versus 60,000 cells per lobe, respectively). Cells were collected from all the thymic lobes, and the cells were analyzed for the expression of the Thy1.1 and Thy1.2 markers. We found[16] relatively lower levels of cells of the old only when the cells were seeded in saturating amounts. In explants colonized with the mixtures applied in limiting amounts, the thymocytes that developed from the young and old donor cells were in the same ratio as in the original inoculum. Hence, under conditions of clonal seeding in which colonization of individual thymic lobes was achieved in all probability by a single bone marrow cell, either young or old, there was no manifestation of developmental preference.

Patterns of Developmental Preference under Sequential Seeding of Young and Old Bone Marrow Cells onto the Thymic Explants

Another explanation of the aging effect observed was that binding of the old mouse bone marrow to homing markers on the thymic stroma is of lower affinity than that of the young, so that the young cells settling in the thymic microenvironment gain a developmental advantage. To examine this possibility we incubated the fetal thymuses with old mouse bone marrow cells for 24 hrs, then rinsed the explants to remove any old cells that did not settle in the tissue. Finally, we applied the cells from the young donors. We used a similar protocol to seed first young cells and subsequently old, or cells from two different young donors. As previously, in all of these experiments, the donor pairs were Thy1 congenic mice, to enable identification of the origin of the developing thymocytes. The results showed that cells that were seeded first, whether from young or from old donors, expressed a developmental advantage.[16]

The results appeared to agree with the idea that the initial interaction of thymocyte progenitors with the thymic stroma leads to a stable contact, and that cells of old and young age groups may compete at this stage of colonization for homing markers.

However, when we seeded the competing cells simultaneously measuring the Thy1$^+$ cells after the first incubation period of 72 hrs, we found that at this stage there was no advantage to either age group. This suggested that although the nature of the primary contact of the cells with the thymic stroma may be critical for ultimate differentiation, additional age-related changes may underlie the developmental inferiority of cells from the old.

Kinetics of Thymocyte Development from Bone Marrow Cells

An additional mechanism that we considered was linked to a possible difference in levels of sequential replication in the thymus. Manifestation of lower levels of sequential replication in lymphocytes of the old have been documented.[17-19] We thus examined whether a similar phenomenon may be manifested also within the colonized fetal thymus. We approached this question by analyzing the kinetics of emergence of Thy1.1$^+$ and Thy1.2$^+$ cells in the thymuses reconstituted simultaneously with bone marrow cells of Thy1 congenic young and old mice. During the first week of culture, the levels of Thy1$^+$ cells from both origins were similar (FIG. 1A), but from the 7th day through the 10th day of culture there was a marked exponential increase in the numbers of cells originating from the young, whereas cells of the old manifested a limited increase. The ultimate result was a significantly higher proportion of thymocytes of the young as compared with the old. Regarding the kinetics of development of Thy1$^+$ cells in fetal thymuses reconstituted by cells from each age group on its own, here too, we found that ultimately lower levels of cells developed from the old (FIG. 1B), yet, this was less pronounced than under the competitive colonization.

Experiments were then designed to determine whether cell replications that may occur at the initial phase of colonization of the thymus were important in determining subsequent colonization events.

We seeded the cells of old mouse bone marrow first in a two-step colonization protocol, and incubated them for 48 hrs with, or without, cytosine arabinoside (2.5×10^{-6} M). At the end of this period the explants were rinsed, and colonized with cells of the young. The idea was to examine whether colonization of the thymus in absence of cell division during the initial 48-hr period would eliminate the advantage of the cells seeded first. The results (TABLE 1) showed that the levels of Thy1$^+$ cells of old origin were lowered as a result of exposure to the cytosine arabinoside, to levels observed when the young and old cells were seeded simultaneously. Thus, inhibition of cell replication by cytosine arabinoside resulted in a disadvantage of the old.

Self Recognition by Thymocyte Progenitors

Recent studies from our laboratory have shown that the initial interaction of bone marrow cells with the thymic stroma involves MHC recognition.[20] When cells from donors syngeneic and allogeneic to the thymus were admixed and simultaneously seeded onto the thymic stroma, under saturating conditions, cells of the syngeneic origin exhibited a significant developmental advantage. On the other hand, bone marrow cells seeded into an allogeneic thymus on their own, gave rise to thymocytes expressing the Thy1 allotype of their donor. Thus we maintained that the homing receptor might be associated with MHC markers. However, when thymic colonization was performed under noncompetitive conditions, the influence of the MHC markers could be uncoupled from that of homing receptor. These studies led us to investigate whether aging affects this early manifestation of MHC recognition in bone marrow cell interaction with the thymic stroma.

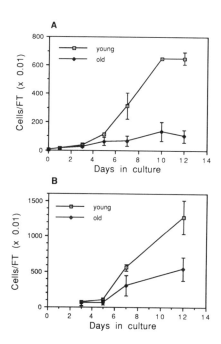

FIGURE 1. Kinetics of Thy1+ cell development in fetal thymus explants colonized with bone marrow cells from young and old mice seeded either together in each individual explant **(A)** or in separate explants **(B)**. Mixtures consisted of cells from Thy1 congenic donors, to enable identification of the donor origin of developing cells. Results are calculated from three experiments in which reciprocal combinations (young Thy1.1 and old Thy1.2 and vice versa) were employed.

When old or young mouse bone marrow cells were seeded onto an allogeneic thymic stroma, in a mixture with bone marrow cells syngeneic with that stroma, the cells which developed were mainly of the syngeneic origin. Similarly, when the seeding mixture contained cells from old or young mice syngeneic with the thymus, and allogenic cells from young donors, the syngeneic cells exhibited a developmental advantage. However, under these conditions there were quantitative differences in the levels of thymocytes developing from the old as compared with those from the young (TABLE 2).

To determine whether these differences were due to the age factor per se, or

TABLE 1. Colonization of FT-Stroma by Sequential Incubation with BM Cells with or without CA[a]

Source of Reconstituting Cells			% Positive Cells[b]	
0–48 Hrs	48–96 Hrs	Treatment	Young	Old
Young[c] + old[d]	young + old	—	67 ± 13	19 ± 4
Young + old	young + old	CA	66 ± 1	15 ± 4
Young	old	—	70 ± 14	10 ± 5
Young	old	CA	63 ± 15	21 ± 8
Old	young	—	32 ± 6	55 ± 1
Old	young	CA	55 ± 9	16 ± 1
Young	young	—	86 ± 7	5 ± 3
Young	young	CA	78 ± 11	4 ± 1
Old	old	—	6 ± 2	81 ± 5
Old	old	CA	6 ± 2	64 ± 6

[a] Cytosine arabinoside (2.5×10^{-6} M) added at 0–48 hrs then washed out.
[b] Calculated as follows:
  [(% Thy1[+] − background)/(100 − background)] × 100.
[c] C57BL/6J, 3 months, Thy1.2.
[d] C57BL/Ka, 2 years, Thy1.1.

whether they indicated an age-related decline in the capacity for MHC recognition by cells of the old, we seeded mixtures of cells from syngeneic and allogeneic old donors. Under these conditions the syngeneic preference diminished (TABLE 2).

Thus, MHC-linked syngeneic preference declines with aging and it remains to be determined whether this is in any way associated with increased autoreactivity in aging.

Bone Marrow Myeloid Progenitors and Thy1[+] Cells in Aging and Their Status versus the Peripheral Lymphoid Tissues

The aging mouse bone marrow was found to contain increased levels of Thy1[+] and Ig[+] cells.[21] Functional analyses have suggested that at least some of these cells represented mature T and B lymphocytes. In view of the fact that the Thy1

TABLE 2. Colonization of FT-Stroma[a] with Allogeneic Young and Old BM Cells Seeded in a Mixture with Syngeneic Cells

Origin of Donor Cells		% Positive Cells	
Syngeneic	Allogeneic	Syngeneic Thy1.1	Allogeneic Thy1.2
Old$_1$[b]	old$_2$[c]	47 ± 2	43 ± 4
Young$_1$[d]	old$_2$	63 ± 5	20 ± 5
Young$_1$	young$_2$[e]	69 ± 3	11 ± 1
Young$_1$	—	89 ± 2	0 ± 0
—	young$_2$	0 ± 0	88 ± 2
—	old$_2$	0 ± 0	87 ± 3

[a] Recipient FT explants were of C57BL/6J or C57BL/Ka origin.
[b] C57BL/Ka, 24 months, Thy1.1.
[c] BALB/c, 24 months, Thy1.2.
[d] C57BL/Ka, 3 months, Thy1.1.
[e] BALB/c, 3 months, Thy1.2.

marker is also expressed on hemopoietic cells,[22,23] we decided to find out whether the increased Thy1[+] cell values related to T lymphocytes or to hemopoietic cells.

Bone Marrow Myeloid Progenitors in Aging

We measured levels of spleen colony-forming units (CFUs) and granulocyte-macrophage colony forming units (GM-CFUs) in cells from young and old mice. Values obtained for the two age groups were similar.[24] However, when we cultivated the cells in liquid culture enriched with colony-stimulating factors, we found increased rates of proliferation in cells of the old. In addition, bone marrow cells of young and aging donors were cultured over an adherent layer of bone marrow stroma cells of the line 14F1.1, which consists of endothelial adipocytes,[25] and the nonadherent cells were collected weekly and examined for cell number and for their capacity to produce GM-CFU colonies. Cells of the old manifested higher levels of proliferation and of GM-CFU formation than cells of the young. In contrast, when the cells harvested from these cultures were analyzed for the presence of thymocyte progenitors, by seeding into fetal thymus explants, they exhibited a decline in the capacity to generate thymocytes.[24]

Thus, myeloid progenitors in the old bone marrow manifest a higher capacity for self renewal and differentiation than in the young. This is in contrast to the status of the thymocyte progenitors. Therefore the age-related changes in thymocyte progenitors do not reflect a general decline in the lymphohemopoietic potential of the stem cell compartment.

Analysis of Thy1[+] Cells in Bone Marrow

We examined bone marrow cell samples for cell surface lymphocyte phenotypes and found[26] a significant age-related increase in Thy1[+] and Ig[+] cell levels, as previously reported.[21] An analysis of T cell responses to conA stimulation, performed by measuring both proliferation and cytotoxic reactions, showed increased T cell functions in the old. In terms of kinetics and peak level, the response patterns in cells of the old, showed an early, acute reaction, which diminished earlier than in the young. Similar observations[26] were recorded on the frequency of cytotoxic T lymphocyte precursors (CTLp).

In view of these results we investigated whether old bone marrow contains an increased level of cells that enter mitosis in response to conA stimulation. Indeed, when we measured the conA-induced proliferation in the presence of colchicine, we found that the number of cells entering the first mitotic cycle was higher in the old.[26]

A direct analysis of Thy1[+]-enriched, or Thy1[+]-depleted cell populations showed a positive correlation between the expression of Thy1[+] cells and the extent of conA-induced response, and no correlation between Thy1 expression and the frequency of myeloid precursors.

These various experiments suggest that the higher levels of Thy1[+] cells in the bone marrow of the old reflect an increase in the number of functional T cells. In view of the fact that the function of the T cells in peripheral lymphoid tissues declines with aging, we have suggested that the bone marrow acts as a compensatory T cell organ in aging.[26] It was of interest to examine whether in the intact organism there is any compensatory mechanism for the decline in thymocyte progenitors originating in the bone marrow. This led us to investigate the spleen, which is a hemopoietic organ in the mouse. However, when splenocytes from young and old mice were seeded into a fetal thymus explant, either each one on its own, or in mixture, or in competition with bone marrow cells, we found that levels of thymocytes developing from cells of the aging mouse spleen were actually lower than those from the young.[27]

TABLE 3. T Cell Subsets in Peripheral Blood, Spleen, and Lymph Nodes of Young and Old Mice[a]

Membrane Marker	Cells	% Positive Cells		P Value
		Young	Old	
Thy1	bone marrow	6.9 ± 0.5	12.0 ± 0.8	0.00001
	spleen	40.6 ± 2.0	39.4 ± 8.8	NS
	lymph nodes	82.2 ± 2.2	74.0 ± 1.3	NS
	PBL	44.0 ± 16.0	33.6 ± 10.0	NS
CD4	bone marrow	3.1 ± 0.7	4.3 ± 0.5	NS
	spleen	25.0 ± 2.0	16.7 ± 2.9	NS
	lymph nodes	47.9 ± 3.2	23.4 ± 4.8	NS
	PBL	30.0 ± 4.3	16.3 ± 2.4	0.002
CD8	bone marrow	2.8 ± 0.5	5.7 ± 1.0	0.01
	spleen	16.4 ± 2.0	22.1 ± 1.9	NS
	lymph nodes	35.1 ± 1.3	45.5 ± 3.7	NS
	PBL	13.4 ± 2.3	23.7 ± 3.8	NS

[a] Prepared from data reported,[27,28] as well as unpublished observations representing 2–4 independent experiments.

Compartmentalization of Thy1⁺ Cells in the Peripheral Lymphoid Tissues

Our observations on the age-related increase in functional T lymphocytes in bone marrow raised the possibility that aging is associated with an altered compartmentalization of T lymphocytes in the peripheral lymphoid tissues. We examined T lymphocyte functions in the spleen as well as in the lymph nodes and peripheral blood of individual young and old mice. Our results[28] showed different age-associated patterns of change in these tissues, with respect to the various T cell parameters that we measured. This was reflected in the distribution of Thy1⁺ cells and the CD4 and CD8 subsets, as well as in the results of functional analyses. As shown in TABLE 3, whereas Thy1⁺ and CD8 cell levels in bone marrow of the old increased significantly, their values did not change in the peripheral lymphoid tissues. On the other hand, levels of CD4 cells decreased in the peripheral tissues, with no significant change in the bone marrow.

Regarding reactivity to conA, the decline of response to mitogen (conA) as measured by standard proliferation assays was more pronounced in the spleen than in the peripheral blood.[28] However, the frequencies of proliferative T cell precursors (PTLp), which decline with aging,[29] were similar in the different anatomic compartments in each of the age groups (TABLE 4) and values in the old were significantly lower than in the young. Evidently, manifestations of aging are not necessarily symmetrical in the different lymphoid compartments in the same individual.

CONCLUDING REMARKS

Our study represents an analysis of the effects of aging on the T lymphocyte compartment in bone marrow from the developmental angle. Hence, decline in the capacity of thymocyte progenitors to differentiate was found following seeding of bone marrow cells from young and old donors onto the same fetal thymus. By this procedure, effects of aging on thymocyte progenitors could be dissociated from those exerted on the thymic stroma. Analysis of the basis for the altered developmental potential of the bone marrow thymocyte progenitors indicated quantitative and qualitative changes at the different stages, from the initial process of interaction with the thymic stroma and colonization, to ultimate T cell development. It appears that the ability of cells of old donors to replicate sequentially is limited. This limitation is more pronounced in the presence of cells from young donors. It could be due to an a priori lower potential for sequential replications or to suppression exerted by the young cells. Such suppression may take place when saturating amounts of cells are used for reconstitution and not when limiting amounts of cells are used. Whatever the mechanism, these results point to a variety of age-related changes in the developmental capacity of bone marrow cells which settle in the thymus.

TABLE 4. Frequency of Proliferating T Lymphocyte Precursors (PTLp $\times$ 10^{-3}) in Young and Old Mice[a]

Cells	Young	Old
Spleen	20.5 ± 4.4	2.3 ± 0.6
Lymph nodes	39.8 ± 12.0	2.2 ± 1.7
PBL	36.0 ± 13.0	4.9 ± 3.6

[a] Calculated from 2 experiments performed on 5 young (2–3 m) and 5 old (24 m) C57BL/6J or C3H/ebJ × C57BL/6J mice. Values were determined by a limiting dilution assay on cells cultured in the presence of conA for 7 days and labelled with ^{3}H-thymidine for the final 16 hrs.

On the other hand, the developmental capacity of the myeloid compartment of bone marrow was not reduced, but exhibited an increased potential for cell replication.

We investigated whether the increase in proportion of Thy1$^+$ cells in bone marrow of aged mice might represent an increase in myeloid progenitors that express this membrane marker, or whether they are T lymphocytes, and found that this fraction includes functional T cells. The source of these cells in bone marrow is, as yet, not critically elucidated. Determining whether they represent an influx from the peripheral lymphoid tissues, or whether they differentiate within the bone marrow will have to await further analysis. Our observations suggest that the bone marrow microenvironment may enable maintenance of Thy1$^+$ cells. This is in line with our recent observations that the 14F1.1 bone marrow stroma cell line supported the development of thymocytes under *in vitro* conditions.[30]

In addition, we have demonstrated that the status of T lymphocytes is changed in aging to a different extent in the various peripheral lymphoid tissues. Bone marrow seemed to compensate for the decline of T lymphocytes in other anatomic sites.

Thus, different mechanisms may underlie the altered developmental potential of thymocyte progenitors and of Thy1$^+$ cells in the peripheral lymphoid tissues. Whether all or part of these processes are controlled by one central mechanism remains to be elucidated.

ACKNOWLEDGMENT

The editorial assistance of Mrs. M. Baer is gratefully acknowledged.

REFERENCES

1. GOLDSTEIN, A. L., J. A. HOOPER, R. S. SCHULOF, G. H. COHEN, G. B. THURMAN, M. C. MCDANIEL, A. WHITE & M. DARDENE. 1974. Thymosin and the immunopathology of aging. Fed. Proc. **33:** 2053–2056.
2. FRIEDMAN, D., V. KEISER & A. GLOBERSON. 1974. Reactivation of immunocompetence in spleen cells of aged mice. Nature **251:** 545–546.
3. FABRIS, N., E. MOCCHEGIANI, L. AMADIO, M. ZANNOTTI, F. LICASTRO & C. FRANCESCHI. 1984. Thymic hormone deficiency in normal ageing and Down's syndrome: Is there a primary failure of the thymus? Lancet **1:** 983–986.
4. HIROKAWA, K. 1977. The thymus and aging. *In* Immunology and Aging. T. Makinodan & E. Yunis, Eds. 51–72. Plenum Press, New York.
5. HIROKAWA K., K. SATO & T. MAKINODAN. 1982. Influence of age of thymic grafts on the differentiation of T cells in nude mice. Clin. Immunol. Immunopathol. **24:** 251–262.
6. TYAN, M. L. 1977. Age-related decrease in mouse T cell progenitors. J. Immunol. **118:** 846–851.
7. HARRISON, D. E. 1983. Long-term erythropoietic repopulating ability of old, young and fetal stem cells. J. Exp. Med. **157:** 1007–1010.
8. OGDEN, D. A. & H. S. MICKLEM. 1976. The rate of serially transplanted bone marrow cell populations from young and old donors. Transplantation **22:** 237–293.
9. GOZES, Y., T. UMIEL & N. TRAININ. 1982. Selective decline in differentiating capacity of immunohemopoietic stem cells with aging. Mech. Ageing Dev. **18:** 251–259.
10. GLOBERSON, A. 1984. Developmental aspects of altered immunoregulatory mechanisms in aging. *In* Lymphoid Cell Functions in Aging. Topics in Aging Research in Europe. A. L. deWeck, Ed. Vol. 3: 17–27. EURAGE. The Netherlands.
11. GLOBERSON, A. & R. AUERBACH. 1965. *In vitro* studies on thymus and lung differentiation following urethane treatment. Wistar Inst. Monogr. **4:** 3–19.
12. JENKINSON, E. J., L. FRANCHI, R. KINGSTON & J. J. T. OWEN. 1982. Effect of deoxyguanosine on lymphopoiesis in the developing thymus rudiment *in vitro:* application in the production of chimeric thymus rudiments. Eur. J. Immunol. **12:** 583–587.
13. EREN, R., D. ZHARHARY, L. ABEL & A. GLOBERSON. 1987. Ontogeny of T cells: development of pre-T cells from fetal liver and yolk sac in the thymus microenvironment. Cell. Immunol. **108:** 76–84.
14. EREN, R., D. ZHARHARY, L. ABEL & A. GLOBERSON. 1988. *In vitro* development of T cells from old and young mouse bone marrow. Cell. Immunol. **112:** 449–455.
15. EREN, R., A. GLOBERSON, L. ABEL & D. ZHARHARY. 1990. Quantitative analysis of bone marrow thymic progenitors in young and aged mice. Cell. Immunol. **127:** 238–246.
16. SHARP, A., T. KUKULANSKY & A. GLOBERSON. *In vitro* analysis of age-related changes in the developmental potential of bone marrow thymocyte progenitors. Eur. J. Immunol. In press.

17. HEFTON, J. M., G. J. DARLINGTON, B. A. CASSAZZA & M. E. WEKSLER. 1980. Immunological studies of aging. V. Impaired proliferation of PHA responsive human lymphocytes in culture. J. Immunol. **125:** 1007–1010.

18. TICE, R. R., E. L. SCHNEIDER, D. KRAM & P. THORN. 1979. Cytokinetic analysis of the impaired proliferative response of peripheral lymphocytes from aged humans to phytohemagglutinin. J. Exp. Med. **149:** 1029–1041.

19. GUTOWSKI, J. K., J. B. INNES, M. E. WEKSLER & S. COHEN. 1986. Impaired nuclear responsiveness to cytoplasmic signals in lymphocytes from elderly humans with depressed proliferative response. J. Clin. Invest. **78:** 40–43.

20. EREN, R., L. ABEL & A. GLOBERSON. 1989. Syngeneic preference manifested by thymic stroma during development of thymocytes from bone marrow. Eur. J. Immunol. **19:** 2087–2092.

21. FARRAR, J., B. E. LONGHMAN & A. A. NORDIN. 1974. Lympho-hemopoietic potential of bone marrow cells from aged mice: comparison of the cellular constituents of bone marrow from young and aged mice. J. Immunol. **112:** 1244–1249.

22. SCHRADER, J. W., F. BATTYE & R. SCOLLAY. 1982. Expression of Thy-1 antigen is not limited to T cells in cultures of mouse hemopoietic cells. Proc. Natl. Acad. Sci. USA **79:** 4161–4165.

23. BOSWELL, H. S., P. M. WADE & P. J. QUESENBERRY. 1984. Thy-1 antigen expression by murine high proliferative capacity hematopoietic progenitor cells. J. Immunol. **133:** 2940–2949.

24. SHARP, A., D. ZIPORI, J. TOLEDO, S. TAL, P. RESNITZKY & A. GLOBERSON. 1989. Age related changes in hemopoietic capacity of bone marrow cells. Mech. Ageing Dev. **48:** 91–99.

25. ZIPORI, D. & F. LEE. 1988. Introduction of interleukin-3 gene into stromal cells from the bone marrow alters hemopoietic differentiation but does not modify stem cell renewal. Blood **71:** 586–596.

26. SHARP, A., T. KUKULANSKY, Y. MALKINSON & A. GLOBERSON. 1990. The bone marrow as an effector T cell organ in aging. Mech. Ageing Dev. **52:** 219–233.

27. GLOBERSON, A., R. EREN, L. ABEL & D. BEN-MENAHEM. 1989. Developmental aspects of T lymphocytes in aging. In Biomedical Advances in Aging. A. L. Goldstein, Ed. Chapter 34. 363–373. Plenum Press, New York.

28. BRILL, S., D. BEN-MENAHEM, T. KUKULANSKY, E. TAL & A. GLOBERSON. 1990. Do peripheral blood T lymphocytes reflect splenic T lymphocyte functions in individual young and old mice? Aging Immunol. Infect. Dis. In press.

29. MILLER R. A. & D. E. HARRISON. 1987. Clonal analysis of age associated changes in T-cell reactivity. In Aging and the Immune Response: Cellular and Hormonal Aspects. E. A. Goidl, Ed. 1–26. Marcel Dekker, Inc. New York.

30. TAMIR, M., R. EREN, A. GLOBERSON, E. KEDAR, E. EPSTEIN, N. TRAININ & D. ZIPORI. 1990. Selective accumulation of lymphocyte precursor cells mediated by stromal cells of hemopoietic origin. Exp. Hematol. **18:** 332–340.

Survey of Thymic Hormone Effects on Physical and Immunological Parameters in C57BL/6NNia Mice of Different Ages[a]

V. K. GHANTA,[b,c] N. S. HIRAMOTO,[b] S-J. SOONG,[d] AND
R. N. HIRAMOTO[b]

*Departments of [b]Microbiology, [c]Biology, and [d]Biostatistics
University of Alabama at Birmingham
Birmingham, Alabama 35294*

INTRODUCTION

The consequences of aging on the immune system are quite predictable. The thymus gland involutes, immune capacity decreases, autoimmunity and cancer increase.[1-3] Attempts have been made to prevent these changes by restorative means such as: passive transfer of lymphoid cells, grafting of young thymus glands to old mice, use of diets and chemical treatment with 2-mercaptoethanol (2-ME) or hormones.[4-7] Presently, dietary restriction is the only known and proven mode which extends mean and maximum survival times.[5-7] Diet also decreases the incidence and/or delays the onset of several diseases of old age.[8-11] To be effective, dietary restriction has to be instituted early, at about the age of weaning (3 to 6 weeks). However, Weindruch and Walford[11] reported a significant increase in the mean survival time for the longest lived 10% of the restricted population of B10C3F1 and C57BL/6J strains where dietary restriction was started at 12 to 13 months of age. Significantly higher survival was observed for the restricted mice when compared to the unrestricted mice. Concomitantly, a decrease in the incidence of spontaneous lymphoma in the food-restricted group was also observed.[11]

Thymic hormone preparations have been used to reconstitute and augment the immune response in immunodeficient situations.[12-17] They are known to induce surface markers, allow maturation and differentiation of T-cells, and regulate immune response.[18-20] However, no one has reported the studies of thymic hormone preparations on the life span. Walford has proposed the immunologic basis for the aging process to be due to loss of regulation and minor histocompatibility reactions arising in the host.[21] If hormone therapy can prevent such occurrences, one might postulate that animals treated with hormones might live longer disease free.

[a] This work was supported by a contract from the National Institute on Aging, N01-AG-9-2100.

RESULTS

Effect of Thymic Hormone Treatment on Life Span in Longitudinal Studies in C57BL/6 Mice

Initial studies were done to see if thymic hormone treatment could affect longevity. Twenty-five mice per group were treated with thymic hormone as follows: FTS, 1 μg and 10 ng 3×/wk; TP5, 1 μg 1×/wk; TP5, 10 ng 3×/wk; TM4, 1 ng 1×/wk; thymosin TF5, 10 and 1 μg 1×/wk; and saline 1×/wk. Treatments were continued for the life of the animal in a longitudinal study.

The effect on maximum life span in the C57BL/6 mice was shorter than generally expected because of failure of heating equipment during the winter, which occurred during the second year of the study when the mice were 16 months old. There was a drop in temperature for a period of 24 hr in the facility. All animals in this study were subject to the effect. Despite this setback the thymic hormone treatment appears to have a protective effect in that survival was significantly greater in the groups treated with TM4 (1 ng), and TF5 (10 and 1 μg) than the saline control (FIG. 1, TABLE 1).

Since animals treated with thymic hormones appear to have a survival advantage under "stressed" conditions it was of interest to investigate whether various normal parameters such as weight; hematocrit; PBL, spleen, and thymus cell numbers; PBL and spleen mitogen stimulation index (SI) to PHA, ConA, and LPS; IgM hemolysin autoantibody levels per mouse;[22,23] and cell-mediated cyto-

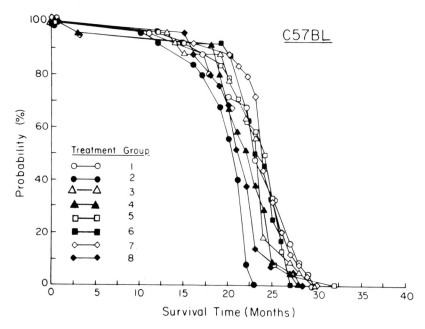

FIGURE 1. The probability of survival of long-term treatment of C57BL/6 mice with different thymic hormone preparations. FTS, 1 μg (○); FTS, 10 ng (●); TP5, 1 μg (△); TP5, 10 ng (▲); TM4, 1 ng (□); TF5, 10 μg (■); TF5, 1 μg (◇); and saline (◆). (From Hiramoto *et al.*[85] Reprinted by permission from Marcel Dekker.)

TABLE 1. Analysis of Survival of C57BL/6 Mice Treated with Thymic Hormones

Treatment/Dose	Median Survival Time (Months)	% Surviving > 25 Months	Maximum Survival Time (Months)	p^a
FTS 1 μg	23	32	30	0.08
FTS 10 ng	20	0	23	0.14
TP5 1 μg	23	16	30	0.07
TP5 10 ng	22	8	28	0.35
TM4 1 ng	24	32	32	0.05
TF5 10 μg	23	24	27	0.02
TF5 1 μg	24	32	30	0.03
Saline	21	8	28	—

[a] Compared with saline control according to the overall survival based on the generalized Wilcoxon test. (From Hiramoto *et al*.[85] Reprinted by permission from Marcel Dekker.)

toxicity to P815 allogeneic cells are modulated by hormone treatment. These parameters can be assessed by cross-sectional studies only. C57BL/6NNia female mice of specific ages were obtained from the National Institute on Aging animal models program. Mice of ages 4 wk (1 m), 26 wk (6 m), 52 wk (12 m), 78 wk (18 m), and 104 wk (24 m) were obtained and allowed to acclimate for one week prior to the treatment. Mice were injected with the hormones 5×/wk for 3 wk and assayed two days after the last injection. The hormones used were Facteur Thymic Serique (FTS) which is a nonapeptide, Glu-Ala-Lys-Ser-Gln-Gly-Gly-Ser-Asn-OH; Thymopentin (TP5), Arg-Lys-Asp-Val-Tyr, which is the active site of thymopoietin residues 32–36; TM4, an enzyme resistant variant of FTS, Sar-Lys-Sar-Gln-NH$_2$; and Thymosin Fraction 5 (TF5) which has been shown to consist of 40–60 polypeptides of 1000 to 15,000 daltons. In the cross-sectional studies, 5 mice/group were injected ip 5×/wk with FTS (1 μg or 10 ng), TP5 (1 μg or 10 ng), TM4 (1 ng), TF5 (10 or 1 μg) and compared with a saline-treated (0.1 ml) control group.

Effect of Hormone Treatment on Weight

TABLE 2 shows the effect of hormone treatment in all age groups from 4 to 104 wk. Short-term hormone treatment did not significantly increase or decrease weight compared to control. Only the TM4 group had lower weight at 78 wk. The weight of control mice increased from 16.5 g at 4 wk to 30 g at 78 wk and remained stable. The longitudinal studies showed mice treated with TF5 (10 μg) increased weight between 20 and 50 wk. FTS (1 μg & 10 ng) depressed weight between 50 and 80 wk. The results indicate long-term treatment produces different results from short-term treatments.

Effect of Hormone Treatment on Hematocrit

Hematocrit gradually declined normally with age (TABLE 3, see saline control). However, significant decline in hematocrit occurred only with TF5 at 10 μg in 26- and 52-wk-old mice. There were no other significant changes in the other groups. Thymic hormone treatment did not show any restorative effect or induce

TABLE 2. Effect of Thymic Hormone Treatment on Weight of C57BL/6 Mice[a]

Treatment/ Dose	(Age) Weeks				
	4	26	52	78	104
FTS 1 μg	16.0 ± 0.1	21.7 ± 0.9	26.5 ± 0.6	28.1 ± 1.4	29.6 ± 2.2
FTS 10 ng	16.6 ± 0.4	24.5 ± 1.4	28.2 ± 2.1	29.3 ± 0.9	29.1 ± 1.9
TP5 1 μg	16.1 ± 0.5	23.9 ± 1.4	26.7 ± 1.2	28.3 ± 2.0	28.0 ± 0.7
TP5 10 ng	15.9 ± 0.6	24.0 ± 0.7	26.0 ± 1.3	28.6 ± 1.9	29.1 ± 2.2
TM4 1 ng	16.6 ± 0.5	25.5 ± 1.2	25.6 ± 0.7	26.2 ± 0.6 ↓	31.4 ± 2.1
TF5 10 μg	15.5 ± 0.2	26.0 ± 1.2	25.4 ± 0.6	28.5 ± 1.2	31.1 ± 3.6
TF5 1 μg	15.2 ± 0.8	22.9 ± 0.4	27.0 ± 1.2	27.0 ± 1.3	33.4 ± 2.9
Saline	16.5 ± 0.6	23.9 ± 1.1	25.7 ± 0.3	30.3 ± 0.4	30.6 ± 0.3

[a] Mean ± SE. Arrow (↓) indicates statistically significant value $p < 0.05$.

hematopoietic stem cells to produce more erythrocytes. In the longitudinally treated mice FTS and TP5 had a tendency to elevate the hematocrit between 10 and 40 wk.

Effect of Hormone Treatment on PBL Numbers

The PBL numbers fluctuated somewhat depending on the cohort of animals received from the vendor (see saline controls). Generally higher at 4 wk of age, PBL numbers stabilized after 26 wk of age. Hormone treatment had a slight effect in 4-wk-old mice (TABLE 4). Only TP5 (10 ng) significantly affected PBL numbers at 4 wk. No effect was seen in 26-, 52-, or 104-wk-old mice. However, FTS (1 μg) and TF5 (10 and 1 μg) significantly increased PBL numbers at 78 wk. FTS, TP5, and TF5 consistently showed suppression of PBL numbers between 54 and 80 wk in animals on longitudinal studies.

Effect of Hormone Treatment on Spleen Cell Numbers

Spleen cell numbers increased from 4 to 26 wk of age and remained relatively stable in the different age groups. There were some hormonal effects in 4-, 26-, and 52-wk-old mice (TABLE 5). TM4 caused an increase at 4 wk but FTS (1 μg)

TABLE 3. Effect of Thymic Hormone Treatment on the Hematocrit of C57BL/6 Mice[a]

Treatment/ Dose	(Age) Weeks				
	4	26	52	78	104
FTS 1 μg	52.4 ± 1.0	49.5 ± 1.0	49.3 ± 0.4	46.2 ± 0.5	48.0 ± 0.9
FTS 10 ng	52.1 ± 0.4	47.9 ± 0.8	48.7 ± 0.5	45.8 ± 0.7	46.3 ± 1.3
TP5 1 μg	51.5 ± 0.7	47.4 ± 0.5	48.4 ± 1.2	46.3 ± 1.8	46.7 ± 1.5
TP5 10 ng	50.8 ± 1.2	47.9 ± 0.3	46.8 ± 0.5	46.0 ± 0.4	46.3 ± 2.3
TM4 1 ng	49.5 ± 0.7	48.1 ± 0.7	46.3 ± 0.6	47.4 ± 0.5	47.0 ± 0.7
TF5 10 μg	49.9 ± 0.7	46.3 ± 0.3 ↓	43.3 ± 1.2 ↓	44.8 ± 1.2	45.8 ± 2.2
TF5 1 μg	50.6 ± 0.5	48.7 ± 0.6	49.2 ± 0.6	47.5 ± 0.4	45.9 ± 1.8
Saline	50.9 ± 0.5	48.3 ± 1.0	48.2 ± 0.5	46.7 ± 1.4	45.0 ± 3.5

[a] Mean ± SE. Arrow (↓) indicates statistically significant value $p < 0.05$.

TABLE 4. Effect of Thymic Hormone Treatment on the Peripheral Blood Lymphocytes (PBL × 10⁶) of C57BL/6 Mice[a]

Treatment/ Dose	(Age) Weeks				
	4	26	52	78	104
FTS 1 μg	8.8 ± 0.7	7.5 ± 0.9	10.1 ± 1.2	8.9 ± 1.9 ↑	7.4 ± 1.2
FTS 10 ng	8.3 ± 1.0	5.7 ± 0.5	10.8 ± 1.5	8.3 ± 0.8	9.0 ± 2.2
TP5 1 μg	10.6 ± 0.9	7.3 ± 0.4	7.6 ± 0.9	6.5 ± 1.1	9.2 ± 1.3
TP5 10 ng	7.7 ± 1.0 ↓	6.8 ± 0.5	8.5 ± 1.4	7.3 ± 0.5	6.9 ± 0.4
TM4 1 ng	10.8 ± 1.0	6.7 ± 0.4	9.7 ± 1.2	6.7 ± 0.4	7.2 ± 0.9
TF5 10 μg	11.1 ± 1.5	6.7 ± 0.6	9.8 ± 0.9	9.5 ± 0.6 ↑	6.5 ± 1.0
TF5 1 μg	8.5 ± 1.0	5.1 ± 1.1	10.2 ± 0.8	10.4 ± 0.7 ↑	8.1 ± 1.0
Saline	11.1 ± 1.4	6.6 ± 0.4	8.5 ± 1.1	6.1 ± 0.2	7.2 ± 1.2

[a] Mean ± SE. Arrows (↓, ↑) indicate statistically significant values $p < 0.05$.

and TP5 (10 ng) caused a decrease in 26-wk-old mice. In 52-wk-old mice FTS (10 ng), and TF5 (10 and 1 μg) increased the spleen cell number. There were no consistent patterns that reflected the progressive effect of hormone treatment with age. It appears that the hormones act differently in different age groups (age specific effects).

Effect of Hormone Treatment on Thymus Cell Numbers

Surprisingly, we recovered relatively high numbers of cells from the cohorts of different ages. The reason for this is unclear. There were isolated cases of suppression of thymus cell numbers. TF5 (10 μg) caused a decrease in 4-wk-old mice and TP5 (10 ng) and TF5 (10 μg) caused a decrease in thymus cell numbers in 78-wk-old mice (TABLE 6). The relatively high numbers of thymus cells recovered from old mice was of concern, but we do not believe this is an error in tissue selection.

Effect of Hormone Treatment on PBL and Spleen Mitogen Response

The peripheral blood lymphocyte stimulation by PHA, ConA, and LPS showed no significant difference in any of the hormone-treated groups from the saline control (data not shown). In mice in the longitudinal studies treatment with

TABLE 5. Effect of Thymic Hormone Treatment on Spleen Cell Numbers (× 10⁸ per Mouse) of C57BL/6 Mice[a]

Treatment/ Dose	(Age) Weeks				
	4	26	52	78	104
FTS 1 μg	0.76 ± 0.10	1.0 ± 0.10 ↓	1.2 ± 0.20	1.4 ± 0.20	1.1 ± 0.20
FTS 10 ng	0.67 ± 0.04	1.1 ± 0.20	1.4 ± 0.10 ↑	1.1 ± 0.02	1.2 ± 0.10
TP5 1 μg	0.86 ± 0.04	1.1 ± 0.10	1.0 ± 0.10	1.4 ± 0.20	1.8 ± 0.90
TP5 10 ng	0.78 ± 0.10	0.93 ± 0.07 ↓	1.2 ± 0.04	1.5 ± 0.20	1.4 ± 0.30
TM4 1 ng	1.1 ± 0.2 ↑	1.3 ± 0.20	1.2 ± 0.04	1.0 ± 0.10	1.5 ± 0.20
TF5 10 μg	0.92 ± 0.06	1.1 ± 0.10	1.3 ± 0.10 ↑	1.3 ± 0.10	1.4 ± 0.10
TF5 1 μg	0.74 ± 0.10	1.3 ± 0.08	1.3 ± 0.10 ↑	1.6 ± 0.30	1.8 ± 0.10
Saline	0.72 ± 0.10	1.4 ± 0.10	0.98 ± 0.06	1.3 ± 0.30	1.0 ± 0.10

[a] Mean ± SE. Arrows (↓, ↑) indicate statistically significant values $p < 0.05$.

TABLE 6. Effect of Thymic Hormone Treatment on Thymus Cell Number ($\times$ 10^6 per Mouse) of C57BL/6 Mice[a]

Treatment/ Dose	(Age) Weeks			
	4	52	78	104
FTS 1 μg	67.4 ± 10.4	56.2 ± 14.0	28.9 ± 5.1	20.6 ± 2.5
FTS 10 ng	61.6 ± 8.3	52.6 ± 10.1	30.1 ± 6.0	40.5 ± 15.5
TP5 1 μg	59.0 ± 19.8	49.2 ± 3.6	34.6 ± 6.2	22.2 ± 5.3
TP5 10 ng	85.7 ± 14.9	53.8 ± 12.2	24.3 ± 4.0 ↓	35.5 ± 6.1
TM4 1 ng	48.6 ± 11.6	63.0 ± 7.6	31.3 ± 8.1	32.4 ± 8.0
TF5 10 μg	34.2 ± 9.0 ↓	43.8 ± 4.8	25.8 ± 6.1 ↓	30.6 ± 8.9
TF5 1 μg	48.6 ± 6.1	46.4 ± 7.9	28.6 ± 3.4	28.7 ± 5.8
Saline	67.6 ± 7.4	61.4 ± 8.4	47.2 ± 2.2	25.7 ± 7.0

[a] Mean ± SE. Arrow (↓) indicates statistically significant value p <0.05.

FTS, TP5, and TF5 produced suppressive effects on the PHA, ConA, and LPS response between 54 and 80 wk. The saline control group as expected shows an age-related decline in the response to PHA by spleen cells (TABLE 7). FTS (1 μg) seems to show some effect; it elevated the PHA response in 26-wk-old mice and suppressed it in 104-wk-old mice. TM4 also suppressed the PHA response. The ConA response showed a general decline with age but there were definite differences among the cohorts of animals (TABLE 8). The ConA response was elevated in 26-wk-old mice treated with FTS (1 μg) and TP5 (1 μg) and suppressed by FTS (1 μg), TP5 (1 μg), and TF5 (10 and 1 μg) in 78-wk-old mice. The LPS response showed elevation in 4- and 52-wk-old mice treated with FTS (10 ng) (TABLE 9). The response declined in 78-wk-old mice treated with FTS (1 μg).

TABLE 10 summarizes the effect seen for the mitogen responses by the various hormones. Statistically significant responses are depicted by arrows indicating whether the response was enhanced (↑) or suppressed (↓) compared to the stimulation index for the saline control groups. Different hormones seem to enhance different responses up to 52 wk and suppress them at 78 and 104 wk. The effect of hormone treatment on the mitogen response appears sporadic and elusive. We saw no consistent or progressive effect of the hormone in the different age groups. 1) FTS seems to be consistently involved in response to PHA, ConA, and LPS. 2) The effect of the hormone treatment appears scattered among the

TABLE 7. Effect of Thymic Hormone Treatment on Spleen PHA Stimulation Index of C57BL/6 Mice[a]

Treatment/ Dose	(Age) Weeks				
	4	26	52	78	104
FTS 1 μg	44.0 ± 19.8	41.4 ± 12.6 ↑	9.8 ± 1.4	2.8 ± 0.6	1.4 ± 0.1 ↓
FTS 10 ng	35.1 ± 13.3	20.8 ± 4.1	10.4 ± 2.3	5.3 ± 0.8	2.7 ± 1.1
TP5 1 μg	30.7 ± 10.9	30.0 ± 8.1	7.7 ± 2.1	4.8 ± 0.8	2.5 ± 0.5
TP5 10 ng	22.2 ± 6.3	21.9 ± 5.4	5.1 ± 1.2	6.2 ± 1.9	2.2 ± 0.2
TM4 1 ng	25.6 ± 4.3	13.1 ± 2.2	5.3 ± 0.9	9.0 ± 4.4	1.3 ± 0.2 ↓
TF5 10 μg	22.1 ± 2.0	13.5 ± 6.2	3.7 ± 0.4	2.8 ± 0.6	4.3 ± 1.0
TF5 1 μg	12.8 ± 2.9	25.1 ± 4.6	9.3 ± 1.7	3.3 ± 0.5	7.5 ± 2.4
Saline	28.4 ± 7.6	19.2 ± 5.1	7.4 ± 1.3	7.4 ± 4.7	5.7 ± 2.6

[a] Mean ± SE. Arrows (↓ , ↑) indicate statistically significant values p <0.05.

TABLE 8. Effect of Thymic Hormone Treatment on Spleen ConA Stimulation Index of C57BL/6 Mice[a]

Treatment/ Dose	(Age) Weeks				
	4	26	52	78	104
FTS 1 μg	150.0 ± 24.2	49.8 ± 13.6 ↑	26.8 ± 3.3	1.5 ± 0.3 ↓	2.6 ± 0.7
FTS 10 ng	155.3 ± 23.7	19.0 ± 4.4	23.9 ± 8.8	5.7 ± 0.8	10.5 ± 3.2
TP5 1 μg	161.7 ± 39.7	22.2 ± 6.7 ↑	18.1 ± 4.3	2.6 ± 0.7 ↓	9.7 ± 6.3
TP5 10 ng	88.8 ± 12.6	16.0 ± 5.1	29.7 ± 8.2	5.7 ± 1.4	6.9 ± 1.9
TM4 1 ng	130.2 ± 7.9	7.0 ± 0.8	22.1 ± 6.5	6.0 ± 1.8	4.4 ± 1.3
TF5 10 μg	110.8 ± 6.4	4.8 ± 2.3	10.6 ± 2.7	2.5 ± 0.3 ↓	7.6 ± 3.4
TF5 1 μg	61.6 ± 4.4	13.8 ± 3.5	19.6 ± 2.2	2.4 ± 0.7 ↓	6.7 ± 2.1
Saline	103.3 ± 10.8	10.9 ± 3.5	21.0 ± 4.5	7.1 ± 2.18	5.7 ± 2.1

[a] Mean ± SE. Arrows (↓, ↑) indicate statistically significant values $p < 0.05$.

different groups; even when selected for those that showed some activity there remained large gaps among the age groups where no effect was seen. 3) There was a tendency to enhance response in younger mice and suppress it in older mice. And 4) at no time was restoration seen of T-cell response to PHA or ConA in 78- or 104-wk-old animals.

Effect of Hormone on IgM Hemolysin Autoantibody

The hormonal effect on IgM autoantibody seems to be the most consistent of all of the data observed. In mice treated with thymic hormones, the IgM hemolysin autoantibody titer as measured in optical density of hemoglobin released had a tendency to be elevated over the saline control groups (compare 4-wk-old vs 52- and 78-wk-old mice, TABLE 11). Treatment of the different age animals for a period of 3 wk showed elevation of autoantibodies by FTS, TP5, and TF5. While hemolytic antibodies were significantly elevated in some of these groups, loss of red blood cells as measured by the hematocrit was significantly lower only in the 26- and 52-wk-old groups treated with TF5 (10 μg). Thymic hormone treatment appears to provoke the early appearance of IgM hemolytic antibodies to erythrocytes. These results were partially confirmed in mice on the longitudinal studies.

TABLE 9. Effect of Thymic Hormone Treatment on Spleen LPS Stimulation Index of C57BL/6 Mice[a]

Treatment/ Dose	(Age) Weeks				
	4	26	52	78	104
FTS 1 μg	48.7 ± 10.4	41.2 ± 5.4	23.3 ± 1.8	12.0 ± 1.0 ↓	13.2 ± 1.1
FTS 10 ng	62.9 ± 7.9 ↑	36.4 ± 2.3	25.1 ± 2.1 ↑	22.1 ± 4.7	16.4 ± 1.8
TP5 1 μg	58.1 ± 15.4	32.8 ± 11.0	22.0 ± 2.1	22.5 ± 4.0	15.1 ± 3.1
TP5 10 ng	43.0 ± 2.9	39.4 ± 5.6	20.2 ± 2.7	22.5 ± 4.0	16.4 ± 2.7
TM4 1 ng	46.8 ± 2.0	40.9 ± 7.6	23.0 ± 1.6	28.5 ± 6.2	13.3 ± 1.6
TF5 10 μg	36.7 ± 2.6	44.8 ± 9.2	14.1 ± 1.0	15.1 ± 2.6	12.5 ± 2.4
TF5 1 μg	33.4 ± 5.4	45.9 ± 2.6	22.7 ± 3.2	21.0 ± 5.2	18.5 ± 2.4
Saline	38.9 ± 3.6	40.9 ± 5.4	19.1 ± 1.5	25.4 ± 7.0	12.1 ± 3.1

[a] Mean ± SE. Arrows (↓, ↑) indicate statistically significant values $p < 0.05$.

TABLE 10. Effect of Thymic Hormone on Spleen Mitogen Response (SI)

Treatment/		(Age) Weeks				
	Dose	4	26	52	78	104
Spleen	FTS 1 μg	—	↑	—	—	↓
PHA	TM4 1 ng	—	—	—	—	↓
	Saline	28.4 ± 7.6	19.2 ± 5.0	7.4 ± 1.2	7.3 ± 4.7	5.2 ± 2.5(SE)
Spleen	FTS 1 μg	—	↑	—	↓	—
ConA	TP5 1 μg	—	↑	—	↓	—
	TF5 10 μg	—	—	—	↓	—
	TF5 1 μg	—	—	—	↓	—
	Saline	103.3 ± 10.8	10.9 ± 3.5	21.0 ± 4.5	7.1 ± 4.8	5.7 ± 4.6
Spleen	FTS 1 μg	—	—	—	↓	—
LPS	FTS 10 ng	↑	—	↑	—	—
Spleen						
Saline	Saline	38.9 ± 7.9	40.9 ± 12.1	19.1 ± 3.2	25.4 ± 15	12.1 ± 7.0

FTS, TP5, and TF5 generally caused elevation of IgM hemolysin autoantibodies between 40 and 80 wk.

Effect of Hormone Treatment on CTL Activity

Cross-sectional studies for CTL activity were carried out on a separate cohort of animals. Mice of ages 4, 26, 52, 78, and 104 wk were brought into our facilities. After a 1-wk adjustment period mice were treated with the different doses of hormones 5×/wk, ip for 3 wk. During the hormone treatment, 10 days prior to assay (day 11 post onset of hormone treatment) mice were immunized with 8 × 10^7 P-815 cells and sacrificed on day 21 (2 days after the last treatment) and assayed for spleen cell mediated target cell cytotoxicity at E : T ratios of 200 : 1, 100 : 1, 50 : 1, and 25 : 1. There were 5 animals/group, each animal was assayed individually. TABLE 12 shows CTL activity at 200 : 1 E : T ratio only. The 78-wk cohort was not included because the saline control values for CTL were faulty.

In general CTL activity declined after 26 wk (see saline control). In 4-wk-old

TABLE 11. IgM Autoantibody (Hemolysin) Measured in OD Units of C57BL/6 Mice Treated with Thymic Hormone[a]

Treatment/	(Age) Weeks				
Dose	4	26	52	78	104
FTS 1 μg	0.09 ± 0.01	0.07 ± 0.02	0.16 ± 0.06	0.34 ± 0.10	0.10 ± 0.04
FTS 10 ng	0.08 ± 0.01	0.10 ± 0.04	0.12 ± 0.02	0.24 ± 0.11	0.43 ± 0.21 ↑
TP5 1 μg	0.11 ± 0.01	0.04 ± 0.02	0.23 ± 0.12	0.37 ± 0.20	0.18 ± 0.06
TP5 10 ng	0.13 ± 0.03 ↑	0.17 ± 0.07	0.21 ± 0.13	0.52 ± 0.05 ↑	0.11 ± 0.04
TM4 1 ng	0.10 ± 0.01	0.24 ± 0.05	0.22 ± 0.07	0.33 ± 0.17	0.25 ± 0.07
TF5 10 μg	0.09 ± 0.02	0.26 ± 0.08	0.59 ± 0.13 ↑	0.36 ± 0.09	0.31 ± 0.07
TF5 1 μg	0.08 ± 0.01	0.09 ± 0.05	0.21 ± 0.04	0.38 ± 0.08	0.34 ± 0.04
Saline	0.07 ± 0.01	0.15 ± 0.06	0.06 ± 0.01	0.05 ± 0.01	0.12 ± 0.03

[a] Mean ± SE. Arrow (↑) indicates statistically significant value $p < 0.04$.

mice TP5 (10 ng) enhanced CTL activity whereas TM4 (1 ng) suppressed it. TF5 (1 μg) suppressed it at 26 wk, FTS (1 μg) suppressed it at 26 and 52 wk, and TP5 (1 μg) and TF5 (10 μg) suppressed it at 104 wk. Some of the thymic hormone treatment had a strong tendency to suppress CTL generation over the saline control group, but this effect was not consistently observed for all of the hormones over all age groups. Thymic hormone treatment did not prevent the age-related decline in CTL activity, nor did the treatment restore CTL activity to the levels seen in young mice.

TABLE 12. Cytotoxic Lymphocyte Activity (E : T Ratio 200 : 1) in C57BL/6 Mice Treated with Thymic Hormone[a]

Treatment/	(Age) Weeks			
Dose	4	26	52	104
FTS 1 μg	61.0 ± 7.7	23.3 ± 8.5 ↓	16.1 ± 8.3 ↓	18.4 ± 4.9
FTS 10 ng	61.1 ± 15.7	39.4 ± 13.1	29.3 ± 10.0	28.1 ± 8.1
TP5 1 μg	61.0 ± 11.5	47.6 ± 7.0	30.7 ± 9.8	5.9 ± 6.0 ↓
TP5 10 ng	65.7 ± 9.7 ↑	48.8 ± 14.2	37.7 ± 12.8	23.7 ± 5.5
TM4 1 ng	27.2 ± 6.4 ↓	64.8 ± 5.7	49.1 ± 6.0	32.4 ± 9.7
TF5 10 μg	42.2 ± 15.3	41.6 ± 13.6	29.7 ± 12.2	6.9 ± 6.5 ↓
TF5 1 μg	43.1 ± 13.8	29.5 ± 13.8 ↓	27.3 ± 11.4	31.7 ± 4.5
Saline	48.6 ± 11.0	51.3 ± 9.5	31.1 ± 10.4	22.3 ± 11.2

[a] Mean ± SD. Arrows (↓ , ↑) indicate statistically significant values $p \leq 0.04$.

DISCUSSION

FTS is a thymic hormone purified from pig blood.[24] It is present in man,[24,25] and in normal but not in thymectomized mice,[26] and can induce differentiation of thymocytes through induction of cAMP.[25] FTS production can be upregulated by administration of prolactin or triiodothyronine (T3). Prolactin when injected daily (20–100 μg/20 g) in young or old C57BL/6 mice induced a specific increase in thymulin (FTS) synthesis and secretion. When hypoprolactinemia was induced in mice with bromocriptin (100–200 μg/20 g), a dopamine receptor agonist that inhibits pituitary PRL secretion, a significant decrease in thymulin secretion occurred.[27]

Fabris *et al.*[28] have shown that there is a positive correlation between plasma thymulin levels and serum thyroid hormone T3 but not T4 concentrations. Low serum thyroid hormone concentrations are frequently found in premature newborn infants, and administration of T3 caused a significant increase in thymulin. In addition to prolactin and T3, zinc (Zn) is important in regulating thymus growth and thymulin activity. The activity of thymulin is dependent on the presence of zinc in the molecule. Oral treatment with Zn increased both total and Zn bound thymulin and reversed the age-related dimunition of thymic activity in patients with chronic renal failure.[29] When mild Zn deficiency was induced in man, an increase in cells lacking in T-cell markers and SIg⁻ cells occurred with a concomitant decrease in T4/T8 ratio, and decrease in IL-2 activity. Administration of Zn corrected all of these changes.[30]

The effect of thymus gland on wound healing has also been tested. FTS and TP5 were injected (1 μg/day/IM) daily into euthymic and nude athymic mice in which a dorsal skin incision was made. Both thymic hormones impaired wound-breaking strength and reparative collagen synthesis in normal and athymic mice. The thymus has an inhibitory effect on wound healing.[31] On the other hand, in rheumatoid arthritis, treatment with 5 mg/day produced significant clinical improvement, but the beneficial effects were not associated with clear changes in immunological parameters.[32] Therefore, the effects of hormone treatment are not consistently predictable or reproducible. Hormone treatment may or may not cause measurable changes in immune parameters. In other studies occasionally conflicting results are observed. For example, thymulin levels were reported to be in the normal range in all children with allergic asthma.[34] These results are not in agreement with the low thymulin activity reported by Garaci et al.[33] The reason for this difference is not clear as both studies used similar populations and the same bioassays for testing.

Thymosin acting through the neuroendocrine circuits might cause the release of prolactin and growth hormone from the anterior pituitary.[35] This suggests that thymosin may act in concert with FTS. It appears clear that thymic hormones not only act through the neuroendocrine circuit but are also modulated by the neuroendocrine network, i.e., by the pituitary, thyroid, adrenals and gonads.[36]

Thymosin fraction 5, a fetal calf thymus extract, is one of several immunorestorative agents that has received widespread attention. Its immunorestorative[37] and antitumor activity in animal models[38,39] has been demonstrated. Thymosin was shown to improve cellular immune response in children with thymic deficiencies[40] and to increase the absolute T-cell count in cancer patients.[41] Thymosin fraction 5 consists of 40–60 peptides which vary in molecular weight from 1,000 to 15,000 and may be mixtures of potential antagonists. In some trials TF5 has been combined with cytotoxic agents or steroids. Such agents may kill or affect lymphocyte function and response to the thymic hormone. Because of the heterogeneity of TF5 it is not always clear what response it might elicit in different test models. TF5 has been shown to enhance spontaneous NK cell activity. In mitogen-stimulated large granular lymphocytes, TF5 enhanced IL-2 production, IL-2 receptor expression, and γIFN production. Thymosin α1, a synthetic polypeptide of 28 amino acid residues, originally isolated in its native form from TF5, also exhibited enhancing effects on LGL activities suggestive that it is the active species in TF5. TF5 presumably regulates NK cell activity through the induction of lymphokine production and expression of receptors in lymphoid populations.[42]

While thymosin appears to be effective in restoring cellular immunity[43–45] and resistance to some animal neoplasm,[39,46,47] it can also induce suppressor cells and may be useful in certain autoimmune diseases.[48] However, a danger with using thymosin concerns the possibility that administration of thymosin to immunocompetent animals could activate T-cells with suppressor activity. In this regard administration of thymosin (40 mg/m^2) to immunocompetent melanoma patients initiated relapses earlier than in patients that were immunoincompetent. Therefore, thymosin may have detrimental effects in immunocompetent patients and beneficial effects in immunoincompetent patients.[49] On the other hand, in one report TF5 with combination chemotherapy prolonged survival of patients with small-cell lung cancer.[50] However, more recently a randomized trial of thymosin fraction 5 (60 mg/m^2 s.c. twice weekly) given during induction chemotherapy and radiation therapy was performed in 91 patients with small cell carcinoma of the lung by Sher et al.[51] A comparison of the thymosin vs no thymosin treated patients revealed no difference in the response rate, response duration, or survival whether analyzed as a whole or by extent of disease. An analysis based on pretreatment immune function and total white blood cell and absolute lymphocyte count revealed no difference in the survival distributions. The addition of thymosin fraction 5 during induction chemotherapy and consolidation radiotherapy produced no beneficial effects.

Thymic hormone production declines with age, and recent strategies for enhancing immune function in elderly people include the administration of various thymic preparations. In *Macaca Mulatta* aged 18–25 years, a 7-day course of either thymosin α1 or placebo was given and *in vivo* immunologic analyses were performed. The relative percentage of T-cells and T-cell subsets declined during treatment in both the thymosin and placebo group. The mitogen-induced proliferation and NK-cell function were increased in most monkeys that received thymosin, a trend that was apparent but not statistically significant. The antibody response to tetanus toxoid vaccine was not any greater in the thymosin compared to the placebo group.[52] Contrarily, in elderly men aged 77 years and older thymosin α1 treatment augmented the influenza antibody response.[53]

Injection of old mice with thymosin α1 increases the frequency of T-cell precursors. A single ip injection of thymosin α1 increased the frequency of response T-lymphocytes in old (19–20-m-old) but not young (3-m-old) mice. In the old immunodeficient mice the peptide amplified the pool of mitogen-responsive and IL-2-producing T-cells.[54] Similarly, a reduction of responsiveness of thymocytes to PHA during bladder tumor induction was restored when the lymphocytes were preincubated with TF5 *in vitro*.[55]

Primus *et al.*[56] have reported that thymosin could not restore the mitogen response of spleen cells and tumor allograft rejection in adult thymectomized mice. Martinez *et al.*[57] also reported that thymopoietin, ubiquitin, and FTS, all of which induce T-cell markers on lymphocytes, failed to restore either resistance to Ib leukemia or responses to PHA or ConA in T-cell-deficient C58 mice.

It is becoming apparent that animal models must be developed which can assess in reproducible fashion the activity of thymic hormones. It may be that in many instances the models being used are not optimal for showing the activity of these preparations. Ohta *et al.*[58] have tested for the restoration of cell-mediated immunity by thymosin fraction 5 and thymosin α1 in 5-FU-immunosuppressed mice. In this animal model, delayed footpad reactions (DTH) against nucleated chicken rbc is assessed. Thymosin α1 peptide showed activity at a low dose of 5–50 μg/kg which was 100–1000 times less than that required for TF5. Thymosin showed no enhancing effect on the DTH response in normal mice without 5-FU injection; therefore, immunosuppression was a necessary condition for demonstrating thymosin effect. In addition, thymosin α1 or TF5 activity was not readily measurable in 5-FU immunosuppressed young animals as in immunosuppressed mature animals. In a separate study C3H mice receiving 1200 rad (12 Gy) of head and neck irradiation showed significant depression of delayed-type hypersensitivity, peripheral blood lymphocyte counts, spleen cell counts, and spleen cell production of IL-2. Treatment with optimal dosages of thymosin α1 produced significant increases in all these values, in some instances to levels higher than in the nonirradiated controls. Importantly, the dose response of thymosin α1 showed only a limited dose range for immune restoration.[59] Above or below the critical dose the hormone had no effect. Therefore, the optimum dose of the hormone for each age group could be different; this might be why we observe only sporadic age-specific effects. Moreover, normal mice might not be the best model in which to assess the effects of hormone treatment.

TP5 is a synthetic pentapeptide that contains the biological function of the 49 amino acid thymic hormone thymopoietin. Goldstein and Hoffmann[60] showed thymic extracts could delay impairment of neuromuscular transmission as measured by electromyographic techniques. Using this assay to monitor the purification of thymus extracts, Goldstein[61] isolated thymopoietin I and II from bovine thymus. From their amino acid sequence,[62,63] it was determined that a synthetic pentapeptide corresponding to residues 32–36 in both thymopoietin I and II reproduced the biological activity of thymopoietin.[64] TP5 has been used *in vitro* and *in vivo* to study the effects of thymopoietin.[65] Thymopoietin is rapidly degraded by proteolytic enzyme present in the plasma[66] and can be degraded by human lymphocytes into two main fragments, the tetrapeptide Lys-Asp-Val-Tyr and the tripeptide Asp-Val-Tyr.[67] Despite this degradation it appears to have long-lived effects presumably by triggering long-lived cascades.[68] Thymopoietin like the other thymic hormones affects the development and regulation of the immune system and has been shown to induce phenotypic differentiation of T-cells,[69–71] and functional maturation of suppressor[72] and helper cells.[73] TP5 *in vitro* and *in vivo* enhanced the frequency of cytotoxic lymphocyte precursor units (CLP-U), but this effect was detected only under conditions where antigenic stimulation was suboptimal. TP5 in higher amounts *in vitro* and *in vivo* suppressed the development of CLP-U.[74,75] TP5 can also inhibit B-cell phenotype differentiation.[70] Thymopoietin has been used extensively in clinical trials to modulate immunity in various diseases in man. In DiGeorge syndrome, TP5 treatment elevated E rossettes, and lymphocyte response to PHA was restored to normal[76] or remained suppressed.[77] TP5 treatment improved NK cell activity and increased the number of T-cells in a patient with severe combined immunodeficiency,[78] suppressed clinical manifestation of rheumatoid arthritis,[79,80] and restored the impaired lymphocyte stimulation in the elderly.[81]

TP5 treatment has been extended to other clinical situations where immune deficits occur. Impaired immunologic reactivity following major surgery is an important consideration in the elderly who are subject to severe opportunistic infections. Treatment with TP5 before or before and after surgery induced improvements in the impaired postoperative *in vitro* lymphocyte proliferation and the *in vivo* DTH responses. IL-2 synthesis remained impaired regardless of whether patients were treated with TP5.[82]

A randomized double-blind study has been done in 24 burned patients to see if TP5 (50 mg daily for 2 wk) can correct postburn immunologic abnormalities and prevent infectious morbidity and mortality. The burned patients were evaluated for WBC counts, T4/T8 ratios, lymphocyte blastogenesis, and neutrophil bactericidal index. There were no differences noted in patient mortality or infectious complications. TP5 treatment caused a decrease in the lymphocyte blastogenic response two weeks after the injury with no change in the T4/T8 ratios, and less leukopenia during the first week after injury.[83]

Long-term thymopentin treatment in patients with HIV-induced lymphadenopathy syndrome has been initiated to correct immunologic derangement caused by this infection. Patients with HIV infection secrete larger amounts of immunoglobulin with reduction of polyclonal Ig synthesis after stimulation with PWM. A decrease in thymic hormone levels with defect in T-cell maturation have been observed. In patients under long-term treatment there was a general though variable increase in the number of T4 from 300 cells/mm³ to 500 cells/mm³ with reduction in T8 cells from 600 cells/mm³ to about 400 cells/mm³. PWM which stimulates normal cells to secrete Ig, reduces Ig secretion by B-cells obtained from patients with HIV infections. PWM stimulation from patients with lymphadenopathy syndrome who received treatment with TP5 resulted in synthesis of both IgA and IgM that were significantly greater than those measured before therapy. Transitory disappearance of symptoms such as weight loss, diarrhea, and night sweats occurred in some receiving treatment. The increase in T4-cells suggests maturation under the influence of thymopentin and the important changes in Ig isotype expression with PWM indicate restoration of T helper functional activity on B-cells.[84]

An attempt was made to simultaneously compare the effects of FTS, TF5, and TP5 in normal C57BL/6, CFW, and A/HeN strains of mice in longitudinal fashion in a study sponsored by the National Institute on Aging. It was clearly evident that the different thymic hormones altered immune parameters in mice. However, the hormones did not always produce the same effects in different strains of mice. The effects were age specific in that hormone treatment did not consistently produce the same results in all age groups tested. While an age-related decline in immune parameters occurred, hormonal treatment did not restore immune activity of old mice to the level of young mice, nor did it increase the maximum life span of the animal. As expected there was a difference in response for short-term vs long-term (lifetime) treatment with hormones.[85] In retrospect, one major concern which is often not considered is the effect of "stress" which is inherent in the treatment protocol. Exposure of the animals to repeated injections and how handling might alter the animals' response to hormonal effects is unknown.

One of the criteria used to classify materials as thymic hormones has been their capacity to induce T-cell surface markers on lymphocytes. The induction of surface markers does not necessarily reflect functional maturation of the T-cell, since many unrelated substances including non-thymic tissue extracts, ubiquitin, poly A : U, endotoxin, prolactin, glucagon, prostaglandin E and histamine, all have the ability to induce the same cell surface markers.[86–88] The activities of FTS, TP5, and thymosin have been evaluated in various types of *in vivo* and *in vitro* immunological assay systems. However, most of these assays are complicated and are influenced by a number of factors, the results are variable and often conflicting, and both the identity and the mechanism of action of various factors that might possibly be ascribed to the thymus still remain uncertain.

The effect of hormone treatment in disease is not always clear cut. In some cases hormone treatment causes measurable changes in immune parameters. In other cases beneficial effects occur with no apparent changes in immune parameters. Currently hormone therapy is being used for almost any situation where immunodeficiency is noted, and there are sufficient variations in the protocols such that reported results have not always been easily duplicated. The time is long overdue for an active working group to 1) redefine goals and specific objectives for hormone therapy; 2) determine the state of the art of hormone therapy; 3) evaluate current methods of testing hormones; 4) review the results of hormone therapy in mice and man and resolve conflicting results seen for different models; and 5) determine what advances must be made for this mode of treatment to be made successful.

SUMMARY

Immunosenescence occurs with aging, which is seen in decline in response to mitogens PHA, ConA, decline in cell-mediated immunity, increase in anemia, and increase in autoimmune antibodies to erythrocytes and DNA. These studies compared FTS, TP5, TM4, and TF5 in C57BL/6NNia mice. Mice aged 4, 26, 52, 78 and 104 wk were treated with various hormones 5×/wk for 3 wk and monitored for hormonal effects on weight; hematocrit; peripheral blood, spleen, and thymic cell numbers; spleen and peripheral blood cell mitogen responses to PHA, ConA, LPS; IgM hemolysin autoantibody; and cell-mediated cytotoxicity to P815 allogenic cells. Hormone treatments altered mitogen responses, enhanced IgM hemolysin autoantibody production, and modulated cell-mediated immune responses. The effects were not consistent for every hormone. There was a tendency for enhancement in younger mice and suppression in older animals. Treatment with FTS showed the greatest changes in either enhancing or suppressing the different parameters measured. The hormonal effects appeared to be age specific in that certain activities were altered for certain age groups but not in others. Hormone treatment did not restore any immune parameters in old mice to the level of young animals. In general, the different hormones did not consistently produce the same effects in C57BL/6NNia mice of different age groups. Even though all animals received from National Institutes on Aging (NIA) animal models program were held under strictly controlled conditions, intrinsic variations between cohorts of different ages are difficult to control. Cohorts of aging animals tested at different times might be intrinsically different. This inherent variability in the cohorts could affect the range of activity, specificity and reproducibility of hormone effects *in vivo*. Most importantly, it should be emphasized that cross-sectional data identifies age differences rather than age changes. There is no assurance that age changes in any individual or in all subpopulations follow this pattern. In our studies only healthy animals were used. Old, sick, or tumor-bearing animals were culled out prior to being sent to us. Therefore, the 78- and 104-wk-old mice represent selected healthy cohorts. The age changes that take place can be answered only from repeated measurements made in the same individual over time.

REFERENCES

1. BOYD, E. 1932. Am. J. Dis. Child **43:** 1162–1214.
2. ANDREW, W. 1952. *In* Cellular Changes With Age. C. C. Thomas, Ed. 3–74. C. Thomas. Springfield, IL.
3. SANTISTEBAN, G. A. 1960. Anat. Rec. **136:** 117–126.
4. MAKINODAN, T. & M. M. B. KAY. 1980. Adv. Immunol. **29:** 287–330.
5. McCAY, C. M., M. F. CROWELL & L. A. MAYNARD. 1935. J. Nutr. **10:** 63–79.
6. ROSS, M. H. 1961. J. Nutr. **75:** 197–210.
7. CHENEY, K. E., R. K. LIU, G. S. SMITH, R. E. LEUNG, M. R. MICKEY & R. L. WALFORD. 1980. Exp. Gerontol. **15:** 237–258.
8. BERG, B. N. & H. S. SIMMS. 1960. J. Nutr. **71:** 255–263.
9. ROSS, M. H. & G. BRAS. 1971. J. Natl. Cancer Inst. **47:** 1095–1113.
10. FERNANDES, G., E. J. YUNIS & R. A. GOOD. 1976. Nature (London) **263:** 504–507.
11. WEINDRUCH R. & R. L. WALFORD. 1982. Science **215:** 1415–1418.
12. GOLDSTEIN, A. L., A. GUHA, M. M. ZATZ, A. HARDY & A. WHITE. 1972. Proc. Natl. Acad. Sci. USA **69:** 1800–1803.
13. SCHEINBERG, M. A., A. L. GOLDSTEIN & E. S. CATHCART. J. Immunol. **116:** 156–158.
14. LAU, C. & G. GOLDSTEIN. 1980. J. Immunol. **124:** 1861–1865.
15. WEKSLER, M. W., J. B. INNES & G. GOLDSTEIN. 1978. J. Exp. Med. **148:** 996–1006.
16. BACH, J. F., M. DARDENNE & J. C. SALOMON. 1973. Clin. Exp. Immunol. **14:** 247–256.
17. BACH, M. A. & P. NIAUDET. 1976. J. Immunol. **117:** 760–764.
18. SCHEID, M. P., M. K. HOFFMANN, K. KOMURO, U. HÄMMERLING, J. ABBOTT, E. A. BOYSE, G. H. COHEN, J. A. HOOPER, R. S. SCHULOF & A. L. GOLDSTEIN. 1979. J. Exp. Med. **138:** 1027–1032.
19. BASCH, R. S. & G. GOLDSTEIN. 1974. Proc. Natl. Acad. Sci. USA **71:** 1474–1478.
20. DARDENNE, M., J. CHARREIRE & J. F. BACH. Cell. Immunol. **39:** 47–54.

21. WALFORD, R. L. 1969. The Immunologic Theory of Aging. 104–111. Munksgaard. Copenhagen.
22. LORD, E. M. & R. W. DUTTON. 1975. J. Immunol. **115:** 1199–1205.
23. HIRAMOTO, R. N., V. K. GHANTA & S-J. SOONG. 1977. Cancer Res. **37:** 365–368.
24. BACH, J. F., M. DARDENNE, J. M. PLEAU & M. A. BACH. 1975. Ann. N.Y. Acad. Sci. **249:** 186–210.
25. ASTALDI, A., G. C. B. ASTALDI, P. THA SCHELLEKENS & V. P. EIJSVOOGEL. 1976. Nature (London) **260:** 713–715.
26. BACH, J. F. & M. DARDENNE. 1972. Transplant. Proc. **4:** 345–350.
27. DARDENNE, M., W. SAVINO, M. C. GAGNERAULT, T. ITOH & J. F. BACH. 1989. Endocrinology **125:** 3–12.
28. FABRIS, N., E. MOCCHEGIANI, S. MARIOTTI, G. CARAMIA, T. BRACCILI, F. PACINI & A. PINCHERA. 1987. J. Clin. Endocrinol. Metab. **65:** 247–252.
29. TRAVAGLINI, P., P. MORIONDO, E. TOGIN, P. VENEGONI, D. BOCHICCHIO, A. CONTI, G. AMBROSO, C. PONTICELLI, E. MOCCHEGRANI & N. FABRIS. 1989. J. Clin. Endocrinol. Metab. **68:** 186–190.
30. PRASAD, A. S., S. MEFTAH, J. ABDALLAH, J. KAPLAN, G. J. BREWER, J. F. BACH & M. DARDENNE. 1988. J. Clin. Invest. **82:** 1202–1210.
31. BARBUL, A., T. SHAWE, H. L. FRANKEL, J. E. EFRON & H. L. WASSERKRUG. Surgery **106:** 373–376.
32. AMOR, B., M. DOUGADOS, C. MERY, M. DARDENNE & J. F. BADI. 1987. Ann. Rheum. Dis. **46:** 549–554.
33. GARACI, E., R. RONCHETTI, V. DEL GROBBO, G. TRAMULTOLI, C. RINALDI-GARACI & C. IMPERATO. 1978. J. Allergy Clin. Immunol. **62:** 357–362.
34. LURIE, A., M. CHAUSSAIN, F. RAYNAUD, G. deMONTIS, G. STRAUCH, A. LOCKHART, J. MARSAC & M. DARDENNE. 1989. J. Allergy Clin. Immunol. **84:** 386–390.
35. SPANGELO, B. L., A. M. JUDD, P. C. ROSS, I. S. LOGIN, W. D. JARVIS, M. BADAMCHIAN, A. L. GOLDSTEIN & R. M. MACLEOD. 1987. Endocrinology **121:** 2035–2043.
36. HALL, N. R., J. P. McGILLIS, B. L. SPANGELO & A. L. GOLDSTEIN. 1985. J. Immunol. **135:** 806s–811s.
37. GOLDSTEIN, A. L., G. B. THURMAN, J. L. ROSSIO & J. J. COSTANZI. 1977. Transplant. Proc. **9:** 1141–1144.
38. HARDY, M. A., M. ZISBLATT, M. LEVINE, A. L. GOLDSTEIN, F. LILLY & A. WHITE. 1971. Transplant. Proc. **3:** 926–928.
39. KHAW, B. A. & A. H. RULE. 1973. Br. J. Cancer **28:** 288–292.
40. WARA, D. W., A. L. GOLDSTEIN, N. E. DOYLE & A. J. AMMANN. 1975. N. Engl. J. Med. **292:** 70–74.
41. GOLDSTEIN, A. L., G. H. COHEN, J. L. ROSSIO, G. B. THURMAN, C. N. BROWN & J. T. ULRICH. 1976. Med. Clin. North Am. **60:** 591–606.
42. SERRATE, S. A., R. S. SCHULOF, L. LEONDARIDIS, A. L. GOLDSTEIN & M. B. SZTEIN. 1987. J. Immunol. **139**(7): 2338–2343.
43. ASANUMA, Y., A. L. GOLDSTEIN & A. WHITE. 1970. Endocrinol. **86:** 600–606.
44. THURMAN, G. B., J. L. ROSSIO & A. L. GOLDSTEIN. 1977. *In* Regulatory Mechanisms in Lymphocyte Activation. D. O. Lucas, Ed. 629–631. Academic Press. New York.
45. DAUPHINEE, M. J., N. TALAL, A. L. GOLDSTEIN & A. WHITE. 1974. Proc. Natl. Acad. Sci. USA **71:** 2637–2641.
46. FORGER, J. M. III & J. CERNY. 1976. Cancer Res. **36:** 2048–2052.
47. ZISBLATT, M., A. L. GOLDSTEIN, F. LILLY & A. WHITE. 1970. Proc. Natl. Acad. Sci. USA **66:** 1170–1174.
48. HOROWITZ, S., W. BORCHERDING, A. V. MOORTHY, R. CHESNEY, H. SCHULTE-WISSERMAN, R. HONG & A. GOLDSTEIN. 1977. Science **197:** 999–1001.
49. PATT, Y. Z., E. M. HERSH, L. A. SCHAFER, T. L. SMITH, M. A. BURGESS, J. U. GUTTERMAN, A. L. GOLDSTEIN, & G. M. MAVLIGIT. 1979. Cancer Immunol. Immunother. **7:** 131–136.
50. COHN, M. H., P. B. CHRETIEN, D. C. IHDE, B. E. FOSSIECK, R. MAKUCH, P. A. BUNN, A. V. JOHNSTON *et al.* 1979. J. Am. Med. Assoc. **241:** 1813–1815.
51. SCHER, H. I., B. SHANK, R. CHAPMAN, N. GELLER, C. PINSKY, R. GRALLA,

D. KELSEN, G. BOSL, R. GOLBEY, G. PETRONI *et al.* 1988. Cancer Res. **48:** 1663–1670.
52. ESHLER, W. B., C. L. COE, N. LAUGHLIN, R. G. KLOPP, S. GRAVENSTEIN, E. B. ROECKER & K. T. SCHULTZ. 1988. J. Gerontol. **43:** 142–146.
53. GRAVENSTEIN, S., E. H. DUTHIE, B. A. MILLER, E. ROECKER, P. DRINKA, K. PRATHIPATI & W. B. ERSHLER. 1989. J. Am. Geriatr. Soc. **37**(1): 1–8.
54. FRASCA, D., L. ADORINI & G. DORIA. 1987. Eur. J. Immunol. **17**(5): 727–730.
55. WADA, S., Y. KINOSHITA, Y. OZAKI, S. NISHIO, S. KIMURA & M. MAEKAWA. 1987. J. Natl. Cancer Inst. **78:** 303–306.
56. PRIMUS, F. J., L. DEMARTINO, R. MACDONALD & H. J. HANSON. 1978. Cell. Immunol. **35:** 25–33.
57. MARTINEZ, D., A. K. FIELD, H. SCHWAM, A. A. TYTELL & M. R. HILLEMAN. 1978. Proc. Soc. Exp. Biol. Med. **159:** 195.
58. OHTA, Y., K. SUEKI, Y. YONEYAMA, E. TEZUKA & Y. YAGI. Cancer Immunol. Immunother. **15:** 108–200.
59. GRAY, W. C., B. J. HASSLINGER, C. M. SUTER, C. L. BLANCHARD, A. L. GOLDSTEIN & P. B. CHRETIEN. 1986. Arch. Otolaryngol. Head Neck Surg. **112:** 1185–1190.
60. GOLDSTEIN, G. & W. W. HOFFMAN. 1968. J. Neurol. Neurosurg. Psychiat. **31:** 453–459.
61. GOLDSTEIN, G. 1974. Nature **247:** 11–14.
62. SCHLESINGER, D. H. & G. GOLDSTEIN. Cell **5:** 319–340.
63. AUDHYA, T., D. H. SCHLESINGER & G. GOLDSTEIN. 1981. Biochem. **20:** 6195–6200.
64. GOLDSTEIN, G., M. P. SCHEID, E. A. BOYSE, D. H. SCHELSINGER & J. VAN WAUWE. 1979. Science **204:** 1309–1310.
65. GOLDSTEIN, G. & C. LAU. 1980. J. Supramol. Struct. **14:** 397–403.
66. TISCHIO, J. P., J. E. PATRICK, H. S. WEINTRAUB, M. CHASIN & G. GOLDSTEIN. 1979. Int. J. Peptide Protein Res. **14:** 479–484.
67. AMOSCATO, A. A., A. BALASUBRAMANIAM, J. W. ALEXANDER & G. F. BABCOCK. 1988. Biochem. Biophys. Acta **955:** 164–174.
68. AUDHYA, T. & G. GOLDSTEIN. 1983. Int. J. Peptide Protein Res. **22:** 187–193.
69. BASCH, R. S. & G. GOLDSTEIN. 1975. Ann. N.Y. Acad. Sci. **249:** 290–297.
70. SCHEID, M. P., G. GOLDSTEIN & E. BOYSE. 1978. J. Exp. Med. **148:** 1727–1743.
71. SCHEID, M. P., G. GOLDSTEIN & E. BOYSE. 1975. Science **190:** 1211–1213.
72. LAU, C. Y., J. A. FREESTONE & G. GOLDSTEIN. 1980. J. Immunol. **125:** 1634–1638.
73. WEKSLER, M. E., J. B. INNES & G. GOLDSTEIN. 1984. J. Exp. Med. **148:** 996–1006.
74. LAU, C. Y. & G. GOLDSTEIN. 1980. J. Immunol. **124:** 1861–1865.
75. LAU, C. Y., E. Y. WANG & G. GOLDSTEIN. 1982. Cell. Immunol. **66:** 217–232.
76. AIUTI, F., L. BUSINCO, P. ROSSI & I. QUINTI. 1980. (Letter) Lancet **1:** 91.
77. JOFFE, M. I., E. SOCHETT, J. M. PETTIFOR & A. R. RABSON. 1982. J. Clin. Lab. Immunol. **8:** 69–73.
78. FIORILLI, M., M. C. SIRIANNI, F. PANDOLFI, I. QUINTI, U. TOSTI, F. AIUTI & G. GOLDSTEIN. 1981. Clin. Exp. Immunol. **45:** 344–351.
79. VEYS, E. M., E. C. HUSKISSON, M. ROSENTHAL, T. L. VISCHER, H. MIELANTS, P. A. THROWER, J. SCOTT, H. OTT, H. SCHEIJGROND & J. SYMOEN. 1982. Ann. Rheum. Dis. **41:** 441–443.
80. KANTHARIA, B. K., N. J. GOLDING, N. D. HALL, J. DAVIES, P. J. MADDISON, P. A. BACON *et al.* 1989. Br. J. Rheumatol. **28:** 118–123.
81. VERHAEGEN, H., W. DECOCK, J. DECREE & G. GOLDSTEIN. 1981. J. Clin. Lab. Immunol. **6:** 103–105.
82. FAIST, E., W. ERTEL, B. SALMEN, A. WEILER, C. RESSEL, K. BOLLA & G. HEBERER. 1988. Arch. Surg. **123:** 1449–1453.
83. WAYMACK, J. P., M. JENKINS, B. D. WARDEN, J. SOLOMKIN, E. LAW JR., R. HAMMEL, A. MILLER & J. W. ALEXANDER. 1987. Surg. Gynecol. Obstet. **164:** 423–430.
84. SILVESTRIS, F., A. GERNONE, M. A. FRASSANITO & F. DAMMACCO. 1989. J. Lab. Clin. Med. **113:** 139–144.
85. HIRAMOTO, R. N., V. K. GHANTA & S-J. SOONG. 1987. *In* Aging and the Immune Response. E. A. Goidl, Ed. Vol. 31: 177–198. Marcel Dekker. New York.

86. GOLDSTEIN, G., M. SCHEID, U. HAMMERLING, E. A. BOYSE, D. H. SCHLESINGER & H. D. NIALL. 1975. Proc. Natl. Acad. Sci. USA **72:** 11–15.
87. SINGH, U. & J. J. T. OWEN. 1976. Eur. J. Immunol. **6:** 59–62.
88. SCHEID, M. P., G. GOLDSTEIN, U. HAMMERLING & E. A. BOYSE. 1975. Ann. N.Y. Acad. Sci. **249:** 531–538.

Pituitary-Adrenocortical and Pineal Activities in the Aged Rat

Effects of Long-Term Treatment with Acetyl-L-Carnitine

S. SCACCIANOCE, S. ALEMÀ, G. CIGLIANA,
D. NAVARRA, M. T. RAMACCI,[a] AND L. ANGELUCCI

Istituto di Farmacologia Medica 2a Cattedra
Università "La Sapienza"
Piazzale A. Moro, 2
00185 Rome, Italy

and

[a]Istituto di Ricerca sulla Senescenza
Sigma-Tau
Via Pontina, km 30.400
00040 Pomezia, Italy

INTRODUCTION

In the rat, as well as for some aspects in humans, the aging process produces modifications in pituitary-adrenocortical and pineal activities. In our studies, these modifications were assumed as markers of senescence on which the effects of a long-term treatment with acetyl-l-carnitine (ALCAR) were investigated. ALCAR, the acetylic derivative of L-carnitine is a physiological substance that plays a crucial role in the mitochondrial metabolism of fatty acids through reversible acylation of carnitine,[1] and likewise in the maintenance of the lipid structure of the neuronal cell membrane.[2]

This paper will present a broad overview of the work carried out in our laboratory on the sensitiveness of the above-mentioned markers toward ALCAR. For the sake of clarity, adrenocortical activity and pineal activity will be treated separately bearing in mind that a relationship between the two has been postulated on the basis that: (a) pinealectomy of the young rat is followed by modification in glucocorticoid hormone secretion resembling that occurring in the old one;[3] (b) melatonin has been suggested as a factor that inhibits ACTH secretion[4] and increases the sensitivity of hypothalamic glucocorticoid receptors to corticoids,[5] and (c) injurious effects of glucocorticoid can be prevented by melatonin.[6]

Effects of a Long-Term Treatment with Acetyl-L-Carnitine on Pituitary-Adrenocortical Activity in the Aged Rat

Aging in the rat is characterized by an increase in circulating levels of glucocorticoid hormone.[7-11] Elevated plasma corticosteroid levels can contribute to many phenomena, such as muscle weakening and decline in mass, osteoporosis and disruption of the immune system, all of which are associated with biological aging.

The increased activity of the hypothalamo-pituitary-adrenocortical (HPA) axis in the aged rat might be ascribed to a substantial decrease in negative hormonal feedback inhibition sensitiveness, as demonstrated by the reduced susceptibility of the aged rat to the suppressive effect of dexamethasone.[12,13] Moreover, it is unlikely that this reduced sensitivity is attributed to the pituitary. In fact, we have demonstrated that corticosterone is able to inhibit ACTH secretion from pituitaries removed from both young and old rats in the same degree.[14] The hippocampus might be the anatomical site in which the aging process produces the loss of hormonal inhibitory control. This brain area exerts an inhibitory control on the activity of the HPA axis,[15–18] and a prominent effect of corticosterone uptake by the pyramidal cells of the hippocampus is an inhibition of their spontaneous activity.[19] Several studies have reported that in the course of aging the hippocampal glucocorticoid receptors density progressively decreases.[11,20] This conspicuous loss of receptors could reduce the ability of the hippocampus to exert its inhibitory control on HPA axis. This is confirmed by the finding that in the aged rat an *in vitro* hypothalamic hyperactivity, associated with normal *in vitro* activity and reactivity of the adrenal and pituitary, was found.[14]

Although it has been reported that prolonged (3 weeks) elevation of circulating levels of corticosterone does not produce any apparent change in hippocampal glucocorticoid receptors,[21] it has been proposed that excessive glucocorticoid secretion could damage the hippocampus, either directly or indirectly.[22]

The issue of the damaging impact of glucocorticoid hormone on hippocampal neurons is complicated in that while adrenalectomy in 12-month-old rats prevents the loss of hippocampal neurons[23] typical of senescence, the absence of adrenal steroids rapidly produces a massive cell death in the granule cell layer of the dentate gyrus.[24] However, from these studies the indication emerges that a loss of hippocampal glucocorticoid receptors and an increase in adrenocortical activity are markers of senescence. Therefore, one would expect these markers to be responsive to the effect of treatments aiming to retard or ameliorate the aging process. In aged rats the activity of the HPA axis was beneficially affected by long-term treatment with ALCAR. As shown in TABLE 1, for example, plasma corticosterone level in resting conditions in the aged male Fischer 344 rats treated with ALCAR was greatly reduced in comparison to that found in controls. As previously stated, the aged HPA axis is less sensitive to the negative glucocorticoid feedback control. This was determined using the synthetic glucocorticoid dexamethasone.[12,13] However, in addition to this pharmacological test, there is a more physiological way to test the presence of a feedback inhibition. In fact, we have demonstrated[25] that the application of a psychic stressor 45 minutes after the cessation of a 90-min cold exposure does not produce any adrenocortical activation in adult rats, indicating that a negative feedback is in play. This tonic control is lost in the aged rat, but is partially preserved in rats treated with ALCAR.[26] In addition, an altered regulation of the HPA axis in the aged rat is also revealed in the increased psychic stress response, an increase that is blunted in rats undergoing long-term treatment with ALCAR.[26] This improved control of adrenocortical activity is accompanied by a reduction in the age-dependent loss of hippocampal glucocorticoid receptors, as shown in TABLE 2; brain autoradiography studies evidenced that the dentate gyrus and the CA2 region are the areas most sensitive to amelioration with ALCAR.[27] Moreover, ALCAR treatment was able to attenuate in the old rat the decrease of Nissl-reactive tigroid substance and the deposition of fluorescent aging pigments in the hippocampus.[26] Finally, one should

TABLE 1. The Effect of ALCAR (100 mg/kg/Day in Drinking Water for 8 Months) on the Activity of the HPA Axis in Aged Male Fischer 344 Rats

	Plasma Corticosterone μg/100 ml
Young (3 months)	2.43 ± 0.66
Old (24 months) control	10.36 ± 1.99[a]
Old (24 months) ALCAR	6.40 ± 0.95[a,b]

Mean value ± SEM; n = 6–9.
[a] $p < 0.001$ vs young; [b] $p < 0.05$ vs old control.

TABLE 2. The Effect of ALCAR (50 mg/kg/Day in Drinking Water for 6 Months) on ³H-Corticosterone Binding Capacity in the Hippocampus of Aged Male Sprague-Dawley Rats

	³H-B Binding Capacity fmoles/mg Protein
Young (6 months)	503.0 ± 27.2
Old (24 months) control	206.3 ± 66.7[a]
Old (24 months) ALCAR	448.4 ± 23.7

Mean value ± SEM; n = 5–12.
[a] $p < 0.05$ vs all other groups.

TABLE 3. The Effect of ALCAR (100 mg/kg/Day in Drinking Water for 8 Months) on Plasma Melatonin Levels in Aged Male Fischer 344 Rats

	Plasma Melatonin pg/ml	
	Day (1000 h)	Night (2400 h)
Young (3 months)	17.1 ± 1.3	43.2 ± 3.0
Old (24 months) control	18.7 ± 2.7	35.8 ± 1.9[a]
Old (24 months) ALCAR	18.1 ± 1.3	43.6 ± 2.4

Mean value ± SEM; n = 8–15.
[a] $p < 0.05$ vs all other groups.

TABLE 4. The Effect of ALCAR (100 mg/kg/Day in Drinking Water for 8 Months) on Pineal Melatonin Content in Aged Male Fischer 344 Rats

	Melatonin Content pg/Gland	
	Day (1000 h)	Night (2400 h)
Young (3 months)	52.7 ± 10.7	386.3 ± 57.4
Old (24 months) control	56.9 ± 8.8	197.9 ± 52.8[a]
Old (24 months) ALCAR	45.7 ± 7.2	324.9 ± 51.4

Mean value ± SEM; n = 6–12.
[a] $p < 0.05$ vs young.

expect a behavioral counterpart of the protecting effect of ALCAR on the hippocampus. This is actually occurring as indicated by the ALCAR ameliorating effect on performance in discrimination and spatial memory tests.[28,29]

Effects of a Long-Term Treatment with ALCAR on Pineal Activity in the Aged Rat

The nocturnal rise in the production of melatonin by the pineal gland, producing an increase in circulating melatonin, constitutes a signal generated in the organism by the changing in the environmental lighting cycle. In the rat,[30,31] as well as in humans,[32] a reduction in plasma and pineal melatonin levels, especially during darkness, is associated with the aging process.

The mechanisms involved in the reduction in pineal melatonin synthesis are still unknown. One proposed possibility involves the decline with age of β-adrenergic receptors on the rat pinealocyte membrane.[33] This would impair the noradrenaline stimulation, via β-receptors, of melatonin production. In addition to that, a reduction in pineal N-acetyltransferase activity, the rate limiting enzyme that N-acetylates serotonin to form melatonin,[34] has been demonstrated in the aged rat.[30]

We recently studied in the 24-month-old male Fischer 344 rat the effect produced by a long term treatment with ALCAR on plasma and pineal melatonin levels at day (1000 h) and night time (2400 h). As shown in TABLE 3, no differences were found in plasma melatonin levels during the light period between young (3 months) and old rats, while at night a reduction of about 17% was found in the old group; ALCAR treatment completely prevented this reduction. As shown in TABLE 4, the pineal melatonin content while unaffected during the light period by aging, was reduced at night. This reduction was not present in the old rats treated with ALCAR.

The mechanism by which ALCAR produces this effect remains to be studied; we propose, however, that this effect might be involved in the ability of ALCAR to retard age-dependent changes in the CNS.

REFERENCES

1. FRITZ, I. B. 1963. Carnitine and its role in fatty acid metabolism. Adv. Lipid Res. **1:** 285–334.
2. RIZZA, V., M. C. MORALE, V. GUARCELLO & F. GUERRERA. 1986. The effect of L-carnitine and acetyl-L-carnitine on lipid metabolism in rat brain. *In* Biological Psychiatry. C. Shagess, R. C. Josiassen, W. H. Bridger, K. J. Weiss, D. Stoff & G. P. Simpson, Eds. Development in Psychiatry. Vol. **7:** 1346–1348. Elsevier. New York.
3. OXENKRUG, G. F., I. M. MCINTYRE & S. GERSHON. 1984. Effects of pinealectomy and aging on the serum corticosterone circadian rhythm in rats. J. Pineal Res. **1:** 181–185.
4. WETTEMBERG, L. 1983. The relationship between the pineal gland and the pituitary adrenal axis in health, endocrine and psychiatric conditions. Psychoneuroendocrinology **8:** 75–80.
5. DILMAN, V., I. LAPIN & G. OXENKRUG. 1979. Serotonin and aging. *In* Serotonin in Health and Disease. W. Essman, Ed. Vol. **5:** 111–123. Spectrum Press. New York.
6. AOYAMA, H., W. MORI & N. MORI. 1986. Anti-glucocorticoid effects of melatonin in young rats. Acta Pathol. Jpn. **36:** 423–428.
7. LANDFIELD, P. W., D. K. SUNDBERG, M. S. SMITH, J. C. ELDRIDGE & M. MORRIS.

1980. Mammalian aging: theoretical implications of changes in brain and endocrine system during mid- and late life. Peptides **1:** 185–188.

8. WEXLER, B. C. & J. P. McMUTRY. 1983. Cushingoid pathophysiology of old, massively obese, spontaneously hypertensive rats (SHR). J. Gerontol. **38:** 148–154.

9. SAPOLSKY, R. M., L. C. KREY & B. S. McEWEN. 1983. The adrenocortical stress-response in the aged male rat: impairment of recovery from stress. Exp. Gerontol. **18:** 55–64.

10. DEKOSKY, S. T., S. W. SCHEFF & C. W. COTMAN. 1984. Elevated corticosterone levels. Neuroendocrinology **38:** 33–38.

11. ANGELUCCI, L., P. VALERI, E. GROSSI, H. D. VELDHUIS, B. BOHUS & R. DE KLOET. 1980. Involvement of hippocampal corticosterone receptors in behavioral phenomena. *In* Progress in Psychoneuroendocrinology. F. Brambilla, G. Racagni & D. De Wied, Eds. 177–185. Elsevier, New York.

12. OXENKRUG, G., M. McINTYRE, M. STANELY & S. GERSHON. 1984. Dexamethasone suppression test: experimental model in rats, and effect of age. Biol. Psychol. **19:** 413–417.

13. RIEGLE, G. & G. HESS. 1972. Chronic and acute dexamethasone suppression of stress activation of adrenal cortex in young and aged rats. Neuroendocrinology **52:** 150–155.

14. SCACCIANOCE, S., A. DI SCIULLO & L. ANGELUCCI. 1990. Age-related changes in hypothalamo-pituitary-adrenocortical axis activity in the rat. Neuroendocrinology **52:** 150–155.

15. KNIGGE, K. M. & M. HANS. 1963. Evidence of inhibitive role of hippocampus in neuronal regulation of ACTH release. Proc. Soc. Exp. Biol. Med. **114:** 67–69.

16. CASADY, R. L. & A. N. TAYLOR. 1976. Effect of electrical stimulation of the hippocampus upon corticosteroid levels in freely-behaving, non stressed rat. Neuroendocrinology **20:** 68–78.

17. SHADE J. P. 1980. The limbic system and the pituitary-adrenal axis. *In* Pituitary Adrenal and the Brain. D. De Wied & J. A. M. Weijnen, Eds. 1–11. Elsevier. Amsterdam.

18. CONFORTI, N. & S. FELDMAN. 1976. Effects of dorsal fornix section and hippocampectomy on adrenocortical response to sensory stimulation in the rat. Neuroendocrinology **22:** 1–7.

19. PFOFF, D. W., M. T. A. SILVA & J. M. WEISS. 1971. Telemetered recording of hormone effects on hippocampal neurons. Science **172:** 394–395.

20. SAPOLSKY, R., L. KREY & B. S. McEWEN. 1983. Corticosterone receptors decline in a site-specific manner in the aged rat brain. Brain Res. **289:** 235–240.

21. SPENCER, R. L. & B. S. McEWEN. 1990. Adaptation of the hypothalamic-pituitary adrenal axis to chronic ethanol stress. Neuroendocrinology **52:** 481–489.

22. SAPOLSKY, R., M. ARMANINI, D. PACKAN & G. TOMBAUGH. 1987. Stress and glucocorticoid in aging. Endocrinol. Metab. Clin. **16:** 965–980.

23. LANDFIELD, P. W., R. K. BASKIN & T. A. PITLER. 1981. Brain-aging correlates: retardation by hormonal-pharmacological treatments. Science **214:** 581–584.

24. GOULD, E., C. S. WOOLEY & B. S. McEWEN. 1990. Short-term glucocorticoid manipulations affect neuronal morphology and survival in the adult dentate gyrus. Neuroscience **37:** 367–375.

25. PATACCHIOLI, F. R., S. SCACCIANOCE & L. ANGELUCCI. 1984. Glucocorticoid and hippocampus: receptors may have found a function. Ann. Ist. Super. Sanità **20:** 119–122.

26. ANGELUCCI, L., F. R. PATACCHIOLI, G. TAGLIALATELA, S. MACCARI, M. T. RAMACCI & O. GHIRARDI. 1986. Brain glucocorticoid receptor and adrenocortical activity are sensitive markers of senescence-retarding treatments in the rat. *In* Modulation of Central and Peripheral Transmitter Function. G. Biggio, P. F. Spano, G. Toffano & G. L. Gessa, Eds. 347–352. Liviana Press. Padova.

27. PATACCHIOLI, F. R., F. AMENTA, M. T. RAMACCI, G. TAGLIALATELA, S. MACCARI & L. ANGELUCCI. 1989. Acetyl-l-carnitine reduces the age-dependent loss of glucocorticoid receptors in the rat hippocampus: an autoradiographic study. J. Neurosci. Res. **23:** 462–466.

28. GHIRARDI, O., S. MILANO, M. T. RAMACCI & L. ANGELUCCI. 1988. Effect of acetyl-l-carnitine chronic treatment on discrimination models in aged rats. Physiol. Behav. **44:** 769–773.
29. CAPRIOLI, A., O. GHIRARDI, M. T. RAMACCI & L. ANGELUCCI. 1990. Age-dependent deficits in radial maze performance in the rat: effect of chronic treatment with acetyl-l-carnitine. Prog. Neuro-Psychopharmacol. & Biol. Psychiatry **14:** 359–369.
30. REITER, R. J., C. M. CRAFT, J. E. JOHNSON, T. S. KING, B. A. RICHARDSON, G. M. VAUGHAN & M. K. VAUGHAN. 1981. Age-associated reduction in nocturnal pineal melatonin levels in female rats. Endocrinology **109:** 1295–1297.
31. LAUDON, M., I. NIR & N. ZISAPEL. 1988. Melatonin receptors in discrete brain area of the male rat: impact of aging on density and on circadian rhythmicity. Neuroendocrinology **48:** 577–583.
32. NAIR, N. P. V., N. HARIHARASUBRAMANIAN, C. PILAPIL, I. ISAAC & J. X. THAVUNDAYIL. 1986. Plasma melatonin—an index of brain aging in humans? Biol. Psychiatry **21:** 141–150.
33. GREENBERG, L. H. & B. WEISS. 1978. β-adrenergic receptors in aged rat brain. Reduced number and capacity of pineal gland to develop supersensitivity. Science **201:** 61–63.
34. AXELROD, J. 1974. The pineal gland: a neurochemical transducer. Science **184:** 1341–1348.

Phospholipase A₂ as a "Death Trigger" in the Aging Process

The Use of PLA₂ Inhibitors as Antiaging Substances[a]

W. REGELSON[a] AND R. FRANSON[b]

Departments of [a]Medicine, [a]Microbiology, Biochemistry, and
[b]Molecular Biophysics
Medical College of Virginia/Virginia Commonwealth University
P.O. Box 273
Richmond, Virginia 23298-0001

Phospholipases, particularly phospholipase A_2 (PLA_2), are key factors in the membrane hypothesis of aging.[1] In this regard, PLA_2 plays a major role in phospholipid membrane destabilization, the synthesis of inflammatory mediators, and the generation of and/or response to free radicals. PLA_2 activation, which results in membrane destruction, is triggered by inflammation, ischemia, or injury.[2] PLA_2 hydrolyzes membrane phospholipid to release free fatty acids such as arachidonate (FIG. 1). These fatty acids are further converted to inflammatory mediators such as leukotrienes and prostaglandins, and in this process, free radicals are formed which in turn can damage more phospholipid membrane to activate more PLA_2 to establish a "breeder reactor" pattern of propagated injury (see FIG. 1). In addition, the lyso derivatives released by PLA_2 action have detergent effects which can also damage cell membranes.[3]

PLA_2s active in inflammation, infection, or injury can be derived from endogenous cells or tissue (i.e., leukocytes)[2] or from exogenous sources such as infectious organisms (i.e., bacteria, or Naegleria), and insect and snake venoms (i.e., bee, scorpion and cobra venom).[4-8] Varying levels of endogenous PLA_2 are found in human cells, tissues, and fluids. As illustrated in TABLE 1, crude extracts of human polymorphonuclear leukocytes (PMNs), platelets, sperm, synovial fluid, and herniated discs have high PLA_2 activity relative to normal plasma. Elevated levels of PLA_2 are associated with the pathology of inflammation.[2,9-11]

PLA_2 is a major component of snake venoms and although other cellular-derived phospholipases can be cytotoxic (i.e., PLC and PLD),[12] PLA_2 is currently the most potent key mediator of an intrinsic cell membrane damaging system that is critical to cell injury and death. However, within homeostatic limits PLA_2 enzymes are vital to cell interaction, differentiation, and membrane-mediated nutrition or signal transduction and, thus, govern the homeostatic balance between normal cell function, injury, and death.[9]

[a] These studies could not have been conducted without the collaboration and efforts of R. S. Sohal, Ph.D., Southern Methodist University who performed the Musca domestica and cardiomyocyte studies, and Joan Smith-Sonneborn, Ph.D., University of Wyoming, for the PGBx studies in Paramecia aurelia. Their studies were conducted under contract to Phoenix Advanced Technology, Inc., Gainesville, FL, administered by Virginia Commonwealth University, Richmond, VA. Independently, some of this work was also supported by the Office of Naval Research and by the Virginia Center for Innovative Technology (Herndon, VA).

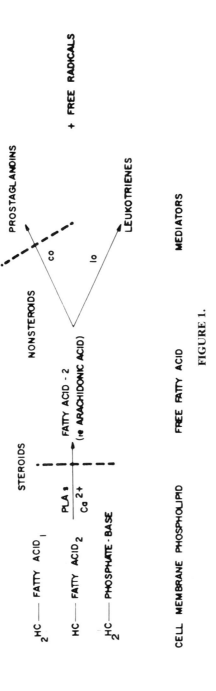

FIGURE 1.

TABLE 1. Comparison of Specific Activities of Nonpancreatic PLA$_2$s Extracted from Various Human Sources[a]

Human Source	Specific Activity (PLA$_2$)[b]
Polymorphonuclear leukocyte	3.2
Platelet	1.4
Sperm	28.0
Plasma	0.006
Synovial fluid	12.1
Mucoid ear infusion	0.3
Herniated disc	833.3

[a] These data show that extracts of human tissues, cells, and fluids have a broad range of enzyme activity. Normal plasma has the lowest specific activity while extracts of inflamed, herniated discs have the most potent Ca^{2++}-dependent and neutral-active PLA$_2$ in crude extracts described to date.

[b] Specific activity = nmol/min/mg (*E. coli* substrate).

In injury and inflammation, endogenous inhibitors such as unsaturated fatty acids, proteins, corticosteroids, and induced lipocortins, as well as other yet unidentified factors regulate the expression of PLA$_2$ activity,[2,13] thus containing or limiting the degree of membrane destruction induced by PLA$_2$s. Clinically, both corticosteroids and nonsteroidal antiinflammatory drugs (NSAIDS) inhibit PLA$_2$ and/or the further metabolism of arachidonic acid[14,15] (see FIG. 1) to relieve inflammation and limit its destructive momentum.[2,13] The importance of PLA$_2$ to aging relates not only to its ability to generate free radicals, but PLA$_2$s and other phospholipases derived from white blood cells or other endogenous cellular or exogenous infectious sources act more effectively to degrade phospholipid already oxidized by previous exposure to free radicals.[12,16]

In the search for a PLA$_2$ inhibiting agent of potential clinical value, our attention was drawn to the work instituted by Polis *et al.* of the Office of Naval Research[14,16–20] who described a prostaglandin B oligomer, PGBx, that protected dogs, cats, and rats from ischemic injury. PGBx also stabilized mitochondrial membranes against a wide range of ischemic insults and direct Ca^{++} ionophore induced swelling or dissolution.[14,21–27] Recently, we reported that PGBx was a potent inhibitor of *in vitro* and *in situ* PLA$_2$ activity.[2,13] Based upon these observations, we proposed that PGBx, as a potent PLA$_2$ inhibitor and therefore membrane stabilizer could modulate the aging process to increase functional survival. This report presents data that support our hypothesis that this potent PLA$_2$ inhibitor blocks inflammation and decreases oxidant related changes to influence aging in model systems.

PGBx

PGBx, the polymeric derivative of prostaglandin B, first synthesized by Polis, has an average molecular weight of 2400.[22,28–31] PGBx is an oil, but its sodium salt is water soluble, and it is autoclavable, filterable, and shelf stable. PGBx and PGB trimer were generously provided by Drs. George Nelson (St. Joseph's University, Philadelphia, PA) and Thomas M. Devlin (Hahnemann Medical College, Philadelphia, PA) and by the Office of Naval Research (Dr. Jeannine Majde, Arlington, VA).

Phospholipase A₂ Inhibition Assay

Phospholipase A_2 activity was measured by established methods using $[1\text{-}^{14}C]$ oleate-labelled autoclaved *Escherichia coli* as substrate.[13] PGBx inhibits calcium-dependent and neutral-active phospholipase A_2 extracted from human synovial fluid, human neutrophils, human platelets, and human sperm (not shown). The effect of the PGB1 monomer, and the base-catalyzed oligomer, PGBx, on phospholipase A_2 activity in extracts from human neutrophils is shown in FIGURE 2. PGBx, an oligomer with an average of 6 monomeric units, inhibited neutral-active and calcium-dependent phospholipase A_2 activity in a dose-dependent manner with an $ID_{50} = 5$ μM. The monomer, PGB1, inhibited activity only at concentrations greater than 10 μM. Comparable inhibitory activity was noted with PGBx as an oil, in DMSO or as a water soluble sodium salt.[2]

As reported by us,[2] PGBx also inhibits agonist-induced arachidonic acid mobilization in human PMNs and endothelial cells at concentrations equal to those inhibiting *in vitro* phospholipase A_2 activities. Thus, PGBx directly inhibited *in vitro* PLA₂s regardless of the enzyme source[13] (TABLE 1, FIG. 2) and enzyme activity was inhibited both *in vitro* and *in vivo*.

PGBx as an Antioxidant

The carbon-carbon double bonds of unsaturated fatty acids found predominantly in the 2 position of mammalian phospholipids are particularly susceptible to attack by molecular oxygen and free radicals. The fact that PGBx inhibited *in vitro* and *in situ* phospholipase activities and contains peroxidizable double bonds itself, suggested that PGBx might also influence the susceptibility of phospholipid to autooxidation. In confirmation of this, we found that PGBx protected phospholipids from autooxidation in the concentration range in which it inhibits phospholipase activity *in vitro* and *in situ*. The demonstration that PGBx is a powerful antioxidant is shown in TABLE 2, which compares the antioxidant activ-

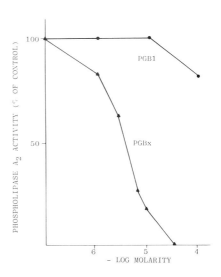

FIGURE 2. Effect of PGB1 monomer and PGBx on Ca^{2+}-dependent phospholipase A_2 extracted from human PMNs. The details of this assay have been reported previously.[13]

TABLE 2. Effect of PGBx and Na-Metabisulfite on Autooxidation of Phosphatidylethanolamine at 37°C for 24 Hours

Treatment	% Peroxidized PE	% Protection
Control	51.5	0
Control + PGBx 10 μM	29.2	23.9
Control + PGBx 100 μM	14.7	71.5
Control + NaMBS 1 mM	41.3	19.8
Control + NaMBS 5 mM	36.1	29.9

ity of PGBx with sodium metabisulfite, a widely used commercial antioxidant. In these experiments, phosphatidylethanolamine was incubated for 24 hrs at 37°C at pH 5.0 with and without PGBx or bisulfite; 51.5% of the phospholipid was peroxidized by this treatment in the absence of antioxidant. Both PGBx and bisulfite inhibited peroxidation of phospholipid, but PGBx was at least 100 times more effective as an antioxidant than bisulfite (TABLE 2); 10 μM PGBx provided 23.9% protection while 1000 μM bisulfite afforded 19.8% protection. Protection was dose related, and in similar experiments PGBx was a more effective antioxidant than vitamin E succinate.

PGBx as an Antiinflammatory Agent

In vitro and *in situ* experiments demonstrated that PGBx has a dual action. It inhibits PLA_2s (FIG. 2) and should therefore block the formation of free radicals generated as arachidonic acid is converted to oxidative metabolites, prostaglandins, hydroxy fatty acids, and leukotrienes (FIG. 1).[2,12,13] Whole animal antiinflammatory studies were done using carrageenan injected into rat limbs as an *in situ* mediator of inflammation (TABLE 3a). These results show that PGBx has antiinflammatory activity when given intraperitoneally; edema was inhibited 50% by IP administration of 1.5 mg/kg PGBx.

To test oral antiinflammatory activity, PGBx, at 10 and 60 mg/kg was delivered to the GI tract by intubation 1 hour prior to injecting human synovial PLA_2 directly into the mouse foot pad. PGBx reduced the edema in a dose-dependent manner (TABLE 3b). Similar antiinflammatory results were obtained with PGBx when cobra venom PLA_2 was used to induce paw edema. These results demonstrate that PGBx has oral antiinflammatory activity in a PLA_2-induced model of inflammation. More recent studies show that oral administration of PGBx inhibited PLA_2 in horse synovial fluid, and PGBx suppressed the acute and chronic

TABLE 3a. Antiinflammatory Activity of PGBx Using Carrageenan-Induced Rat Paw Edema

	Foot Width (mm)	% of Control
Control	4.2 (n = 10)	100
Control + carrageenan	8.7 (n = 8)	207
Control + carrageenan + PGBx[a]	6.4 (n = 5)	152

[a] PGBx (1.5 mg/kg) injected IP 1 hr prior to irritant.

TABLE 3b. Oral Antiinflammatory Activity of PGBx vs Human Synovial Fluid PLA$_2$-Induced Mouse Paw Edema[a]

Treatment Mouse Footpad	PGBx (oral)[b]	% Increased Edema[c]	% Protection
Human synovial fluid PLA$_2$	—	45.7 ± 2.1	0
Human synovial fluid PLA$_2$	10 mg/kg	35.8 ± 3.5	20
Human synovial fluid PLA$_2$	60 mg/kg	17.7 ± 2.0	61

[a] PGBx was given 1 hour prior to injection of the mouse foot pad with PLA$_2$. Edema was measured by monitoring by caliper measurement (Table IIIa) or by paw weight relative to controls (Table IIIb).
[b] Gastric intubation.
[c] Data are means ± SD, n = 6.

phases of Freund's adjuvant induced carpitis in horses. The ability of PGBx to inhibit PLA$_2$ activity *in vivo* may be important clinically because elevated levels of serum PLA$_2$ correlate with lethal prognosis related to sepsis in horses.[32]

Antiaging Activity

The above results demonstrate the clinical potential of PGBx (and related PLA$_2$ inhibitors) as effective antiinflammatory agents; properties which should contribute to cytoprotective action and may influence cell viability and life span. We, therefore, studied the potential antiaging action of PGBx.

Antioxidant Effects on Houseflies (Musca domestica)

Malonyldialdehyde (MDA), measured as thiobarbituric acid reactive substances, is an index of lipid peroxidation.[34] TABLE 4a shows that PGBx, when incubated with homogenates of whole house fly tissue at 37°C for 24 hours, inhibited MDA accumulation. In similar experiments, not reported here, PGBx also inhibited MDA production using rat liver homogenates. These studies indicate that PGBx has *in vitro* antioxidant activity and may preserve tissue homogenates.

TABLE 4a. Effect of PGBx on Lipid Peroxidation of Whole Tissue Homogenates *In Vitro* of Houseflies

PGBx (μM)	nmols MDA[a]/gm Wet Weight	% Protection
0	4.10	0
10	4.10	0
20	2.05	50
30	1.54	64
40	1.02	85

[a] MDA = malonyldialdehyde.

TABLE 4b. Effect of Feeding PGBx via Drinking Water for 15 Days on Endogenous Lipid Peroxide Content in Houseflies

Group	nmols MDA/gm Wet Weight	% Inhibition
Control	3.97 ± 0.25	—
PGBx 20 μM	2.56 ± 0.72	36%

To demonstrate *in vivo* antioxidant activity, houseflies were fed PGBx (20 μM) in sucrose-containing drinking water for 15 days and were sacrificed, and the total endogenous peroxide content was measured as MDA. A 36% reduction of MDA content was observed in the test group fed PGBx in drinking water (TABLE 4b). Thus, PGBx has both *in vitro* and *in vivo* antioxidant as well as anti-PLA$_2$ activity.

Effect on Life Span of Houseflies

TABLE 5 and FIGURE 3 show the effect of feeding graded concentrations of PGBx on the life span of male houseflies. Houseflies, like mammals, orally absorb PGBx. In these experiments, PGBx was given with sucrose in drinking water. As measured by survival, the average life span is prolonged by almost 30%, at non-toxic (20 μM) concentration of PGBx as compared to controls. Absolute survival was increased up to 9 days, or 28%. Methods regarding the evaluation of aging in houseflies have been presented by Sohal's group[33–35] who performed these studies.

Effect of PGBx on Mitochondrial Respiration

The effect of PGBx on the life span of houseflies could relate to such factors as ambient temperature[33,34,36–38] or physical activity,[35] which affect free radical generation.[33,37,38] Alternatively, it is possible that PGBx could directly or indirectly affect metabolic or motor activity via an effect on mitochondrial function, particularly since PGBx was originally reported to have profound effects on the stabilization and recovery of mammalian mitochondria to *in vitro* or ischemic injury.[14,22–27] For this reason, we examined the effects of PGBx on the functional state of mitochondria in houseflies.[34] PGBx had no influence on the rate of state 3 or state 4 mitochondrial respiration *in vivo* or *in vitro* with isolated mitochondria from 14-day-old male houseflies. There was no significant decline in total O$_2$ consump-

TABLE 5. Effect of Feeding PGBx via Drinking Water on Life Spans of Adult Male Houseflies

PGBx (μM)	Average Life Span (Days)	Maximum Life Span (Days)
0	22.1 ± 7.7	45
10	24.9 ± 5.2	47
20	29.0 ± 6.1	52
40	22.0 ± 7.6	54

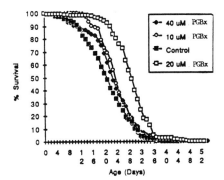

FIGURE 3. The effect of PGBx feeding at different concentrations on the percent survival over time.

tion on prolonged PGBx feeding. These preliminary studies suggest that PGBx does not act by lowering the metabolic rate, but may work through its reduction of oxidative stress.

Effect on Rat Cardiomyocytes

In an effort to demonstrate cytoprotective effects of PGBx in mammalian cells, lipofuscin accumulation, contractibility, and cell survival were studied in cardiomyocytes under increased oxygen tension. Sohal et al.[38] and Marzabadi et al.[39] have established methods to study the survival and accumulation of lipofuscin in postmitotic heart muscle cells using 3-day-old Sprague-Dawley rat myocardial cells. Using these methods, the results in TABLE 6 show that cells exposed to PGBx, at 6 days of age and 20% O$_2$, contained significantly less lipofuscin than controls. However, at 12 days no protective effect is noted. PGBx is not protective in 40% oxygen (6 days) except at the highest concentration (100 nM).

The average rate of pulsatile contraction in control myocytes in 20% oxygen, increased from 1 to 12 days of age and decreased thereafter. During 1 to 6 days of age, the rate of contraction was rhythmic but became arrhythmic thereafter. In cardiomyocytes exposed to 1 nM PGBx and 20% oxygen, the rate of contraction

TABLE 6. Effect of PGBx on Lipofuscin Accumulation in Cultured Mouse Cardiomyocytes Exposed to High Oxygen Tension

Groups	% O$_2$ Concentration	Lipofuscin Concentration (Units, ± SEM)	
		6 Days	12 Days
Control	20	161 ± 9	309 ± 19
1 nM PGBx	20	144 ± 9	296 ± 27
10 nM PGBx	20	131 ± 9	328 ± 34
100 nM PGBx	20	126 ± 8	308 ± 20
Control	40	178 ± 11	361 ± 23
1 nM PGBx	40	165 ± 12	277 ± 21
10 nM PGBx	40	170 ± 12	346 ± 21
100 nM PGBx	40	139 ± 19	350 ± 23

remained relatively steady for a longer period than in the controls, and after 15 days, cells exposed to PGBx clearly continued to show higher rates of pulsatile contraction than controls. Contraction remained rhythmic for a longer period of cardiomyocyte life span in PGBx-exposed cells than in the controls (TABLE 7).

The contractile ability of myocytes stops about 1 day before death. Relatively few cells were contractile at 21 days of age in control groups (20% oxygen), and cell death was evident in focal areas around 15 days of age. Virtually no cells were alive at 22 days of age. By contrast, in cardiomyocytes exposed to 1 nM PGBx (20% oxygen), focal areas of degeneration appeared 6 days later (at 21 days of age), and extensive cell death occurred around 23 days of age.

TABLE 7. Effect of PGBx on the Rate and Pattern of Contraction of Rat Heart Myocytes in 20% Ambient Oxygen

% O$_2$ Concentration	In Vitro Age of Myocytes (Days)	Rate and Pattern of Contraction[a]	
		Control	PGBx (1 nM)
20	1	60 (R)	60 (R)
20	3	57 (R)	60 (R)
20	6	67 (R)	64 (R)
20	9	69 (R)	65 (R)
20	12	71 (Ar)	65 (R)
20	15	60 (Ar)	65 (Ar)
20	18	38 (Ar)	54 (Ar)
20	21	5 (Ar)	20 (Ar)
20	24	0	0

[a] R = rhythmic; Ar = arrhythmic.

The decrease in lipofuscin deposition and the enhancement of survival of isolated cardiomyocytes despite high oxygen tension suggests that PGBx protects against prooxidant injury, and this property may contribute to PGBx's antiaging effects previously noted (TABLE 5, FIG. 3).

Effect on Cell Viability Using Paramecia

The protozoan, *Paramecia aurelia* has been used by Joan Smith-Sonneborn and developed by the Environmental Protection Agency (EPA) as an *in vitro* screen for environmental carcinogens[40,41] and for antiaging studies.[42] In this model, a combination of blue light (photodynamic action) and a chemical sensitizer, benzpyrene, interact to induce cell death, though either alone does not kill. The photodynamic toxicity of 3,4-benzpyrene to these free living single cells involves a preincubation with the benzpyrene in the dark, followed by an irradiation phase with blue light.[40,41]

PGBx protected stock 51 paramecia from the immediate concentration-dependent phototoxic effects of the interaction of 3,4-benzpyrene and ultraviolet irradiation (TABLE 8a). Paramecia were incubated in the dark with 1.0 μg/ml benzpyrene. To determine whether the PGBx protective action was mediated via an ultraviolet light (UV) screening action or by direct interaction with the paramecia, the culture was surrounded by a cuvette acting as a shield which contained water

TABLE 8a. Effect of PGBx on the Survival of Irradiated Paramecia in the Presence of 3,4-Benzpyrene (Percent Survival)

Time (Min)	3,4-Benzpyrene 1.0 μg/ml	PGBx 1 mM	PGBx 0.5 mM	PGBx 0.25 mM
5	100	100	100	100
10	0	100	100	100
15	0	100	80	70
20	0	100	20	20
30	0	62	0	0
60	0	22	0	0

± 1 mM PGBx. The cuvette containing the water control or test agent (PGBx) as a shield was interposed between the UV light and the cuvette containing the paramecia (10 or 20) living in their nutritive medium, with or without PGBx. Paramecia were UV-radiated at 5- or 10-minute intervals at a distance of 3.4 centimeters, and the survival of the paramecia was evaluated.

TABLE 8b shows that cells shielded externally by PGBx in solution showed a significant increase in survival relative to the water shield control alone. After 5 minutes of UV irradiation, no significant increase in survival between PGBx-shielded cells and those directly suspended in PGBx could be detected. When the duration of irradiation increased to 10 minutes significant differences between control, PGBx shield, and cells suspended in PGBx-containing media were noted. These results indicate that PGBx acts to reduce exposure to UV light by functioning to absorb light, but also has a direct protective effect when cells interact with PGBx in the medium.

We also examined the effect of PGBx on cytotoxicity and mutagenicity of paramecia exposed to the carcinogen/mutagen, 4-nitroquinoline-N-oxide (NQ). A protective effect of PGBx was found for both cytotoxicity and viability of survivors (data not shown). After 3 hours of exposure to 1.0 μg/ml of NQ, survival was 13% for controls versus 66% with PGBx and at cytotoxic NQ levels, the survivors protected by PGBx are mutated while the unprotected cohorts are dead. These preliminary results suggest that PGBx protects against the acutely lethal action of mutagens.

DISCUSSION

PLA₂ is a potent source of inflammatory activity that can lead to the development of free radicals as membrane phospholipid is digested or hydrolyzed. Our theoretical justification for this enzyme having a vital place in aging is its unique

TABLE 8b. *In Situ* PGBx versus PGBx Shielding Resulting in Photodynamic Protection of UV Irradiated Paramecia (Percent Survival)[a]

Time Interval (Min)	Control	PGBx Shield Only	In Situ	PGBX Shield and In Situ
5	32.5 ± 27(40)	76 ± 9.4(50)	88 ± 9.8(50)	100 ± 0(20)
10	22.5 ± 13.6(80)	43.3 ± 18(100)	74.3 ± 9.0(70)	88 ± 12(20)
10			81.5 ± 9.4(20)	91.5 ± 5.8(20)

[a] The number in the parenthesis are the number of paramecia used.

functional role in bridging both the direct membrane damage hypothesis of aging and aging as a phenomenon of dysdifferentiation resulting from alterations in genetic expression or surface-mediated informational exchange.[1] Our focus on the potential antiaging application for antiinflammatory PLA_2 inhibitors is also based on the practical clinical application of these inhibitors, as part of a dual strategy: First, as aging is not thought to be a disease, by the Food and Drug Administration (FDA) and our clinical colleagues, one must develop antiaging drugs that focus on clinical syndromes or diseases such as inflammation that can be successfully treated, and which provide a measurable disease response. Subsequently these agents can be tested in aging models. Secondly, inflammation as a concomitant of injury and infection results in the mobilization of numerous mediators from effector cells, *i.e.,* pyrogens and free radicals that promote phospholipid, protein and/ or nucleic acid oxidation and degradation to accelerate the aging process. Because antiinflammatory drugs produce measurable effects of immediate clinical value, we sought to develop nontoxic, antiinflammatory agents, suitable for chronic administration that could provide ancillary benefit as antiaging drugs.

PGBx is a potent direct inhibitor of PLA_2 enzyme activity[2,13] (FIG. 2). We have demonstrated that the inhibitory effect of PGB_1 oligomers increases with polymer size and in recent studies to be reported, we have established a structural activity relationship between newly developed specific agents and broad spectrum PLA_2 inhibition. As such, PGBx is the first of a series of synthetic or naturally derived compounds that possess antiinflammatory and cytoprotective activity.

PGBx not only inhibits peroxidation itself, but also intervenes in the injury process after initiation of the oxidative insult. Thus, we have demonstrated that phospholipase activity in canine myocardial sarcoplasmic reticulum preferentially hydrolyzes autooxidized phospholipid[12] and, in studies to be reported, have shown that this activity is inhibited by PGBx. This observation is significant to membrane injury or senescence where oxidative changes may predispose cell membranes to attack by phospholipases to alter function or viability. In this regard, PLA_2 can act as a "death trigger" to digest previously oxidized membranes to further alter their integrity. These deleterious and self-propagating events may be arrested by administration of effective phospholipase inhibitors and/or antioxidants such as PGBx.

In previous studies, PGBx protected against anoxic and ischemic stress in heart,[14,17,19,20,43] cord,[44] and brain.[14,18] It also prevented and/or restored degenerative changes which inhibited phosphorylation in mitochondria.[30] Of interest to aging, PGBx normalized high blood glucose, obesity and excessive appetite in hereditary diabetic mice.[43-45] PGBx also maintained the integrity of the gastric mucosa in stress-induced ulcers in rats[46] and prevented sickling in -SS- red blood cells.[47] Collectively, these observations with PGBx suggest that their specific application as PLA_2 inhibitors in clinical disease, leads to a generalized preventive or reparative role that will be particularly beneficial in the aging syndrome.

In related studies, we have shown that PGBx blocks the formation of superoxide from f-Met-Leu-Phe stimulated human PMN's (B. Susskind, work in progress, cited REF. 2). Thus, PGBx may inhibit injury propagated by activated phagocytes. These cells induce vascular and tissue damage via singlet oxygen formation to contribute to tissue injury.[2,13] Since ischemia in aging is a process promoted by endothelial injury and associated with platelet adhesion, thrombosis and atherosclerosis, it is of interest that PGBx also enhances the storage life of human platelets.[48] We have found that PGBx inhibits platelet activating factor (PAF) generation,[2] prevents platelet aggregation, and has anticoagulant activity at high concentrations (work in progress).

Pertinent to its antiaging effects, as presented in this paper (TABLE 5, FIG. 3), PGBx in drinking water inhibits the formation of malonyldialdehyde (TABLE 4b), suggesting that it can alter oxidation of lipids and/or carbohydrates, proteins, and nucleic acids *in vivo*. This is not surprising in that *in vitro*, PGBx is 100 times more effective than sodium metabisulfite in protecting phosphatidylethanolamine from autoxidation (TABLE 2). PGBx was more effective as an antioxidant than α tocopherol succinate which, distinct from α tocopherol itself, we have found to inhibit *in vitro* phospholipase A$_2$.

PGBx feeding delayed age-related death in houseflies. Although a preliminary finding, PGBx is competitive and/or superior to vitamin E or other antioxidant supplementation[49] (TABLE 5; FIG. 3). Sohal *et al.,* have reported that ascorbate, β-carotene, or α-tocopherol in sucrose feeding have no effect on enhanced survival of houseflies.[49] In contrast, in the fruit fly, drosophila,[50] the antioxidants, vitamin E (α-tocopherol) and nordihydroguaiaretic acid (NDGA) and thiazolidine carboxylic acid (thioproline) increased both the mean and maximum life span. The increase in life span ranged from 12% and 14% for NDGA and vitamin E, to 31% for thioproline and is associated with a 20% decline in oxygen consumption in male drosophila melanogaster. This decline in O$_2$ consumption was not associated with a decline in functional behavior as there was a marked enhancement of age-related sexual activity in these treated flies. Miquel and Lindseth[50] suggest that this enhancement of survival may be associated with the maintenance of mitochondrial integrity and energy efficiency induced by these antioxidants. More recently, Wadhwa[51] has reported that sodium hydrophosphate feeding, as an antioxidant, increased the life span of another dipteran (*Z. paravittiger*) by 27–34%.

The protective effect of PGBx on age-related housefly survival does not appear to be due to a simple decline in mitochondrial function, or housefly activity. We believe that it is due to the diminution of endoperoxides which are known to accumulate with age. In that regard, PGBx protects mammalian mitochondria from injury[17,22–30] and can restore damaged mitochondrial function following *in vitro* aging[24,25,28] or exposure to hypotonic media.[24,25] The restoration of oxidative phosphorylation capacity by PGBx,[25,26] is most likely due to stabilization of the mitochondrial membrane. We hypothesize that PGBx treatment results in stabilization and/or restoration of mitochondrial function via PLA$_2$ inhibitory and/or antioxidant activity. PGBx's action might be similar to that reported by Miquel and Lindseth[50] for antioxidant life extension in drosophila.

There is an extensive literature on aging as an oxidative event. For example, there is increased hepatic oxidation with resultant MDA formation in the liver of mice with progressive age,[52] and this is associated with a decline in mitochondrial oxidative metabolism.[53] MDA formation, or that of related peroxidants, may have profound effects on the functional state of proteins, nucleic acids, and lipids which are damaged by the oxidative effects of this metabolite. Thus, aging is associated with a decline in mitochondrial oxidative phosphorylation and concomitant changes in mitochondrial phospholipid composition which might be favorably affected by PGBx.[54]

Aging in the housefly is associated with oxidative stress as seen in a rise in H$_2$O$_2$, a decline in reduced glutathione (GSH), and an increase in superoxide generation.[34,36] The latter is associated with enhanced state 4 mitochondrial respiration, something that was not observed in our PGBx-fed houseflies. The decrease in MDA formation with an increase in life span by PGBx may be mediated by an enhanced ability to manage or respond to oxidative stress. Sohal *et al.*[57] have also shown that short-lived houseflies generate more MDA than long-lived strains, suggesting that the ability to maintain lower levels of oxidant product is associated with longevity.

Interestingly, exercise generates MDA and lipid hydroperoxides in skeletal muscle,[59] and Cutler et al.[60] have shown a distinct difference in the spontaneous autooxidation of tissue as measured by MDA with rapid tissue autolysis following homogenization of kidneys and brains of short-lived versus long-lived mammalian species. MDA formation is rapid in autolyzing brains of short-lived mice and rats, and slower in brain tissue of long-lived mammals such as humans. It would be of interest to determine in tissue autolysis or injury, if MDA generation correlates with PLA_2 activity in the brain and kidney, and whether this process could be altered by PGBx administration.

The significance of life prolongation in houseflies by feeding PGBx in drinking water (TABLE 5, FIG. 3) is strengthened by the in vitro observations of an effect of PGBx in mammalian tissue culture. Mouse cardiomyocytes show a decrease in lipofuscin with an increase in functional survival (TABLES 6 and 7). Lipofuscin is a biomarker for aging in insects and mammals as it increases intracellularly with age,[50,61,62] and antioxidants that prolong survival of drosophila decrease lipofuscin formation[50] in similar fashion to our experience with cardiomyocytes. The linear rate of lipofuscin accumulation may depend on total life span energy expenditure,[62,63] which may have a bearing on the PGBx life extension effect, although no decline in O_2 consumption or energy output for PGBx has been reported.

Further support for the cytoprotective action of PGBx which has a bearing on aging, is seen in the protozoan paramecium model wherein PGBx protected against benzpyrene ultraviolet mediated injury (TABLE 8 a,b) and the lethal action of the mutagen, nitroquinoline (NQ). In this regard, Newton et al.[64] have reported that the DNA repair capacity of houseflies relates to strain-related survival differences. Flies with longer life expectancy have greater capacity to reverse DNA single-strand breakage, as compared to short-lived cohorts. Although PGBx protects paramecia from the lethal action of the mutagen NQ, we have no data in regard to PGBx's effects on strand breakage and DNA repair except as an inference related to PGBx enhancement of the survival of mutagen exposed paramecia. PLA_2 inhibitors are now being evaluated for their effects on carcinogenesis in mammalian systems.

In summary, we hypothesize that the chemical stability of cell membranes, and particularly the cell envelope governs cell responsiveness and survival in the aging process. Damage to membranes, with particular emphasis on lipid peroxidation, and the activation of phospholipases modulate cellular integrity, resistance to injury, repair, and the ability of the host to respond to environmental change. Phospholipases, particularly PLA_2, may act as "death triggers" to digest, destabilize and destroy cell membranes when activated beyond the constraints of homeostatic control mechanisms where PLA_2 propagates injury by inducing a cascade of cell membrane changes.

PGBx is the first in a series of compounds which inhibit PLA_2 activity and are effective antiinflammatory agents in mice, rats, and horses. Our studies indicate that PGBx and future PLA_2 or phospholipase inhibitors, with and without antioxidant activity, will maintain the integrity of cell membranes to promote functional survival and longevity, and hopefully will have clinical applicability to the aging process.

REFERENCES

1. ZS-NAGY, I., R. G. CUTLER & I. SEMSEI. 1988. Ann. N.Y. Acad Sci. **521:** 215–225.
2. ROSENTHAL, M. D. & R. C. FRANSON. 1989. Biochim. Biophys. Acta **1006:** 278–286.

3. PHILLIPS, G. B., P. BACHNER & D. C. MCKAY. 1965. Proc. Soc. Exp. Biol. Med. **119:** 846–885.
4. DOER, Y. H. M., B. J. MAGNUSSUM, J. GALASEKHARAM & J. F. PEARSON. 1956. J. Gen. Microbiol. **40:** 283–296.
5. MACFALANE, M. C. & B. C. KNIGHT. 1941. Biochem. J. **35:** 884–902.
6. VAN DEN BOSCH, H. 1981. Biochim. Biophys. Acta **604:** 191–246.
7. WAITE, M. 1987. In Handbook of Lipid Research. Vol. 5: 243–281. Plenum Press. New York.
8. HYSMITH, R. M. & R. C. FRANSON. 1982. Biochim. Biophys. Acta **711:** 26–32.
9. VAN DEN BOSCH, H. & G. VAN DEN BESSELAAR. 1978. Adv. Prostaglandin Thromboxane Res. **3:** 69–75.
10. VADAS, P. & PRUZANSKI. 1984. Adv. Inflammation Res. **7:** 751–757.
11. PUOTONEU-REINERT, A. & M. SANDHOLM. 1986. Proc. Equine Vet. J. **18:** 143–148.
12. GAMACHE, D. A., A. A. FAWZY & R. C. FRANSON. 1988. Biochim. Biophys. Acta **958:** 116–124.
13. FRANSON, R. C. & M. D. ROSENTHAL. 1989. Biochim. Biophys. Acta **1006:** 272–277.
14. VON LUBITZ, K. J. E. & D. J. REDMOND. 1989. Eur. J. Pharmacol. **164:** 405–414.
15. FRANSON, R. C., D. EISEN, R. JESSE & C. LANNI. 1980. Biochem. J. **186:** 633–636.
16. SERVANIAN, A., S. F. MUAKKASSAH-KELLY & S. MONTRESTRUQUE. 1983. Arch. Biochem. Biophys. **223:** 441–452.
17. ANGELAKOS, E. T., R. L. RILEY & B. D. POLIS. 1980. Physiol. Chem. Phys. **12:** 81–96.
18. KOLATA, R. J. & B. D. POLIS. 1980. Physiol. Chem. Phys. **12:** 545–550.
19. POLIS, E. & F. W. COPE. 1983. Aviat. Space Environ. Med. **54:** 420–424.
20. ARONSON, C. E. & N. H. GUERRENO. 1979. Gen. Pharmacol. **10:** 301–308.
21. JACOBS, T., J. HALLENBECK, T. DEVLIN & G. FEVERSTEIN. 1987. Pharm. Res. **4:** 130–132.
22. POLIS, B. D., E. POLIS & S. KWONG. 1979. Proc. Natl. Acad. Sci. USA **76:** 1598–1602.
23. OHNISHI, S. T. & T. M. DEVLIN. 1979. Biochem. Biophys. Res. Commun. **89:** 240–245.
24. SCHMUKLER, H. W., E. SOFFER, M. G. ZAWRYT et al. 1982. Physiol. Chem. Phys. **14:** 445–476.
25. SCHMUKLER, H. W., M. G. ZAWRYT, E. F. SOFFER et al. 1982. Physiol. Chem. Phys. **14:** 471–486.
26. KREUTTER, D. K. & T. M. DEVLIN. 1983. Arch. Biochem. Biophys. **221:** 216–226.
27. URIBE, S., S. OHNISHI, C. ISRAELITE & T. DEVLIN. 1987. Biochim. Biophys. Acta **924:** 87–98.
28. POLIS, B. D., S. KWONG, E. POLIS & G. L. NELSON. 1980. Physiol. Chem. Phys. **12:** 167–177.
29. SCHMUKLER, H. W., S. F. KWONG & E. POLIS. 1980. Physiol. Chem. Phys. **12:** 557.
30. POLIS, B. D., E. POLIS & S. F. KWONG. 1981. Physiol. Chem. Phys. **13:** 531–548.
31. NELSON, G. L. 1988. Adv. Exp. Biol. **238:** 359–382.
32. PURTUNEN-REINERT, A. & M. SANDHOLM. 1986. Proc. Equine Vet. J. **18:** 143–148.
33. SOHAL, R. S., A. MULLER, B. KOLETZKO & H. SIES. 1985. Mech. Ageing Dev. **29:** 317–326.
34. FARMER, K. J. & R. S. SOHAL. 1989. Free Radical Biol. Med. **7:** 23–29.
35. FARMER, K. J. & R. S. SOHAL. 1987. Exp. Gerontol. **22:** 59–65.
36. SOHAL, R. S., R. G. ALLEN & K. J. FARMER. 1985. Mech. Ageing Dev. **31:** 329–336.
37. SOHAL, R. S. & J. H. RUNNELS. 1986. Exp. Gerontol. **21:** 509–514.
38. SOHAL, R. S., M. R. MARZABADI, D. GALARIS & V. T. BRUNK. 1989. Free Radical Biol. Med. **6:** 23–30.
39. MARZABADI, M. R., R. S. SOHAL & V. T. BRUNK. 1988. Mech. Ageing Dev. **46:** 145–157.
40. SMITH-SONNEBORN, J., G. L. FISHER, A. PALIZZI & C. HERR. 1981. Environ. Mutagen. **3:** 239–252.
41. SMITH-SONNEBORN, J. 1983. Use of a ciliated protozoan as a model system to detect toxic and carcinogenic agent. In In Vitro Toxicity Testing of Environmental Agents. Pt. A. R. Kaber, T. K. Wong & L. D. Grant, Eds. 113–137. Plenum Publ. Corp. New York.
42. SMITH-SONNEBORN, J., P. D. LIPETZ & R. E. STEPHENS. 1983. Paramecium bio-

assay of longevity modulating agent. *In* Intervention in the Aging Process. Pt. B. W. Regelson & M. Sinex, Eds. 253–273. Alan R. Liss, New York.
43. POLIS, D. B. & E. POLIS. 1976. Physiol. Chem. Phys. **8:** 429–436.
44. JACOBS, T. P., J. M. HALLENBECK, T. M. DEVLIN & G. Z. FEURSTEIN. 1987. Pharm. Res. **4:** 130–132.
45. POLIS, D. B. & E. POLIS. 1979. Physiol. Chem. Phys. **11:** 3–8.
46. KUMASHIRO, R., T. M. DEVLIN, M. KOLOUSSY & T. MATSUMOTO. 1985. Int. Surg. **70:** 247–250.
47. DEVLIN, M. T., T. M. DEVLIN & S. T. OHNISHI. 1981. Biophys. J. **33:** 81.
48. SMITH, D. J., D. G. ODOM & B. A. CHENEY. 1989. Transfusion **29:** 153–158.
49. SOHAL, R. S., R. G. ALLEN, K. J. FARMER *et al.* 1985. Mech. Ageing Dev. **31:** 329–36.
50. MIQUEL, J. & K. LINDSETH. 1983. Determination of biological age in anti-oxidant treated drosophila and mice. *In* Intervention in the Aging Process. Pt. B. Basic Research and Preclinical Screening. W. Regelson & M. Sinex, Eds. 317–358. Alan R. Liss. New York.
51. WADHWA, R. 1987. Arch. Gerontol. Geriatr. **6:** 101–106.
52. UYSAL, M., S. SECKIN, N. KOCAK-TOKER & H. OZ. 1989. Mech. Ageing Dev. **48:** 85–89.
53. DARNOLD, J. R., M. L. VORBECK & A. P. MARTIN. 1990. Mech. Ageing Dev. **53:** 157–167.
54. KIM, J. W. & B. P. YU. 1989. Mech. Ageing Dev. **50:** 277–287.
55. SOHAL, R. S., P. L. TOY & K. J. FARMER. 1987. Arch. Gerontol. Geriatr. **6:** 95–100.
56. SOHAL, R. S., P. L. TOY & R. G. ALLEN. 1986. Mech. Ageing Dev. **36:** 71–77.
57. SOHAL, R. S. 1988. Exp. Gerontol. **23:** 211–216.
58. SOHAL, R. S., R. G. ALLEN, K. J. FARMER & R. K. NEWTON. 1985. Mech. Ageing Dev. **32:** 33–38.
59. AL ESSIO, H. M., A. H. GOLDFARM & R. G. CUTLER. 1988. Am. J. Physiol. **255:** PC 874–877.
60. CUTLER, R. G. 1985. Proc. Natl. Acad. Sci. USA **82:** 4798–4802.
61. NAKANO, M., T. MIZUNO & S. GOTOH. 1990. Mech. Ageing Dev. **52:** 93–106.
62. NAKANO, M., T. MIZUNO, H. KATON & S. GOTOH. 1989. Mech. Ageing Dev. **49:** 41–48.
63. SOHAL, R. S., I. SVENSSON, B. H. SOHAL & T. BRUNK. 1989. Mech. Ageing Dev. **49:** 129–135.
64. NEWTON, R. K., J. M. DUCORE & R. S. SOHAL. 1989. Mech. Ageing Dev. **49:** 259–270.

The Decline of the Immune Response during Aging: the Role of an Altered Lipid Metabolism[a]

GEORG WICK,[b,c,d] LUKAS A. HUBER,[c] XU QING-BO,[d]
ELMAR JAROSCH,[e] DIETHER SCHÖNITZER,[f] AND
GÜNTHER JÜRGENS[g]

[c] Institute for General and Experimental Pathology
University of Innsbruck Medical School
Fritz-Pregl-Strasse 3/IV
6020 Innsbruck, Austria

[d] Immunoendocrinology Research Unit of the Austrian Academy
of Sciences
Fritz-Pregl-Strasse 3/IV
6020 Innsbruck, Austria

[e] Central Laboratory and [f] Blood Transfusion Unit
University Hospital
Anichstrasse 35
6020 Innsbruck, Austria

[g] Institute of Medical Biochemistry
University of Graz Medical School
Harrachgasse 21/III
8010 Graz, Austria

INTRODUCTION

The immune system is endowed with the potential to differentiate self from nonself and to tolerate the former. This ability is gradually lost during aging concomitantly with a general decline of the immune response. The overall reactivity of the immune system is regulated by intrinsic control mechanisms and by extensive modulatory factors. In this article we shall first briefly discuss the intrinsic principles of control and then focus on the immunoregulatory role of lipids with special emphasis on the altered immune reactivity in the elderly.

The capacity for self recognition is acquired by T cells during their sojourn in the thymus.[1] Those capable of self major histocompatibility complex (MHC) class I and class II restriction are sorted out by positive selection, while those potentially reacting with high affinity with self-MHC in association with non-MHC self antigens seem to be deleted by negative selection.[2,3] The exact site(s) where these selection processes take place is (are) unknown but we have recently found exper-

---

[a] This work was supported by the Austrian Research Council (projects No. S-41/01 and 7341), the Austrian Ministry of Science and Research, the Sandoz Foundation for Gerontological Research, Basel, Switzerland, and a donation by Mr. Hermann Mayer, Paris. Xu Qing-Bo is a recipient of a fellowship from the Boehringer Ingelheim Fund.
[b] Corresponding author.

imental evidence that peculiar large complexes of thymic epithelial cells, the so called thymic nurse cells,[4] with internalized intact T cells, may play a crucial role in this respect.[5,6] Thus, it may be of relevance that an animal model with a spontaneously occurring, Hashimoto-like autoimmune thyroiditis has a significant deficit of thymic nurse cells, while also showing an increased humoral and cellular autoreactivity against thyroid and various nonthyroid autoantigens.[7] The T cell repertoire of an individual is finally made up by a majority of cells that react with foreign antigens with high affinity in a MHC-restricted fashion. There is also a minority of T cells that react with low affinity with non-MHC self antigens associated with autologous MHC molecules.[8] These latter cells maintain tolerance by various immunoregulatory mechanisms, such as antiidiotypic suppression, hormonal factors, etc. On the other hand, potentially autoantibody-producing B cells seem to occur in rather high frequency but they do not exert their autoreactivity due to functional inactivation of appropriate T helper cells.[9]

The subtle tuning of the immune system providing protection against foreign invaders and tolerance to the body's own components is defective in patients with autoimmune diseases and gradually lost during aging. It is known that T cell function deteriorates with age, while B cells and macrophages seem to maintain normal reactivity throughout the life span. Paradoxically, the general decline of the immune response against exogenous antigens in the elderly is paralleled by increased autoreactivity.[10] The latter is, however, not synonymous with an increase of autoimmune disease, i.e., organ-specific or systemic lesions that lead to clinical symptoms. It is attractive to reflect on the parallels of the these phenomena with age-dependent loss of cognitive function of the brain resulting in the inability to appropriately deal with external and internal intellectual stimuli and the subsequent failure to communicate with the environment as well as the loss of the ability for self recognition, e.g., in Alzheimer patients.

Thus, murine cytotoxic T lymphocytes (CTL) from young (3 months) donors with a given H-2 haplotype a stimulated in a mixed lymphocyte reaction with cells of haplotype b show strong alloreactivity against b, but not against a (self) or c (unrelated third party) cells. On the other hand, CTLs from old (24 months) mice of haplotype a will show significantly lower cytotoxicity against target cells carrying haplotype b (original stimulators), but additionally react with cells of haplotype c (loss of specificity) and, to a certain extent, with cells of haplotype a (autoreactivity).[11] The reasons for this paradoxical behavior of the immune system with senescence are not yet clear. One theory postulates that nonspecific T suppressor cells increase during aging, thus leading to a generally lower immune response. On the other hand, the number and/or function of certain clones of antigen-specific T suppressor cells are decreased, thus permitting the proliferation of certain autoreactive T cell clones.[12] Furthermore, the life-long exposure of the body's constituents to external and internal stress and damage may result in increased altered self antigens that are taken care of by the immune system as a "pitting" mechanism in the sense of Grabar's "transporteur" theory.[13] Another possibility for the augmented autoreactivity in the elderly would be polyclonal activation due to the known surge of viral, bacterial and parasitic infections.

In addition to these intrinsic changes, the immune system is, of course, also subject to general age-dependent metabolic changes. In this respect, the known alterations of the lipid metabolism with age seems to be of special importance, a fact largely neglected in studies of the aging immune system.[14] Lymphocytes and macrophages, like all other cells of the organism, require cholesterol for proper function. This cellular constituent can either be produced by the cells themselves or provided from the environment by lipoproteins.[15] These lipoproteins, especially low density (LDL) and high density (HDL) lipoproteins, are taken up via specific high affinity receptors or low affinity nonspecific binding. LDL[16] and HDL receptors are subject to downregulation by increasing environmental concentrations of the respective lipoproteins. The expression of the rate limiting enzyme of intercellular cholesterol synthesis, hydroxymethylglutaryl-coenzymeA reductase (HMG-CoAR), is downregulated by the uptake of external cholesterol. In this communication we shall first briefly discuss the role of lipids in the normal immune response in general, and then focus on the possible significance of an altered lipid metabolism to the decline of the immune response in the elderly.

The Role of Lipids in the Normal Immune Response

Cholesterol is transported in plasma in a packaged form. LDL are considered to be responsible for delivery of cholesterol to the cells ("bad" cholesterol) while HDL remove cholesterol from the cell surface and turn it to the liver for excretion ("good" cholesterol). The latter phenomenon is called reverse cholesterol transport.[18] Cholesterol is taken up via receptor-mediated endocytosis of LDL and, to a certain extent, also by the receptor-independent mechanisms that result in equilibration of free cholesterol between lipid constituents of cell membranes and lipoproteins. The structure of the LDL receptor is known, and it has recently been cloned.[19] High LDL concentrations in the cellular environment entails downregulation of the LDL receptor and inhibition of HMG-CoAR. The degree of LDL receptor expression reflects cellular requirement for cholesterol in a given functional state. Thus, resting peripheral blood lymphocytes (PBL) need very little cholesterol, express very low levels of LDL receptors and show little HMG-CoAR reactivity.[20,21] In an activated state, however, or after *in vivo* or *in vitro* cholesterol deprivation a significant upregulation of LDL receptor expression takes place.[22] Very high concentrations of plasma LDL, unfortunately, override this intricate regulatory mechanism, and uptake of cholesterol via the nonspecific predominates over the receptor-mediated pathway.

Lymphocytes were the first cells on which **LDL receptors** were demonstrated using classical *in vivo* biochemical methods, *i.e.*, isotope-labeled LDL as a ligand. We have, surprisingly for the first time in such detail, analyzed LDL receptor expression on lymphocytes using flow cytometry with a fluorescent-labeled LDL preparation.[23] For this purpose, purified LDL from normal human plasma was labeled with the red fluorescent dye dioctadecylindocarbocyanine (DiI). PBL were incubated with this ligand and subjected to fluorescence activated cell sorter (FACS) analysis. Relative quantitation of fluorescence was achieved by assessment of the fluorescence intensity (FI), equivalent to the respective FACS channel, of the 50th or 75th percentiles of either positively stained cells or the total cell population. FIGURE 1 shows that this technique is more sensitive than the classical isotope-labeling method, since an, albeit low, FI can already be measured in freshly isolated PBL, *i.e.*, with downregulated LDL-receptor expression. After several days of cholesterol starvation *in vitro*, a significant upregulation of LDL receptor expression can be observed.[24] Furthermore, this method also allows for the determination of the classical receptor characteristics saturation, inhibition and affinity, as demonstrated in FIGURE 2. The association constants (K_d) were calculated from double-reciprocal plots (Lineweaver-Burke plots) of the specific binding data.[24] Applying double fluorescence with DiI-LDL (red) and a panel of monoclonal antibodies recognizing PBL subpopulations (green), it was shown that T cells make up the majority of LDL receptor positive cells with a CD4/CD8

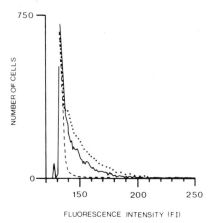

FIGURE 1. Upregulation of LDL receptors on PBL during incubation in serum-free medium. *Dashed line*, 1×10^6 PBL labeled with 12.5 mg/ml DiI-LDL immediately after plastic depletion of monocytes; *solid line*, incubated 16 h and *dotted line*, 40 h in Iscoves modified Dulbeccos medium before DiI-LDL labeling. (Adapted from Traill *et al.*[24])

ratio of approximately 3.0.[24] The highest degree of LDL receptor expression, and thus cholesterol requirement, was observed on mitogen-activated T cells, T cell lines and leukemia cells. PBL of patients with familial hypercholesterolemia (FH), a hereditary deficiency of LDL receptors, show no expression of LDL receptors.[24] Measuring the receptor activity of single (living) cells in cultures of resting lymphocytes by flow cytometry reveals a large spread among healthy donors in the percentage of lymphocytes that upregulate their LDL receptor levels during a 3-day period of cholesterol deprivation, but the receptor activity of receptor-bearing cells does not differ among healthy subjects. This difference has obviously been overlooked in conventional assays of receptor binding/internalization/degradation where the results were only expressed for a whole cell population. Thus, although LDL receptor expression has been amply documented, our original contribution in this area was the exact characterization of such receptors on *single living* cells by FACS analysis and the demonstration of the classical receptor characteristics based on this methodology. The higher sensitivity of FACS analysis as compared to classical isotope methodology is underlined by the fact that LDL receptors can clearly be demonstrated also on resting, freshly isolated PBL.

With respect to the demonstration of classical **HDL receptors** the situation was less unequivocal. Although high affinity ($K_d = 1-5 \times 10^{-8}$ M) binding sites for HDL were described on different cell types, such as macrophages,[25] fibroblasts[26] and hepatocytes,[27] their nature and physiological significance were unknown. Their requirement for the exchange of free cholesterol and/or cholesterol ester on the cell surface or intercellularly after receptor-mediated retrograde transport is still controversial. We[28] and Schmitz *et al.*[29] first reported a high-affinity HDL binding site, but others have not found such evidence.[30] Using FACS methodology, we then clearly proved that this binding site has all the above-mentioned characteristics of a classical receptor, *i.e.*, is saturable, specific and of high affinity. HDL binding is mediated via the apoprotein AI and can be blocked by an apoAI-staphylococcal proteinA hybrid molecule (apoAI alone is unstable). The binding can also be inhibited by specific anti-apoAI antibodies, but not by antibodies against the apoprotein B that serves as a receptor attachment site for LDL.[31]

Data on the **role of lipoproteins in immune function** are still scarce. It is known that none of the lipoprotein fractions seems to be mitogenic for lymphocytes but that they can either enhance or suppress immune reactivity under different conditions. It is not yet clear which lipid components have stimulatory or suppressive properties, respectively. We have focused our attention on cholesterol because this is the main molecule transported by lipoproteins.

To clarify the functional role of lipoproteins, we performed mitogen stimulation tests on PBL, the HMG-CoAR reactivity of which had been blocked by preincubation with the drug mevinolin.[31] Such cells cannot synthesize their own cholesterol and their proliferation and survival are, therefore, dependent on an exogenous source. As shown in FIGURE 3, LDL can rescue mevinolin-treated lymphocytes and even enhance the response to over 100% of the original value at concentrations that are still within saturation limits, *i.e.*, where binding occurs via specific high affinity LDL receptors. At higher concentrations, *i.e.*, where uptake takes place via nonspecific, receptor-independent mechanisms, LDL have a suppressive effect. Surprisingly, HDL was also shown to function as an exogenous source of cholesterol; in other words, we found no evidence for HDL dependent reverse cholesterol transport in the lymphocytic system. The rescuing effect of HDL was, however, only observed at concentrations above saturation, *i.e.*, did

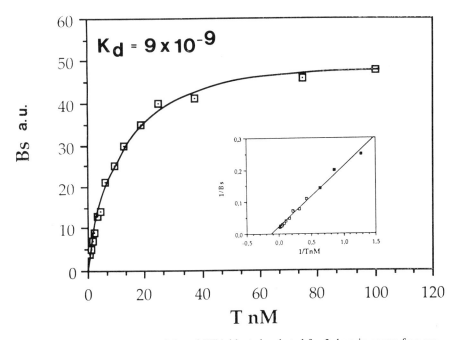

FIGURE 2. LDL receptor activity of PHA-blasts incubated for 3 days in serum-free medium. 1×10^6 cells were incubated with the indicated concentrations of DiI-LDL (T nM = total added in nM) for 2 h at 37°C. Nonspecific binding was assessed in the presence of 12.5 mM EDTA in the incubation medium. DiI-LDL uptake was measured in a flow cytometer. Fluorescence intensity (FI) is expressed in arbitrary units. Specific uptake (Bs) was assessed by subtracting nonspecific binding from total binding for each DiI-LDL concentration. *Inset*: Lineweaver-Burke plot of specific binding data. K_d and Bmax (in arbitrary units) are obtained from these curves. However, these experiments were not designed to provide an absolute, or even comparative Bmax but rather to afford accurate binding curves.

not seem to be mediated by specific receptors. Furthermore, suppression was never found with HDL, even at very high concentrations.

In addition to cholesterol there are, of course, also numerous other lipid fractions that affect immune function. Thus, responses are enhanced by tryglycerides, phospholipids and various individual fatty acids. As a matter of fact, fatty acids can also be delivered by lipoproteins of various density, including apoE-free HDL 2 and HDL 3.[31,32] It should be emphasized that all these effects can only be observed under strictly controlled experimental conditions, notably serum-free or appropriately supplemented tissue culture medium.

The exact biochemical basis for the immunosuppressive activity of LDL is not yet known. Curtiss and Edgington[33] have, however, described a special LDL fraction denoted LDL_{In}, "inhibitory" LDL, that was later shown to be the intermediate density lipoprotein (IDL). LDL_{In} inhibits cellular and humoral immune responses in mice, and its effect is mediated via binding to low affinity lymphocyte surface receptors ($K_d = 1.5 \times 10^{-7}$ M). The active principle of LDL_{In} has recently been identified as apoE, a product of monocytes and macrophages and thus considered a potent immunoregulatory monokine.[34]

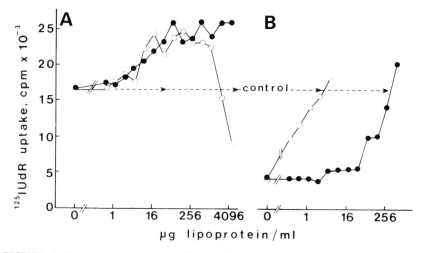

FIGURE 3. Immunoregulation by LDL and HDL. PBL were stimulated with PHA in medium (**A**) or in medium containing 0.56 μM mevinolin (**B**) together with the indicated concentrations of LDL (*open symbols*) or apoE-free HDL₃ (*closed symbols*) expressed as mg lipoprotein/ml. Cultures were pulsed with ^{125}IUdR for 3 h on day 4; data expressed as counts per minute (cpm). Note suppressive effect of LDL in high concentrations (above saturation of specific receptors) in (A) and rescuing potential of both LDL and HDL, albeit with lower efficiency of the latter.

Because several groups have proposed that the immunosuppressive activity of LDL may be mediated via interference with the uptake of the iron transport protein **transferrin** by lymphoid cells,[35] we shall briefly consider this concept. These authors postulate the existence of a low affinity "immunoregulatory receptor" specific for apoB/E but distinct from the classical high-affinity receptor and also different from the above-mentioned LDL$_{In}$ receptor. Harmony *et al.* (for review see REF. 36) believe that this "immunoregulatory receptor" is actually a low affinity receptor for transferrin that is not essential for lymphocyte activation, but is indispensible for regulation of activation by transferrin in plasma lipoproteins. Transferrin exerts positive control and lipoproteins negative control by interaction with this receptor. The role of transferrin via this immunoregulatory receptor pathway consists of inducing production of a factor necessary for cell recruitment into the cell cycle. Transferrin receptors become expressed during the G1 phase of the cell cycle, and transferrin is synthesized by T helper cells in an autocrine fashion similar to that of interleukin-2 (IL-2).[37] LDL and transferrin receptors are localized in the same coated pits, but seem to be sufficiently dispersed to abrogate transferrin blockade of LDL binding. LDL, on the other hand, does not interfere with the binding of a monoclonal antibody against the transferrin receptor.[35] As a matter of fact, anti-transferrin receptor monoclonal antibodies have recently been shown to detect two types of transferrin binding sites, only one of which is active in binding and internalizing the iron transport protein.[38] Both receptors are expressed on phytohemagglutinin (PHA) activated blasts, but only the inactive receptor is found on cells stimulated with Ca^{++} ionophore and phorbol ester.[22] Based on this concept, we were able to show that transferrin can rescue cells from LDL suppression of the response to the Ca^{++} ionophore A23187 or phorbol ester. However, our own flow cytometric and functional data do not support the concept that lymphocytes possess a separate low affinity receptor for apoprotein B and E, which could serve as an immunoregulatory receptor. Careful analyses led us to conclude that this receptor shares all characteristics with the classical high affinity cholesterol transport receptor and, in addition, cannot be demonstrated on freshly isolated T cells from homozygous, high affinity LDL receptor-defective FH patients. Comparison of the concentration dependence of immunosuppression with binding curves for freshly isolated lymphocytes confirmed that suppression is not receptor- (high or low affinity) mediated. Finally, since this type of suppression is only demonstrated by very high concentrations of transferrin, it may be irrelevant under physiological conditions.[22,39]

To conclude this part of our discussion on immunoregulation by lipid, it should be mentioned that Cuthbert and Lipsky[35] have shown that cholesterol *per se* is also immunosuppressive, and that this effect could be alleviated by transferrin. It is now clear, however, that the suppressive activity of cholesterol depends on oxysterol contamination of the assay preparation. This may also explain some of the differences reported between experiments performed with different preparations of lipoproteins or cholesterol. Heavily **oxydized LDL** is actually cytotoxic for lymphocytes and a variety of other cells, an effect that can be reversed by addition of HDL to the tissue culture medium.[40] *In vivo*, these particles are bound to the so-called scavenger receptor on macrophages, and are thus rapidly removed from circulation[40] without having the opportunity to exert an immunosuppressive effect. Less heavily oxydized LDL may, however, escape this clearance process and be responsible for the observed differences in immunosuppressive potency of different LDL preparations.

We conclude that immunoregulation is not only dependent on the widely known intrinsic cellular interactions and mediators briefly described in the Introduction of this paper, but that a multitude of other modulating factors must be considered among which the lipid metabolism is perhaps the most important in view of the crucial role of membrane composition in the activity of all kinds of cellular achievements, from mobility to adhesion, and the function of different receptors with respect to ligand binding and signal transduction.

Lipids and Lymphocyte Function in the Elderly

Admission Criteria for Immunogerontological Studies

Data on the senescent immune function are often contradictory, primarily due to the large variation of proband admission criteria that different groups of investigators apply for such studies. With this in mind, the *European Economic Community Concerted Action on Aging Research*, EURAGE, has devised the so called SENIEUR protocol that contains the definition criteria for old (and, by analogy, also young control) person as being "healthy".[41] These criteria include:

    (a) an exact case history,
    (b) laboratory values, and
    (c) information on drug consumption.

Adherence to this protocol should permit determination of age-dependent decline of immune responsiveness or, if the observed alterations are only due to underlying diseases, the influence of immunosuppressive drugs, etc. Thus, probands treated with steroids as a therapy for rheumatoid diseases must be excluded from an aging study, as are young female controls who take oral contraceptives. On the other hand, persons with recent vaccinations that precipitate a general stimulation of the immune system must also be excluded.

There is no doubt that establishment of the SENIEUR protocol has two great merits: 1) to draw attention of workers in the field to the fact that data can only be compared when the same admission criteria for the study groups are implemented, and 2) the necessity of excluding the factors that lead to skewed results on immunological function.

We have performed a total of 3 extensive studies[24,42,43] based on the application of the SENIEUR protocol and thus can look back on ample experience with this mode of selection. In spite of the merits of this approach, several criticisms have emerged that can be summarized as follows:

    (a) The different parameters listed in the protocol cannot be given equal weight. Therefore, our first study attempted to compare the effect of strict compliance with the protocol with a more differentiated approach, and found the latter to be very useful.[42]

    (b) Some important laboratory values are missing in the original protocol, and it should be amended in this respect. Based on what was said earlier in this paper, we would like to suggest that the parameters relating to the lipid metabolism be added.

    (c) An elaborate statistical cluster analysis comparing young (mean age 25 years) and old (mean age 82 years) females revealed a considerable overlap and redundancy of various values presently included in the protocol that could be deleted.[43]

    (d) We are now performing a third study that includes determination of all parameters contained in the original protocol and additional values to provide the basis for discussion with other laboratories who rely on the protocol for subsequent revision or extension.

    (e) Since testing of lymphocyte function, including determination of membrane viscosity on a single cell basis, pheontyping, mitogen stimulation, etc. can only be done on a limited number of samples per day and must always include cells from both old and young donors in a given test, it was important to show that frozen *vs* fresh lymphoid cells can be used for such studies without compromising the results.[24]

(f) Finally, one important aspect that has not been sufficiently considered during the establishment and reassessment, respectively, of the SENIEUR protocol are the costs involved per sample.

One argument raised against the principle of selecting donors as being "normal healthy" is that this does not reflect the overall population. This is certainly true, and the present studies using the protocol should, therefore, only be considered as a mean to provide baseline values on the immune function of the elderly, which then can serve as a reference for more extensive projects involving unselected study groups. As a spinoff of our own SENIEUR-based investigations, we were, surprisingly for the first time, able to determine exact age-dependent values for a variety of routine parameters (but also more specialized determinations, such as serum neopterin) for an Austrian population.[43]

The Role of the Lipid Metabolism for an Altered Immune Reactivity in Old Age

Our interest in this field was, in addition to our long-standing work on autoimmunity, stimulated by a study from the Weizmann Institute of Science, Rehovot, Israel, which showed that the diminished *in vitro* responsiveness of lymphocytes from the elderly correlates with decreased plasma membrane fluidity.[44,45] We found this idea attractive because it is easily conceivable that the accessibility and function of surface receptors depends, among other things, on their mobility within the plasma membrane. Plasma membrane fluidity depends on chemical factors, such as the ratio between free cholesterol/phospholipids (C/PI), the sphingomyelin/lecithin, the protein/phospholipid ratio and the content of saturated and polyunsaturated fatty acids. Physical factors that affect membrane fluidity include temperature, pressure (osmotic and ambient), pH, Ca^{++} content of the surrounding milieu, etc. In the above-mentioned study and in our own laboratory, membrane fluidity is measured by fluorescence depolarization, where in the lipophylic probe 1,6-diphenyl-1,3,5-hexatriene (DPH) partitions into the plasma membrane and emits a blue fluorescence upon excitation with polarized UV light. The degree of depolarization of the emitted *vs* excitation light is a measure for the intramembrane mobility of DPH, and thus membrane fluidity. Such measurements are usually performed on "bulk" preparations of PBL in cuvettes using an appropriate fluorometer. We have adapted this method to single cell membrane viscosity measurements in a FACS.[46]

In vitro analyses clearly show that membrane viscosity is inversely correlated to mitogen responsiveness. Since membrane fluidity has been shown to depend on the molar C/PI ratio, we investigated whether modulation of this ratio resulted in altered mitogen responsiveness. An increase of the C/PI ratio was accomplished by incubation of PBL in cholesterol-enriched medium, a decrease by *in vitro* depletion of membrane cholesterol. This treatment clearly showed that higher plasma membrane fluidity is reflected by better mitogen responsiveness. We have also assessed a "membrane fluidizing" mixture[47] of neutral glycerides, phosphatidylcholine and phosphatidylethanolamine in a proportion of 7 : 2 : 1 (active lipid 721-AL721) and were able to show that this compound, also recommended as a therapeutic agent in elderly and AIDS patients, has no fluidizing potential but rather exerts its enhancing effects by supplying lymphocytes or monocytes with a source of lipids required for optimal growth.[48] Thus, AL721 has to be present during the whole culture period in order to have an ameliorating effect on the mitogen response; preincubation of PBL with AL721 and washing prior to mitogen stimulation abrogates its effect.

FIGURE 4 illustrates two points: 1) the above-mentioned inverse correlation between membrane viscosity and mitogen responsiveness, and 2) the age-dependent increase of membrane viscosity that can also be demonstrated on a single cell basis with the FACS method.

We next addressed the question of whether an altered lipid metabolism of lymphocytes from old donors can explain the observed physical and chemical changes of the plasma membrane. Using the above-mentioned FACS method, we were surprised to find an *increased* expression of LDL receptors on resting T cells from old *vs* young donors.[24] Since the old donors also showed the well-known increased serum LDL levels, this latter observation was paradoxical; LDL receptor expression should be downregulated by increased LDL concentrations in the environment.

TABLE 1 gives the LDL serum levels, LDL membrane receptor density, and ConcanavalinA (ConA) response in a group of young and old donors selected on the basis of the SENIEUR admission criteria. Thus far, we do not know the biochemical and molecular biological basis for the statistically significant correlations shown in this table. Thus, the upregulation of LDL receptors upon cholesterol deprivation in tissue culture seems to function normally in lymphocytes of the elderly. Furthermore, we have no evidence that the composition of serum LDL in SENIEUR protocol compatible elderly donors differs significantly from that of young people and thus could be responsible for inappropriate binding to the receptors: In competition studies LDL from old donors is equally efficient as that of young donors, and mevinolin-intoxicated lymphocytes can be functionally rescued in mitogen stimulation tests to the same degree when LDL from young or old donors is added.[49] Using our approach, *i.e.*, applying the SENIEUR protocol, there is obviously a large overlap between individuals in the young and old group regarding plasma membrane viscosity, lymphocyte function, etc. There is always a considerable number of elderly who immunologically respond as young, and

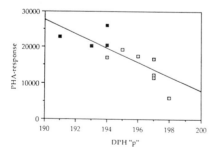

FIGURE 4. Example of the inverse correlation between mitogen responsiveness (PHA) and an age-related decrease of membrane fluidity: DPH"p". Young males, aged 20 to 35 years (n = 4), *closed symbols*, old males, aged 65 to 85 years (n = 7), *open symbols*. PHA response in serum-free medium was measured by pulsing day 4 cultures for 3 h with ^{125}IUdR. Data are expressed as counts per minute (cpm). Membrane viscosity was determined by FACS DPH depolarization measurement (DPH"p"). Frequency histograms for the groups were calculated from the median fluorescence intensity (FI) for each individual donor. Data expressed in arbitrary FACS channel units. (From Traill *et al.*[49] Reprinted by permission from Academic Press.)

TABLE 1. Age-Related Differences in Serum LDL Levels, DiI-LDL Uptake and Mitogen Responsiveness of PBL[a]

	Total		SENIEUR Compatible	
	Young (n = 46)	Old (n = 27)	Young (n = 23)	Old (n = 11)
DiI-LDL (FI)	154 ± 1	[b]163 ± 1	154 ± 1	[b]166 ± 2
Serum LDL (mg/dl)	225 ± 8	[b]336 ± 14	236 ± 13	[c]306 ± 21
ConA-response (cpm × 10⁻²)	120 ± 7	[b]71 ± 8	111 ± 11	[d]67 ± 16

[a] Data expressed as mean ± SE. DiI-LDL (FI): LDL uptake measured during a 2-h incubation at 37°C with DiI-LDL (2.5×10^6 PBL/ml, 50 μg DiI-LDL/ml). Fluorescence intensity measured by flow cytometry (in arbitrary FACS channel units). ConA response: ^{125}IUdR uptake during a 3-h pulse on day 2 of culture. (Adapted from Wick *et al.*[11])

[b] $p < 0.001$ (Student t test).

[c] $p < 0.01$.

[d] $p < 0.05$.

vice versa, reflecting the fact that the SENIEUR protocol is identifying "normal, healthy" old and young individuals.

An interesting and unexplained phenomenon is the finding that the age-dependent increase of LDL binding is paralleled by increased expression of HDL binding sites.[50]

We are now addressing the following questions:

(a) Is the biochemical composition of the PBL plasma membrane from old donors, especially with respect to saturated and unsaturated fatty acids as well as various types of phospholipids, altered with age?

(b) Are there subtle differences, *e.g.*, oxidation, between lipoproteins from old and young donors, that may be responsible for an abnormal regulation of lipoprotein receptor expression beyond the sensitivity of our analytic methods?

(c) Is the structure of lipoprotein receptors changed during aging?

(d) Is the regulatory feedback mechanism between uptake of cholesterol via LDL and expression of HMG-CoAR disturbed?

(e) Are there differences in the susceptibility to LDL- and HDL-mediated rescue of mitogen responsiveness of mevinolin-treated lymphocytes from old and young donors? This problem is addressed using cDNA probes for the human LDL receptor and HMG-CoAR (HDL receptor probes are not yet available) for evaluation of our most recently established cell bank.

(f) Are there differences in membrane lipid homeostasis of lymphocytes as compared to nonlymphoid cells, *e.g.*, fibroblasts, from the same donors?

CONCLUSIONS

Aging is a multifacetted process, but the deterioration of immune function is certainly one of the central theoretical and practical issues. Paradoxically, the immune response in the elderly is decreased against exogenous antigens, but at the same time autoimmune reactivity is increased.

One aim of our investigations was to study immune function under exactly defined conditions of "normal, healthy" aging applying the original and modified versions of the EURAGE SENIEUR protocol admission criteria. Furthermore, we are specifically interested in the possible role of an altered lipid metabolism as one of the factors that affect the immune system during aging. We have shown clearcut positive and negative correlations, respectively, between serum LDL levels, plasma membrane viscosity, LDL and HDL receptor expression and mitogen responsiveness. In the course of these studies we have developed two methodological improvements for the determination of lipoprotein receptor expression and function and the measurement of plasma membrane viscosity on single living cells by flow cytometry. We are currently trying to elucidate the biochemical and molecular biological basis for the altered lipid metabolism of cells of the immune system and thus age-dependent changes of the immune reactivity. The ultimate goal of these studies is, of course, the elaboration of possible ways to interfere with the immune response of the elderly by behavioral, dietary or pharmacological means to modulate the lipid metabolism.

ACKNOWLEDGMENTS

We would like to acknowlege the contributions of our former colleague K. N. Traill, the discussions with and constructive criticism of H. A. Dresel and the technical help by Ms. Anya Mair.

REFERENCES

1. OWEN, J. J. T., E. J. JENKINSON & R. KINGSTON. 1986. Thymic stem cells. Their interaction with the thymic stroma and tolerance induction. Curr. Top. Microbiol. Immunol. 126: 35–41.
2. ZINKERNAGEL, R. M. 1978. Thymus and lymphohemopoietic cells: their role in T-cell maturation, in selection for T-cell H-2 restriction specificity and in H-2 linked Ir gene control. Immunol. Rev. 42: 224–270.
3. VON BOEHMER, H., H. S. TEH & P. KISIELOW. 1989. The thymus selects the useful, neglects the useless and destroys the harmful. Immunol. Today 10: 17–61.
4. WEKERLE, H. & U. P. KETELSEN. 1980. Thymic nurse cells: Ia bearing epithelium involved in T-lymphocyte differentiation. Nature 183: 402–405.
5. WICK, G. & G. OBERHUBER. 1986. Thymic nurse cells: a school for alloreactive and autoreactive cortical thymocytes? Eur. J. Immunol. 16: 855–858.
6. PENNINGER, J., K. HÁLA & G. WICK. 1990. Intra-thymic nurse cell lymphocytes can induce a specific graft-versus-host-reaction. J. Exp. Med. In press.
7. BOYD, R. L., G. OBERHUBER, K. HÁLA & G. WICK. 1984. Obese strain (OS) chickens with spontaneous autoimmune thyroiditis have a deficiency in thymic nurse cells. J. Immunol. 132: 714–718.
8. MARRACK, P. & J. KAPPLER. 1988. The T-cell repertoire for antigen and MHC. Immunol. Today 9: 308–315.
9. ZANETTI, M. & D. H. KATZ. 1985. Self-recognition, auto-immunity, and internal images. Curr. Top. Microbiol. Immunol. 119: 111–126.
10. HIJMANS, W., J. RADL, G. F. BOTTAZZO & D. DONIACH. 1984. Autoantibodies in highly aged humans. Mech. Ageing Dev. 26: 83–89.
11. WICK, G., L. A. HUBER, F. OFFNER, U. WINTER, G. BÖCK, K. SCHAUENSTEIN, G. JÜRGENS & K. N. TRAILL. 1989. In Immunodeficiency in Old Age. Immunodeficiency and the Skin. P. Fritsch, G. Schuler & H. Hinter, Eds. Curr. Probl. Dermatol. 18: 120–130.
12. RITTERBAND, M. & A. GLOBERSON. 1982. Developmental aspects of T-suppressor cells induced by hapten-carrier conjugates. Adv. Exp. Med. Biol. 149: 725–730.
13. GRABAR, P. J. 1975. Hypothesis, auto-antibodies and immunological theories: an analytical review. Clin. Immunol. Immunopathol. 4: 453–466.

14. TRAILL, K. N. & G. WICK. 1984. Lipids and lymphocyte function. Immunol. Today **5:** 70–76.
15. GOTTO, A. M., H. J. POWNALL & R. J. HAVEL. 1986. Introduction to the plasma lipoproteins. Methods Enzymol. **128:** 3–41.
16. BROWN, M. S. & J. L. GOLDSTEIN. 1975. Regulation of the activity of the low density lipoprotein receptor in human fibroblasts. Cell **6:** 307–316.
17. BROWN, M. S., S. E. DANA & J. L. GOLDSTEIN. 1974. Regulation of 3-hydroxymethylglutaryl coenzymeA reductase activity in cultured human fibroblasts: comparison of cells from a normal subject and from a patient with homozygous familial hypercholesterolaemia. J. Biol. Chem. **249:** 789–796.
18. HAMBITZER, R., I. MELZNER & O. HAFERKAMP. 1987. Relationships between lymphocyte cholesterol homeostasis and LDL-cholesterol. Clin. Biochem. **20:** 97–104.
19. MIYAKE, Y., S. TAJIMA, T. FUNAHASHI & A. YAMAMOTO. 1989. Analysis of a recycling impaired mutant of low density lipoprotein receptor in familial hypercholesterolaemia. J. Biol. Chem. **264:** 16584–16590.
20. HO, Y. K., M. S. BROWN, D. W. BILHEIMER & J. L. GOLDSTEIN. 1976. Regulation of low density lipoprotein receptor activity in freshly isolated human lymphocytes. J. Clin. Invest. **58:** i465–1474.
21. HO, Y. K., J. R. FAUST, D. W. BILHEIMER, M. S. BROWN & J. L. GOLDSTEIN. 1977. Regulation of cholesterol synthesis by low density lipoprotein in isolated human lymphocytes. Comparison of cells from normal subjects and patients with homozygous familial hypercholesterolaemia and abetaliproteinaemia. J. Exp. Med. **145:** 1531–1549.
22. HUBER, L. A., G. BÖCK, G. JÜRGENS, K. N. TRAILL, D. SCHÖNITZER & G. WICK. 1990. Increased expression of high affinity LDL receptors on human T-blasts. Submitted for publication.
23. TRAILL, K. N., G. BÖCK, U. WINTER, M. HILCHENBACH, G. JÜRGENS & G. WICK. 1986. Simple method for comparing large numbers of flow cytometry histograms exemplified by analysis of the CD4 (T4) antigen and LDL receptor on human peripheral blood lymphocytes. J. Histochem. Cytochem. **34:** 1217–1221.
24. TRAILL, K. N., G. JÜRGENS, G. BÖCK, L. A. HUBER, D. SCHÖNITZER, K. WIDHALM, U. WINTER & G. WICK. 1987. Analysis of fluorescent low density lipoprotein uptake by lymphocytes. Paradoxical increase in the elderly. Mech. Ageing Dev. **40:** 261–288.
25. SCHMITZ, G., H. ROBINEK & G. ASSMANN. 1985. Interaction of high density lipoproteins with cholesterylester laden macrophages: biochemical and morphological characterization of cell surface receptor binding endocytosis and resecretion of high density lipoproteins by macrophages. EMBO J. **4:** 613–622.
26. MENDEL, C. M. S. T. KUNITAKE, J. P. KANE & E. S. KEMPER. 1988. Radiation inactivation of binding sites for high density lipoproteins in human fibroblast membranes. J. Biol. Chem. **263:** 1314–1319.
27. MONACO, L., H. M. BOND, K. E. HOWELL & R. CORTESE. 1987. A recombinant apo A1 protein A hybrid reproduces the binding parameters of HDL to its receptor. EMBO J. **6:** 3253–3260.
28. TRAILL, K. N., G. JÜRGENS, G. BÖCK & G. WICK. 1987. High density lipoprotein uptake by freshly isolated human peripheral blood T lymphocytes. Immunobiol. **175:** 447–454.
29. SCHMITZ, G., G. WULF, T. BRÜNIG & G. ASSMANN. 1987. Flow cytometric determination of high-density lipoprotein binding sites on human leukocytes. Clin. Chem. **33:** 2195–2203.
30. CUTHBERT, J. A. & P. E. LIPSKY. 1987. Provision of cholesterol to lymphocytes by high density and low density lipoproteins. Requirement for low density lipoprotein receptors. J. Biol. Chem. **262:** 7808–7818.
31. JÜRGENS, G. QING-BO XU, L. A. HUBER, G. BÖCK, H. HOWANIETZ, G. WICK & K. N. TRAILL. 1989. Promotion of lymphocyte growth by high density lipoproteins (HDL). Physiological significance of the HDL binding site. J. Biol. Chem. **264:** 8549–8556.
32. CUTHBERT, J. A. & P. E. LIPSKY. 1989. Lipoproteins may provide fatty acid necessary for human lymphocyte proliferations by both low-density lipoprotein receptor-dependent and independent mechanisms. J. Biol. Chem. **264:** 13468–13474.

33. CURTISS, L. K. & T. S. EDGINGTON. 1976. Immunoregulatory serum lipoproteins. Regulation of lymphocyte stimulation by a species of low density lipoprotein. J. Immunol. **116:** 1452–1458.
34. PEPE, M. G. & L. K. CURTISS. 1986. Apo lipoprotein E is a biologically active constituent of the normal immunoregulatory lipoprotein LDL-Im. J. Immunol. **136:** 3716–3723.
35. CUTHBERT, J. A. & P. E. LIPSKY. 1984. Immunoregulation by low density lipoproteins in man. Inhibition of mitogen induced T-lymphocyte proliferation by interference with transferrin metabolism. J. Clin. Invest. **73:** 992–1003.
36. HARMONY, J. A. K., A. L. AKESON, B. M. MCCARTHY, R. E. MORRIS, D. W. SCUPHAM & S. A. GRUPP. 1986. Immunoregulation by plasma lipoproteins. *In* Biochemistry and Biology of Plasma Lipoproteins. A. N. Scanu & A. A. Spector, Eds. 403–451. Marcel Dekker Inc. New York.
37. LUM, J. B., A. J. INFANTE, D. M. MAKKER, F. YANG & B. H. BOWMAN. 1986. Transferrin synthesis by induced T lymphocytes. J. Clin. Invest. **77:** 841–849.
38. BOLDT, D. J., J. L. PHILIPS & O. ALCANTARA. 1987. Disparity between expression of transferrin receptor ligand binding and non ligand binding domains on human lymphocytes. J. Cell. Physiol. **132:** 331–336.
39. TRAILL, K. N., L. A. HUBER, G. WICK & G. JÜRGENS. 1990. Lipoprotein interaction with T-lymphocytes: An update. Immunol. Today **11:** 411–417.
40. JÜRGENS, G., H. F. HOFF, G. M. CHISHOLM & J. ESTERBAUER. 1987. Modification of human serum low density lipoprotein by oxidation, characterization and pathophysiological implication. Chem. Physics Lipids **45:** 315–336.
41. LIGHART, G. J., J. X. CORBERAND, C. FOURNIER, E. GALANAUD, W. HIJMANS, B. KENNES, H. K. MÜLLER-HERMELINK & G. G. STEINMANN. 1984. Admission criteria for immunogerontological studies in man: the SENIEUR PROTOCOL. Mech. Ageing Dev. **28:** 47–55.
42. TRAILL, K. N., D. SCHÖNITZER, G. JÜRGENS, G. BÖCK, R. PFEILSCHIFTER, M. HILCHENBACH, A. HOLASEK, O. FÖRSTER & G. WICK. 1985. Age-related changes in lymphocyte subset proportions, surface differentiation antigen density and plasma membrane fluidity: application of the Eurage SENIEUR PROTOCOL admission criteria. Mech. Ageing Dev. **33:** 39–66.
43. REIBNEGGER, G., L. A. HUBER, G. JÜRGENS, D. SCHÖNITZER, E. R. WERNER, H. WACHTER, G. WICK & K. N. TRAILL. 1988. Approach to define ''normal aging'' in man. Immune function, serum lipids, lipoproteins and neopterin levels. Mech. Ageing Dev. **46:** 67–82.
44. RIVNAY, B., A. GLOBERSON & M. SHINITZKY. 1979. Viscosity of lymphocyte plasma membrane in aging mice and its possible relation to serum cholesterol. Mech. Ageing Dev. **10:** 71–79.
45. RIVNAY, B., S. BERGMAN, M. SHINITZKY & A. GLOBERSON. 1980. Correlations between membrane viscosity, serum cholesterol, lymphocyte activation and aging in man. Mech. Ageing Dev. **12:** 119–126.
46. BÖCK, G., L. A. HUBER, G. WICK & K. N. TRAILL. 1989. Use of a FACS III for fluorescence depolarization with DPH. J. Histochem. Cytochem. **37:** 1653–1658.
47. LYTE, M. & M. SHINITZKY. 1985. A special lipid mixture for membrane fluidization. Biochim. Biophys. Acta **812:** 133–138.
48. TRAILL, K. N., F. OFFNER, U. WINTER, F. PALTAUF & G. WICK. 1988. Lipid requirements of human T lymphocytes stimulated with mitogen in serum-free medium. Membrane ''fluidity'' changes are an artefact of lipid (AL721) uptake by monocytes. Immunobiol. **176:** 450–464.
49. TRAILL, K. N., L. A. HUBER, G. BÖCK, G JÜRGENS & G. WICK. 1988. Lipoprotein and immune function in the aged. *In* Crossroads in Aging. M. Bergener, M. Ermini & H. B. Stäherlin, Eds. Academic Press. London. 129–139.

The Pineal Control of Aging

The Effects of Melatonin and Pineal Grafting on the Survival of Older Mice

WALTER PIERPAOLI,[a] ANTONELLA DALL'ARA,[a]
ENNIO PEDRINIS,[b] AND WILLIAM REGELSON[c]

[a]Institute for Biomedical Research
Via Luserte, 2
6572 Quartino-Magadino, Switzerland

[b]Istituto Cantonale di Patologia
6604 Locarno, Switzerland

[c]Medical College of Virginia
Virginia Commonwealth University
Box 273, MCV Station
Richmond, Virginia 23298

Melatonin modulates the seasonal "Zeitgeber" which is largely affected by day length and/or temperature and which governs avian and mammalian nesting, fat deposition, molting and sexual cycling. Melatonin production may govern sexual maturity, and it has been observed that levels of melatonin decline with age.[1,2] Melatonin secretion is largely circadian and produced and derived from the pineal gland during the dark (scotophase) circadian cycle.[3,4]

As melatonin production may govern sexual maturity and declines clinically with age,[1,2] and as recent data suggests that it may also have an immunoregulatory role,[5,6] we felt that its multiple roles may govern the pattern of aging and senescence. For this reason, melatonin was given in drinking water to syngeneic mice during the dark cycle to see if it would influence patterns of survival or disease. In initial studies, we found in C3H/He female mice, 12 months of age, that melatonin *shortened* survival by inducing ovarian cancer. In contrast, initial results in older mice showed enhancement of longevity by 20% as compared to age-matched controls.[5-7] Based on these early results, experiments with circadian (night) administration of melatonin were replicated. We also homologously transplanted the pineal gland, the primary source of melatonin, from young to older mice to determine if there would be effects on mouse longevity when a youthful intact pineal was grafted into older mice.

We used the thymus as the graft recipient site, as the thymus and the pineal gland share a common adrenergic innervation via the superior cervical ganglion.[8] Pineal function is also associated with thyrotropin releasing hormone (TRH) production, and we have shown that TRH restores thymic function.[9]

For these reasons, as well as for surgical anatomic convenience, a thymic placement of the "young" (3–4 months) pineal grafts was thought to provide the best approach for homologous pineal engraftment.

We also examined survival, changes in thyroid production (T3, T4), immune response and lipid levels in treated and untreated mice in an attempt to derive insights into mechanisms of melatonin and pineal-modulated response in aging mice.

Both models used resulted in a significant enhancement of survival, suggesting that both melatonin and pineal function may play a role in mouse longevity.

METHODS

Melatonin Exposure

Mice were fed ad libitum using commercial mouse chow (NAFAG 890, 10 mm, Gossau, Switzerland). Darkness and light exposure were controlled by a fixed timer governing 2 standard fluorescent fixtures (Philips TLD 36W/84) 7 pm light-off, 7 am light-on. Melatonin (10 μg per ml tap water) was administered in the drinking water with a fixed darkness cycle and the control and melatonin-containing, opaque bottles were removed from 8:30 am to 6:00 pm. We examined survival, and the mice were individually weighed monthly to determine if the effects seen related to dietary intake. Mice were housed 4–10 to a cage.

The mouse strains studied and the ages at which melatonin was administered are presented below in FIGURES 1–3.

Pineal Implantation into the Thymus

Donor mice were 3- to 4-month-old, post pubertal BALB/c or C57BL/6. Recipients were groups of aging, BALB/c, C57BL/6 or C57BL/6 × BALB/c F1 hybrid female mice, 16 to 22 months old, depending on the experiment. The donor mice were killed by cervical dislocation and the skull fragment to which the pineal gland adheres was removed and immersed in cooled TC 199 medium with antibiotics (penicillin-streptomycin). The three main radial ligaments were dissected under a dissection microscope and the pineal was carefully displaced with fine scissors and removed, *in situ,* contained in its original membranes. The maintenance of original supporting membranes around the pineal appears to aid the engraftment with vascularization.

The aging graft recipient was anesthetized by ip injection of barbiturate (Vetanarcol, Veterinaria Inc., Zürich, Switzerland). The shaven chest was sterilized with Merfen and the skin above the jugulum was cut for 5–8 mm. The sternum was medially excised from the jugulum for a length of 2–3 mm by using bent scissors. After cutting the muscles, the mediastinal tissue was exposed and the residual, generally atrophic or involuted thymus was exposed by exerting moderate pressure on the abdomen. A single pineal gland in its membranes was positioned on the tip of a needle and introduced into it by gentle aspiration with a one-ml syringe under the dissection microscope. The pineal gland was rapidly injected into a lobe of the exposed thymus after introduction of the needle for 1–2 mm under the capsule. Occasionally, when a successful transplantation of the pineal was doubtful because of displacement of the pineal from the thymus, a second pineal gland was injected. The sternum, muscles and skin were then sutured and a protective plastic film (Nobecutan, Bofors, Sweden) was sprayed on the wound. Postoperative mortality was negligible, but in a few cases the operation produced the immediate rapid death of the mouse due to hemorrhage or pneumothorax.

The recipient mice were females of uniform age, housed 3 to 7 per cage. They were prepared for surgery and studied in groups, as indicated in TABLE 1. Weight changes of control and pineal-transplanted animals were also recorded monthly.

TABLE 1. Implantation of a Pineal Gland from Young 3- to 4-Month-Old Donors into the Thymus of Old Aging, Strain- and Sex-Matched Mice Postpones Aging and/or Prolongs the Life of the Pineal-Implanted Recipients

Groups	Strain and Treatment	Age at Implant or S.O. (Months)	No. of Mice[b]	No. of Surviving Mice (Months of Age)																
				17	18	19	20	21	22	23	24	25	26	27	28	29	30	31	32	33
A	Implanted C57BL/6	16	7	7	7	7	7	7	6	6	5	4	3	3	2	1	1	1	0	
B	Control C57BL/6	16	7	6	6	6	4	4	2	1	1	0	0	0	0	0	0	0		
C	Implanted hybrids[a]	19	5	—	—	—	5	5	5	5	5	5	5	5	5	5	4	3	2	1
D	Control hybrids	19	6	—	—	—	6	6	4	3	2	1	0	0	0	0	0			
E	Implanted BALB/cJ	22	3	—	—	—	—	—	—	3	3	3	3	3	3	3	3	1	0	
F	Control BALB/cJ	22	5	—	—	—	—	—	—	5	5	5	2	0						

[a] C57BL/6XBALB/cJ female hybrids.
[b] All donor and recipient mice used were inbred females. For details on the method and technique, see text.
A versus B: $p < 0.05$ (Mann-Whitney "U" test).
C versus D: $p < 0.01$ (Mann-Whitney "U" test).
E versus F: $p < 0.05$ (Mann-Whitney "U" test).

Pinealectomy

Pinealectomy was performed in young, 3- to 4-month-old C57BL/6 female mice by transcranial galvanocauterization under barbiturate anaesthesia (Vetanarcol).

Determination of Thyroid Hormones

For triiodothyronine (T3) or thyroxin (T4) determinations, the mice were bled from the retroorbital plexus under acute ether anaesthesia at 1 am under dim red light illumination.

Sera from individual mice were kept separate and frozen at $-30°C$ until the hormones were measured by radioimmunoassay (T4-Amerlex-M and T3-Bridge, Serono).

Assessment of Delayed-Type Hypersensitivity (DTH) Response

DTH response to oxazolone was assessed by application of 4 μl of 5% oxazolone (Aldrich Chem. Co., Milwaukee, WI) dissolved in acetone/oil (1/1) to the clipped skin of the chest and upper abdomen. Four days later, the mice were challenged by topical application of 25 μl 0.5% oxazolone on both sides of the right ear. DTH response was assessed by measuring the increase in ear thickness of oxazolone-sensitized mice 48 hours after challenge, with a modified micrometer dial gauge (Verdict Gauge Ltd, Dartford, Kent, UK).

Determination of Lipids in Plasma

The mice under investigation were selected randomly and bled under acute ether anaesthesia from the retroorbital plexus between 0:30 and 1:30 am. The plasma from individual mice was kept separate. Cholesterol, phospholipids and triglycerides were measured with an Hitachi 737 Analyser.

Light Microscopy

Fresh specimens for histological examination were fixed in 8% buffered formalin, embedded in paraffin and stained with haematoxylin-eosin.

RESULTS

Chronic Administration of Circadian (Night) Melatonin to One-Year-Old Mice Does Not Postpone Aging but Induces a High Incidence of Tumors

In preliminary studies, exogenous, night administration of melatonin prolonged the life of mice when the treatment started at the age of 18–20 months.[5–7] In order to verify whether the onset of melatonin treatment at an *earlier* age in mice might affect aging and thus prolong their life span beyond that observed when treatment was started in older mice, two identical experiments were performed in which melatonin treatment was started in one-year-old C3H/He female mice. The results illustrated in FIGURE 1 show that melatonin not only failed to prolong the life span of the mice, but, on the contrary, induced a high number of tumors primarily affecting the reproductive tract (lympho- or reticulosarcoma, carcinoma of ovarian origin; histology not shown here) and thus adversely affected the health and survival of melatonin-treated mice. These data suggest that at concentrations of 10 µg per ml in the drinking water, melatonin administration by the oral route in relatively "younger" female mice may produce derangements of the neuroendocrine pineal-piloted regulation of sexual organs, this resulting in onset of tumors of the reproductive tract.

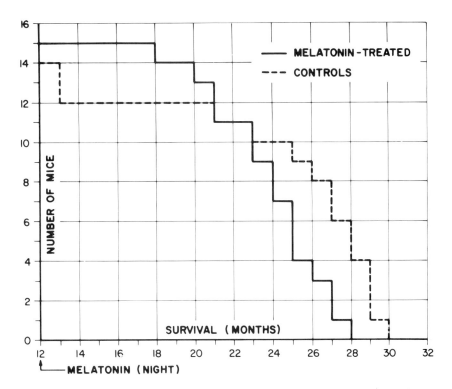

FIGURE 1. Chronic administration of exogenous (night) melatonin to one-year-old female C3H/He mice shortens their life span.

Chronic Administration of Circadian (Night) Melatonin to Young, Autoimmune Disease-Prone New Zealand Black (NZB) Female Mice Prolongs Their Life

As shown in FIGURE 2, a remarkable prolongation of life was seen when NZB mice were chronically given melatonin in the drinking water at night, while no effect was seen when melatonin was given during the day. In spite of the effect of melatonin, the common causes of death in all melatonin-treated or control NZB

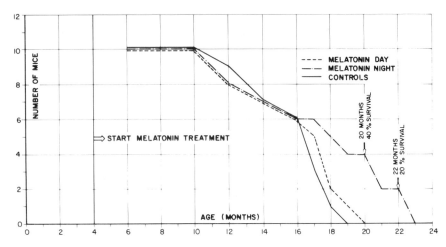

FIGURE 2. Circadian (night) administration of melatonin prolongs life of New Zealand black (NZB) female mice.

mice were autoimmune haemolytic anemia, nephrosclerosis and development of systemic or localized type A or B reticulum cell neoplasia.

Night Administration of Melatonin to Old, Aging C57BL/6 Mice Retards Their Senescence

A repetition of our experiments by night administration of melatonin in older, aging C57BL/6 male mice resulted again in a significant prolongation of their survival and confirmed thus our earlier preliminary findings (FIG. 3). Melatonin treatment starting at 19 months of age prolonged the absolute duration of their life by 6 months when compared to untreated controls. There was no significant weight loss or gain in the melatonin-treated mice as compared with controls. Therefore, a decreased food intake or anorexia, with resultant caloric restriction to explain the improvement in survival of the treated mice, does not explain the survival prolongation.

Implantation of a Pineal from Young Donors into the Thymus of Aging Recipients Greatly Prolongs Their Survival and Maintains Juvenile Conditions

TABLE 1 shows the pattern of survival in pineal-implanted C57BL/6, BALB/c × C57BL/6 hybrids and BALB/c females, pineal-engrafted at 16, 19 and 22 months. There was a striking difference in survival between controls and pineal homografted animals. All untreated animal controls were dead at 26 months while several pineal/thymus-transplanted animals were still alive at 31 months. No significant weight loss was seen in pineal-grafted mice. It is significant that this procedure improves survival in mice well along in their life cycle and beyond their reproductive estrous cycle. As seen in FIGURE 4, pineal implantation from young to older mice resulted in a remarkable prolongation of juvenile body conditions (pelage, skin, activity).

In order to ascertain whether this new method permitted proper, clear engraftment of the whole, intact pineal gland into the thymus, and whether the engrafted gland was vascularized and accepted with no visible alterations of its structure and cell (pinealocyte) function (nuclear or cytoplasmatic changes), a few pineal-implanted mice were sacrificed 3, 4 and 6 weeks after implantation. Serial 5 μm sections of all the thymuses were prepared and examined. As can be seen in the example of FIGURE 5, the pineal gland was clearly found in the thymic cortex. The pineals appeared in excellent condition, apparently intact and functioning, with no significant signs of cellular alterations. However, in spite of the clear life-prolonging effects of pineal implantation in old mice (TABLE 1), it is still unknown whether or not the grafted pineal is also innervated and able to produce and secrete melatonin in the blood circulation.

A more detailed investigation of cell viability and function of the engrafted pineal gland in the thymus of aging, surviving mice is in progress, combined with a study on the effect of pineal engraftment on the preservation of thymus size and cellularity.

Melatonin Treatment Modifies Night Levels of Thyroid Hormones and Preserves Cell-Mediated Immunity in Aging Mice

As shown in TABLE 2, in surviving mice at 19 and 23 months, melatonin treatment resulted in a significant decrease in night levels of T3 and T4 after 7 months and maintained an efficient cellular immune response to oxazolone sensitization.

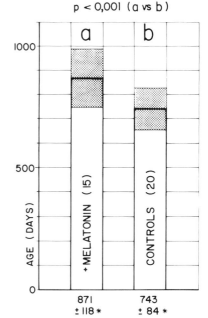

FIGURE 3. Aging postponement and/or life prolongation in C57BL/6 male mice consequent to night administration of melatonin.

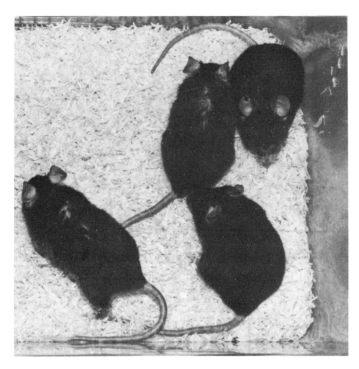

FIGURE 4. Young-to-old pineal implantation into the thymus delays aging and prolongs a juvenile status in mice. In this group of C57BL/6, 20-month-old female mice, the two mice on the *right-hand side* have been implanted with a pineal gland from a 3-month-old strain- and sex-matched donor at the age of 16 months. Notice maintenance of a healthy and luxuriant fur coat and youthful conditions in these two pineal-grafted mice. The mice in the picture correspond to Groups A and B of TABLE 1. One pineal-grafted mouse is still alive (31 months old).

Early Pinealectomy in Mice Results in Increased Levels of Lipids in Blood

As seen in TABLE 3, removal of the pineal gland in 4-month-old C57BL/6 mice resulted in an alteration of lipid metabolism. Pinealectomized mice, in contrast to sham-operated animals, showed a rise in cholesterol, triglycerides and circulating phospholipids.

DISCUSSION

We have shown that in early ontogeny the developing thymic, hypothalamic-pituitary and thyroid functions are functionally interdependent.[10] The thymus programs the immature neuroendocrine system by affecting the maturation of still modifiable hormonal feedback mechanisms.[11] The thymus is thus functionally linked to the thyroid gland. On the other hand, we have suggested and partially demonstrated that the melatonin-pineal effects observed in aging mice may be

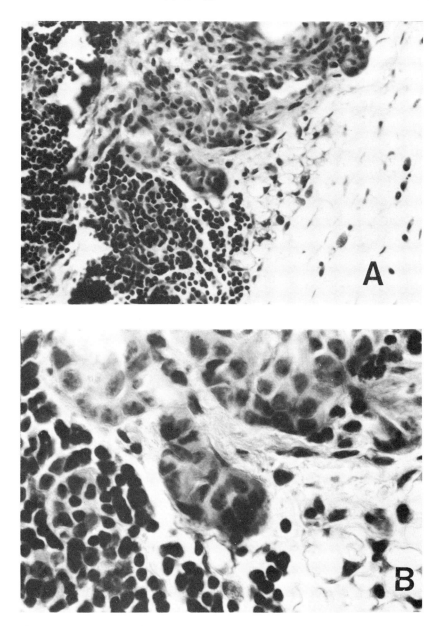

FIGURE 5. Young-to-old pineal implantation in the thymus: pineal gland of a 3-month-old donor mouse grafted in the thymic cortex of a 6-month-old recipient, at four weeks after transplantation; **(A)** × 400, **(B)** × 1000. Donor and recipient were inbred, histocompatible C57BL/6 mice. Typical, normal and viable clusters of pinealocytes are assembled in the context of the intact, transplanted pineal gland, which closely maintains its original structure. On the *left-hand and lower side* of the picture, packed, normal thymocytes of the thymic cortex are visible. Haematoxylin-eosin.

TABLE 2. Chronic (Night) Treatment with Melatonin Modifies Night Levels of Thyroid Hormones in Serum and Maintains the Delayed-Type Hypersensitivity (DTH) Response of Aging C57BL/6 Male Mice

Groups	No. of Surviving Mice	Age (M)	Melatonin (M of Treatment)	T3 (ng/ml)	T4 (μg/100 ml)	Oxazolone Response	
						Before or	After Challenge
A. Untreated	10	19	—	0.854 ± 0.165	5.48 ± 1.09	—	—
B. Melatonin-treated	10	19	3	0.873 ± 0.160	5.46 ± 1.51	—	—
C. Untreated	4	23	—	0.850 ± 0.028	4.94 ± 1.10	32.44 ± 4.52[c]	34.72 ± 3.21 (+7%)[a]
D. Melatonin-treated	8	23	7	0.682 ± 0.049[e] (−25%)	3.79 ± 1.37[d] (−30%)	27.75 ± 0.99	33.33 ± 4.00 (+16%)[b]

[a] Not significant (after challenge compared with before challenge).
[b] $p < 0.005$ (analysis of variance; two-tailed t test for unpaired normal samples).
[c] Mean ear thickness (mm^{-2}) ± SD.
[d] Not significant (D versus C).
[e] $p < 0.001$ (D versus C).

TABLE 3. Early Pinealectomy Results in an Increase of Lipid Levels in the Peripheral Blood of Aging C57BL/6 Female Mice[a]

Groups	No. of Mice	Age[b] (Months)	Months after Pinealectomy	Cholesterol (nMol/l)	Triglycerides (nMol/l)	Phospholipids (nMol/l)
Pinealectomy	8	23	19	$1.91 \pm 0.35 \ (+30\%)$[c]	$1.03 \pm 0.28 \ (+26\%)$[d]	$2.21 \pm 0.27 \ (+21\%)$[e]
Sham-operated	6	23	19	1.47 ± 0.11	0.82 ± 0.13	1.82 ± 0.60

[a] The mice were bled individually from the retroorbital plexus under light, acute ether anaesthesia and dim red light between 0.30 and 1.30 a.m.
[b] When bleeding and measurements of lipids were performed.
[c] $p < 0.01$.
[d] Not significant.
[e] Not significant.

mediated via the thyrotropin-releasing hormone-TSH-thyroid-thymus axis.[9] In regard to the above, there may also be a true anatomical connection between these apparently unrelated organs and tissues. It has been shown in similar fashion to the thymus, that the innervation of the pineal gland is derived mainly from the superior cervical ganglia, although direct innervation from the CNS also exists.[12] The pineal gland also contains a large number of lymphocytes closely linked to its rich perivascular, perifollicular and intrafollicular nerves and terminals. From this point of view, the pineal gland closely resembles the thymus, which is also richly innervated by, and directly connected with, the superior cervical ganglion.[8,13] Thus, independent of their functional significance, the thymus, the pineal gland and the thyroid[8] share common adrenergic innervation, possibly for short-range communication. However, the presence of lymphocytes within the pineal as a neuroendocrine organ is still an enigma. These functional and anatomical connections suggested that the thymus could be a suitable transplantation site for the pineal gland, offering the possibility of rich and rapid vascularization, and, thus, the growth of viable pineal glandular tissue with such transplantation.

If aging is a programmed event governed by a neuroendocrine clock, the role of the pineal in governing circadian and circannual rhythms, pubertal development and seasonal sexual cycling suggests that it may have a place in the programming or prevention of senescence. This is supported by our results as can be seen in FIGURE 3 and TABLE 1. Most importantly, pineal engraftment was performed in aging and in 16-, 19- and 22-month-old mice. The engrafted mice, in some cases, lived for an increased life span of 5 to 6 months, with a median of 4.2, 4.5 and over 6.5 months longer than controls (TABLE 1). The effect of pineal engraftment from young to old resulted in a 17, 21 and 27% increase in absolute survival suggesting the possibility that engraftment of a young pineal may have a rejuvenating effect, reversing patterns of intrinsic pathology associated with aging.

Our interest in pineal engraftment was based on our studies reported here using melatonin, in which melatonin given during the dark cycle of circadian rhythm in BALB/c female (data not shown here) and C57BL/6 male mice prolonged survival in treated animals when administered in the drinking water beginning at 15 and 19 months throughout their remaining life. The gain in average survival is from 743 to 871 days (TABLE 3). In contrast, when melatonin was given to one-year-old female C3H/He mice, the results were calamitous, with premature death due to the development of ovarian tumors in the melatonin-treated mice. It was not surprising, in this study, that ovarian tumors developed following chronic melatonin administration, as Kikuchi et al.[14] found that melatonin stimulated in vitro proliferation of a human ovarian KF cell line. It has been shown that human and rat ovaries contain receptors for melatonin which can modulate ovarian function[15] and/or steroidogenesis[16] and, in turn, ovarian function can affect melatonin levels.[17]

Our data on the development of ovarian tumors in C3H/He mice on melatonin feeding, beginning at 12 months, contradicts studies in which chronic melatonin administration has been shown to inhibit hormonally dependent prostatic and breast cancer.[18,19] In other experiments (data not shown here), either because of strain differences or because melatonin administration was begun at 15 months in BALB/c and at 18 months in C57BL/6 female mice, late in the sexual cycling of these female mice, early induction of tumors was not observed and there was a 20% prolongation in survival. Experiments must be carried out in which melatonin treatment starts later at 18–20 months of age in female C3H/He mice.

Although the role of the pineal and its major hormone melatonin are not fully defined,[1-3] if aging is a programmed event governed by a neuroendocrine clock, the mechanism of action may relate to the reported binding action of melatonin to the suprachiasmatic nucleus.[20,21] Our pineal engraftment and melatonin observations logically relate to the key role of the pineal and its hormones in governing circadian rhythm, pubertal development and seasonal sexual cycling, suggesting that the pineal may have an important place in the programming or prevention of senescence.[22] Certainly, there is evidence that the length of sexual life in a species appears to govern the median and absolute levels of survival. This is seen in animals as diverse as nematodes, drosophila, rodents and primates.

Related to the above, the age of melatonin administration is critical, as neonatal melatonin administration can stimulate sexual maturity in the rat.[23] Thus, melatonin must be viewed as a time-keeping hormone[24] wherein its major source, the pineal, functions as a neuroendocrine transducer interacting with the suprachiasmatic nuclei of the hypothalamus[21,22,25] and the reproductive system.[26,27]

In regard to physiologic mechanisms, the pineal gland (epiphysis cerebri), as a vertebrate endocrine organ, receives impulses from neural sympathetic sources which govern melatonin production. Melatonin (N-acetyl-methoxy-tryptamine) is derived primarily from the pineal gland, although the retina, the GI tract and, in rodents, the harderian glands contribute.

As mentioned previously, the timekeeping role for the pineal is seen in the delay in sexual maturation induced by melatonin in male rats, where it decreases pituitary binding and the hypothalamic synthesis of gonadotrophin-releasing hormone.[28] It would be of interest if this phenomenon were one key to melatonin's antiaging effect. However, pinealectomy, which reduces melatonin production, produces varied results on sexual maturity depending on the photoperiod governing the sexual response in the animal.[29]

The major physiologic role for the pineal is in governing seasonal adaptation, critical for species survival, particularly in seasonal breeders and in small rodents subject to harsh winters where short day length modulates winter adjustment. Pineal function modulates weight loss, molting of winter coat and can induce torpor, changes in thermogenic capacity and reproductive regression. In the clinic, aspects of depression seen with age have been related to melatonin circadian levels or decreased pineal sensitivity with exposure to light.[30] In this regard, total light deprivation reduces serum thyroxin (T4). This effect is prevented by pinealectomy. In contrast, pinealectomy induces thyroid hypertrophy, an effect reversed by melatonin.[31,32] A progressive derangement of overall thyroid function and thyroid-mediated adaptation mechanisms (*e.g.*, motor activity, thermoregulation, sleep, decline of cell-mediated immunity) are typical of the aging syndrome.[33] In evaluating the aging-postponing effects of circadian melatonin, we considered the "thyroid system" as a main route by which melatonin may exert its correcting immunopotentiating and antidistress effects.[5,9] We therefore measured night levels of thyroid hormones in the blood of aging, melatonin-treated mice. We also measured a parameter which expresses impairment or decrease of thyroid function and its liver-related oxidative mechanisms, namely, lipid levels in the peripheral blood of pinealectomized mice. It can be seen that chronic night treatment with melatonin in the drinking water in aging mice significantly lowers night levels of T3 and T4 in peripheral blood (TABLE 2) and thus affects aging-related thyroid dysfunction by a mechanism yet to be elucidated. However, as thyroid hormones are involved in the synthesis and degradation of cholesterol and in the detoxication processes of the liver, removal of the main source of circadian (night) melatonin through pinealectomy may affect both production of thyroid hormones and levels of lipids in peripheral blood. In fact, as shown in TABLE 3, levels of cholesterol, triglycerides and phospholipids are remarkably increased in

the peripheral blood of 23-month-old, aging C57BL/6 mice which had been pinealectomized at the age of four months. In contrast, chronic treatment with night
melatonin in aging mice corrects age-related increase of lipids in blood (data not
shown here) even though thyroid hormonal production is decreased (TABLE 2).
The above effects of melatonin on thyroid function may be pertinent to Denckla's
observations regarding the rejuvenating action of hypophysectomy in rat models.
In Denckla's studies, hypophysectomy enhances thyroid hormonal action[33] with
apparent evidence of functional reversal of age-related physiologic changes, including reversal of nephrosclerosis, restoration of immune response and return to
a youthful hepatic functional profile. In support of possible melatonin or pineal
influence in thyroid function, recent work by Puig-Domingo et al.[34] in the Richardson Ground Squirrel has shown that thyroxine 5'-deiodinase is found in the frontal
cortex, cerebellum, pineal gland and brown adipose tissue (BAT). In these hiber-
nators, melatonin administration produced a 7-fold increase in BAT thyroxine
deiodinase with an enhancing effect for both BAT and the pineal deiodinase upon
exposure to cold. The modulation of the thermogenic capacity of BAT by melatonin suggests that melatonin may be pertinent to both temperature and energy
utilization changes that occur with age. Of interest as to this and to the effect of
dietary restriction on life extension, there is a loss of thermogenic response with
overfeeding beyond 26 weeks of age in rats.[35]

Supporting the validity of our studies are data showing the decline of melatonin circadian values with age in rats and hamsters.[1,2,36,37] Although response to
light-dark cycling remains intact, there is an age-related decrease in melatonin
values in the pineal itself and in the circulating levels of melatonin.[38]

Clinically, Touitou et al.[39] found that levels of plasma melatonin in elderly
institutionalized patients showed a decline. Clinical correlates with disease or
pathology have been attempted but have not been significantly defined. Similarly,
Grinevich and Labunetz[40] found an age-related decrease in 6-oxymelatonin excretion in 140 normal male subjects over 30 years of age, although this was not seen
in women. Of interest to our pineal thymic grafting, this study described an age-
related decrease in thymic serum factor (TSF) while blood cortisol levels rose
with age.

Nair et al.[41] and Sack et al.[42] have shown a clinical age-related 24-hour decrease in serum melatonin as measured by radioimmunoassay and a lag in circadian melatonin peaking. They suggest that this could be used as a clinical
biomarker of aging. Waldhauser et al.[43] confirmed a nocturnal decline with lowest
serum levels in the 70–90 year old group.

In a search for mechanisms of age-related melatonin effects, Sharma et al.[44]
reviewed the literature regarding melatonin and corticosteroid changes with age.
Their data, from normal individuals (44 men, 27 women) divided into three age
groupings, show an age-related decline in melatonin and corticosteroid production. With age, there was a later diurnal onset of melatonin production with an
earlier daily output of cortisol. These observations have been confirmed in a
smaller series by Thomas & Miles.[45] Pertinent to this, Gupta[46] found an inverse
relationship between growth hormone releasing factor (GRF) and melatonin levels
in male rats. Similar clinical results, which may be pertinent to aging, were also
found in children and adults.

Waldhauser & Wurtman[47] reviewed the literature regarding pineal modulation
of hypothalamic function. Recent Soviet data suggest that a pineal polypeptide
may reduce sensitivity to dexamethasone.[48] This pineal product was involved in
stimulating increased transcortin binding of corticosteroids[49] which decreases
with age. The action of hydrocortisone in neonatal rats delays maturation of

pineal noradrenergic uptake and Yuwiler[50] suggests that steroids directly affect the pineal's response to noradrenergic stimulation by actions distal to β-receptor response. Chronic steroid exposure reduces noradrenergic stimulation of pineal N-acetyltransferase (NAT) activity and the formation of N-acetylated indols.

Rivest et al.[51] have shown clinical melatonin values to be highest when corticosteroid values were lowest. Rebuffat et al.[52] report that long-term melatonin administration causes hypertrophy of adrenal zona glomerulosa with a rise in serum aldosterone in rats. Wurtman et al.[53] also found adrenal enlargement subsequent to surgical pinealectomy or increased exposure to darkness. This makes sense, as Demisch et al.[54] have found that as little as 1 mg of evening dexamethasone suppresses nocturnal melatonin production.

Of interest to distress-mediated injury and the presence of melatonin in the GI tract, melatonin protects the rat stomach from serotonin and ethanol-induced ulceration which is thought to relate, in turn, to a reduced gastrointestinal glandular mucosal flow.[55]

In regard to the above, De Fronzo & Roth[56] have also suggested that there was a relationship between pineal function and the adrenals. Troiani et al.[57] found that saline injection in rats inhibited melatonin synthesis, probably via enhanced corticosteroid output, inasmuch as hypophysectomy blocked this response. Again, these results are important to Denckla's observation, and others', that hypophysectomy can reverse or delay aging in mice and rats.[33] In that regard, Denckla postulated that hypophysectomy removed "DECO", a "death hormone" that governs aging. What may have been involved in Denckla's observations was the action of a block to distress-mediated pineal inhibition of melatonin production.

In the search for an explanation pertinent to our effects on prolonging survival in mice, Maestroni & Pierpaoli[58] showed that functional (constant light) or pharmacological β-adrenergic blockage produced not only impairment of body growth but caused thymolymphatic atrophy and a decline in antibody production. In further support of this, Csaba et al.[59,60] had earlier shown that pinealectomy exerted profound effects on thymic morphology and function. In this regard, melatonin seems to upregulate immune response and antagonize the immunosuppressive effects of acute distress.[5]

Distinct from melatonin, Pierpaoli and Yi[9] have shown that TRH has remarkable thymus stimulating and immunoenhancing effects. However, in the case of TRH, its upregulating action is reported to antagonize endorphin effects[61] distinguishing it from melatonin. Furthermore, pineal function seems to be responsible for TRH production. In fact TRH is nocturnally elevated in a circadian fashion similar to melatonin.[62] TRH, as a tripeptide, is found in porcine, ovine and rodent pinealocytes. In addition, B and T lymphocytes are found in pineal parenchyma of the 3–4-week-old chicken.[13] This indicates that the pineal may have lymphoproliferative capacity. Vede et al.[63] reported that T cells increase with age in the rat pineal. Olath and Glick[64] suggest that the ectodermal origin of pinealocytes indicate that the pineal may influence thymic function in similar fashion to thymic keratinocytes.[65,66] Hume et al.[67] found that endocrine glands contain significant macrophage populations and that the pineal contains sinusoidal perivascular F4/80, antigenically identifiable phagocytic cells which could process antigen to modulate immune responses.[67]

The modulating effects of pineal engraftment in our study may also relate to the fact that the pineal contains peptide hormones found in the hypothalamic-neurohypophyseal system, i.e., oxytocin, vasopressin and vasotocin-like peptides in addition to melatonin or serotonin-related indoles. Prechel et al.[68] showed that these neuropeptides are not seasonally completely dependent on superior cervical ganglion sympathetic control and Schroder et al.[69] showed that vasopressin inhibits nocturnal melatonin production.

In a search for mechanisms of age-related melatonin decline, Tang et al.[70] showed that there was a decline in mid-dark pineal serotonin, norepinephrine and dopamine production in 18-month-old rats. As an explanation, they suggested that sympathetic activity enhanced conversion of serotonin to melatonin in the pineal.[70] An age-related decline in pineal response might reflect a pineal functional decline in sympathetic tone and, in that regard, there is delayed recovery of β-adrenergic downregulation induced by desmethylimipramine in 20–26-month-old rats.[71] This was confirmed by Greenberg[72] who showed that aged (24-month-old) mice lose their capacity to develop β-adrenergic hypersensitivity during the light cycle or following reserpine administration, where noradrenaline production is decreased or inhibited. As reported above, the pineal loses its capacity to upregulate both β and α receptors as a function of age because of delayed recovery from adrenergic downregulation.[72] In support of this, in vivo studies show that noradrenergic sensitivity declines with age and that there is an inverse relationship between corticosteroids and melatonin present in clinical depression.[73] In this regard, reduced melatonin production is found in elderly patients suffering from orthostatic hypotension.[74] This indicates a possible association between melatonin synthesis and sympathetic tone. In support of this, cold immobilization stress in rats causes a marked rise in pineal melatonin. This is accompanied by inhibition of monoamine oxidase which is ascribed to a brain-associated peptide, identified as "tribulin."[75]

Wu et al.[76] report that swimming stress enhances melatonin output at night or in the presence of desmethylimipramine, a norepinephrine blocker. As mentioned previously, the pineal contains high concentrations of monoamine oxidase. Agents like clorgyline and deprenyl, which inhibit the decrease of norepinephrine[77] induced by monoamine oxidase degradation, enhance melatonin production,[78] and there is recent work suggesting that deprenyl may enhance longevity and sexual performance in male rodents.

In another related area, Wright et al.[79] showed an age-related decline in superior cervical ganglion and pineal nerve growth factor (NGF) content. This change was sex related, NGF being higher in males or following testosterone treatment. Reuss et al.[80] also showed an age-related decline in pineal night-time melatonin excretion in 18-month-old rats correlating with decreased spontaneous pineal electrical activity in older animals.

As discussed earlier, in our study the thymus was used as the graft site, as both the innervation of the pineal gland and the thymus is derived mainly from the superior cervical ganglia,[8] although there is additional direct innervation from the CNS to the pineal.[12]

In the search for age-related mechanisms, Dax and Sugden[81] suggest that the major reason for decline in pineal melatonin synthesis with age is not receptor related in the Wistar rat, but due to a decline in pineal hydroxyindole-o-methyltransferase.

In another aspect of mechanisms of aging, one action of melatonin is the regulation of forebrain dopaminergic function.[82] L-dopa given to rats increases melatonin pineal content,[83] and there is a mixed clinical literature regarding the benefits of melatonin in Parkinson's disease and other movement disorders. As L-dopa administration enhances the life expectancy and motor responses of mice, it would be of interest if, in our melatonin or pineal transplantation studies, the results seen were mediated through the dopaminergic system.

In support of the above, Zisapel and Laudon[84] have shown that melatonin blocks the stimulated release of 3H-dopamine from the rat hypothalamus *in vitro*. Inhibition of dopamine release by melatonin has been observed in the ventral hippocampus, medulla-pons preoptic area and median and posterior hypothalamus, but not in the striatum or other areas.[85] In view of the above and the dopaminergic inhibition of prolactin secretion, it is of interest that melatonin causes a decrease in prolactin secretion in pituitary-grafted male rats. In addition, melatonin is reported to increase serotonin and decrease dopamine turnover in intact rats. Friedman *et al.*[86] have shown pineal indoles to decrease with age in old rats that were sensitive to imipramine β-adrenergic receptor, and also found serotonin receptor reduction with age.

The action of pinealectomy on prolactin production has been reviewed by Stanisiewski *et al.*[87] and Boissin-Agasse *et al.*[88] In mink, prolactin production following pinealectomy varies independent of its yearly photoperiods, and Kennaway *et al.*[89] have observed a heightened prolactin level in pinealectomized ewes. It would be of interest to investigate whether the rise in prolactin with age is a function of pineal changes with age, related to declining nocturnal melatonin production. In this regard, the role of melatonin in the induction of adrenarche is confused, as is the role of prolactin: dopaminergic blockade can hasten puberty in dogs.[90]

In another area, Haldar-Misra and Pevet[91] developed a concept that 5-methoxy indoles, including melatonin produced by the pineal, can affect the secretion of protein/peptides by the pineal. This would explain potential value of pineal engraftment from young to old mice as a method of maintaining pineal secretory integrity in older animals.

One of the biomarkers of aging is a change in polyamine ratios, and there is an increase in spermine over polyamines. In this regard, pinealectomy induces a decrease in ornithine decarboxylase.[92] Polyamines are key intracellular cations that are modulators of DNA and RNA synthesis.

Kahan[93] cites his work with pineal transplantation into the anterior eye chamber of the "rd" rat which develops spontaneous retinal degeneration. Pineal transplantation from normal animals prevented retinal dystrophy in these animals by supplying melatonin. He states in his review that patients with retinitis pigmentosa were "transitorily improved by melatonin injections" but provides no data.

One clinical potential of melatonin reflects upon its capacity to suppress ventral prostatic hyperplasia in rats.[94] These effects depend upon dosage. High dosages inhibited acinar proliferation, while lower dosages resulted in reduced stroma and epithelium. Based on this, one must ask if benign prostatic hypertrophy might relate to declining clinical melatonin levels with age.

As discussed previously, melatonin has direct inhibitory effects on human breast cancer cells in tissue culture which relates to the observation of a direct lethal action on this estrogen-sensitive cell line.[19] In addition, melatonin exerts direct inhibitory action on the Dunning prostatic adenocarcinoma.[18]

Our results in prolonging survival in aging mice did not concern dietary deprivation. No relevant difference in body weight was observed between control and melatonin-treated mice. It is in fact known that daily melatonin injections in male Syrian hamsters increase body weight.[95,96] Feeding melatonin increases plasma concentration of melatonin and increases fat deposition in the carcass of heifers.[97] Melatonin peaks at a point of lowest body temperature. The role of dietary deprivation in extending life expectancy has been related to a fall in body temperature. The decline in thyroid hormone production on nocturnal administration of melatonin (TABLE 2) suggests that this may be an important parallel effect to caloric restriction. In this regard, short-term fasting has been associated with a rise in norepinephrine and serum melatonin.[98,99] Others[100] describe underfeeding as a pineal-function-potentiating-factor in the rat. In addition, there is evidence that melatonin can modulate magnesium and zinc cationic levels.[101] This is of interest because of evidence that Mg^{++} enhances melatonin synthesis.[102] In this regard, Morton[101,102] suggests the possibility, based on work of Zaboni et al.[103] and Karppanen et al.[104] that pineal function could be a factor in hypertension. Alternatively, Landfield[105] has shown that Mg^{++} supplementation enhances CNS behaviour in aging mice, which may be due to a melatonin-magnesium relationship. If zinc levels are modulated by melatonin, this could be a factor in thyroid function and aging as discussed by Fabris et al.[106] and Travaglini et al.[107]

In summary, the two most important factors for species survival and maintenance of "identity" are gonadal and immunologic.[11] Based on this, we felt that the pineal is the developmental pacemaker which in the course of neuroendocrine ontogeny plays a major role in translating and modulating environmental cues to govern the developmental and functional integration of the hypothalamic-pituitary-gonadal-adrenal-TRH-thyroid system.[5,7,9] The pineal is constantly translating external stimuli (light, temperature, magnetism, pheromones, antigens) as well as internal messages (neuroendocrine, autonomic, psychic) into circadian and seasonal responses necessary for individual and species survival.

We feel the results in this study, which suggest that melatonin nocturnal administration or youthful pineal transplantation into older mice prolongs median and absolute survival, indicate that we must explore the mechanisms involved which may include trophic factors related to pineal peptides or indoles.

ACKNOWLEDGMENTS

We thank Ms. M. Hämmerli and CIBA-GEIGY AG, Animal Farm, Sisseln, for the generous supply of animals and helpful suggestions; Dr. K. Dixon and Mr. K. Rotach, WANDER AG, Bern, for the determinations of T3 and T4 and Ms. D. Malpangotti and Ms. M. Bacciarini for technical help. We are indebted to Dr. A. Giuliani, SIGMA-TAU INC., Pomezia, Italy, for his help in the statistics studies.

REFERENCES

1. REITER, R. J., C. M. CRAFT, J. E. JOHNSON et al. 1981. Age associated reduction in nocturnal pineal melatonin levels in female rats. Endocrinology 109: 1295–1297.
2. HOFFMANN, K., H. ILLNEROVA & I. VANECEK. 1985. Comparison of pineal melatonin rhythms in young adult and old djungarian hamsters (phodopus sungorus) under long and short photoperiods. Neurosci. Lett. 56: 39–43.
3. ERLICH, S. S. & M. L. J. ADUZZA. 1985. The pineal gland: anatomy, physiology and clinical significance. J. Neurosurg. 63: 321–341.
4. BREZEZINSKI, A. & R. J. WURTMAN. 1988. The pineal gland: its possible roles in human reproduction. OB Gyn. Survey 43: 197–207.
5. PIERPAOLI, W. & G. J. M. MAESTRONI. 1987. Melatonin: a principal neuroimmunoregulatory and anti-stress hormone: its anti-aging effects. Immunol. Lett. 16: 355–362.
6. MAESTRONI, G. J. M., A. CONTI & W. PIERPAOLI. 1988. Pineal melatonin, its fundamental immunoregulatory role in aging and cancer. Ann. N.Y. Acad. Sci. 521: 140–148.
7. PIERPAOLI, W. & C. X. YI. 1990. The pineal gland and melatonin: the aging clock? A

concept and experimental evidence. *In* Stress and Aging Brain. Raven Press. New York. In Press.

8. BULLOCH, K. 1985. Neuroanatomy of lymphoid tissue: a review. *In* Neural Modulation of Immunity. R. Guillemin, M. Cohn & T. Melnechuk, Eds. 111–141. Raven Press. New York.

9. PIERPAOLI, W. & C. X. YI. 1990. The involvement of pineal gland and melatonin in immunity and aging. I. Thymus-mediated, immunoreconstituting and antiviral activity of thyrotropin-releasing hormone. J. Neuroimmunol. **27:** 99–110.

10. PIERPAOLI, W. & H. O. BESEDOVSKY. 1975. Role of the thymus in programming of neuroendocrine functions. Clin. Exp. Immunol. **20:** 323–338.

11. PIERPAOLI, W. 1981. Integrated phylogenetic and ontogenetic evolution of neuroendocrine and identity-defence, immune functions. *In* Psychoneuroimmunology. R. Ader, Ed. 575–606. Academic Press. New York.

12. MOORE, R. Y. 1978. Neural control of pineal function in mammals and birds. J. Neural Transm. Suppl. **13:** 47–58.

13. COGBURN, L. A. & B. GLICK. 1983. Functional lymphocytes in the chicken pineal gland. J. Immunol. **130:** 2109–2112.

14. KIKUCHI, Y., T. KITA, M. MIYAUCHI *et al.* 1989. Inhibition of human ovarian cancer cell proliferation *in vitro* by neuroendocrine hormones. Gyn. Oncol. **32:** 60–64.

15. SCHMIDT, T. J. & M. LIPPMAN. 1978. Evidence for cytoplasmic melatonin receptor. Nature **274:** 894–895.

16. MACPHEE, A. A., F. E. COLE & B. F. RICE. 1975. The effect of melatonin on steroidogenesis by the human ovary *in vitro*. J. Clin. Endocrinol. Metab. **40:** 688–696.

17. WEBLEY, G. E. & F. LEINBENBERGER. 1986. The circadian pattern of melatonin and its positive relationship with progesterone in women. J. Clin. Endocrinol. Metab. **63:** 323–328.

18. PHILO, R. & A. S. BERKOWITZ. 1988. Inhibition of dunning tumor growth by melatonin. J. Urol. **139:** 1099–1102.

19. HILL, S. M. & D. E. BLASK. 1988. Effect of the pineal hormone melatonin on the proliferation and morphological characteristics of human breast cancer cells (MCF7) in culture. Cancer Res. **48:** 6121–6126.

20. REPPERT, S. M., D. R. WEAVER, S. A. RIVKEES & E. G. STOPA. 1988. Putative melatonin receptors in a human biological clock. Science **242:** 78–81.

21. REDMAN, J., S. ARMSTRONG & K. T. NG. 1983. Free-running activity rhythms in the rat: entrainment by melatonin. Science **219:** 1080–1081.

22. SIZONENKO, P. C., U. LANG, R. W. RIVEST & M. L. AUBERT. 1985. The pineal and pubertal development. *In* Photoperiodism, Melatonin and the Pineal. Ciba Foundation Symp. **117:** 208–225.

23. ESQUIFINO, A. I., M. A. VILLANUA & C. AGRASAL. 1987. Effect of neonatal melatonin administration on sexual development in the rat. J. Steroid Biochem. **27:** 1089–1093.

24. REITER, R. J. 1987. The melatonin message: duration versus coincidence hypothesis. Life Sci. **40:** 2119–2131.

25. WEAVER, D. R., J. T. KEOHAN & S. M. REPPERT. 1987. Definition of a prenatal sensitive period for maternal-fetal communication of day length. Am. J. Physiol. 253 (Endocrinol. Metab. 16): E701–E704.

26. REITER, R. J. 1980. The pineal and its hormones in the control of reproduction in mammals. Endocr. Rev. **1:** 109–131.

27. GOLDMAN, B. D., D. S. CARTER, V. D. HALL *et al.* 1982. Physiology of pineal melatonin in three hamster species. *In* Melatonin Rhythm Generating System. C. Klein, Ed. 210–231. Karger. Basel.

28. RIVEST, R. W., P. SCHULZ, S. LUSTENBERGER *et al.* 1989. Differences between circadian and ultradian organization of cortisol and melatonin rhythms during activity and rest. J. Clin. Endocrinol. Metab. **68:** 721–729.

29. MASSON-PEVET, M., P. PEVET & B. VIVIEN-ROELS. 1987. Pinealectomy and constant release of melatonin or 5-methoxytryptamine induce testicular atrophy in the European hamster (*Cricetus cricetus*). J. Pineal Res. **4:** 79–88.

30. SOUETRE, E., N. E. ROSENTHAL & J-P. ORTONNE. 1988. Affective disorders, light and melatonin. Photodermatology **5:** 107–109.
31. DAVIS, L. & J. MARTIN. 1940. Results of experimental removal of pineal gland in young mammals. Arch. Neurol. Psychiatr. **43:** 23–45.
32. HOUSSAY, A. B. & J. H. PAZO. 1968. Role of pituitary in the thyroid hypertrophy of pinealectomized rats. Experientia **24:** 813–814.
33. REGELSON, W. 1983. The evidence for pituitary and thyroid control of aging: is age reversal a myth or reality? The search for a "death hormone". *In* "Interventions in the Aging Process. W. Regelson & F. M. Sinex, Eds. 3–52. Alan R. Liss. New York.
34. PUIG-DOMINGO, M., J. M. GUERRERO & R. J. REITER. 1988. Thyroxine 5′-deiodination in brown adipose tissue and pineal gland: implications for thermogenic regulation and the role of melatonin. Endocrinology **123:** 677–680.
35. STOCK, M. J. & N. J. ROTHWELL. 1986. The role of brown fat in diet induced thermogenesis. Int. J. Vitam. Nutr. Res. **56:** 205–210.
36. REITER, R. J., L. Y. JOHNSON, R. W. STEGER *et al.* 1980a. Pineal biosynthesis and neuroendocrine physiology in the aging hamster and gerbil. Peptides **1**(Suppl. 1): 69–77.
37. REITER, R. J., B. A. RICHARDSON, L. Y. JOHNSON *et al.* 1980b. Pineal melatonin rhythm; reduction in aging syrian hamsters. Science **210:** 1372–1373.
38. PANG, S. F. & P. L. TANG. 1983. Decreased serum and pineal concentrations of melatonin and NAT in aged male hamsters. Horm. Res. **17:** 228–234.
39. TOUITOU, Y., M. FEVRE-MONTAGNE, J. PROUST *et al.* 1985. Age- and sex-associated modification of plasma melatonin concentrations in man. Relationship to pathology, malignant or not, and autopsy findings. Acta Endocrinol. **108:** 135–144.
40. GRINEVICH, Y. A. & I. F. LABUNETZ. 1986. Melatonin, thymic serum factor and cortisol levels in healthy subjects of different age and patients with skin melanoma. J. Pineal Res. **3:** 263–275.
41. NAIR, N. P. V., N. HARIHARASUBRAMANIAN, C. PILAPIL *et al.* 1986. Plasma melatonin—an index of brain aging in humans? Biol. Psychiatr. **21:** 141–150.
42. SACK, R. L., A. J. LEWY & D. L. ERB *et al.* 1986. Human melatonin production decreases with age. J. Pineal Res. **3:** 379–388.
43. WALDHAUSER, F., G. WEISSENBACHER, E. TATZER *et al.* 1988. Alterations in nocturnal serum melatonin levels in humans with growth and aging. J. Clin. Endocrinol. Metab. **66:** 648–652.
44. SHARMA, M., J. PALACIOS-BOIS, G. SCHWARTZ *et al.* 1989. Circadian rhythms of melatonin and cortisol in aging. Biol. Psychol. **25:** 305–319.
45. THOMAS, D. R. & A. MILES. 1989. Melatonin secretion and age. Biol. Psychol. **25:** 365–367.
46. GUPTA, D. 1986. Neuropeptide neurotransmitter interaction due to GRF and CRF stimulation in experimental and clinical conditions during development. Monogr. Neural Sci. **12:** 128–141.
47. WALDHAUSER, F. & R. J. WURTMAN. 1983. The secretion and action of melatonin. *In* Biochemical Actions of Hormones. C. Litwack, Ed. 187–225. Academic Press. New York.
48. DILMAN, V. M. 1983. Endokrinologicheskaya Onkologiya. Medicina. Leningrad.
49. GOLIKOV, P. P. 1973. Influence of pinealectomy on transcortin binding ability in rats. Prob. Endocrinol. **19:** 100–102.
50. YUWILER, A. 1985. Neonatal steroid treatment reduces catecholamine-induced increases in pineal serotonin N-acetyltransferase activity. J. Neurochem. **44:** 1185–1193.
51. RIVEST, R. W., M. E. E. JACONI, N. GRUAZ *et al.* 1987. Short term and long term effects of melatonin on GnRH stimulated gonadotropin secretion in pituitaries of sexually maturing rats. Neuroendocrinology **46:** 379–386.
52. REBUFFAT, P., G. MAZZOCCHI, A. STACHOWIAK *et al.* 1988. A morphometric study of the effects of melatonin on the rat adrenal zona glomerulosa. Exp. Clin. Endocrinol. **91:** 59–64.

53. WURTMAN, R. J. M. D. ALTSCHULE & U. HOLMGREN. 1959. Effects of pinealectomy and of a bovine pineal extract in rats. Am. J. Physiol. **197**: 108–110.
54. DEMISCH, L., J. DEMISCH & T. NIKELSEN. 1988. Influence of dexamethasone on nocturnal melatonin production in healthy adult subjects. J. Pineal Res. **5**: 317–322.
55. CHO, C. H., S. F. PANG, B. W. CHEN & C. J. PFEIFFER. 1989. Modulating action of melatonin on serotonin induced aggravation of ethanol ulceration and changes of mucosal blood flow in rat stomachs. J. Pineal Res. **6**: 89–97.
56. DEFRONZO, R. A. & W. D. ROTH. 1972. Evidence for the existence of a pineal-adrenal and pineal-thyroid axis. Acta Endocrinol. **70**: 31–42.
57. TROIANI, M. E., R. J. REITER, M. K. VAUGHAN *et al.* 1988. The depression in rat pineal melatonin production after saline injection at night may be elicited by corticosteroid. Brain Res. **450**: 18–24.
58. MAESTRONI, G. J. M. & W. PIERPAOLI. 1981. Pharmacologic control of the hormonally mediated immune response. *In* Psychoneuroimmunology. R. Ader, Ed. 405–425. Academic Press. New York.
59. CSABA, G., M. BODOKY, J. FISHER & T. ACS. 1966. The effect of pinealectomy and thymectomy on immune capacity of the rat. Experientia **22**: 168–169.
60. CSABA. B. & P. BARATH. 1975. Morphological changes of thymus and the thyroid gland after postnatal extirpation of pineal body. Endocrinol. Exp. (Bratisl.) **9**: 59–65.
61. FADEN A. I. 1984. Opiate antagonists and thyrotropin-releasing hormone. J. Am. Med. Assoc. **252**: 1177–1180.
62. VANHAELST, C., E. VAN CAUTER, J. DEGAUTE & J. GOLDSTEIN. 1972. Circadian variations of serum thyrotropin levels. J. Clin. Endocrinol. Metab. **35**: 479–482.
63. VEDE, T., Y. ISHII, A. MATSUME *et al.* 1981. Immunohistochemical study of lymphocytes in rat pineal gland: Selective accumulation of T lymphocytes. Anat. Rec. **199**: 239–247.
64. OLAH, I. & B. GLICK. 1984. Lymphopoietic tissue in the chicken. Dev. Comp. Immunol. **8**: 855–862.
65. RUBENFELD, M., A. SILVERSTONE, D. KNOWLES *et al.* 1981. Induction of lymphocyte differentiation by epidermal cultures. J. Invest. Dermatol. **77**: 221–225.
66. LUGER, T. A., B. M. STAPLER, S. I. KATZ & J. J. OPPENHEIM. 1981. A thymocyte activating factor produced by a murine keratinocyte cell line. J. Immunol. **127**: 1493–1498.
67. HUME, D. A., D. HALPIN, H. CHARLTON & S. GORDON. 1984. The mononuclear phagocyte system of the mouse defined by immunohistochemical localization of antigen F4/80: macrophages of endocrine organs. Proc. Natl. Acad. Sci. USA **81**: 4174–4177.
68. PRECHEL, M. M., T. K. AUDHYA, R. SENSON *et al.* 1989. A seasonal pineal peptide rhythm persists in superior cervical ganglionectomized rats. Life Sci. **44**: 103–110.
69. SCHRODER, H., E. WEIIFE, D. NOHR & L. VOLLRATH. 1988. Immunohistochemical evidence for the presence of peptides derived from proenkephalin, prodynorphin and proopiomelanocortin in the guinea pig pineal gland. Histochemistry **88**: 333–341.
70. TANG, F., M. HADJI CONSTANTINOU & S. F. PANG. 1985. Aging and diurnal rhythms of pineal serotonin, 5-hydroxyindolacetic acid, norepinephrine, dopamine and serum melatonin in the male rat. Neuroendocrinology **40**: 160–164.
71. GREENBERG, L. H., P. J. BRUNSWICK & B. WEISS. 1985. Effect of age on the rate of recovery of β-adrenergic receptors in rat brain following desmethylimipramine-induced subsensitivity. Brain. Res. **328**: 81–88.
72. GREENBERG, L. H. 1986. Regulation of brain adrenergic receptors during aging. Fed. Proc. **45**: 55–59.
73. BECK-FRIIS, J., B. F. KJELLMAN, B. APERIA *et al.* 1985. Serum melatonin in relation to clinical variables in patients with major depressive disorder and a hypothesis of a low melatonin syndrome. Acta Psychiatr. Scand. **71**: 319–330.
74. TETSUO, M., R. J. POLINSKY & S. P. MARKEY. 1981. Urinary 6-hydroxymelatonin in hypotension. J. Clin. Endocrinol. Metab. **53**: 607–609.

75. BHATTACHARYA, S. K., V. GLOVER, I. MCINTYRE et al. 1988. Stress causes an increase in endogenous monoamine oxidase inhibitor (tribulin) in rat brain. Neurosci. Lett. **92:** 218–221.
76. WU, W., Y-C. CHEN & R. J. REITER. 1988. Day-night differences in the response of the pineal gland to swimming stress. Proc. Soc. Exp. Biol. Med. **187:** 315–319.
77. DELEO, F., P. RUGGERI & A. VALENTI. 1983. Monoamino-oxidase activity in rat pineal gland. Histochemical studies. Bas. Appl. Histochem. **27:** 211–217.
78. OXENKRUG, G., I. MCINTYRE, R. MCCAULEY & A. YUWILER. 1988. Effect of selective monoamine oxidase inhibitors on rat pineal melatonin synthesis in vitro. J. Pineal Res. **5:** 99–109.
79. WRIGHT, L. L., C. BECK & J. R. PEREZ-POLO. 1987. Sex differences in nerve growth factor levels in superior cervical ganglia and pineals. Int. J. Dev. Neurosci. **5:** 383–390.
80. REUSS, S., J. OLCESE & L. VOLLRATH. 1986. Electrophysiological and endocrinological aspects of aging in the rat pineal gland. Neuroendocrinol. **43:** 466–470.
81. DAX, E. M., & D. SUGDEN. 1988. Age associated changes in pineal adrenergic receptors and melatonin synthesizing enzymes in the Wistar rat. J. Neurochem. **50:** 468–472.
82. BRADBURY, A. J., M. E. KELLY & J. A. SMITH. 1985. Melatonin action in the midbrain can regulate dopamine function both behaviorally and biochemically. *In* The Pineal Gland: Endocrine Aspects. G. M. Brown & S. D. Wainwright, Eds. 327–332. Pergamon Press. Oxford.
83. LYNCH, H. J., P. WANG & R. J. WURTMAN. 1973. Increase in rat pineal melatonin content following L-dopa administration. Life Sci. **12:** 145–151.
84. ZISAPEL, N. & M. LAUDON. 1982. Dopamine release induced by electrical field stimulation of rat hypothalamus in vitro: inhibition by melatonin. Biochem. Biophys. Res. Commun. **104:** 1610–1616.
85. ZISAPEL, N., Y. EGOZI & M. LAUDON. 1982. Circadian variations in the inhibition of dopamine by melatonin regional distribution in the rat brain. Brain Res. **246:** 161–164.
86. FRIEDMAN, E., T. COOPER & F. YOCCA. 1986. The effect of imipramine treatment on brain serotonin receptors and β-adrenoreceptors and on pineal β-adrenergic function in adult and aged rats. Eur. J. Pharmacol. **123:** 351–356.
87. STANISIEWSKI, E. P., N. K. AMES, L. T. CHAPIN, C. A. BLAZE & H. A. TUCKER. 1988. Effect of pinealectomy on prolactin, testosterone and luteinizing hormone concentration in plasma of bull calves exposed to 8 or 16 hours of light per day. J. Anim. Sci. **66:** 464–469.
88. BOISSIN-AGASSE, L., J. M. JACQUET, A. LA-CROIX & J. BOISSIN. 1988. Long term effects of pinealectomy on testicular function, luteinizing hormone-releasing hormone hypothalamic system, and plasma prolactin levels in the mink, a short day breeder. J. Pineal Res. **5:** 358–396.
89. KENNAWAY, D. J., E. A. DUNSTAN, T. A. GILMORE & R. F. SEAMARK. 1983. Effects of shortened daylength and melatonin on plasma prolactin and melatonin levels in pinealectomized and sham operated ewes. Anim. Reprod. Sci. **5:** 287–294.
90. PEREZ-FERNANDEZ, R., F. FACCHINETTI, A. BEIRAS et al. 1987. Morphological and functional stimulation of adrenal reticularis zone by dopaminergic blockage in dogs. J. Steroid Biochem. **28:** 465–470.
91. HALDAR-MISRA, C. & P. PEVET. 1983. The influence of different 5-methoxyindoles on the process of protein/peptide secretion characterized by the formation of granular vesicles in the mouse pineal gland. Cell Tissue Res. **230:** 113–126.
92. FRASCHINI, F., M. E. FERIOLI, R. NEBULONI & G. SCALABRINO. 1980. Pineal gland and polyamines. J. Neural Transm. **48:** 209–221.
93. KAHAN, A. 1985. Developmental implication of ocular pharmacology. Pharmacol. Ther. **28:** 163–226.
94. SRIUILAI, W. & B. WITHYACITUMROARNKU. 1989. Stereological changes in rat ventral prostate induced by melatonin. J. Pineal Res. **6:** 111–119.
95. HOFFMAN, R. A., K. DAVIDSON & K. STEINBERG. 1982. Influence of photoperiod and

temperature on weight gain, food consumption, fat pads, and thyroxine in male golden hamsters. Growth **46**: 150–162.

96. HOFFMAN, R. A. 1983. Seasonal growth and development and the influence of the eyes and pineal gland on body weight of golden hamsters (M. Auratus). Growth **47**: 109–121.

97. ZINN, S. A., L. T. CHAPIN, W. J. ENRIGHT *et al.* 1988. Growth, carcass composition and plasma melatonin in postpubertal beef heifers fed melatonin. J. Anim. Sci. **66**: 21–27.

98. BEITINS, I. Z., A. BARKAN, A. KLIBANSKI *et al.* 1985. Hormonal responses to short term fasting in post menopausal women. J. Clin. Endocrinol. Metab. **60**: 1120–1126.

99. VAUGHAN, M. K., M. NORDIO, P. J. CHENOWITH *et al.* 198. Underfeeding and exposure to short photoperiod alters rat pineal and harderian gland lysosomal enzyme activities. Proc. Soc. Exp. Biol. Med. **189**: 211–216.

100. BLASK, D. E., J. NODELMAN, C. A. LEADEM *et al.* 1980. Influence of exogenously administered melatonin on the reproductive system and prolactin levels in underfed male rats. Biol. Reprod. **22**: 507–512.

101. MORTON, D. J. 1989. Effect of methoxyindole administration on plasma cation levels in the rat. J. Pineal Res. **6**: 141–147.

102. MORTON, D. J. & M. F. M. JAMES. 1985. Effects of magnesium ions on rat pineal N-acetyltransferase activity. J. Pineal Res. **3**: 387–391.

103. ZABONI, A., A. FORNI, W. ZABONI-MUSIACCIA & C. ZANUSSI. 1978. Effect of pinealectomy on arterial blood pressure and food and water intake in the rat. J. Endocrinol. Invest. **2**: 125–130.

104. KARPPANEN, H., H. VAPARTALO, S. LAHOVAARA & M. K. PAASONONONN. 1970. Studies with pinealectomized rats. Pharmacology **3**: 76–84.

105. LANDFIELD, P. W., R. K. BASKIN & T. A. PITLER. 1981. Brain aging correlates: retardation by hormonal-pharmacological treatments. Science **214**: 581–584.

106. FABRIS, N., E. MOCCHEGGIANI, L. AMADIO *et al.* 1984. Thymic hormone deficiency in normal aging and Down's syndrome: is there a primary failure of the thymus? Lancet **1**: 983–986.

107. TRAVAGLINI, P., P. MORIONDO, E. TOGNI *et al.* 1989. Effect of oral zinc administration on prolactin and thymulin circulating levels in patients with chronic renal failure. J. Clin. Endocrinol. Metab. **68**: 186–190.

The Role of Zinc in Neuroendocrine-Immune Interactions during Aging

N. FABRIS, E. MOCCHEGIANI, M. MUZZIOLI,
AND M. PROVINCIALI

Chair of Immunology, Medical Faculty
University of Pavia

and

Italian National Research Centers on Aging (INRCA)
Via Birarelli, 8
60121 Ancona, Italy

INTRODUCTION

Among the more than fifty elements identified in mammalian tissues, some of them, called trace elements because present in extremely small amounts, play a fundamental role in various enzymatic and hormonal functions. Most relevant in this context are copper, iron, nickel, manganese, zinc, selenium and fluoride.

The possibility that trace elements may play a role in physiological aging processes was originally hypothesized following the observation that with advancing age, at least in humans, alimentary habits consistently vary and defective intake of various micronutrients is almost unavoidable.

This assumption seems to be particularly true for zinc, whose intake is much more reduced in old age when compared with the Recommended Dietary Allowance (RDA), than the intake of other trace elements (TABLE 1).

This is reflected by the relatively low concentration of plasma zinc in elderly, though it should be taken into account that present technology, largely based on physicochemical determination of the trace element concentration in different body fluids and tissues, does not indicate the quality of the mineral-bound proteins, their binding affinity, or the free-fraction of the mineral which may be of even higher relevance than the bound fraction.

Due to these considerations, the determination of the total concentration of minerals may not reflect the real requirement, and even marginal mineral deficiencies might play a relevant role in age-associated pathologies.

The relevance of the age-dependent decline in zinc turnover is not, at present, completely clarified. It does not seem, however, a purely temporal coincidence that some of the known zinc-dependent functions, such as wound healing, skin-cell turnover, taste acuity and immune efficiency,[1] are all found depressed in old individuals and that in some instances the age-dependent deterioration can be reversed by zinc supplementation.[2]

This presentation aims to review the relevance of zinc for the immune-neuroendocrine function and, particularly, for the immune-endocrinological disorders associated with advancing age.

314

Zinc Turnover in Aging

With regard to zinc intake and turnover in old individuals, information is still incomplete. According to one of the major surveys, performed by the USDA, zinc intake appears to be reduced in old age.[3] Plasma level of zinc was reduced while, however, no definite information was available on intracellular zinc content.

The assumption that alterations of zinc turnover are common findings in old age requires confirmation in species other than humans. In this context, very little data are available. Recent findings from our laboratory have demonstrated that also in mice and rats plasma zinc levels are significantly reduced with age and in spite of the fact that, at least in laboratory animals, food intake is not modified.[4]

TABLE 1. Recommended Daily Allowances (RDA) or Estimate of Safe and Adequate Daily Intake of Some Trace Elements and Actual Intake in Elderly

Trace Elements	RDA (mg)	Daily Intake (mg)	References
Copper (RDA)	2–3	1.0–2.2	Gibson *et al.* 1983[41]
Zinc (RDA)	15	7.0–10	Wager *et al.* 1983[42]
Manganese[a]	2.5–5.0	2.5–3.5	Gibson *et al.* 1983[41]
Chromium[a]	0.05–0.2	0.005–0.11	Levine *et al.* 1968[43]
Iron (RDA)	10	9.2–14.1	DHEW 1979[44]
Selenium[a]	0.05–0.2	0.05–0.2	Gibson *et al.* 1983[41]

[a] Estimated safe and adequate intake.

The causes for such a progressive reduction of zinc turnover in aging are still unknown. Zinc is absorbed at intestinal level by transportation across the mucosal brush border and basolateral membranes to the portal circulation. The process probably requires ATP. Zinc is then transferred to high molecular weight proteins, to metallothioneins or to the plasma, where it binds to albumin, alpha2-macroglobulin, transferrin, coeruloplasmin, haptoglobulin: only a small fraction (2–3%) exists as ultrafiltrable fraction, largely bound to aminoacids or in an ionic form.[1] No data are presently available on which of these steps are altered with advancing age. But, at least in humans, it has been shown that both zinc absorbtion and zinc losses through urine and feces are reduced with advancing age. The last phenomenon has been considered as compensatory in nature, though not sufficient to prevent progressive reduction of zinc plasma levels.[5] With regard to absorption rate, it should be taken into account that zinc is available primarily from animal proteins,[6] whose intake is generally reduced in old age, but also other dietary habits may interfere with zinc absorbtion. Phytate, inorganic phosphate, fibre, iron, tin and oxalic acid have all been reported to modify zinc requirement.[7]

The conditions characterized by zinc deficiency are quite numerous in human pathology (TABLE 2): in addition to congenital diseases, such as acrodermatitis enteropathica and sickle cell anemia, a good number of acquired diseases are characterized by alterations in zinc turnover, and it is conceivable that subclinical aspects of some of these diseases, usually present in elderly, may further contribute to the alteration of the trace element absorbtion or excretion. Of particular relevance in this context, there may be malabsorbtion syndromes, renal disease, alcoholism and the use of drugs capable of interfering with zinc metabolism (chelating agents, diuretics, glucocorticoids, etc.).

Although further investigations are required in order to establish the physiological and pathological components of the altered zinc turnover in elderly, it is clear from this short illustration that a large proportion of aged individuals may be at risk in not consuming or retaining adequate amounts of zinc.

Furthermore, the fact that a large proportion of zinc is bound to proteins with quite different Kd, ranging from 10^{-11} for NGF to 10^{-3} for metalloaldolase (TABLE 3), adds an additional source of interference, according to the rate of synthesis and the distribution in tissues and body fluids of the different zinc-binding proteins, which may also be changed in the elderly and may, therefore, modify the quota of free-zinc or its distribution among the various zinc-requiring proteins. This consideration may account for the fact that signs of zinc deprivation may also appear in marginal zinc deficiencies when the plasma level of zinc is reduced by less than 20% of normal values.[8] In this case it might be assumed that not all zinc-dependent functions are altered but just those which are due to molecules with lower binding affinity for zinc, as may happen for thymulin within the immune system, or those which may be more crucial in a given period of life such as during brain development in early life or during sexual maturation at puberty.

TABLE 2. Potential Causes of Zinc Deficiency

Genetic and congenital diseases	Infections
Acrodermatitis enteropathica	Active tuberculosis
Sickle cell anemia	Parasitic infections
Celiac sprue	Pulmonary infections
Cystic fibrosis	Urinary tract infections
Down's syndrome	Acquired immunodeficiency syndrome
Duchenne's syndrome	(AIDS)
Reduced intake and absorption	Endocrine disorders
Pancreatic insufficiency	Hyperprolactinemia
Inflammatory bowel disease	Pregnancy
Regional enteritis (Crohn's disease)	Diabetes
Ulcerative colitis	Introgenic causes
Alcoholism	Antianabolic drugs
Alcoholic cirrhosis	Antimetabolite drugs
Hepatitis	Chelating drugs (Penicillamine, EDTA)
Starvation	Corticosteroids
Cancer	Diuretic drugs
Intestinal diverticuli or blind loops	Oral contraceptives
Anorexia nervosa	
Chronic severe depression	
Reumathoid arthritis	
Excessive loss	
Postsurgical	
Burns	
Collagen-vascular disease	
Acute myocardial infarction	
Renal failure	
Nephrotic syndrome	
Massive tissue injury	

TABLE 3. Different Binding Affinity of Various Proteins for Zinc

Compounds	Kd	References
Angiotensin-converting-enzyme (ACE)	2.3×10^{-3} M	Reeves *et al.* 1986[45]
Superoxide dismutase	5.0×10^{-4} M	Coleman 1974[46]
Alcohol deydrogenase	1.0×10^{-5} M	Coleman 1974[46]
Alkaline-phosphatase	1.0×10^{-6} M	Coleman 1974[46]
Metalloproteins (α, β)	$10^{-6}/10^{-7}$ M	Baudier *et al.* 1983[47]
Thymulin (ZnFTS)	$5 \pm 2 \times 10^{-7}$ M	Gastinel *et al.* 1984[48]
Metallotioneins	1.5×10^{-8} M	Phylipps 1979[49]
Nerve growth factor (NGF)	$10^{-10}/10^{-11}$ M	Dunn *et al.* 1980[50]

The Role of Zinc in the Neuroendocrine-Immune System

The involvement of zinc in immunocompetence in man and other animals is probably the best known at present. Zinc deficiency in laboratory animals causes thymic and lymphonode atrophy and impaired cell-mediated cutaneous hypersensitivity reactions.[9] Lymphocytes isolated from zinc-deficient animals show impaired response to phytohaemagglutinin (PHA) and depression of T cell-dependent antibody production.[10] Furthermore zinc-deficient diet in experimental animals causes impaired T helper and T suppressor function and decreased T killer and natural killer activity.[11]

In humans the effect of zinc deficiency on the immune function has been studied in congenital diseases such as acrodermatitis enteropathica, sickle cell anemia[1] and Down's syndrome[12] and in conditions characterized by acquired altered zinc turnover such as in malabsorption syndromes. Depending on the severity and duration, zinc deficiency causes hypoplasia of the thymus, spleen, lymphonodes and Peyer's paches.[13] Alterations in lymphocyte population including reduced helper T lymphocyte function, reduced natural killer activity, decreased number of total T lymphocytes with increased B lymphocytes, are a common and constant aspect in zinc-deficiency diseases.[2,14]

The mechanism by which zinc may affect the immune system is certainly multifaceted, due to the widespread action of zinc on different enzymes and hormones involved in various physiological steps of immune development and response.

Zinc is required for the nucleoside phosphorylase, a purine enzyme which is required also by T cell for its functioning,[15] and it has been shown that it is also a potent *in vitro* T lymphocyte mitogen for both man and animals over a narrow range of concentrations.[16]

These observations, however, should be reconsidered in the light of the findings that zinc is involved in the production of at least two cytokines, IL-1 and IL-6 and that the first one is an obligatory step in T cell proliferation.[17]

Zinc is required also for conferring biological activity to one of the best known thymic peptides, *i.e.*, the *facteur thymique serique* (FTS), more recently called *thymulin* in its zinc-bound form,[18] whereas the zinc-unbound peptide is able to bind to target sites but is inactive and likely prevents the active form exerting its action.[12] The presence of inactive hormone molecules in biological fluids may be revealed by measuring their capacity for inhibiting known amounts of synthetic active thymulin,[9,12] and indirectly by measuring thymulin activity in biological samples before and after *in vitro* addition of zinc ions, which may unmask the presence of inactive hormone.[20]

It has in fact been demonstrated that in conditions characterized by more or less deep zinc deficiencies, such as those associated with physiological aging or Down syndrome[12] or with congenital diseases such as acrodermatitis entero-pathica, cystic fybrosis, and Duchenne syndromes,[8] with infectious diseases, such as AIDS,[21] or with renal failure[22] a reduction of the circulating level of active thymulin is observed with a concomitant appearance of inactive zinc-unbound FTS molecules. The *in vitro* addition of zinc ions to plasma samples is able to unmask inactive circulating FTS molecules, showing that the total amount of the thymic hormone (zinc bound + zinc unbound FTS) is frequently much higher than the active fraction in all the above-reported zinc marginal deficiencies.

The mechanism of action of zinc on the immune system may not be restricted to directly activate thymic peptides or to influence some peripheral immune functions. Zinc-deficient diets cause alterations in various neurohormonal profiles, involving hormones and neurotransmitters which have been shown to modulate the immune system and, in particular, the rate of synthesis and/or secretion of thymic peptides.

Thus, reduction of plasma levels of growth hormone, of thyrotropic hormone, of thyroid hormones as well as of enkephalins has been reported to occur in the course of zinc-deprivation;[1] all these humoral factors positively influence various immune parameters. In addition, zinc-deficiency causes increased plasma level of glucocorticoids, epinephrine and norepinephrine, which, on the contrary, have an immunosuppressive effect.

Following these considerations it cannot be excluded that the action exerted by zinc on the immune system might be mediated through the modulation of immune-promoting or immunosuppressing hormones and neurotransmitters.

Zinc and Neuroendocrine-Immunological Aging: Effect of Zinc Supplementation

The observation of age-associated alterations in zinc turnover together with the knowledge of its involvement in neuroendocrine-immune efficiency has led to the investigation of the effect that a zinc supplementation may have on the age-related decline of immune functions.

Experiments performed in rodents, by applying dietary zinc supplementation during the whole life span, have demonstrated that in these conditions many of the known age-related immune modifications, including decreased thymic hormone production, reduced T helper and T suppressor activity and depressed NK cyto-toxicity could be prevented by such treatment.[11]

Furthermore, when this regimen was applied to autoimmune-susceptible NZB mice, zinc supplementation was able to delay the time of appearance of autoag-gressive reactions.[23] These findings have been interpreted in the light of a possible prevention of age-related alterations. A major question raised by these data has been whether age-related immune deterioration could be corrected, even after the immune alterations had occurred.

Trials performed in aged humans have shown that, in fact, zinc supplementa-tion might be able to increase the cutaneous sensitivity to various antigens and the antibody response to tetanus toxoid,[24] and to improve thymic endocrine activity.[25]

Recent experiments from our laboratory have attempted to elucidate the mech-anism of such an action and, in particular, have been addressed to investigate whether zinc supplementation acts only on discrete immune functions or is exerted also at the neuroendocrine level. At present, only two experimental designs have been followed. The first one was based on zinc supplementation given to subjects affected by Down's syndrome, a syndrome which is considered one of the best syndromes of accelerated aging.

Down's syndrome is the most frequent human chromosomal aneuploidy, being characterized by the presence of an extra chromosome 21.[26] This is quite a complex clinical syndrome, where cardiopathies, high incidence of leukemia, and increased susceptibility to infectious diseases[27] are frequent cause of death.

We have shown that a marginal but biologically relevant zinc deficiency is usually present in children with DS.[12] The alteration in the bioavailability of this trace element plays an important role in the pathogenesis of some immune defects associated with the syndrome.[28] In particular, thymic endocrine function and T cell-dependent immunity appear to be affected by zinc deficiency in subjects with DS.[29,12,28] On the other hand, zinc supplementation positively affects some immune parameters, such as the activation of thymulin,[28] T cell subsets, and neutrophil chemotaxis function,[29] and decreases the incidence of infectious diseases in children with DS[30] (TABLE 4).

Recently, a peculiar abnormality of thyroid hormone pattern was described. In fact, an excess of TSH with normal levels of T3 and T4 and decreased levels of rT3 appear to be frequently associated with the syndrome.[31,32,33]

In our study, we found that the abnormal levels of both TSH and rT3 could be corrected in a group of children with DS after zinc supplementation.[30]

The second model is based on experimental animals.

Oral zinc supplementation, when given to aged mice, is able to induce a regrowth of the thymus (TABLE 5) with increased thymic hormone production and augmented percentage of thymulin-producing cells, a complete recovery of the reduced number of Thy 1.2^+ and Lyt$^-1^+$ cells in the spleen and a partial reconstitution of PHA response and NK cytotoxic activity of spleen cells.[4]

The increased thymulin plasma level depends primarily on the peripheral reactivation of zinc-unbound FTS, although a modest effect on the rate of production of thymic hormones by the thymus seems also to be achieved after oral zinc supplementations. Concomitantly, zinc supplementation in old mice recovers the abnormally low serum level of triiodothyronine, a hormone which can directly modulate the thymic peptide synthesis by the thymic epithelial cells[34] (TABLE 5).

The interpretation of all these findings is at present not so easy, essentially because of the still unclear pattern of the bidirectional interaction existing between the immune and the neuroendocrine system.

Zinc and Neuroendocrine-Immunological Aging: Theorical Implications

There is substantial evidence that hormones and neurotransmitters may modulate immune functioning,[35,36] and consistent data support the idea that immune-derived factors also modulate neuroendocrine function and particularly pituitary efficiency. Thus a bidirectional interdependence seems to exist between the two systems and such an interdependence seems to operate even in old age, as revealed by the fact that experimental manipulation on one of the two systems modifies and sometimes restores the function of the other one.[36]

Thus treatment of old animals with exogenous thyroxine, with growth hormone, or with analogues of LH-RH induces regrowth of the thymus, recovery of its endocrine function as measured by circulating level of thymulin and restoration

TABLE 4. Effect of Oral Zinc Supplementation in Down's Syndrome Subjects on Endocrine and Immune Parameters[a]

Parameters	Source	I Cycle			II Cycle		
		Before	After	p	Before	After	p
Zinc (μg/dl)	S	85.8 ± 4.5	126.9 ± 9.2	<0.01	71.3 ± 3.4	100.2 ± 5.3	<0.01
T_3 (ng/dl)	P	146.1 ± 13.1	157.7 ± 12.1	n.s.	148.9 ± 8.9	136.2 ± 7.2	n.s.
T_4 (μg/dl)	P	10.1 ± 0.9	9.5 ± 0.4	n.s.	8.35 ± 0.3	8.0 ± 0.4	n.s.
Active thymulin (Log_{-2})	P	1.1 ± 0.2	4.3 ± 0.3	<0.01	2.1 ± 0.3	4.2 ± 0.2	<0.01
Total thymulin (Log_{-2})	P	5.0 ± 0.3	5.8 ± 0.3	n.s.	5.1 ± 0.3	5.6 ± 0.3	n.s.
Inactive thymulin (pg/ml)	P	45.0 ± 9.6	0.6 ± 0.2	<0.001	33.5 ± 10.0	0.5 ± 0.1	<0.001
Total peripheral blood lymphocytes (absolute n°/mm³)	B	2115 ± 205	3220 ± 210	<0.05	2100 ± 209	2917 ± 215	<0.05
CD3 (absolute n°/mm³)	B	1530 ± 325	2320 ± 210	<0.05	1335 ± 307	2225 ± 210	<0.05
CD4 (absolute n°/m³)	B	N.D.	N.D.		508 ± 203	1107 ± 203	<0.05
CD8 (absolute n°/mm³)	B	N.D.	N.D.		610 ± 310	750 ± 213	n.s.

[a] Mean ± SEM; p calculated by paired Student t test. Zinc (1 mg Zn^{++}/Kg b.w./day) was administered through two cycles (two months each) separated by a period of 10 months. S = serum; P = plasma; B = blood.

TABLE 5. Effect of Oral Zinc Supplementation in Old Mice on Endocrine and Immune Parameters[a]

Parameters	Source	Before	After	p
Zinc (μg/dl)	P	81.0 ± 2.0	91.30 ± 3.58	<0.05
T3 (ng/dl)	P	54.0 ± 2.07	86.60 ± 1.76	<0.01
T4 (μg/dl)	P	1.36 ± 0.21	1.23 ± 0.23	n.s.
Active thymulin (Log_{-2})	P	1.50 ± 0.2	4.3 ± 0.3	<0.01
Total thymulin (Log_{-2})	P	4.0 ± 0.3	5.8 ± 0.3	n.s.
Inactive thymulin (pg/ml)	P	65.0 ± 3.5	0.6 ± 0.2	<0.001
Thymulin-producing cells (n° cells/100 fields)	Th	250 ± 30	435 ± 27	<0.01
THY 1.2+ cells (%)	Sp	12.2 ± 0.7	25.7 ± 1.4	<0.01
LYT-1+ cells (%)	Sp	11.8 ± 1.1	14.1 ± 0.51	<0.05
LYT-2+ cells (%)	Sp	8.3 ± 0.5	6.59 ± 0.13	n.s.
LYT-1+/LYT-2+ ratio (%)	Sp	1.39 ± 0.09	1.81 ± 0.17	<0.01
PHA response (c.p.m. × 10^{-3})	Sp	20.13 ± 2.3	42.25 ± 3.3	<0.01
ConA response (c.p.m. × 10^{-3})	Sp	73.5 ± 3.8	78.85 ± 4.5	n.s.
NK activity (% lysis)	Sp	2.8 ± 0.21	7.35 ± 0.33	<0.05

[a] Mean ± SEM; p calculated by paired Student t test. Zinc (25 μg/day/mouse) was administered by oral route for 30 days. P = plasma; sp = spleen; Th = thymus.

of some age-associated peripheral immune disfunctions. In old humans the hyper-thyroid and the acromegalic state is associated with a young-like performance of thymic endocrine activity. On the other hand, transplant of newborn thymuses into old animals corrects the age-associated alterations in the blood levels of thyroxine and insulin, in the responses to beta-adrenergic stimuli, in the expression of beta-adrenergic receptors in different tissues, including brain, and in the rate of polyploidy of the liver.[36]

These last data confirm and extend our original observation that the lymphoid system has extraimmunological functions and is deeply involved in the aging process.[37]

These findings clearly demonstrate that at least some age-related alterations of the nervous, the neuroendocrine, and the immune network are not *per se* intrinsic and irreversible and that the definition of the temporal priority in age-related deterioration is quite difficult to assign to either one or other homeostatic apparatus.

These considerations oblige to review, at a theorical level, both the "nervous-neuroendocrine",[38] and the "immune" hypothesis of aging insofar proposed.[39]

Without going into the details of the experimental and clinical data in support of one or the other of these theories, a common conceptual approach of both of them is, in fact, represented by the assumption that there exists a genetically determined hierarchy among the three homeostatic systems of the body and that the deterioration of one of them, according to each single theory, is a primary, intrinsic and irreversible event, the age-associated alterations of the other systems being an obliged consequence.

As an alternative to either "neuroendocrine" or "immune" theories of aging, we would hypothize that, due to the strict interactions existing between the nervous, the neuroendocrine and the immune system during the whole life of the organism, it is the disruption of such interactions in old age which is responsible for most of the age-associated dysfunctions.[35,40] FIGURE 1 schematically illustrates this concept. We may assume that the genetic background of an organism is set up in order to assure a physiologically correct interaction between the nervous, the neuroendocrine and the immune systems. Such a potentiality is continuously checked during life by external stressors which may be either cognitive (psychoemotional, social, etc.) or noncognitive (chemical, antigenic, etc.) and, accordingly, undergo a progressive exhaustion, which may vary in dependence on the quality and quantity of stressor events that each individual had suffered from. The individual diversity of life experience may explain the different involvement of a single homeostatic mechanism both in early ontogeny and in aging in different individuals, but the interaction with the other network, may justify the global alterations usually observed in these situations. In other words, hierarchy among the three major homeostatic systems is not a strictly genetically determined phenomenon, but it develops at individual level according to personal life experience. This assumption might explain the increased incidence of diseases either in otogeny, most likely due to defective development of the interactions among the three homeostatic systems or to abnormal stressor events, or in aging, due to the accumulation of individually different "collages" of various noncognitive or cognitive stressor consequences.

As an alternative to a stochastic approach of the theory, the existence of a single biological event can also be hypothized as being responsible for the disruption of the nervous-neuroendocrine-immune interactions in old age. In this context the role played by zinc may become crucial. Zinc, due to its wide-range action and to the common finding of age-related alteration of its turnover, together with the observation that zinc supplementation in old age is able to recover thymic endocrine activity, various immune parameters and probably also some age-related hormonal defects, may represent a putative crucial element to causally explain the disruption of the nervous-neuroendocrine-immune interactions in old age and consequently might offer a new key to understand aging processes.

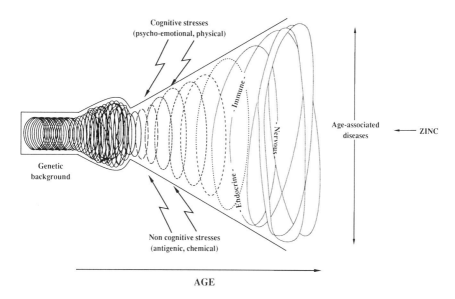

FIGURE 1. Disruptions of nervous-neuroendocrine-immune interactions in old age.

ACKNOWLEDGMENTS

All studies on Down's syndrome have been pursued in collaboration with Dr. C. Franceschi (University of Modena), and Dr. F. Licastro, Dr. M. Chiricolo, Dr. M. Zannotti, and Dr. M. Masi (University of Bologna).

We thank Mrs. N. Gasparini and Mr. M. Marcellini for their excellent technical assistance and Ms. Monica Glebocki for reading the text.

REFERENCES

1. PRASAD, A. S. 1985. Clinical, endocrinological and biochemical effects of zinc-deficiency. Clin. Endocrinol. Metab. **14**(3): 567–589.
2. CHANDRA, R. K. 1985. Trace element regulation of immunity and infection. J. Am. Coll. Nutr. **4**: 5–16.
3. USDA. 1980. Science and Education Administration, Food and Nutrient Intakes of Individuals in 1 Day in the United States, Spring 1977 Prelim. Rep. N. 2. 40–45. U.S. Department of Agriculture (USDA). Washington, DC.
4. FABRIS, N., E. MOCCHEGIANI, M. MUZIOLI & M. PROVINCIALI. 1990. Zinc, immunity and aging. *In* Biomedical Advances in Aging. A. L. Goldstein, Ed. 271–281. Plenum Press. New York.

5. TURNLUND, J. R., N. DURVIN, F. COSTA & S. MARGEN. 1986. Stable isotope studies of zinc absorption and retention in young and elderly men. J. Nutr. 116(7): 1239–1247.
6. SANDSTEAD, H. H. 1982. Availability of zinc and its requirements in human subjects. In Clinical, Biochemical, and Nutritional Aspects of Trace Elements. A. S. Prasad, Ed. 83–102. Alan R. Liss. New York.
7. SOLOMONS, N. W. 1983. Competitive mineral-mineral interactions in the intestine: implications for zinc absorption in humans. In Nutritional Bioavailability of Zinc. G. E. Inglett, Ed. 247–271. American Chemical Society. Washington, DC.
8. FABRIS, N., E. MOCCHEGIANI & R. PALLONI. 1988a. Zinc-dependent failure of thymic hormones in human pathologies. In Trace Elements in Man and Animals. L. S. Hurtley, Ed. 315–317. Plenum Press. New York.
9. FERNANDES, G., M. NAIR, K. ONOE, T. TAMAKA, R. FLOYAL & R. A. GOOD. 1979. Impairment of cell-mediated immunity functions by dietary zinc deficiency in mice. Proc. Natl. Acad. Sci. USA 76: 457–461.
10. GROSS, R. L., N. OSDIN, L. FOUG & P. M. NEWBERNE. Depressed immunological function in zinc-deprived rats as measured by mitogen response of spleen, thymus and peripheral blood. Am. J. Clin. Nutr. 32: 1260–1266.
11. IWATA, T., G. S. INCEFY, T. TANAKA, G. FERNANDES, C. I. MENENDEZ-BOTET, K. PIH & R. A. GOOD. 1979. Circulating thymic hormone levels in zinc deficiency. Cell. Immunol. 47: 100–105.
12. FABRIS, N., E. MOCCHEGIANI, L. AMADIO, M. ZANNOTTI, F. LICASTRO & C. FRANCESCHI. 1984. Thymic hormone deficiency in normal aging and Down's syndrome: is there a primary failure of the thymus? Lancet 1: 983–986.
13. McCLAIN, C. S. 1985. Zinc metabolism in malabsorption syndromes. J. Am. Coll. Nutri. 4: 49–64.
14. ALLEN, J. I., E. N. KAY & C. S. McCLAIN. 1981. Severe zinc deficiency in humans. Association with a reversible T-lymphocyte dysfunction. Ann. Intern. Med. 95: 154–157.
15. UNDERWOOD, E. J. 1977. Trace elements in human and animal nutrition, 4th edit. 1–302. Academic Press. New York.
16. FRAKER, P. J., S. HAAS & R. M. LUECKE. 1977. Effect of zinc deficiency on the immune response of the young adult A/Jax mouse. J. Nutr. 107: 1889–1895.
17. SCUDERI, P. 1990. Differential effect of copper and zinc on human peripheral blood macrocyte cytokine secretion. Cell. Immunol. 126: 391–405.
18. DARDENNE, M., J. M. PLEAU, B. NABAMA, P. LEFANCIER, M. DENIEN, J. CHOAY & J. F. BACH. 1982. Contribution of zinc and other metals to the biological activity of the serum thymic factor. Proc. Natl. Acad. Sci. USA 79: 5370–5373.
19. BACH, M. A. & G. BEAURAIN. 1979. Respective influence of extrinsic and intrinsic factors on the age-related decrease of thymic secretion. J. Immunol. 122: 2505–2507.
20. FABRIS, N., E. MOCCHEGIANI, S. MARIOTTI, F. PACINI & A. PINCHERA. 1986. Thyroid function modulates thymus endocrine activity. J. Clin. Endocrinol. Metab. 62: 474–478.
21. FABRIS, N., E. MOCCHEGIANI, M. GALLI, L. IRATO, A. LAZZARIN & M. MORONI. 1988b. AIDS, zinc deficiency, and thymic hormone failure. J. Am. Med. Assoc. 259(6): 839–840.
22. TRAVAGLINI, P., P. MORIONDO, E. TOGNI, P. VENEGONI, D. BOCCHICCHIO, G. FAGLIA, G. AMBROSO, C. PONTICELLI, E. MOCCHEGIANI & N. FABRIS. 1989. Effect of oral zinc administration on prolactin and thymulin circulating levels in uremic patients. J. Clin. Endocrinol. Metab. 68: 186–190.
23. BEACH, R. S., M. E. GERSHWIN & L. S. HURLEY. 1981. Nutritional factors and autoimmunity. 1. Immunopathology of zinc deprivation in New England mice. J. Immunol. 126: 1999–2006.
24. DUCHAETEU, J., G. DELESPESSE, R. VRIJEN & H. COOLET. 1981. Beneficial effects of oral zinc supplementation on the the immune response of old people. Am J. Med. 70: 1001–1004.
25. CHANDRA, R. K. 1989. Nutritional regulation of immunity and risk of infection in old age. Immunology 67: 141–147.

26. LeJeune, J., M. Gautier & R. Turpin. 1959. Les chromosomes humains en culture de tissues. CRC Acad. Sci. Paris. **248:** 602–603.
27. Baird, P. A. & A. D. Sadovnick. 1988. Causes of death to age 30 in Down's syndrome. Am. J. Hum. Genet. **43:** 239–248.
28. Franceschi, C., M. Chiricolo, F. Licastro, M. Zannotti, M. Masi, E. Mocchegiani & N. Fabris. 1988. Oral zinc supplementation in Down's syndrome: restoration of thymic endocrine activity and of some immune defects. J. Ment. Defic. Res. **32:** 169–181.
29. Bjorkstein, B., O. Back, H. Gustavson, G. Hallmans, B. Hagglof & A. Tarnvik. 1980. Zinc and immune function in Down's syndrome. Acta Paediatr. Scand. **69:** 183–187.
30. Licastro, F., E. Mocchegiani, M. Zannotti & N. Fabris. 1990. Normalization of thyroid stimulating hormone and reversal of triiodothyronine plasmic levels by dietary zinc supplementation in children with Down's syndrome: evaluation of clinical impact. Submitted.
31. Pueschel, S. M. & J. C. Pezzullo. 1985. Thyroid dysfunction in Down syndrome. Am. J. Dis. Child. **139:** 636–639.
32. Cutler, A. T., R. Benezra-Obeiter & S. J. Brink. 1986. Thyroid function in young children with Down syndrome. Am. J. Dis. Child. **140:** 479–483.
33. LeJeune, J., M. Peeters, M. C. De Blois, M. Berger, A. Grillot, M. O. Rethore, G. Vallee, M. Izembart & J. P. Devaux. 1988. Fonction thiroidienne et trisomie 21. exces de TSH et deficit en rT3. Ann. Genet. **31:** 137–143.
34. Mocchegiani, E. & N. Fabris. 1990. Neuroendocrine-thymus interactions. I. "In vitro" modulation of thymic factor secretion by thyroid hormones. J. Endocrinol. Invest. **13:** 139–147.
35. Fabris, N. 1986. Pathways of neuroendocrine-immune interactions and their impact with aging processes. *In* Immunoregulation in Aging. A. Facchini, J. J. Haaijman & G. Labò, Eds. 117–130. Eurage.
36. Fabris, N., E. Mocchegiani, M. Muzzioli & M. Provinciali. 1988. Neuroendocrine-thymus interactions: perspectives for intervention in aging. Ann. N. Y. Acad. Sci. **521:** 72–87.
37. Fabris, N., W. Pierpaoli & E. Sorkin. 1972. Lymphocytes, hormones and aging. Nature. **240:** 557–559.
38. Meites, J., R. Goya & S. Takahashi. 1987. Why the neuroendocrine system is important in aging process, a review. Exp. Gerontol. **22:** 1–15.
39. Walford, R. L. 1969. The immunologic theory of aging. 1–248. Munksgaard. Copenhagen.
40. Fabris, N. 1990. A neuroendocrine-immune theory of aging. Int. J. Neurosci. **51:** 373–375.
41. Gibson, R. A., B. M. Anderson & J. H. Sabry. 1983. The trace metal status of a group of post-menopausal vegetarians. J. Am. Dietet. Assoc. **82:** 246–251.
42. Wager, P. A. *et al.* 1983. Zinc nutriture and cell mediated immunity in the aged. Int. J. Vitam. Nutr. Res. **53:** 94–101.
43. Levine, R. A., D. H. P. Streeten & R. J. Doisy. 1968. Effects of oral chromium supplementation on the glucose tolerance of elderly human subjects. Metabolism **17:** 114–120.
44. DHEW. 1979. Dietary intake source data. Health and nutrition examination surgery, U.S., 1971–1974. DHEW Publ. No. (PHS) 1979, 79-1221. Dept. Health, Education and Welfare. Hyattasville, MD.
45. Reeves, P. G. & B. Dell. 1986. Effects of dietary zinc deprivation on the activity of angiotensin-converting enzyme (ACE) in serum of rats and guinea pigs. Int. J. Nutr. **116:** 128–134.
46. Coleman, J. E. 1974. The reactivities of functional groups of metalloproteins. *In* Biochemistry Series One: Chemistry of Macromolecules. H. Gutfreund, Ed. Vol. 1: 185–260. University Park. Baltimore, MD.
47. Baudier, J. & D. Gerard. 1983. Ions binding to S100 proteins: structural changes induced by calcium and zinc on S100a and S100b proteins. Biochemistry **22:** 3360–3369.

48. GASTINEL, L. N., M. DARDENNE, J. M. PLEAU & J. F. BACH. 1984. Studies on the zinc binding site to the serum thymic factor. Biochim. Biophys. Acta 197: 147–155.
49. PHYLLIPS, J. L. 1979. Zinc-induced synthesis of low molecular weight zinc-binding protein by hormone lymphocytes. Biol. Trace Elem. Res. 1: 359–371.
50. DUNN, M. F., S. E. PATTISON, M. C. STORM & E. QUIEL. 1980. Comparison of the zinc binding domains in the 7S nerve growth factor and the zinc-insulin Hexamer. Biochemistry 19: 718–725.

Effects of Different Regimens of Dietary Restriction on the Age-Related Decline in Insulin Secretory Response of Isolated Rat Pancreatic Islets[a]

E. BERGAMINI, M. BOMBARA, V. FIERABRACCI,
P. MASIELLO, AND M. NOVELLI

Centro di Ricerca Interdipartimentale sull'Invecchiamento
Istituto di Patologia Generale
University of Pisa
Via Roma, 55
56100 Pisa, Italy

INTRODUCTION

It is well known that the process of aging results in a progressive deterioration in most endocrine functions. With regard to the pancreas, there is evidence that the ability of the rat to maintain insulin secretory function decreases with increasing age, since islets from old rats are larger and contain more insulin than islets from young rats, but do not release *in vitro* insulin as rapidly as do these latter islets.[1–4]

In this report, we show that the onset of the functional decline of beta cells can be timed by the age of 6–9 months. The process is likely to be related to rat longevity, since it can be modulated by dietary restriction,[5] the most effective antiaging strategy tested in mammals.[6,7]

In order to increase knowledge about this important topic, we have explored the protective effects against age-related islet secretory impairment of two different types of diet restriction which are highly effective in prolonging the life span of rodents, namely, intermittent feeding[8] and, the most widely used, 60% food restriction. Metabolic fuels such as arginine and 2-ketoisocaproate, the phosphodiesterase inhibitor 3-isobutyl-1-methyl-xanthine and depolarizing concentrations of K^+ have been used as stimulating agents in addition to glucose.

MATERIALS AND METHODS

Animals

Male Sprague-Dawley rats were obtained from Nossan, Milan at 2 months of age and maintained in our facilities until used for the study.

The first set of experiments was performed on 2-, 6-, 9-, 12- or 24-mo-old rats, fed ad libitum with a standard laboratory chow.

[a] This work was supported in part by grants from the Ministero della Pubblica Istruzione and Consiglio Nazionale delle Ricerche (Rome).

For a second study, a number of 2-mo-old animals were subjected for 10 or 16 months to intermittent feeding (IF), *i.e.*, they were fed every other day, food being provided at 10 a.m. and removed on the following morning at the same hour. Rats on IF were taken for experiments at the end of the day of feeding.

In a third study, 2-mo-old rats were divided into three groups and subjected for 10 months to the following dietary regimens: A) ad libitum feeding (controls); B) IF; C) 60% food restriction (60% DR), calculated on the base of daily food intake of controls. The amount of food ingested by each rat was measured daily. The body weight of each rat was measured at 4-week intervals. For each diet regimen, rats were used for isolation of islets of Langerhans both fed and starved on the day prior to the experiment.

Experimental Protocol

Pancreatic islets were isolated by a modification of the method of Lacy and Kostianovsky,[9] according to the suggestions of Trueheart Burch *et al.*[10] and using the same procedure in all cases. After a 60-min preincubation period in modified Krebs-Ringer bicarbonate (KRB) buffer containing 0.5% bovine serum albumin, 10 mM N-2-hydroxy-ethylpiperazine-N^I-2-ethanesulphonic acid (Hepes) (pH 7.4) and 2.8 mM glucose, groups of 7–10 islets were incubated for 30 or 60 min at 37°C in a humidified atmosphere of 5% CO_2 in air, in 1 ml KRB-Hepes buffer, containing 2.8 and 16.7 mM glucose and various other secretagogues (20 mM arginine, 20 mM 2-ketoisocaproate (2-KIC), 1mM 3-isobutyl-1-methyl-xanthine (IBMX) and 30 mM KCl). At the end of the incubation, the medium was collected for insulin determination. Finally, 1 ml of cold acidified ethanol (HCl 0.7 M : ethanol, 1 : 3 v/v) was added to the islets in order to extract their insulin content.

Assay

Insulin was measured by radioimmunoassay according to Herbert *et al.*,[11] using rat insulin as a standard. The sensitivity and the coefficients of variation of the radioimmunoassay were as follows: detection limit 0.13 ng/ml, intraassay variation 3.1%, interassay variation 10.2%.

Chemical Reagents

Arginine, 2-KIC and IBMX were purchased from Sigma, St. Louis, Missouri, USA. Collagenase used for islet digestion was obtained from Serva Feinbiochemica GMBH, Heidelberg, FRG. ^{125}I-insulin was kindly provided by professor R. Navalesi, Cattedra di Malattie del Ricambio, University of Pisa. All reagents were of analytical grade.

Expression of Results and Statistical Analysis

Insulin release from isolated islets has been expressed as percentage of the islet insulin content. In this way it was possible to estimate the efficiency of the secretory response in islets of different sizes, the hormone content usually being a good index of the total beta cell mass.[12] Student *t* test was used for statistical comparisons.

RESULTS AND DISCUSSION

Since defective *in vitro* insulin secretory responses to glucose,[1] leucine[13] and D-glyceraldehyde[14] had been already reported in aging rats, we wanted to extend the previous observations, using other stimuli known to act through different mechanisms, in an attempt to establish the extent and the nature of the hormone secretory defect.

Indeed, FIGURE 1 shows the results of the stimulation by various secretagogues of islets of Langerhans isolated from Sprague-Dawley rats 24 months of age, in comparison to 2-mo-old controls. At 2.8 mM glucose, insulin release, expressed as the percentage of islet insulin content, was similar between young and old animals, with the relevant exception of that stimulated by 2-ketoisoca-proate, which caused a 4-fold enhancement of hormone release in the 2-mo-old rats and only a slight increase in the older ones. At 16.7 mM glucose, the difference between the secretory pattern of the two groups of animals was striking: in the younger animals, as expected, insulin release was stimulated by glucose and further increased by the other secretagogues, whereas in the 24-mo-old rats the response to glucose was weak and no potentiation occurred with arginine, KCl or 2-KIC. In the latter animals, only IBMX was able to enhance significantly glucose-stimulated insulin release, indicating that the islets were still sensitive to an increased availability of cAMP.

In order to time the onset of the age-related defect, incubation experiments were performed on isolated islets from rats of 2, 6, 9 and 12 months of age.

The results are shown in FIGURE 2, where it can be noticed that the insulin secretory response of islets taken from 12-mo-old animals was close to that observed previously in 24-mo-old rats, *i.e.*, much less efficient than in younger animals. Again, the response to glucose was small and other secretagogues did not potentiate this response adequately, with the partial exception of IBMX.

These results confirmed and extended previous observations for glucose- and leucine-stimulated insulin release in 12-mo-old animals.[1,13,15] Indeed, the loss of efficiency in insulin secretion is clearly apparent at 12 months of age, but even at 6 and 9 months there is some decline of the secretory effectiveness in comparison to that of 2-mo-old rats.

Therefore, the onset of the age-related impairment of pancreatic endocrine function should be timed by the age of 6–9 months. This does not imply necessarily that the animals have glucose intolerance, since they develop a compensatory islet hyperplasia (see below).

In the thought that the unlimited food intake of laboratory rodents could be at least partially responsible for the secretory defect, we investigated the effect of dietary restriction on the function of islets of Langerhans *in vitro*. When two different groups of 2-mo-old Sprague-Dawley rats were submitted to a particular diet regimen, such as intermittent feeding, lasting 10 and 16 months respectively, it was observed (TABLE 1) that in both cases there was a clear improvement of the insulin secretory effectiveness of the islets isolated from food-restricted rats in respect to those taken from controls fed ad libitum.

Looking at the insulin content of the islets of Langerhans at various ages (TABLE 2), it should be noticed that mature and older rats have a larger hormonal content than 2-mo-old animals (2-mo-old: 57 ± 1.6 ng/islet; 12-mo-old: 142 ± 5.8; 24-mo-old: 134 ± 7.3), in agreement with the results of Gold *et al.*[2] Therefore, it is likely that islets of animals with unlimited food intake develop hyperplasia and/or hypertrophy to match the excessive demand for insulin. In this respect, it is very interesting that intermittent feeding can largely prevent the development of such adaptive changes, limiting markedly the increase of islet insulin content in 12- and

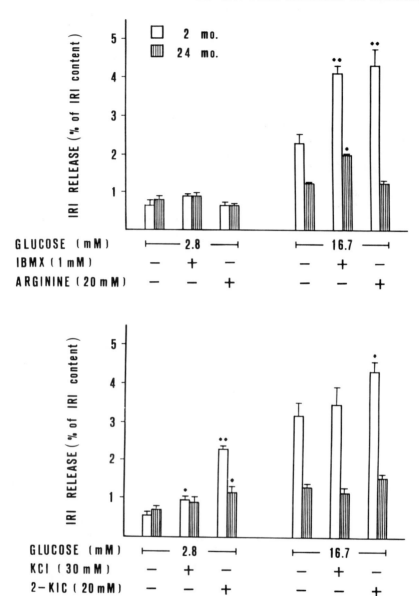

FIGURE 1. Insulin release from isolated islets of 2- and 24-mo-old Sprague-Dawley rats. Islets, freshly isolated by the collagenase method, were incubated for 30 min in the presence of the indicated substances. Results are given as mean ± SEM of five observations. *p <0.05, **p <0.01 versus incubation with glucose alone (unpaired Student t test). IRI = immunoreactive insulin; IBMX = isobutylmethylxanthine; 2-KIC = 2-ketoisocaproate.

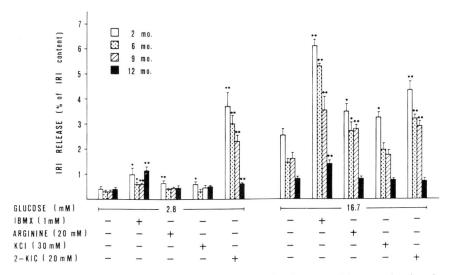

FIGURE 2. Insulin release from isolated islets of rats of various ages. Islets were incubated for 30 min in the presence of the indicated substances. Results are given as mean ± SEM of four to six observations. *p <0.05, **p <0.01 versus incubation with glucose alone (unpaired Student *t* test).

18-mo-old rats (12-mo-old controls: 145 ± 4.9 ng/islet, 12-mo-old IF: 73 ± 3.0; 18-mo-old controls: 242 ± 6.2 ng/islet, 18-mo-old IF: 92 ± 5.1).

The amelioration of the secretory *in vitro* response obtained in rats subjected to intermittent feeding was in contrast with previous observations[16,17] reporting the lack of improvement in islet function of rats subjected to 60% caloric restriction.

Therefore, it was decided to compare directly the effects of these two different

TABLE 1. Insulin Release from Isolated Islets of 12- and 18-Mo-Old Sprague-Dawley Rats on Free (Controls) or Intermittent Feeding (IF) during 30-Min Incubation in KRB-Hepes Buffer[a]

	IRI Release (% of IRI Content)			
	12-Mo-Old Rats		18-Mo-Old Rats	
Incubation Conditions	Controls (N = 5)	IF (N = 5)	Controls (N = 6)	IF (N = 5)
1. Glucose 2.8 mM	0.27 ± 0.05	0.24 ± 0.04	0.41 ± 0.06	0.47 ± 0.11
2. Glucose 16.7 mM	0.93 ± 0.15	3.74 ± 0.52*	1.16 ± 0.10	2.98 ± 0.27*
3. Idem + IBMX 1 mM	2.26 ± 0.23	8.87 ± 1.11*	1.58 ± 0.09	6.06 ± 0.53*
4. Idem + Arginine 20 mM	1.24 ± 0.12	7.13 ± 1.13*	1.34 ± 0.12	4.99 ± 0.59*
5. Idem + KCl 30 mM	1.43 ± 0.21	5.27 ± 0.24*	1.29 ± 0.11	4.05 ± 0.30*
6. Idem + 2-KIC 20 mM	1.69 ± 0.10	5.31 ± 0.42*	1.43 ± 0.10	4.12 ± 0.32*

[a] IRI = immunoreactive insulin, IBMX = isobutylmethylxanthine; 2-KIC = 2-ketoisocaproate. Results are expressed as mean ± SEM. *p <0.01 vs controls (unpaired Student *t* test).

TABLE 2. Insulin Content of Islets Isolated from 12-Mo-Old Sprague-Dawley Rats on Different Diet Regimens Compared to That of 2-Mo-Old Rats[a]

| | Islet IRI Content (ng/Islet) | |
	Fed Rats	Fasting Rats
12-Mo-old rats		
Controls	225 ± 6.0 (30)	184 ± 6.2 (30)*
Intermittent feeding	86 ± 4.6 (30)§	155 ± 6.0 (30)*
60% restriction	88 ± 4.9 (30)§	118 ± 5.6 (30)§*
2-Mo-old rats	96 ± 4.9 (34)	79 ± 3.1 (34)*

[a] IRI = immunoreactive insulin. Mean ± SEM of the number of observations indicated in parentheses. §p <0.01 versus controls; *p <0.01 versus the corresponding fed rats (unpaired Student t test).

diet regimens on the secretory effectiveness of islets taken from 12-mo-old animals, which already show the defective response of older rats. Three groups of randomly divided Sprague-Dawley rats were subjected to IF, or 60% DR, or fed ad libitum, for 10 months before sacrifice and islets were isolated from both fed and fasting animals in order to study the influence of the nutritional status on the changes in islet function.

The body weights and the food intakes of the three groups of animals were measured throughout the interval of the study (FIG. 3). It is worthwhile to notice that the effects of the two different dietary restrictions on these parameters are practically the same, and that with both regimens a 35% decrease in food consumption in respect to controls is paralleled by a 38% reduction in body weight gain.

The circadian variations in blood glucose and insulin levels were also determined in these animals.[18] The results demonstrated that both types of dietary restrictions led to a reduction of the average daily plasma concentrations of glucose and insulin in respect to fed ad libitum controls, likely related to the different rhythm of food intake (in IF rats, there were 18% and 39% reductions of glycemia and insulinemia, respectively, versus controls, as calculated from the areas under

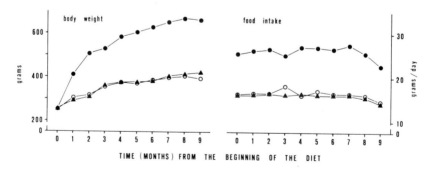

FIGURE 3. Body weight and daily food intake of Sprague-Dawley rats on different diet regimens. ●----● free feeding; ▲----▲ 60% food restriction; ○----○ intermittent feeding.

the curves of two-days observations; in 60% DR rats, reductions were 32% and 10% as calculated from the areas under the curves of one-day observations).

FIGURE 4 shows the insulin release during a 60-min incubation period of isolated islets from fed IF, 60% DR and control 12-mo-old rats, again expressed as percent of islet hormone content to allow the comparison of the secretory efficiencies of islets of different sizes. A scanty sensitivity to glucose and other secretagogues was again apparent in control islets, on account also of the high basal values of insulin secretion. In comparison with controls, responsiveness to most secretagogues was improved in islets from IF rats, whereas in islets from 60% DR rats improvement was found only upon stimulation with 2-KIC.

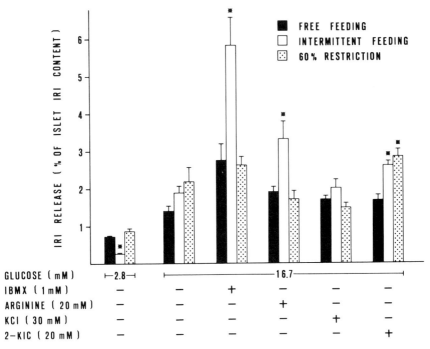

FIGURE 4. Insulin release from isolated islets of fed 12-mo-old rats on different diet regimens. Islets were incubated for 60 min in the presence of the indicated substances. Results are given as mean ± SEM of four observations. *p <0.05 versus corresponding control rats (unpaired Student t test).

When islets were taken from fasting rats (FIG. 5), the percent insulin release from control islets in response to glucose was paradoxically increased, partially due to a decrease in islet hormone content (see TABLE 2), but no potentiation occurred with arginine, 2-KIC or KCl. In islets from both IF and 60% DR rats, insulin release, reduced as a whole in respect to that observed in the "fed" state, was nevertheless stimulated 3-fold over basal by 16.7 mM glucose and further enhanced by IBMX and 2-KIC, but not by KCl (FIG. 5).

In TABLE 2, the insulin contents of the islets are shown. Both dietary restrictions were largely able to prevent the increase in hormone content occurring in control islets, particularly in fed rats, the islet insulin content of these 12-mo-old food-restricted animals being as low as that of 2-mo-old rats. Moreover, it is remarkable that the fasting state influenced the hormonal content of control and food-restricted rats differently. This result suggests that hormone biosynthesis might undergo adaptive changes as well. However, further studies are needed to clarify to which extent dietary restrictions can modify the ratio between insulin biosynthesis and release in the islets.

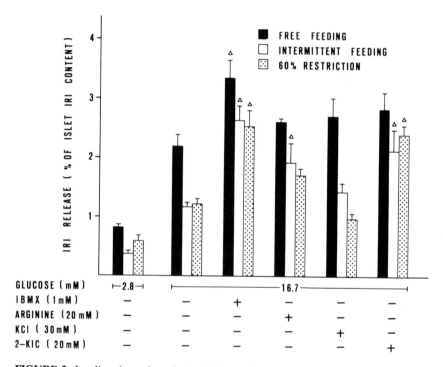

FIGURE 5. Insulin release from isolated islets of fasting 12-mo-old rats on different diet regimens. Islets were incubated for 60 min in the presence of the indicated substances. Results are given as mean ± SEM of four observations. △ $p < 0.05$ versus incubation with 16.7 mM glucose alone (unpaired Student t test).

In conclusion, our findings confirm that there is an age-dependent decline of insulin secretion by isolated islets. Indeed, the data obtained in fasting rats rule out the criticisms raised by Trueheart Burch et al.[10] about the differences in the sensitivity of bigger, "older" islets to injury during the isolation procedure.

With regard to the effects of dietary restrictions, this study shows that they can prevent, to a different extent, the age-related decline in islet secretory efficiency and the age-related islet hypertrophy. Intermittent feeding, in this respect, appears to be more effective than 60% dietary restriction. Moreover, in 12-mo-old animals dietary restrictions appear to modify islet adaptation to fasting.

Presently, work is in progress to ascertain the changes in islet insulin content and secretion as a function of the duration of food restriction.

ACKNOWLEDGMENTS

The precious help of Mr. A. Troilo for the care of the animals and the skillful technical assistance of Mr. E. Madrigali are gratefully acknowledged.

REFERENCES

1. REAVEN, E. P., G. GOLD & G. M. REAVEN. 1979. Effect of age on glucose-stimulated insulin release by the beta-cell of the rat. J. Clin. Invest. **64:** 591–599.
2. GOLD, G., G. M. REAVEN & E. P. REAVEN. 1981. Effect of age on proinsulin and insulin secretory patterns in isolated rat islets. Diabetes **30:** 77–82.
3. MASIELLO, P., V. DE TATA, M. NOVELLI & E. BERGAMINI. 1986. Impaired insulin secretion from isolated islets of aging rats. Diabetologia **29:** 569A.
4. SARTIN, J. L., M. CHAUDHURI, S. FARINA & R. C. ADELMAN. 1986. Regulation of insulin secretion by glucose during aging. J. Gerontol. **41:** 30–35.
5. MASIELLO, P., V. FIERABRACCI, M. NOVELLI, M. BOMBARA & E. BERGAMINI. 1990. Intermittent feeding can prevent the age-related decline in insulin secretory response to secretagogues in isolated pancreatic islets of the rat. *In* Protein Metabolism in Aging. H. L. Segal, M. Rothstein & E. Bergamini, Eds. 269–276. Wiley-Liss. New York.
6. WEINDRUCH, R., R. L. WALFORD, S. FLIGIEL & D. GUTHRIE. 1986. The retardation of aging in mice by dietary restriction: longevity, cancer, immunity and lifetime energy intake. J. Nutr. **116:** 641–654.
7. MASORO, E. J. 1987. Biology of aging. Current state of knowledge. Arch. Intern. Med. **147:** 166–169.
8. GOODRICK, C. L., D. K. INGRAM, M. A. REYNOLDS & J. R. FREEMAN. 1982. Effect of intermittent feeding upon growth and life span in rats. Gerontology **28:** 233–241.
9. LACY, P. E. & M. KOSTIANOVSKY. 1967. Method for the isolation of intact islets of Langerhans from the rat pancreas. Diabetes **16:** 35–39.
10. TRUEHEART BURCH, P., D. K. BERNER, A. LEONTIRE, A. VOGIN, B. M. MATS-CHINSKY & F. M. MATSCHINSKY. 1984. Metabolic adaptation of pancreatic tissue in aging rats. J. Gerontol. **39:** 2–6.
11. HERBERT, V., K. S. LAU, C. W. GOTTLIEB & S. J. BLEICHER. 1965. Coated charcoal immunoassay of insulin. J. Clin. Endocrinol. **25:** 1375–1384.
12. JAHR, H., D. GOTTSCHLING & H. ZUHLKE. 1978. Correlation of islet size and biochemical parameters of isolated islets of Langerhans of rats. Acta Biol. Med. Germ. **37:** 659–662.
13. REAVEN, E. P., G. GOLD & G. M. REAVEN. 1980. Effect of age on leucine-induced insulin secretion by the beta-cell. J. Gerontol. **35:** 324–328.
14. MOLINA, J. M., F. H. PREMDAS & L. LIPSON. 1985. Insulin release in aging: dynamic response of isolated islets of Langerhans of the rat to D-glucose and D-glyceralde-hyde. Endocrinology **116:** 821–826.
15. CURRY, D. L., G. M. REAVEN & E. P. REAVEN. 1984. Glucose-induced insulin secretion by perfused pancreas of 2- and 12-mo-old Fischer 344 rats. Am. J. Physiol. **247:** E385–E388.
16. REAVEN, E. P. & G. M. REAVEN. 1981. Structure and function changes in the endocrine pancreas of aging rats with reference to the modulating effect of exercise and caloric restriction. J. Clin. Invest. **68:** 75–84.

17. REAVEN, E. P., D. WRIGHT, C. E. MONDON, R. SOLOMON, H. HO & G. M. REAVEN. 1983. Effect of age and diet on insulin secretion and insulin action in the rat. Diabetes **32:** 175–180.
18. BERGAMINI, E., G. CAVALLINI, A. DEL ROSO, V. DE TATA, V. FIERABRACCI, P. MASIELLO, M. MASINI, M. NOVELLI & I. SIMONETTI. 1990. Different circadian variation of plasma glucose and insulin concentration in rats submitted to 60% food restriction or intermittent feeding. *In* Protein Metabolism in Aging, H. L. Segal, M. Rothstein & E. Bergamini, Eds. 295–297. Wiley-Liss. New York.

Retardation of the Aging Processes in Rats by Food Restriction

E. J. MASORO, I. SHIMOKAWA, AND B. P. YU

Department of Physiology
The University of Texas Health Science Center
7703 Floyd Curl Drive
San Antonio, Texas 78284-7756

Restricting the food intake of rodents has long been known to extend the life span, both the mean and the maximum length of life.[1] Questions that have been addressed in recent years and are still under investigation are: Does food restriction retard the primary aging processes? Are most age-associated processes influenced? What are the mechanisms underlying these actions? Findings obtained to date on these questions are the subject of this paper. Particular emphasis will be placed on the studies carried out in our laboratory.

Physiological Systems

Our initial reason for studying the influence of food restriction on age-changes in the physiological systems was our belief that this information would provide insights on mechanism of action. The male Fischer 344 rat was the animal model we used. Rats were singly housed to permit an accurate assessment of food intake and were kept in a barrier facility to maintain their specific pathogen-free status. The food restricted rats were provided 60% of the mean food intake of the rats allowed to eat ad libitum and unless otherwise stated food restriction was initiated at 6 weeks of age (2 weeks postweaning). A semisynthetic diet was used.[2]

Food restriction was found to delay and/or blunt most age-changes in the physiological systems. The data of Liepa *et al.*[3] on plasma cholesterol levels (Fig. 1) are a typical example. At 6 months of age, food restricted and ad libitum fed rats had similar plasma cholesterol levels. In ad libitum fed rats, plasma cholesterol levels were markedly higher by 12 months of age reaching a peak concentration by 18 months of age. In contrast, in food restricted rats an increase in plasma cholesterol level did not occur until 18 months of age and the magnitude of the age-related increase was less marked than in ad libitum fed rats. We have observed preventive effects of food restriction with these male Fischer 344 rats in regard to many other age-changes[1] such as the increase in plasma triglyceride concentration, the loss in lipolytic response of adipocytes to hormones, alterations in skeletal muscle structure and function, the increase in serum calcitonin levels, the decline in spontaneous locomotor activity. The studies of other investigators involving many different mouse and rat strains have yielded similar results; examples of the retardation of age-changes include its effects on central nervous system neurotransmitter receptors and neurochemical markers, lens crystallins, female reproductive function, and immune functions to name a few.

The breadth of these effects on age-changes in the physiological systems provides strong support for the view that food restriction retards fundamental primary aging processes. On the other hand, this breadth undermines the usefulness

337

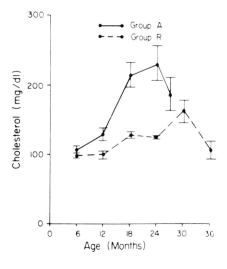

FIGURE 1. Influence of age and food restriction on serum cholesterol concentrations. Group A were ad libitum fed and Group R were fed 60% of the mean food intake of Group A. (From Liepa *et al.*[3] Reprinted by permission from the *American Journal of Physiology*.)

of these actions of food restriction on physiological processes as tools for uncovering the nature of underlying mechanisms.

Disease Processes

The occurrence of age-associated diseases appears to be an almost inevitable consequence of aging. Studies with many different mouse and rat strains have shown that food restriction retards most of these disease processes.[1]

The major age-associated disease processes in male Fischer 344 rats are nephropathy, cardiomyopathy and neoplastic disease. Food restriction was found to influence all three classes of disease processes.[4]

The progression in severity of nephropathy was assessed by sacrificing ad libitum fed and food restricted rats at various ages and examining the kidneys histologically (FIG. 2). The severity of lesions was graded 0 (no lesions), 1, 2, 3, 4, E (end-stage) in the order of increasing severity. The increase in severity with age was significantly greater for ad libitum fed than for food restricted rats.[4] The findings at the time of spontaneous death (TABLE 1) are in accord with this conclu-

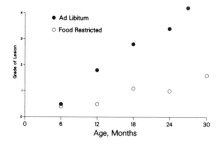

FIGURE 2. Age and the severity of nephropathy. Each point in the graph is the mean value from the analysis of 10 rats. Data on which this graph is based were reported by Maeda *et al.*[4] in which the severity of lesions was assessed using multiple ordered categories and the progression in sacrificed rats analyzed using ridit analysis.

TABLE 1. Severity of Chronic Nephrophy at the Time of Spontaneous Death[a]

Dietary Regimen	Number of Rats Examined	% of Rats with Lesions of Grade:					
		0	1	2	3	4	E
Ad libitum fed	182	0	4	14	14	23	45
Food restricted	145	6	72	15	6	0	1

[a] Data in table are from Maeda *et al.*[4] and Masoro *et al.*[5]

sion.[4,5] At the time of spontaneous death 68% of the ad libitum fed rats had Grade 4 or E lesions compared to 1% of the food restricted rats and 4% of the ad libitum fed rats had Grade 0 and 1 lesions compared to 78% of the food restricted rats. These findings are even more striking when it is also recognized that the food restricted rats are much older at the time of spontaneous death than the ad libitum fed rats.[6]

The progression in severity of cardiomyopathy was also assessed by sacrificing ad libitum fed and food restricted rats at various ages and examining the heart histologically (FIG. 3). The severity of lesions was graded 0 (no lesions) 1, 2, 3 in the order of increasing severity. The increase in severity with age was significantly greater for ad libitum fed than for food restricted rats.[4] The findings at the time of spontaneous death (TABLE 2) agree with this conclusion.[4,5] At the time of spontaneous death 19% of the ad libitum fed rats had Grade 3 lesions compared to 6% of the food restricted rats while 8% of the ad libitum fed rats had no lesions (Grade 0) compared to 21% of the food restricted rats.

The percentage of rats with neoplastic disease at the time of spontaneous death was greater for food restricted than for ad libitum fed rats.[4,5] However, this finding may be due to the fact that food restricted rats live to much older ages than ad libitum fed rats. To assess this possibility, theoretical survival curves (FIGS. 4 and 5) were generated based on all neoplastic diseases or leukemia/lymphoma (a major neoplastic disease in this rat strain) as the sole cause of death. The results show that food restriction delays the occurrence of death due to neoplasia in general or specifically to leukemia/lymphoma to older ages.

Disease and the Physiological Systems

The marked influence on the age-associated diseases raises the possibility that the action of food restriction on the age-changes in physiological systems may be

FIGURE 3. Age and the severity of cardiomyopathy. Each point in the graph is the mean value from the analysis of 10 rats. Data on which this graph is based were reported by Maeda *et al.*[4] in which the severity of lesions was assessed using multiple ordered categories and the progression in sacrificed rats analyzed using ridit analysis.

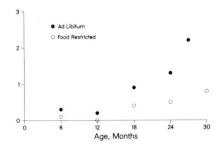

TABLE 2. Severity of Cardiomyopathy at the Time of Spontaneous Death[a]

Dietary Regimen	Number of Rats Examined	% of Rats with Lesions of Grade:			
		0	1	2	3
Ad libitum fed	182	8	33	40	19
Food restricted	145	21	54	19	6

[a] Data in table are from Maeda et al.[4] and Masoro et al.[5]

secondary to the retardation of disease. Assessment of the broad spectrum of data collected in our laboratory on the male Fischer 344 rat indicates that usually such is not the case. Specifically, the time course of age-change in the physiological process is usually dissociated from that of the progression or occurrence of disease. For example, the increase in serum cholesterol concentration starts by 12 months of age with maximum levels being reached by 18 months of age in ad libitum fed rats; in these rats severe nephropathy or cardiomyopathy is rarely seen until well after 18 months of age nor is there evidence of an appreciable amount of neoplastic disease by 18 months of age.[4]

However, some of the actions of food restriction on age-changes in physiological process do appear to be secondary to its effect on disease processes. A case in point is the age-associated increase in serum parathyroid hormone concentration in male Fischer 344 rats. In FIGURE 6, age-changes in serum parathyroid hormone concentrations are compared for male Fischer 344 rats fed ad libitum either the usual casein-containing diet or a similar diet in which soy protein has replaced casein and for food restricted rats.[4] Both food restriction and replacing casein with soy protein in ad libitum fed rats almost totally prevented the age-associated increase in serum parathyroid hormone concentration. These two dietary manipulations also retard the progression of nephropathy.[4,8] These findings suggest that at least in part the blunting by food restriction of the age-associated increase in serum parathyroid hormone is secondary to the retardation of kidney disease.

Primary Aging Processes

The findings obtained in our laboratory as well as the research of others strongly indicate that one or more of the primary aging processes is or are major site(s) of action of food restriction. This conclusion is based on: 1) Food restric-

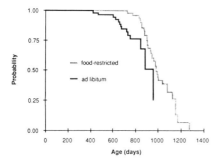

FIGURE 4. Survival curves of ad libitum fed and food restricted rats if neoplastic disease were the sole cause of death. Curves were generated from the data reported by Masoro et al.[5] by the Kaplan-Meier method.

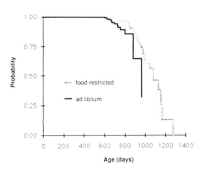

FIGURE 5. Survival curves of ad libitum fed and food restricted rats if leukemia/lymphomas were the sole cause of death. Curves were generated from the data reported by Masoro *et al.*[5] by the Kaplan-Meier method.

tion extends the maximum life span of many different strains of mice and rats. 2) Food restriction retards most age-changes in the physiological systems of rodents indicating an action that is general rather than specifically related to a particular physiological process. 3) Food restriction retards almost all age-associated diseases indicating an action which modulates disease processes in general rather than a specific pathogenesis.

If food restriction acts on the primary aging processes, what is the nature of these processes and how does food restriction influence them? Our recent efforts and those of many other investigators have focused on these two questions.

Mechanism of Action

Specific Nutrient

The possibility that the restriction of a specific nutrient underlies the action of food restriction was investigated in our laboratory. In several of our studies the effects on longevity of restricting a class of nutrients without restricting caloric intake were measured. The results of restricting the mineral component by 40% or the fat component by 40% on survival characteristics are shown in FIGURES 7 and 8. Restriction of neither the minerals nor the fat influenced the life span.[8]

However, restricting the protein component by 40% without restricting caloric intake did increase the median length of life, the age of the tenth percentile

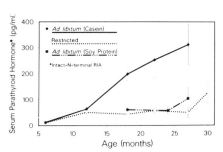

FIGURE 6. Effects of aging and dietary manipulation on serum parathyroid hormone concentration. (From Kalu *et al.*[7] Reprinted by permission from *Endocrinology*.)

survivors and the maximum length of life[6] but much less markedly than when protein restriction was accompanied by a similar reduction in caloric intake (TABLE 3). Moreover, a 40% restriction of caloric intake without restricting protein intake was as effective as caloric restriction which included protein restriction in increasing the median length of life, the age of tenth percentile survivors and the maximum length of life. Our conclusion from these studies is that protein restriction is not a factor in most of the actions of food restriction including its effects on longevity. That protein restriction without caloric restriction decreases the extent of severe nephropathy is probably the major reason for the small increase in longevity. However, caloric restriction with or without protein restriction almost totally prevents the occurrence of severe nephropathy and it is probably for this reason that the level of protein intake has little effect on the longevity of calorically restricted rats.

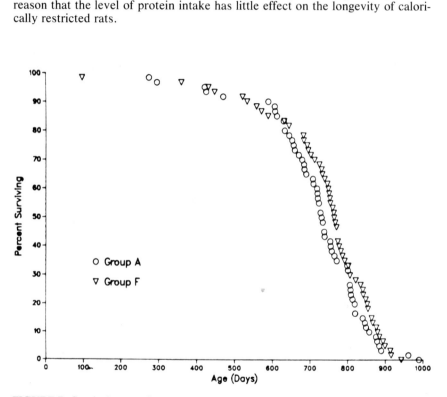

FIGURE 7. Survival curves for rats fed the standard semisynthetic diet (Group A) and rats fed a diet restricting mineral intake by 40% (Group F). The caloric intake of both groups was the same. (From Iwasaki *et al.*[9] Reprinted by permission from the *Journal of Gerontology: Biological Sciences.*)

Thus, our research strongly indicates that the retardation of the aging processes in food restriction is due to the restriction of energy intake rather than a specific nutrient. However, the design of our studies does not completely rule out a possible specific role for the carbohydrate component in this regard.

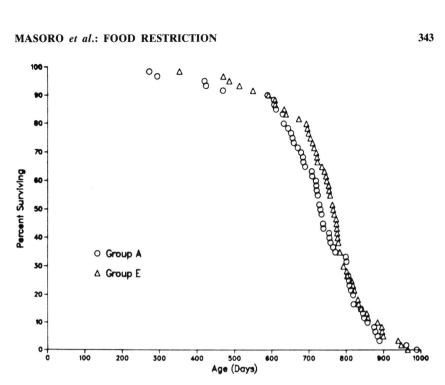

FIGURE 8. Survival curves for rats fed the standard semisynthetic diet (Group A) and rats fed a diet restricting fat intake by 40% (Group E). The caloric intake of both groups was the same. (From Iwasaki *et al.*[9] Reprinted by permission from the *Journal of Gerontology: Biological Sciences*.)

Growth and Development

In 1935, McCay *et al.*[10] postulated that food restriction extends the length of life by slowing growth and development. We directly tested this hypothesis in studies with rats on the following dietary programs:[6,11] Group 1, fed ad libitum throughout life; Group 2, food restricted starting at 6 weeks of age; Group 3, food

TABLE 3. Influence of Caloric Restriction, Protein Restriction and Protein Plus Caloric Restriction on Longevity

% Restriction of Calories	% Restriction of Protein	Median Length of Life Days	Age of 10th Percentile Survivors Days	Maximum Length of Life
0	0	701[a]	822[a]	941[a]
0	40	810[a]	935[a]	969[a]
40	0	956[b]	1158[b]	1295[b]
40	40	936[b]	1121[b]	1275[b]

[a] Data from Yu *et al.*[6]
[b] Data from Masoro *et al.*[5]

restricted from 6 weeks to 6 months of age and thence ad libitum fed; Group 4, food restricted starting at 6 months of age. The results in regard to longevity are summarized in FIGURE 9. Starting food restriction at 6 months of age was found to be as effective as starting at 6 weeks of age in extending the age of the tenth percentile survivors and the maximum length of life. Thus, food restriction is quite effective in the mature rats in which growth is almost complete. Our results are not in accord with the growth and development hypothesis of McCay and his associates.

Body Fat

Food restricted rats have a lower fat content per gram body weight than ad libitum fed rats.[4] It has been proposed that the reduction in body fat contents plays an important role in the life span extending action of food restriction.[12] This hypothesis was tested in our laboratory in studies with the male Fischer 344 rat. The body fat content of ad libitum fed rat was not found to correlate with the length of life and in the case of the food restricted rats there was positive correlation. These findings make it unlikely that reducing the body fat content plays a causal role in the life span extending action of food restriction.

Metabolic Rate

Based on the work of Rubner[13] and his own studies,[14] Pearl postulated that the rate of aging is inversely related to the metabolic rate. Extending this concept, Sacher[15] proposed that food restriction brings about an increase in life span and a slowing of the aging processes by decreasing the metabolic rate. It should be noted that Rubner, Pearl and Sacher viewed metabolic rate in terms of the rate of energy expenditure per unit of body mass.

Our findings with ad libitum fed and food restricted male Fischer 344 rats are not in accord with the hypothesis of Sacher. The data on food intake first alerted us to this. Although food intake per gram body weight decreased by 40% when food intake was reduced by 40%, the changes in body weight in response to food restriction soon resulted in a slightly higher food intake per gram body weight in food restricted than in ad libitum fed rats; these findings were graphically summarized by Masoro[17] in FIGURE 10. This issue was pursued further by McCarter and his associated[18,19] who measured 24 hour oxygen consumption by these rats under usual living conditions. They expressed the data as Kcalories of energy expenditure per Kgram lean body mass per day. Initially, food restriction caused a fall in energy expenditure per unit lean body mass but within 6 weeks of the initiation of food restriction the food restricted and the ad libitum fed rats had similar rates of oxygen consumption per unit of lean body mass. The reason for these findings is that lean body mass is rapidly reduced in proportion to the reduction in energy intake.

These findings make it unlikely that the effects of food restriction are due to a reduction in the intensity of metabolism or to a decreased intake of energy or any other nutrient per unit of lean body mass. Rather they indicate that the antiaging actions of food restriction involve a total organism response possibly involving the nervous system or endocrine system or both.

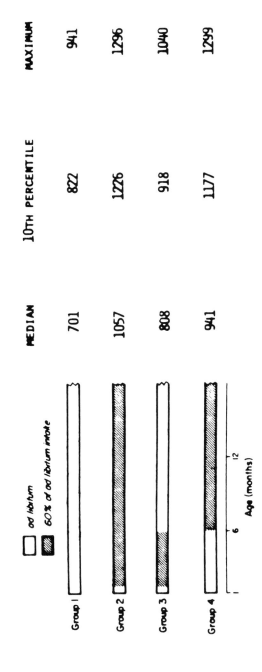

FIGURE 9. The influence of the time of initiation and duration of food restriction (40% reduction in food intake) on longevity. (Data from Yu *et al.*[6] Figure from Masoro.[11] Reprinted by permission from MTP Press Limited.)

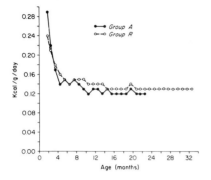

FIGURE 10. Food intake per unit of body mass by ad libitum fed (Group A) and food restricted rats. (Data from Masoro et al.[16] Figure from Masoro.[17] Reprinted by permission from Van Nostrand Reinhold.)

Glucocorticoid Cascade Hypothesis

In considering the specific systems that might be involved, the Glucocorticoid Cascade Hypothesis of Aging proposed by Sapolsky et al.[20] attracted our attention. This hypothesis is based on the concept that hippocampal neurons rich in glucocorticoid receptors are involved in the negative feedback regulation of plasma glucocorticoid concentrations. Increases in plasma glucocorticoid concentration in response to stress are perceived as downregulating these neuron receptors and when coupled with another insult such as ischemia are believed to result in a loss of these neurons. This hypothesis proposes that by this mechanism there is a gradual loss with advancing age of these hippocampal neurons and the ultimate result is a feed-forward cascade of sustained hyperadrenocorticism. Sapolsky et al. further suggested that many of the major detrimental aspects of aging, e.g., immunosuppression, osteoporosis, impaired cognition and many others, are at least in part due to this hyperadrenocorticism.

Studies are being conducted in our laboratory with ad libitum fed and food restricted male Fischer 344 rats to further evaluate the concept of Sapolsky et al. and to explore the possibility that food restriction retards the aging processes by preventing the occurrence of hyperadrenocorticism. The following are being assessed in a longitudinal study: the circadian pattern of plasma corticosterone concentration, the plasma concentration of corticosterone binding globulin (CBG), the mean 24-hour concentration of plasma total corticosterone and free corticosterone. In addition, in a cross-sectional study, the rise in plasma corticosterone concentration in response to restraint stress and its recovery following the stress are being assessed.

The basic characteristics of the circadian plasma corticosterone concentration pattern did not change with age through 25 months of age, the oldest rats studied to date. The mean 24-hour plasma total corticosterone concentration in ad libitum fed rats remained at about 100 ng/ml through 13 months of age; by 15 months of age it increased to 130 ng/ml and remained at that level through 25 months of age. Food restricted rats had mean 24-hour plasma total corticosterone concentrations of about 100 ng/ml through 25 months of age. Plasma CBG concentrations remained at about 1500 nM through 25 months of age in ad libitum fed rats but progressively fell in food restricted from about 1500 nM at 3 to 7 months of age to about 850 nM at 21 to 25 months of age. Over most of the 25 months, the plasma free corticosterone was significantly higher in food restricted rats than in ad libitum fed rats; e.g., in the 21 to 25 month age range the concentration in the food restricted rats was twice that of the ad libitum fed rats.

The rise in plasma corticosterone concentration in response to restraint stress and its recovery following the stress were similar in 5 to 6 months old ad libitum fed and food restricted rats. In both rat groups there was a slower recovery of plasma corticosterone concentration following a restraint stress at 18 to 19 months than at 5 to 6 months of age but no further slowing was observed at 23 to 24 months of age.

A conclusion to be drawn from our findings is that food restriction does not retard the aging processes by preventing the occurrence of hyperadrenocorticism. Rather our findings raise the possibility that increased plasma free corticosterone levels might be a factor in the antiaging actions of food restriction. Further research is required to explore this possibility.

Moreover, in the ad libitum fed rats neither a progressive increase in mean 24 hour plasma corticosterone levels or a progressive slowing in recovery of plasma corticosterone following a restraint stress occurred with advancing age. These findings do not support the Glucocorticoid Cascade Hypothesis as describing a major aspect of aging.

Glycation Theory

The proposal by Cerami[21] that glucose may serve as a mediator of aging pointed to another possible mechanism by which food restriction might influence the aging processes. Research aimed at exploring this possibility is in progress in our laboratory.

Cerami believes that the nonenzymatic glycation of proteins and nucleic acids by glucose may underlie many aspects of aging. The initial reaction is between the aldehyde group of glucose and amino groups of the protein or nucleic acids to form a Schiff base. A series of further reactions occur between the glucose adduct and the macromolecule resulting ultimately in what Cerami calls Advanced Glycation End-Products (AGE). Cerami points out that excessive glycation of proteins and nucleic acid may have detrimental consequences such as the loss of enzymatic activity, altered genetic expression, altered binding of regulatory molecules and inappropriate cross-linking of proteins. It is by these effects that it is postulated that glycation mediates aging.

The extent of glycation of macromolecules relates to many factors. The concentration of glucose (or other sugar) in the environment of the macromolecule and the length of time exposed to this concentration are two of the most important.

The influence of food restriction on sustained levels of plasma glucose is being studied in our laboratory with the male Fischer 344 rat. The diurnal pattern of plasma glucose concentration is shown in FIGURE 11 for ad libitum fed and food restricted rats at 4 to 6 months of age. Except for immediately after feeding the food restricted rats had a significantly lower plasma glucose level than ad libitum fed rats. In a longitudinal study the mean 24 hour plasma glucose concentrations have been determined for ad libitum fed and food restricted rats from 3 to 25 months of age. Through this time period food restricted rats have had sustained mean 24 hour plasma glucose levels approximately 15 mg/dl below that of the ad libitum fed rats.

These findings are consistent with the Glycation Theory of Aging but, of course, further work is needed to establish a causal role for the reduced plasma glucose levels in the action of food restriction on the aging processes. Moreover, a reduction in plasma glucose concentration could influence the aging processes by means other than glycation. It is striking, however, that the rate of glucose utilization per unit lean body mass of food restricted rats is as great as in ad libitum fed rats. This suggests that either glucose effectiveness or insulin sensitivity as defined by Bergman[23] or both is/are increased by food restriction. Whichever be the case this effect of food restriction may be a fundamental mechanism since it permits the effective use of an important but potentially toxic fuel at sustained lower concentrations and thus presumably at less damaging concentrations.

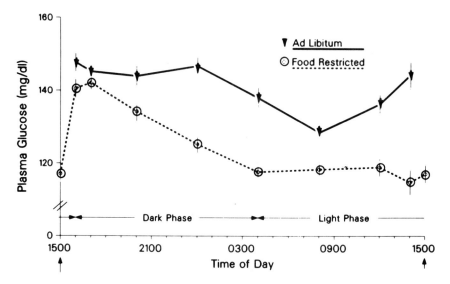

FIGURE 11. Diurnal pattern of plasma glucose concentration in ad libitum fed and food restricted rats in the age range of 4 to 6 months. The *arrow* indicates the time of feeding of the food restricted rats. (From Masoro *et al.*[22] Reprinted by permission from the *Journal of Gerontology: Biological Sciences.*)

Free Radical Theory

Since the free radical theory of aging was proposed in 1956 by Harman,[24] many attempts have been made to relate free radical metabolism to the aging processes. Interventions using antioxidants, free radical scavenging drugs and other agents of this type have been only marginally successful in extending the median length of life and without effect on the maximum life span. This failure does not provide strong evidence against the free radical theory for two reasons: 1) the exogenously administered antioxidant or other drugs may not be distributed to the cellular site of production of the free radicals, and 2) particular antioxidants and other drugs are specific for a particular free radical species and thus are unlikely to have a global effect.

Recently, studies on the effects of food restriction have given new life to the free radical theory. In our laboratory, food restriction of male Fischer 344 rats has been found to modulate free radical production, scavenging enzyme activities, free radical damage and the detoxification of the products of free radical damage.

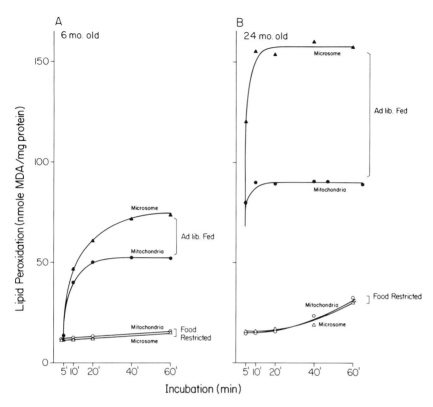

FIGURE 12. *In vitro* enzyme-dependent lipid peroxidation by hepatic membranes. **(A)** 6-month-old rats. **(B)** 24-month-old rats. Peroxidation was performed in the presence of 0.2 mM $FeSO_4$, 5 mM ADP and 1 mM NADPH. (From Laganiere and Yu[25] Reprinted by permission from *Biochemical and Biophysical Research Communications.*)

Lipid peroxidation under *in vitro* conditions by liver microsomal and mitochondrial membranes (FIG. 12) was determined by measuring MDA production.[25] In the case of ad libitum fed rats, MDA production was higher in membranes from 24 month old rats than in those from 6 month old rats. Membranes from food restricted rats generated much less MDA than those from ad libitum fed rats. These *in vitro* findings are in agreement with the hydroperoxide content (TABLE 4)

TABLE 4. Hydroperoxide in Hepatic Membranes (nmoles/mg Protein)[a]

Age (Mos.)	Ad Libitum Fed Mitochondria	Microsomes	Food Restricted Mitochondria	Microsomes
6	1.31 ± 0.38	1.47 ± 0.33	0.44 ± 0.09	0.74 ± 0.12
12	1.57 ± 0.10	2.81 ± 0.15	0.99 ± 0.18	1.64 ± 0.17
24	1.98 ± 0.29	2.42 ± 0.29	1.24 ± 0.23	1.54 ± 0.10

[a] Data from Yu *et al.*[26]

of freshly isolated mitochondria and microsomes.[26] Several hepatic cytosolic anti-oxidants and related enzymatic activities (TABLE 5) were found to be influence by age and food restriction.[26] Glutathione reductase changed little with age but was maintained at significantly higher levels in food restricted than ad libitum fed rats. Reduced glutathione was stable through 18 months of age but fell by 24 months of age in ad libitum fed but not food restricted rats. Catalase activity declined slightly with age but food restriction maintained it at higher levels than in ad libitum fed rats. Mn-Superoxide dismutase and glutathione peroxidase changed little with age.

Food restriction was also found to influence the metabolism of malondialde-hyde, a product of free radical damage.[26] The ability of hepatic mitochondria from ad libitum fed rats to oxidize malondialdehyde decreased with age and this de-crease was partially prevented by food restriction (TABLE 6). This action may at least in part underlie the ability of food restriction to retard the age-associated accumulation of lipofuscin and related substances.

Yu et al.[27] recently postulated a cellular mechanism of action of food restric-tion based on the free radical theory of aging. In this postulation, aging is viewed to result from the continuous oxidative threat inherent from the basic metabolic processes of life; by protecting the cell from this threat, food restriction is felt to maintain the integrity of cellular structure and function even at advanced ages.

CONCLUSIONS

Two of the three questions addressed in the introductory paragraph appear to have been effectively addressed over the past 15 or so years. Are most age-associated processes influenced? The answer is yes. Most age-changes in physio-logical processes that have been studied are delayed or partially prevented by food restriction and almost all age-associated disease processes are retarded by food restriction. Does food restriction retard the primary aging processes? A

TABLE 5. Hepatic Cytosolic Antioxidants and Related Enzymes[a]

	6 Mos.		18 Mos.		24 Mos.	
	Gp. A	Gp. R	Gp. A	Gp. R	Gp. A	Gp. R
Superoxide	4.2	4.8	3.9	4.9	4.7	4.8
dismutase	± 0.3	± 0.2	± 0.1	± 0.1	± 0.4	± 0.3
Catalase	529.4	708.5	590.0	452.0	288.9	666.6
	± 68.7	± 158.6	± 52.0	± 127.2	± 42.0	± 88.1
GSH reductase	41.6	49.8	57.4	67.5	41.0	52.3
	± 2.8	± 4.0	± 2.0	± 2.4	± 2.7	± 3.3
GSH trans-	527.4	708.5	590.0	452.0	473.6	653.2
ferase	± 68.7	± 158.6	± 52.0	± 127.2	± 22.6	± 40.6
GSH peroxidase	262.5	279.6	347.2	249.1	273.4	292.6
	± 14.9	± 30.4	± 217.1	± 87.7	± 26.4	± 20.7
Glutathione	59.8	50.9	56.4	51.5	46.0	62.3
	± 7.7	± 2.9	± 13.1	± 2.0	± 5.0	± 5.2
Ascorbic acid	2249.7	2494.1	2866.8	2394.6	1618.2	1763.6
	± 221.3	± 266.2	± 273.5	± 401.3	± 94.6	± 99.0

[a] Gp. A refers to ad libitum fed and Gp. R to restricted groups. (Data in table are from Yu et al.[26])

TABLE 6. Hepatic Mitochondrial MDA Oxidation (nmol MDA Oxidized/mg Protein/10 Min)[a]

Age (Mos.)	Ad Libitum Fed Group	Restricted Group
6	1.47	1.64
12	1.12	1.33
18	1.01	1.12
22	0.69	—
24	—	1.14

[a] Data in table are from Yu *et al.*[26]

definitive answer must await the identification of the primary aging processes. However, the findings to date strongly indicate that a major site of action of food restriction is the primary aging processes. The salient findings supporting this view are the marked extension of the maximum life span and the breadth of the effects on age-changes in physiological processes and age-associated diseases. Such breadth must be the result of an action on a general fundamental process or processes rather than on a particular physiological event or a specific pathogenic process.

What are the mechanisms underlying the actions of food restriction on the aging processes? This question has proved to be most difficult to effectively explore. The major hypotheses proposed have been ruled out by recent studies. What has emerged from our studies is the concept that food restriction retards the aging processes by enabling the rodent to utilize fuel in less damaging ways than is the case for ad libitum fed rats. Our work has focused on the use of glucose and oxygen, both potentially toxic processes. Our findings indicate that glucose is used at sustained lower concentrations and therefore potentially less toxic levels in food restricted rats and that the generation of oxygen radicals is reduced and the mechanisms protecting the cell from their damaging action enhanced in food restricted rats. However, the exploration of this concept is in its infancy and further studies are needed to establish causality in the antiaging actions of food restriction.

REFERENCES

1. MASORO, E. J. 1988. J. Gerontol.: Biol. Sci. **43:** B59–64.
2. BERTRAND, H. A., F. T. LYND, E. J. MASORO & B. P. YU. 1980. J. Gerontol. **35:** 827–835.
3. LIEPA, G. U., E. J. MASORO, H. A. BERTRAND & B. P. YU. 1980. Am. J. Physiol. **238:** E253–257.
4. MAEDA, H., C. A. GLEISER, E. J. MASORO, I. MURATA, C. A. McMAHAN & B. P. YU. 1985. J. Gerontol. **40:** 671–688.
5. MASORO, E. J., K. IWASAKI, C. A. GLEISER, C. A. McMAHAN, E. SEO & B. P. YU. 1989. Am. J. Clin. Nutr. **49:** 1217–1227.
6. YU, B. P., E. J. MASORO & C. A. McMAHAN. 1985. J. Gerontol. **40:** 657–670.
7. KALU, D. N., E. J. MASORO, B. P. YU, R. R. HARDIN & B. W. HOLLIS. 1988. Endocrinology **122:** 1847–1854.
8. IWASAKI, K., C. A. GLEISER, E. J. MASORO, C. A. McMAHAN, E. SEO & B. P. YU. 1988. J. Gerontol.: Biol. Sci. **43:** B5–12.
9. IWASAKI, K., C. A. GLEISER, E. J. MASORO, C. A. McMAHAN, E. SEO & B. P. YU. 1988. J. Gerontol.: Biol. Sci. **43:** B13–21.
10. McCAY, C., M. CROWELL & L. MAYNARD. 1935. J. Nutr. **10:** 63–79.

11. MASORO, E. J., 1988. Extension of life span. *In* Aging in Liver and Gastrointestinal Tract. L. Bianchi, P. Holt, O. F. W. James & R. N. Butler, Eds. 49–58. MTP Press Limited. Lancaster, Great Britain.
12. BERG, B. N. & H. S. SIMMS. 1960. J. Nutr. **71:** 255–263.
13. RUBNER, M. 1908. Das Problem der Lebensdauer und seine Beziehungen zum Wachstum und Ernabrung. Oldenbourg. Munich.
14. PEARL, R. 1928. The Rate of Living. Alfred Knopf. New York.
15. SACHER, G. A. 1977. Life table modifications and life prolongation. *In* Handbook of the Biology of Aging. C. Finch & L. Hayflick, Eds. 582–638. Van Nostrand Reinhold. New York.
16. MASORO, E. J., B. P. YU & H. A. BERTRAND. 1982. Proc. Natl. Acad. Sci. USA **79:** 4239–4241.
17. MASORO, E. J. 1985. Metabolism. *In* Handbook of the Biology of Aging, 2nd edit. C. E. Finch & E. L. Schneider, Eds. 540–563. Van Nostrand Reinhold. New York.
18. McCARTER, R. J., E. J. MASORO & B. P. YU. 1985. Am. J. Physiol. **248:** E488–492.
19. McCARTER, R. J. & J. R. McGEE. 1989. Am. J. Physiol. **257:** E175–179.
20. SAPOLSKY, R. M., L. C. KREY & B. S. McEWEN. 1986. Endocr. Rev. **7:** 284–301.
21. CERAMI, A. 1985. J. Am. Geriatr. Soc. **33:** 626–634.
22. MASORO, E. J., M. S. KATZ & C. A. McMAHAN. 1989. J. Gerontol.: Biol. Sci. **44:** B20–22.
23. BERGMAN, R. H. 1989. Diabetes **38:** 1512–1527.
24. HARMAN, D. 1956. J. Gerontol. **11:** 298–300.
25. LAGANIERE, S. & B. P. YU. 1987. Biochem. Biophys. Res. Commun. **145:** 1185–1191.
26. YU, B. P., S. LAGANIERE & J. W. KIM. 1989. Influence of life-prolonging food restriction on membrane lipoperoxidation and antioxidant status. *In* Oxygen Radicals in Biology and Medicine. M. G. Simic, K. A. Taylor, J. F. Ward & C. von Sonntag, Eds. 1067–1073. Plenum Pub. New York.
27. YU, B. P., D. W. LEE, C. G. MARLER & J. H. CHOI. Proc. Soc. Exp. Biol. Med. **193:** 13–15.

Food Restriction Slows Down Age-Related Changes in Cell Membrane Parameters

C. PIERI

Cytology Center
Gerontological Research Department
Italian National Research Center on Aging (INRCA)
Via Birarelli, 8
60121 Ancona, Italy

INTRODUCTION

Food restriction is a unique and powerful modulator of the aging process. In rodents, undernutrition imposed for prolonged periods from weaning or adulthood induced a marked extension of life span and delayed the age-dependent decline of some physiological functions.[1] The mechanism through which undernutrition decelerates the rate of aging is obscure, though the widespread effect of this treatment in the animal physiology suggests an involvement of basic age-dependent modifications.

Changes in the physicochemical properties of cell membranes have been found to occur during aging in cells of human and animal origin.[2–6]

These changes may account for the age-dependent modifications occurring in a wide variety of processes including ion transport,[7–9] signal recognition and transduction[10,11] and the regulation of enzyme activities.[12–13]

In spite of this, the physicochemical properties of cell membrane have not yet been investigated in diet restricted animals. The aim of the present paper is to show that undernutrition improves the properties of cellular membranes from different cells, *i.e.,* it slows down age-related changes in membrane parameters.

Animals and Diet Restriction

Most of the studies dealing with the effect of undernutrition on the aging process imposed the treatment from weaning, giving the rodents a diet containing a lower amount of calories as compared to the normal diet.[14–19] However, Yu *et al.*[20] reported that food restriction initiated at 6 months of age was about as effective in extending life span as a restriction started soon after weaning. In a number of experiments, significant life span extension has been demonstrated by restricting feeding to an every-other-day schedule during the entire postweaning life span of rodents.[16,21–23]

In our experiments, diet restriction was applied by feeding female Wistar rats on an every-other-day basis, starting from the age of 3.5 months.[24] Briefly, 120 animals of our own breed were randomly divided into two groups of 60 animals each. One of these groups was diet restricted by feeding on an every-other-day schedule (EOD) with the same laboratory diet given ad libitum (AL) to the control group according to Goodrick *et al.*[16] The chow (Nossan, Italy) contained 41% carbohydrate, 21% protein and 6% fat. For the EOD animals, food was provided in the morning hours and removed on the following morning; the animals of both groups had free access to drinking water and were caged three per cage in plastic cages. By the age of 8 months both EOD and AL rats were divided randomly into two subgroups consisting of 30 animals each. One EOD and the AL subgroups were reserved for the determination of the survival curves, the others were sacrificed for the analysis of different biological parameters.

The animals were weighed weekly in the mornings when EOD rats were given the food and the cages were checked daily for dead animals.

Survival Analysis

Survivorship curves were analyzed by a new procedure using a parametric mathematical model built for the purpose of improving the ground upon which the widespread Gompertzian model was based.

The basic features of the previous model[25,26] and the new version is reported in detail elsewhere.[27] The parametric analysis gave the fitted theoretical curves presented in FIGURE 1.

Female Wistar rats diet restricted according to an EOD schedule showed an increase in median, mean and maximal life span when compared to the AL ones. The increase of these parameters was statistically significant. These findings are in close agreement with the results of other authors which applied the same diet from weaning.[16,21-23]

In the new mathematical model proposed by Piantanelli[27] two parameters entering the model are of importance: the first (ω) represents the ability of a given species to survive in a given environment, low values indicating good environmental conditions and/or genetic background. The other parameter (So) is an indicator of the extent of variability of physiological functions inside the group. Both parameters were lowered in diet restricted rats as compared to the controls.[27] An interpretation of these data could be that undernutrition increases the individual resistance to the environmental insults and decreases the variability among the members of the same group.

FIGURE 2 shows the body weight pattern of both diet restricted and control animals. Each point represents the mean value from all rats surviving at any given

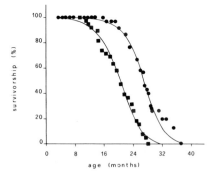

FIGURE 1. Survivorship kinetics of undernourished EOD ($\bullet$) and control AL ($\blacksquare$) rats. Survival analysis, described elsewhere,[24,27] gives the following parameter values for the fitted curves: EOD rats, $\omega = 0.117 \pm 0.001$, $S_0 = 0.441 \pm 0.005$; controls, $\omega = 0.136 \pm 0.002$, $S_0 = 0.538 \pm 0.004$. Both differences between the parameter values from the two curves are statistically significant ($p < 0.01$).

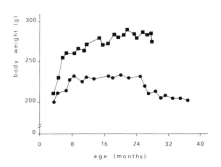

FIGURE 2. Body weight values of under-nourished EOD (●) and control AL (■) rats during the whole life span. Each value is representative of the mean body weight from all animals surviving at any time.

time. In spite of diet restriction, the body weight of EOD animals increased up to the age of 10 months, remained constant until the age of 25 months, and then decreased. A sharp increase was observed in AL fed rats until 6–7 months; then the body weight increase was continuous but of a lower extent during the remaining lifespan.

Membrane Parameters of Splenic Lymphocytes

The effect of food restriction on immune response has been well established. Lymphocytes from undernourished animals responded to polyclonal mitogens better than those from age-matched normally fed ones.[15,21,28] In addition, other studies showed that diet restriction decreased the basal level of natural killer (NK) cell activity but improved the NK activity induced by polyinosinic: poly-cytidylic acid as well as the response of cytotoxic lymphocytes.[29]

In these studies, however, a parameter which may be of great importance was not taken into account, *i.e.,* the decrease of body temperature induced by under-feeding and found to occur both in mice and rats.[15,19,30] Since the incubation temperature affects the response of lymphocytes to mitogens[31,32] as well as the membrane microviscosity,[33] we measured these two parameters at two different temperatures in order to have an indication of the real *in vivo* pattern. TABLE 1 reports results of proliferative responses of splenic lymphocytes.

As was expected, a sharp decrease of the response was observed comparing young and old lymphocyte cultures, and the cells from EOD rats responded much better than those from old AL even if they were incubated at 35°C. Thus a real improvement of lymphocyte response may be suggested also for *in vivo* conditions.

One of the parameters which modulate the response of lymphocytes to mitogens is membrane microviscosity,[34-37] and this parameter has been evaluated in our experiments.

Membrane microviscosity was determined by measuring the fluorescence polarization of the lipid probe 1,6-diphenyl-1,3,5-hexatriene (DPH).[33] The interpretation of fluorescence polarization of DPH as a measure of membrane microviscosity has been questioned.[38-39] However, there is an agreement that polarization of this type of probe reflects local properties of its microenvironment,[40] and in this paper the term "microviscosity" is used only to indicate changes in the local lipid packing.

Membrane microviscosity of lymphocytes measured at 37°C was higher in old AL than in young ones (TABLE 2) and, what is more, the membrane of EOD

TABLE 1. ³H-Thymidine Incorporation in Con A Stimulated Lymphocytes (cpm × 10^{-3} ± SEM)

Temperature (°C)	Young	Old AL	Old EOD
37	102 ± 9	22 ± 4	50 ± 6
35	80 ± 7	20 ± 3	39 ± 5

animals at 35°C was more fluid than that of AL ones measured at 37°C. Considering these data together with the response to Con A, it can be suggested that together with membrane alterations, some other age-dependent modifications, not corrected by diet restriction, are responsible of the impairment of immune response during aging.

Measurements on Liver Plasma Membranes

Changes in lipid composition have been documented in membranes of aging animals. The relative amount of cholesterol increased and the level of unsaturated fatty acid decreased in several tissues during aging.[2] These two parameters together with the temperature are among the factors which deeply influence membrane properties. Indeed they contribute to the maintenance of the cristalline state of membrane lipids which is an essential condition for different membrane functions.[5]

Recently, it was shown that food restriction modified fatty acid composition of mitochondrial and microsomal membrane preparations and suppressed age-related peroxidative deterioration of membranes.[41,42]

In order to get deeper new insight into the effect of food restriction upon various membrane parameters, we analyzed the breakpoint temperatures of the Arrhenius plot of DPH fluorescence polarization as well as of 5'-nucleotidase activity on liver cell membranes from young and old AL and old EOD rats.[43]

Breakpoints of Arrhenius plots, are generally associated with lipid phase transitions in the membranes and the temperatures at which these phenomena occur are closely related to the chemical composition of membranes.[40,44]

The transition temperatures of the fluorescence polarization of DPH in liver plasma membranes from the three experimental models used are shown in TABLE 3. Young and old AL and old EOD animals exhibited well defined breakpoints at 16.3, 19.3 and 16.7°C, respectively. The clear-cut increase in breakpoint temperature observed in old AL as compared with young rats indicated changes in the membrane composition, pointing towards a more rigid state during aging. Importantly enough, undernourished rats showed breakpoints very close to those of young animals, supporting the view that the age-dependent alterations in membrane composition were prevented by diet restriction.

TABLE 2. Membrane Microviscosity of Lymphocytes (n)

Temperature (°C)	Young	Old AL	Old EOD
37	2.03 ± 0.02	2.24 ± 0.02	1.90 ± 0.01
35	2.19 ± 0.02	2.41 ± 0.02	2.04 ± 0.02

TABLE 3. Breakpoints of Arrhenius Plots (°C)

	Young	Old AL	Old EOD
DPH fluorescence polarization	16.3 ± 0.3	19.5 ± 0.6	16.7 ± 1.4
5'-nucleotidase activity	25.1 ± 0.6	28.0 ± 0.7	25.7 ± 0.4

Further support for these conclusions came from the analysis of the break-points of Arrhenius plots of 5'-nucleotidase activity (TABLE 3). This enzyme is a glicoprotein, located primarily in the plasma membrane. It is an ectoenzyme, exposing its active site at the external surface of the membrane.[45] Its activity is regulated by the composition and microviscosity of the external half of the bilayer.[46] Changes in the Arrhenius plot breakpoint temperatures have been related to changes in phospholipid and/or fatty acid composition of the interacting lipids.[47]

The breakpoint temperatures were 25.1, 28.0 and 25.7°C for young and old AL and old EOD animals, respectively, indicating again that food restriction modifies liver plasma membrane composition.

Changes in β-Adrenoceptor Density

Lipid fluidity may modulate the binding of agonists to receptor membrane. When microviscosity of synaptic membranes was increased by in vitro incubation with cholesteryl-hemisuccinate, a fivefold increase of the specific binding of serotonin was observed.[10,11] In parallel, increasing the lipid microviscosity by feeding a cholesterol-enriched diet, lowered cardiac β-adrenergic receptor number in marmoset monkey.[48]

The responsiveness to many hormonal stimulations, which declines during aging and is often associated with reduced hormone receptor density,[49,50] may be at least in part explained with membrane modifications. In particular, the β-adrenoceptor density was reduced in cerebral cortex[51] and cerebellum[52] of senescent rats as compared to the same areas of young animals. It is of interest that membrane preparations from brain cortex[53] and cerebellum[54] showed an age-dependent increase of membrane microviscosity. On the contrary, β-receptor density of lymphocytes which does not seem to be influenced by membrane microviscosity[55] remains unchanged during aging.[56]

The different age-dependent pattern of β-adrenoceptor density in different tissue represents a suitable model to analyze whether diet restriction exerts a generalized effect on this parameter or its action is directed specifically against age-dependent alterations.[57] TABLE 4 shows the β-adrenoceptor density of cere-

TABLE 4. β-Adrenerg Receptor Density (fmol/mg Proteins)[a]

Models	Cerebellum	Kd	Lymphocytes	Kd
Young	67.8 ± 6.2	1.35 ± 0.18	46.8 ± 14.6	0.32 ± 0.06
Old AL	17.2 ± 4.2[b]	0.43 ± 0.18[b]	50.6 ± 5.5	0.47 ± 0.07
Old EOD	38.4 ± 6.8[c,e]	1.30 ± 0.28[d]	41.0 ± 3.9	0.43 ± 0.03

[a] The entries are the mean ± SEM of all six experiments.
Statistically significant from young: [b]p <0.001; [c]p <0.01.
Statistically significant from old AL: [d]p <0.02; [e]p <0.05.

bellar and splenic lymphocyte membranes. In the cerebellum, receptor density was significantly higher in young than in old rats. Compared to 6-month-old rats, 24-month-old AL littermates had 75% reduction of β-adrenoceptor density. Undernutrition strongly influenced this parameter which was almost doubled in EOD old animals as compared to the AL fed ones. Nevertheless, this recovery was partial, the receptor density of EOD rats being only 56% compared to the 6-month-old controls. Recently, the same diet-dependent recovery of the β-adrenoceptor density was observed in membrane preparation from cerebral cortex[58] and from lung.[59]

A completely different picture emerged from the determination of this parameter in lymphocytes. Indeed, neither age nor food restriction influenced the number of β-receptors in the membranes of these cells. Thus, diet restriction was able to modify the β-adrenoceptor density in those tissues in which an age-dependent alteration could be observed, without any general and aspecific effect.

CONCLUSIONS

The main message of present work is that diet restriction preserves the normal physicochemical properties of cell membranes, protecting them from age-dependent alterations.

The view that modifications of membrane properties are of chief importance in the aging process seems to be well established. Indeed, damages induced at membrane levels or an improvement of functional membrane parameters modulate several altered responses related to aging.[8,60–63] This is in good agreement with the hypothesis of Laganiere and Yu[41,42] that undernutrition exerts a positive effect on the whole organism primarily by protecting the cellular membranes from age dependent deterioration.

Although we agree with this hypothesis, we think that another factor of great importance should also be taken into account, *i.e.,* the body temperature, which was lower in undernourished animals as compared to the ad libitum fed ones.[15,19,30] It had already been hypothesized as long as ten years ago that the lowering of body temperature observed in underfed mice could contribute to the lifespan extension.[15]

However, the difficulties, which arose in establishing a chronic nontoxic hypothermia, made this hypothesis difficult to demonstrate in homeotherms. Nevertheless, the existence of a relationship between body temperature and lipid composition of cell membranes has been found not only in poikilothermic animals[64] but in homeotherms, too.[65] As an example of the latter case, the body temperature of genetically obese mice was lower than that of their lean littermates[66] as a result of defective thermogenesis, but the body temperature could be normalized by housing the animals at 34°C or by thyroid hormone treatment.[67]

When the body temperature was normalized, phosphatidylcholine and sphingomyelin composition, breakpoint of Arrhenius plots of DPH polarization and 5'-nucleotidase activity of liver membranes all returned to values close to those observed in the lean control mice of similar body temperature. These data indicated a strong effect of body temperature as modulator of chemical composition of the plasma membranes. Taking into account these findings one can hypothesize that undernutrition induces modifications of membrane lipid composition stimulating the cells to react against the lowering of body temperature, to maintain the cellular membranes in a proper functional state, this way. Together with these, the maintenance of the activity of enzymes which protect against peroxidation is the other key event which prevents the age-dependent deterioration of cell membrane functions.

SUMMARY

The effect of undernutrition on some plasma membrane parameters has been analyzed. Diet restriction was applied to female Wistar rats on every-other-day schedule (EOD), starting from the age of 3.5 months.

Membrane microviscosity of splenic lymphocytes was lower in EOD rats than in the ad libitum (AL) fed ones even if one assumes a decrease of body temperature of 2°C. The decrease of membrane microviscosity due to diet restriction ran parallel with the improvement of proliferative response of lymphocytes. The analysis of Arrhenius plots of 1,6-diphenyl-1,3,5-hexatriene as well as of 5'-nucleotidase activity showed a diet-dependent improvement of membrane properties also of liver plasma membranes.

Diet restriction was able to partially recover the age-dependent decrease of β-adrenoceptor density of cerebellar membranes. On the contrary, β-adrenoceptor density of lymphocytes, which did not show any age-dependent alteration, was not influenced by diet restriction.

Present results support that undernutrition exerted a protective effect on cell membranes of old animals and it was able to improve those alterations which are related to aging.

REFERENCES

1. MASORO, E. J. 1988. Food restriction in rodents: an evaluation of its role in the study of aging. J. Gerontol. **43:** B59–64.
2. SHINITZKY, M. 1987. Pattern of lipid changes in membranes of the aged brain. Gerontology **33:** 149–154.
3. CHOEN, M. B. & M. D. ZUBENKO. 1985. Aging and the biophysical properties of cell membranes. Life Sci. **37:** 1403–1409.
4. KESSLER, A. R., B. KESSLER & S. YEHRUDA. 1985. Changes in the cholesterol level, cholesterol-to-phospholipid mole ratio and membrane lipid microviscosity in rat brain induced by age and plant oil mixture. Biochem. Pharmacol. **34:** 1120–1121.
5. HEGNER, D. 1980. Age-dependence of molecular and functional changes in biological membrane properties. Mech. Ageing Dev. **14:** 101–118.
6. NOKUBO, M. 1985. Physical-chemical and biological differences in liver plasma membranes in aging F-344 rats. J. Gerontol. **40:** 409–414.
7. PIERI, C., I. ZS-NAGY, V. ZS-NAGY, C. GIULI & C. BERTONI-FREDDARI. 1977. Energy dispersive X-ray microanalysis of the electrolytes in biological bulk specimen. II. Age-dependent alterations in the monovalent ion contents of the cell nucleus and cytoplasm in rat liver and brain cells. J. Ultrastruct. Res. **59:** 320–331.
8. PIERI, C., C. GIULI, C. BERTONI-FREDDARI & A. BERNARDINI. 1986. Vitamin E deficiency alters the *in vivo* Rb⁺ discrimination of rat brain cortical cells. Arch. Gerontol. Geriatr. **5:** 21–31.
9. GYENES, M., GY. LUSTYIK, V. ZS-NAGY, F. JENEY & I. ZS-NAGY. 1984. Age-dependent decrease of the passive Rb⁺ and K⁺ permeability of the nerve cell membranes in rat brain cortex as revealed by *in vivo* measurement of the Rb⁺ discrimination ratio. Arch. Gerontol. Geriatr. **3:** 11–32.
10. HERON, D. S., M. SHINITZKY, M. HERSHKOWITZ & D. SAMUEL. 1980a. Lipid fluidity markedly modulates the binding of the serotonin to mouse brain membrane. Proc. Natl. Acad. Sci. USA **77:** 7463–7467.

11. HERON, D. S., M. HERSHKOWITZ, M. SHINITZKY & D. SAMUEL. 1980b. The lipid fluidity of synaptic membranes and the binding of serotonin and opiate ligands. *In* Neurotransmitters and Their Receptors. U. Z. Littauer, Y. Dudai, I. Silman, V. I. Toichberg & Z. Vagel, Eds. 125–136. John Wiley Press. New York.

12. BASS, G. R., L. F. THOMPSON, H. L. SPIELBERG, W. J. PICHLER & J. E. SEEGMILLER. 1980. Age-dependency of lymphocyte ecto-5′-nucleotidase activity. J. Immunol. **125:** 679–682.

13. NOHL, M. 1979. Influence of age on thermotropic kineticks of enzymes involved in mitochondrial energy metabolism. Z. Gerontol. **12:** 9–18.

14. MASORO, E. J., B. P. YU & H. A. BERTRAND. 1982. Action of food restriction in delaying the aging process. Proc. Natl. Acad. Sci. USA **79:** 4239–4241.

15. WEINDRUCK, R. H., J. A. KRISTIE, K. E. CHENEY & R. L. WALFORD. 1979. Influence of controlled dietary restriction on immunologic function and aging. Fed. Proc. **38:** 2007–2016.

16. GOODRICK, C. L., D. K. INGRAM, M. A. REYNOLDS, J. R. FREEMAN & N. L. CIDER. 1982. Effect of intermittent feeding upon growth and lifespan in rats. Gerontology **28:** 233–241.

17. ENESCO, E. M. & J. SAMBROSKY. 1983. Liver polyploidy: influence of age and dietary restriction. Exp. Gerontol. **18:** 79–87.

18. FERNANDES, G., E. J. YUNIS & R. A. GOOD. 1976. Influence of diet on survival of mice. Proc. Natl. Acad. Sci. USA **73:** 1279–1283.

19. DUFFY, P. H., R. J. FEUERS, J. A. LEAKEY, K. D. NAKAMURA, A. TURTURRO & R. HART. 1989. Effect of chronic caloric restriction on physiological variables related to energy metabolism in male Fisher 344 rat. Mech. Ageing Dev. **48:** 117–133.

20. YU, B. P., E. J. MASORO & A. McMAHAN. 1985. Nutritional influences on aging of Fisher 344 rats: physical, metabolic and longevity characteristics. J. Gerontol. **40:** 657–670.

21. GERBASE-DE LIMA, M., R. K. LIU, K. E. CHENEY, R. MICKEY & R. L. WALFORD. 1975. Immune function and survival in long-lived mouse strain subjected to undernutrition. Gerontology **21:** 184–202.

22. CHENEY, K. E., R. K. LIU, G. S. SMITH, R. E. LEUNG, R. MICKEY & R. L. WALFORD. 1980. Survival and disease pattern in C57 BL/6J mice subjected to undernutrition. Exp. Gerontol. **15:** 237–258.

23. BAUCHENE, R. E., C. W. BALES, C. A. SMITH, S. M. TURKER & R. L. MASON. 1979. The effect of food restriction on body composition and longevity of rats. Physiologist (Washington) **22:** 8a.

24. PIERI, C., R. RECCHIONI, F. MORONI, F. MARCHESELLI, M. FALASCA & L. PIANTANELLI. 1990a. Food restriction in female Wistar rats: I. Survival characteristics, membrane microviscosity and proliferative response in lymphocytes. Arch. Geront. Geriatr. **11:** 99–108.

25. PIANTANELLI, L. 1986. A mathematical model of survival kinetics. I. Theoretical basis. Arch Geront. Geriatr. **5:** 107–118.

26. PIANTANELLI, L. 1988. Cancer and aging: from the kinetics of biological parameters to the kinetics of cancer incidence and mortality. Ann. N. Y. Acad. Sci. **521:** 99–109.

27. PIANTANELLI, L., G. ROSSOLINI & R. NISBET. 1990. Modelling survivorship kinetics: a two parameters model. In preparation.

28. FERNANDES, G., P. S. FRIEND, R. A. GOOD & E. J. YUNIS. 1978. Influence of dietary restriction on immunologic function and renal disease in (NZB × NZW) F1 mice. Proc. Natl. Acad. Sci. USA **75:** 1500–1504.

29. WEINDRUCK, R., B. H. DEVENS, H. V. ROFF & R. L. WALFORD. 1985. Influence of dietary restriction and aging on natural killer cell activity in mice. J. Immunol. **130:** 993–996.

30. NELSON, W. &. F. HALBERG. 1983. Meal-timing, circadian rhythms and lifespan of mice. J. Nutr. **116:** 2244–2253.

31. MACCECCHINI, M. L. & M. M. BURGER. 1977. Stimulation of lymphocytes by concanavalin A. Temperature dependent effect of fatty acid replacement. Biochim. Biophys. Acta **469:** 33–44.

32. SMITH, J. B., R. P. KNOWLTON & S. S. AGARWAL. 1978. Human lymphocyte responses are enhanced by culture at 40°C.
33. SHINITZKY, M. & S. BARENHOLTZ. 1978. Fluidity parameters of lipid regions determined by fluorescence polarization. Biochim. Biophys. Acta 515: 367–394.
34. ALDERSON, J. C. E. & C. GREEN. 1975. Enrichment of lymphocytes with cholesterol and its effect on lymphocyte activation. FEBS Lett. 52: 208–211.
35. RIVNAY, B., S. BERGMAN, M. SHINITZKY & A. GLOBERSON. 1980. Correlation between membranes viscosity, serum cholesterol, lymphocyte activation and aging in man. Mech. Ageing Dev. 12: 119–126.
36. SHINITZKY, M., M. LYTE, D. S. HERON & D. SAMUEL. 1983. Intervention in membrane aging. The development and application of active lipid. In Intervention in the Aging Process. Part. B: Basic Research and Preclinical Screening. W. Regelson & F. Linex, Eds. 175–186. Arlan Liss Inc. New York.
37. LUSTYIK, GY., H. M. HALLGREEN, N. BERGH & J. J. O'LEARY. 1989. Effect of preliminary culture on the membrane microviscosity of lymphocytes from young and old donors. Arch. Gerontol. Geriatr. 10: 77–88.
38. KLEINFELD, A., P. DRAGSTEN, R. KLAUSER, W. PJURA & F. MATAYASHI. 1981. The lack of relationship between fluorescence polarization and lateral diffusion in biological membranes. Biochemistry 13: 3699–3705.
39. MCVEY, E., J. YGUERABIDE, D. HAMSON & W. CLARK. 1981. Cooperative nature of bindings of cholesterol onto synaptosomal plasma membrane of dog brain. Biochem. Biophys. Acta 462: 106–118.
40. WUNDERLICH, F., A. RONAI, V. SPETH, J. SEELIG & A. BLUME. 1975. Thermopropic lipid clustering in Tetrahymena membranes. Biochemistry 14: 3730–3735.
41. LAGANIERE, S. & B. P. YU. 1989a. Effect of chronic food restriction in aging rats: I. Liver subcellular membranes. Mech. Ageing Dev. 48: 207–219.
42. LAGANIERE, S. & B. P. YU. 1989b. Effect of chronic food restriction in aging rats: II. Liver cytosolic antioxidants and related enzymes. Mech. Ageing Dev. 48: 221–230.
43. PIERI, C., M. FALASCA, F. MORONI, F. MARCHESELLI & R. RECCHIONI. 1990b. Food restriction in female Wistar rats: III. Thermotropic transition of membrane lipid and 5'-nucleotidase activity in the hepatocytes. Arch. Gerontol. Geriatr. 11: 117–124.
44. LEE, A. G., N. J. N. BIRSDALL, J. C. METCALFE, P. A. TOOM & G. B. WARREN. 1974. Cluster in lipid bilayers and interpretation of thermal effects in biological membranes. Biochemistry 13: 3699–3705.
45. EVANS, W. H. 1974. Nucleotidase pyrophosphatase: a sialoglycoprotein located in the hepatocyte surface. Nature 250: 391–394.
46. DIPPLE, I., L. M. GORDON & M. D. HOUSLAY. 1982. The activity of 5'-nucleotidase in liver plasma membrane is affected by the increase in bilayer fluidity achieved by anionic drugs but not by cationic drugs. J. Biol. Chem. 257: 1811–1815.
47. MERISKO, E. M., G. K. OJAKIAN & C. C. WIDNELL. 1981. Effect of phospholipids on properties of hepatic 5'-nucleotidase. J. Biol. Chem. 256: 1983–1993.
48. MCMURCHIE, E. J. & G. S. PATTEN. 1988. Dietary cholesterol influences cardiac β-adrenergic receptor and adenylate cyclase activity in marmoset monkey by changes in membrane cholesterol status. Biochem. Biophys. Acta 324–332.
49. ROTH, G. S. & G. D. HESS. 1982. Changes in the mechanisms of hormone and neurotransmitter action during aging: current status of the role of receptor and postreceptor alterations. A review. Mech. Ageing Dev. 20: 175–194.
50. PIANTANELLI, L., P. FATTORETTI & C. VITICCHI. 1980. β-adrenoceptor changes in submandibular glands of old mice. Mech. Ageing Dev. 14: 155–164.
51. CIMINO, M., G. VANTINI, S. ALGERI, G. CURATOLA, C. PEZZOLI & G. STRAMENTINOLI. 1984. Age-related modification of dopaminergic and β-adrenergic receptor system: restoration to normal activity by modifying membrane fluidity with 5-adenosylmethionine. Life Sci. 34: 2029–2039.
52. GREENBERG, L. M. & B. WEISS. 1978. β-adrenergic receptors in aged brain: reduced number and capacity of pineal gland to develop supersensitivity. Science 201: 61–63.
53. NAGY, K., P. SIMON & I. ZS-NAGY. 1983. Spin label studies on synaptosomal membranes of rat brain cortex during aging. Biochem. Biophys. Res. Commun. 117: 688–694.

54. PIERI, C., F. MORONI, M. FALASCA, F. MARCHESELLI & R. RECCHIONI. 1990c. Diet restriction decreases the membrane microviscosity of cerebellar membranes of old female Wistar rats. Boll. Soc. Ital. Biol. Sper. **66:** 915–920.

55. PIERI, C., F. MORONI, M. FALASCA, R. RECCHIONI & F. MARCHESELLI. 1990d. Rabbit cholesterol-rich serum decreases the β-adrenergic receptor density of human lymphocytes without altering membrane microviscosity. Med. Sci. Res. **18:** 651–652.

56. ABRASS, I. B. & P. J. SCARPACE. 1982. Catalytic unit of adenylate cyclase: reduced activity in aged human lymphocytes. J. Clin. Endocrinol. Metab. **55:** 1026–1028.

57. PIERI, C., F. MORONI, F. MARCHESELLI, M. FALASCA & R. RECCHIONI. 1990e. Food restriction in female Wistar rats: II. β-adrenoceptor density in the cerebellum and in the splenic lymphocytes. Arch. Gerontol. Geriatr. **11:** 109–115.

58. VITICCHI, C., C. PIERI & L. PIANTANELLI. 1990. Undernutrition retards the age-related decrease of brain cortex β-adrenoceptor density. In preparation.

59. SCARPACE, P. J. & P. B. YU. 1987. Diet restriction retards the age related loss of β-adrenergic receptors and adenylate cyclase activity in rat lung. J. Gerontol. **42:** 442–446.

60. BERTONI-FREDDARI, C., C. GIULI & C. PIERI. 1982. Vitamin E deficiency on the synapses of cerebellar glomerulus of young rats. Mech. Ageing Dev. **9:** 237–246.

61. PIERI, C., C. GIULI & F. MARCHESELLI. 1989. Chronic dietary choline influences the permeability of nerve cell membranes as revealed by *in vivo* Rb+ uptake and release. Arch. Gerontol. Geriatr. **9:** 87–95.

62. BERTONI-FREDDARI, C., R. F. MERVIS, C. GIULI & C. PIERI. 1985. Chronic dietary choline modulates synaptic plasticity in the cerebellar glomeruli of aging mice. Mech. Aging Dev. **30:** 1–9.

63. BERTONI-FREDDARI, C., C. GIULI & C. PIERI. 1982. The effect of acute and chronic centrophenoxine treatment on the synaptic plasticity of old rats. Arch. Gerontol. Geriatr. **1:** 365–372.

64. HAZEL, J. 1979. Influence of thermal acclimatation on membrane lipid composition of rainbow trout liver. Am. J. Physiol. **263:** R91–R101.

65. HOUSLAY, M. D. & R. W. PALMER. 1978. Changes in the form of Arrhenius plots of the activity of glucagon stimulated adenylate cyclases and other hamster liver plasma membrane enzymes occurring on hibernation. Biochem. J. **174:** 909–1009.

66. BRAY, J. A. & D. A. YORK. 1979. Hypothalamic and genetic obesity in experimental animals: an autonomic and endocrine hypothesis. Physiol. Rev. **59:** 719–809.

67. FRENCH, R. R., D. A. YORK, J. N. PORTMAN & K. ISAAC. 1983. Hepatic plasma membranes from genetically obese (ob/ob) mice: studies on fluorescence polarization, phospholipid composition and 5'-nucleotidase activity. Comp. Biochem. Physiol. **76B:** 309–319.

Longevity-Assurance Mechanisms and Caloric Restriction

ANGELO TURTURRO AND RONALD W. HART

National Center for Toxicological Research
United States Public Health Service
Jefferson, Arkansas 72079

INTRODUCTION

Aging is a multifocal phenomenon[1] with a genetic base, modified by environment, as are the many diseases falling under the category called cancer. To understand how to modulate these phenomena, it is important to understand their origins in an evolutionary and comparative sense. It is thus useful to discuss aging in the context of what has been termed longevity-assurance mechanisms.[2]

In the context of longevity assurance mechanisms, instead of the pathology of aging, the focus is on those processes which result in species longevity. Organisms thrive despite constant assault from endogenous and exogenous sources. It is axiomatic that evolutionary selection operates most strongly on factors important to reproduction. It is unlikely that selection pressure was directed at increasing longevity, especially in primates, since animals are unlikely to survive to old age in the wild, and, if they do, they probably contribute few offspring since postreproductive senescence can occur at less than half the maximal life span. It is more likely that the increase in life span that is thought to have occurred in evolution of the advanced primates[3] is a by-product of the protective mechanisms which have arisen to allow humans to survive to the age of reproduction, as well as other genes which result in reproductive success.

Comparative analysis highlights those factors that correlate with species longevity. Better termed Longevity Related Processes, or LRP, it was found that four factors could account for 80% of the variation in species life span:[4] brain weight, body weight, specific metabolism and body temperature. In addition, DNA repair has been shown to be correlated with species lifespan.[5]

Caloric restriction (CR) is the only paradigm which consistently extends mammalian lifespan, also reducing the age-related incidence of chronic diseases.[6] Previous attempts to address CR in the context of LRPs have considered only one genotype, and focused on the relationship of CR to lifetime energy dissipation.[7] This dissipation is greater in the restricted animal than an ad libitum fed one on a per gram lean body weight basis.[8] This paper uses lifetime studies in different genotypes to address CR in a more comparative sense.

METHODS

We conducted lifetime monitoring of a 100/genotype/sex/diet cohort for the B6D2F1, DBA/2NNia, B6C3F1, and C57B16 mouse, and the BROWN-NORWAY (BN), BN X F-344, and F-344 rat, all fed NIH-31, and, additionally, the

C57B16 mouse fed EM-911a and the F-344 rat fed Masoro Diet C.[9] The restriction involved feeding 60% of the ad libitum diet consumed by a control population, with vitamin supplementation of the restricted feed to bring it up to the ad libitum levels. The animals were singly housed in Specific Pathogen Free conditions. The animals were monitored daily and weighed, and food consumption was measured on a weekly or monthly basis depending on the genotype and age. Standard pathology profiles were developed every six months, and organ weights were obtained. Core body temperature, physical activity, metabolism,[10,11] P-450 isoenzymes,[12] and DNA repair[13] were measured on these animals.

RESULTS AND DISCUSSION

Body Weight

One of the most important LRP is body weight. Using only one genotype/diet as an example, the average body weight of the C57B1/6 on the NIH-31 diet at selected ages over its life span is shown in TABLE 1. The drop-off after 21 months is not a result of selective die-off of large individuals. Almost all the surviving males lose between 10 and 20% of their body weight as well as consume less food (data not shown). In other genotype/diet conditions (*e.g.*, the same mouse fed EM-911A), the oldest males are self-restricted, sometimes to the level of the experimental group at advanced ages. A similar trend is seen in the females, although interpretation is complicated by mammary tumors, which increase body weight. This increase to a maximum and drop-off at the older ages occurs in all the mice genotypes/diet combinations tested, as well as the F-344 rat. It is most prominent in the males, which generally acquire more weight than the females.

It has been found, from studies on P-450 isoenzyme patterns,[12] that sex-specific patterns decline with age in rats, a decline which is slowed in CR animals. The mechanism for this may involve changes in male pattern growth hormone secretion, as this has been found to be important in the control of P-450 isozyme expression.[12] Analogously, body weight can be viewed as part of the male sex-specific response, which declines with age in ad libitum fed animals. As with the P-450 isoenzyme patterns, CR reduces the expression of this response, but allows it to persist longer.

When compared to animals fed NIH-31, the same animals, under identical environmental conditions fed EM-911A are heavier and have a shorter life span (TABLE 1). EM-911A, contains 11% fat and 20% protein, and was developed primarily as a diet to assist breeding. NIH-31 is a standard rodent diet with 5% fat and 18% protein. Interestingly, the restricted body weights were similar for the two diets. The animals fed NIH-31 outlive the mice EM911A, although the restricted animals have similar life spans on either diet. In a sense, therefore, CR may be considered an extension of the diet effect of using a diet which inhibits the sex-specific response, and which also limits reproduction.

Thus, the same process which increases breeding success leads to decreased longevity. This is an example of what has been termed pleiotropism.[14] It appears that the mechanism may be a hormonal one, probably through the sex-related hormones. Both males and females lose their sex-specific response with age, and this process is delayed by caloric restriction. Many of the biomarkers which are altered with CR may undergo a similar trend, following this pattern. Interestingly, mice that undergo CR stop breeding during restriction, while rats experience reduced fertility.[15] Direct measurement of the relationship of body weight and longevity is complicated,[16] as pathology, especially since tumors, which increase body weight or inanition, which reduce it, cloud interpretation. However, Ross[17] found that factors such as the time to a particular body weight and consumption during some early ages were important in predicting rat longevity. These observations, as well as Bidder's classical hypothesis about the relationship of growth and aging,[18] may actually be another metric to evaluate the lack of expression of developmentally appropriate sex-specific responses.

TABLE 1. Body Weights and Life Span of C57B1/6 Mice with Different Diets[a]

Age (Mo)	Diet			
	NIH-31		EM-911A	
	A	R	A	R
6	35.5	22.9	37.0	24.0
9	38.2	23.2	45.5	23.5
12	41.2	25.0	49.0	26.5
15	42.2	22.5	47.9	25.5
18	42.2	23.2	47.8	27.0
21	40.8	24.9	49.0	27.5
24	40.2	24.9	46.6	26.8
27	39.6	23.6	39.8	26.9
30	34.8	21.5	29.5	23.0
33	35.5	21.5	24.0	24.0
36	34.0	21.5	x	23.5
39	x	21.4	x	22.8
	Life Span (Mo)			
MnLS	28.5	32.2	25.4	33.6
90LS	33.8	41.1	28.9	40.1

[a] Body weights in grams (standard deviation is less than 10%, and is smaller for restricted animals). MnLS is mean life span, 90LS is time to 90% mortality, in months. A is ad libitum, R is restricted.

Brain Weight

Brain weight is fairly proportional to body weight between species.[7] Within a species, in different genotypes and at different weights, the relationship is more complex. From the measurements done in all the mouse genotype/diet combinations listed in the methods section, the brain weight in the four genotypes at different ages is related to body weight with the equation:

$$\text{Br Weight} = a_1 + a_2 * \text{BW}$$

where values for the constants, and representative values at average body weights, is given in TABLE 2.

The brain weight appears to have a component which is independent of body weight (*i.e.*, is the same for all members) as well as a body weight sensitive component. Using average weights at various ages, as shown in TABLE 3, the body weight sensitive component is approximately 20% of the total brain weight in ad libitum fed animals, and 40–50% of the weight in CR animals. Interestingly, if a CR female mouse weighed as much as the average ad libitum male mouse, its

TABLE 2. Effect of Chronic Caloric Restriction on Some Hepatic Drug Enzymes[a]

Enzyme	Sex	Ad Lib. (9 Mo)	Rest. (9 Mo)	Ad Lib. (22 Mo)	Rest. (22 Mo)
P-450 IIC11	M	2.77	1.70	0.07	0.97
Androgen 5a reductase	F	2.10	4.20	19.9	10.4
Corticosterone Sulfotransferase	F	5.00	18.0	20.8	20.1

[a] Rats are F-344 restricted to 60% of ad libitum diet. All values are means of at least 5 rats. SEMs are less than 20% of mean except for 0.07 value, which is 80%. Enzyme activities are nmol/min/mg microsomal protein except for sulfotransferase which are nmol/min/mg cytosolic protein. (Adapted from Leakey et al.[12])

brain weight would be 30% larger than is found in the male mouse. *Peromyscus leucopus* is a criticid rodent which is about as large as the average ad libitum fed mouse, but has a brain approximately twice as large, as well as a life span that is about twice as long.[19] Our attempts to calorically restrict this animal beyond a 20% restriction have failed, and many of its physiological parameters, such as body temperature regulation are more similar to a CR mouse than an ad libitum fed one.[20] In our breeding colonies, *P. leucopus* does not breed as well as mice. This criticid may be an example of a rodent which utilizes many of the same LRP that are available to small mice-like rodents.

Specific Metabolism

One of the oldest hypotheses, such as Rubner's, in aging relates aging inversely to specific metabolism.[21] On a per mouse or rat basis, CR mice have a lower metabolism, as shown in TABLE 4. However, in agreement with previous work,[8] on a per gram body weight or lean body weight basis, as also shown in TABLE 4, CR rodents have a similar or slightly higher specific metabolism. In retrospect, a slightly higher metabolism is not unexpected since a thinner body fat insulating layer and smaller size (indicating a higher surface area/body weight

TABLE 3. Brain Weight in Mice[a]

Group	Brain Weight = A_1 + A_2 · Body Weight			
	A_1	A_2	Avg. BW	Avg. BrW
Male: ad lib.	0.4025	0.0026	35.90	0.494
Male: rest.	0.2760	0.0086	22.45	0.468
Female: ad lib.	0.3906	0.0041	27.63	0.503
Female: rest.	0.2261	0.0118	20.80	0.472

[a] BW is body weight and BrW brain weight in grams. Fifteen mice are used for each genotype on test, at 6, 12, 18, 24 and 30 months of age (when the genotype lives that long).

ratio) will cause the animals to work harder to keep their body temperature elevated above ambient. There is also an increased physical activity in the CR animals,[11,12] which also leads to increased energy output. The only mitigating factor is the decrease in average body temperature which occurs in CR animals.[11,12]

Body Temperature

Another major physiological parameter correlated with life span was body temperature. Lowering body temperature is the only other mechanism ever found to increase longevity (and only in poikilotherms[21]). Hibernating animals (whose body temperature was lower than normal at times of the year) were compared with nonhibernating sister species, and found to live longer.[7] Given this evidence, it is paradoxical that Sacher's analysis suggests that an increased body temperature is weakly related to increased life span. Correlation of body temperature with other life-style factors may be important. For instance, in an interspecies comparison, species dwelling in cooler climates (which live longer) may require higher internal temperatures to survive the cold. CR decreases body average body temperatures, approximately 0.8°C in F-344 rats and 1.3°C in B6C3F1 mice,[11,12] and may have similar effects in man.[22]

TABLE 4. Specific Metabolism[a]

Animal	Ad Lib.			Rest.		
	/Animal	/g BW	/g LBM	/Animal	/g BW	/g LBM
B6C3F1 (33 Mo)	90.2	2.82	3.34	75.3	3.23	3.44
F-344 (18 Mo)	463.3	1.02	1.35	308.8	1.22	1.37

[a] Metabolism is in the average consumption/day in ml O_2/h, ml O_2/h-g. Number under animal designation is age in months when evaluated. Animals are males, approximately 10/group. (Adapted from Duffy et al.[10] and Duffy et al.[11])

Longevity Equation

The four variables above were related to longevity using Sacher's analysis:

$$L = 8 \cdot E^{0.6}/S^{0.4} \cdot 10^{0.025T}/M^{0.5}$$

where L is longevity in years, E and S are brain and body weight in grams, T is body temperature in °C and M is specific metabolism in watts/g. The brain and body weight are often combined together as encephalization (I), where:

$$I = E/S^{2/3}.$$

By dividing the life span predicted for restricted animals by that predicted for ad libitum fed animals, one derives the equation:

$$L_r/L_a = (I_r/I_a)^{0.6} \cdot 10^{0.025(T_r - T_a)} \cdot (M_a/M_r)^{0.5}$$

where the subscript r denotes restricted and a denotes ad libitum. Values for this encephalization ratio for the species on test, at average weights, are given in TABLE 5.

If we evaluate the encephalization and the metabolism, as shown in TABLE 5 for male F-344 rats, one predicts a 6% increase in longevity for CR. Given the inverse relationship of life span to temperature in intraspecies comparisons such as in poikilotherms, if we consider the Sacher equation without the temperature term, the increase in longevity is predicted to be 12%. If the specific metabolism is put on a per gram lean body weight basis, on the premise that the lean body mass is more appropriate when comparing animals in the wild across species (since animals in the wild are not likely to be maintained similar to laboratory rodents), the predicted life span extension is 16% using the interspecies equation. If temperature is excluded, the predicted extension is 22%, which is what is observed (TABLE 5). In mice, also excluding temperature, the predicted life extensions are approximately a third of those observed.

TABLE 5. Life Extension Predicted by Longevity Equation[a]

Animal	I_d	T_d	M_{dbw}	M_{dlbm}	Lp_t (%)	L_p (%)	L_o (%)
F-344	1.406	−0.82	0.84		7	12	21
(18 Mo)	1.406	−0.82		0.99	16	21	21
B6C3F1	1.25	−1.24	0.87		0	7	37
(33 Mo)	1.25	−1.24		0.97	5	13	37

[a] Longevity equation in text. I_d is ratio of the encephalization of the rest./ad lib., T_d the difference between the rest. and ad lib. body temperatures, M_{dbw}, the ratio of the specific metabolism (per body weight) of the ad lib./rest., M_{dlbm}, the ratio of the specific metabolism (per lbm) of the ad lib./rest., L_{pt}, the % longevity extension using the full equation, L_p, the predicted extension without the temperature term, and L_o, the observed longevity extension, taken as the % of the mean life spans rest./ad lib. Animals are males.

In the context of the equation, in rats, the increase in encephalization more than compensates for any increase in specific metabolism that occurs with CR. The increase in encephalization may suggest that a large brain/body weight is important, or may be an indicator that there has been some selection for a factor associated with a larger encephalization, such as delaying puberty by longer retention of mammalian early growth characteristics (I is elevated in early growth). If the latter is true, it has interesting implications for the evolution of the extended human life span.

In mice, the equations predict a much shorter life span extension. This may be a result of the much lower body temperature seen in the mice. The life span of hibernating animals, which spend part of their life span at lowered body temperatures, is also underpredicted by the physiological equation. For these rodents, CR may have less of an effect on the variable associated with the encephalization, and may have its longevity-extending effects operating though its simulation of hibernation, or lower body temperature. Thus, CR may have a differential effect on different species, depending on what LRPs are most stimulated.

DNA Repair

CR stimulates certain metabolic pathways, physical activity (especially around feeding time) and an apparent direct increase in glucocorticoids,[13] as well

TABLE 6. Age and UV-Induced Repair in Cells Isolated from Male F-344 Rats[a]

Age (Mo)	Hepatocytes[b]		Kidney Cells[c]	
	Ad Lib.	Rest.	Ad Lib.	Rest.
5	5.78	—	—	—
13	4.90	5.72	—	—
22	3.05	4.03	2.01	2.36
28	2.65	3.31	1.34	1.93
34	—	3.02	—	1.33

[a] Rest. is 60% of ad lib. diet. All values are dpm per ug DNA for irradiated/unirradiated cells after one hour. Ratios of rest. and ad lib. are significantly different ($p < 0.01$) at all ages and in both types of cells. (Adapted from Weraarchakull et al.[24])

[b] Irradiated with 877J/m².

[c] Irradiated with 100J/m².

as an increase in the corticosterone sulfotransferase,[13] suggesting a chronic elevation of stress hormone. Given these effects, there may be an increase in DNA damage as a result of CR. This is consistent with the results of Randerrath et al.,[23] who found an increase in their I-spots with CR. It is not clear what the significance is of these spots. However, CR has an effect on limiting proliferation, a mechanism for diluting DNA damage in cells. There may be an increase in the observable DNA damage seen in cells. If one effect of CR is to stimulate DNA damage, one would predict a compensatory increase in DNA repair.

In cells from kidney and liver of Fischer 344 rats, there was a decline in both control and UV stimulated DNA repair with age (TABLE 6).[24] For both tissues, consistent with Licastro et al.,[25] caloric restriction resulted in less of a decline with age.

Skin fibroblasts from Brown Norway, BN, and Brown Norway × Fischer 344 F1 hybrid, BNF1, showed an increase in both rat genotypes of both types of excision repair (TABLE 7).[13] Increased also were the levels of MGAP activity in BN rats. Skin fibroblasts from the B6C3F1 mice were evaluated at different times of day, and their response had circadian changes[13] with the maximum increase less than half the effect seen in the rats (TABLE 7).

Given the differential species response, DNA repair seems to be more related to the parameters in the longevity equation than longevity extension *per se*. An increase in DNA damage would stimulate DNA repair. Another, mutually nonexclusive, possibility is, given the circadian response, that a hormonal or metabolic

TABLE 7. DNA Repair and Caloric Restriction in Rat and Mouse Skin Cells[a]

Inducer of DNA Damage	Brown-Norway		BN X F-344		B6C3F1	
	A	R	A	R	A	R
MMS (0.5 mM)	1.156	1.180	1.404	1.608	n.d.	n.d.
UV (20 J/m²)	1.375	1.412	2.072	2.750	n.d.	n.d.
Spontaneous[b] (MGAP levels)	0.38	0.65	n.d.	n.d.	0.34	0.46

[a] Rest. is 60% of ad lib. diet; all rats are 18 months of age. Ad lib. vs rest. repair values are significantly different ($p < 0.01$) in all cases. Values are ratios of stimulated versus nonstimulated cells except MGAP levels which are in femtomoles/ug DNA of 0^6-methylguanine-acceptor protein activity. n.d. is not determined. (Adapted from Lipman et al.[13])

[b] Mouse levels are at 12 hours post lights on.

adaption triggers this effect. One of the most consistent responses to CR is the decrease in the levels of a number of circulating hormones, especially the gonadotrophins.[15] Available information suggests that hormones can significantly effect DNA repair. An example of this is the effect of the estrous cycle on DNA repair in mammary gland and uterine DNA repair of a nonmetabolically activated agent, excluding hormonal effects on metabolism. It can be seen that the time in the cycle when estrogen is lowest (diestrus) is the time when DNA repair is highest (TABLE 8).[26,27] The mechanism of this is unknown. Thus, an hormonal effect may be important for the elevated DNA repair seen.

CR results in a number of adaptations which contribute to the total effect. Some of these effects may be positive, others, such as perhaps an increase in DNA damage, negative. The total differential response of different strains and species to CR may be a result of the differing weight of the various LRP activated.

TABLE 8. Estrous and DNA Repair in Sprague-Dawley Rats[a]

Organ	Repair Length (hrs)	Diestrous	Stage Proestrous	Estrous
Mammary	1	0.150[b]	0.150	0.160
Epithelium	8	0.123	0.150	0.162
Uterus	1	0.122[b]	0.072	0.073
	8	0.079	0.086	0.062
Liver	1	0.111	0.077	0.088
	8	0.122	0.097	0.102

[a] 50–53-day-old virgin female Sprague-Dawley rats were given a 50 mg/kg b.w. dose of N-methyl-nitrosourea. Values are ratios of 0^6-methylguanine to N^7-methylguanine. (Adapted from Braun et al.[26] and Ratko et al.[27])

[b] Repair differences between stages are significant at $p < 0.05$.

CONCLUSIONS

CR seems to trigger many of the LRPs that appear to be significant for species longevity in the animals tested. It is also interesting that the state which CR induces, a hypogonadathrophic, hypothermic, low body weight one, is the same that occurs both at early ages and in long-lived members of the species eating ad libitum. These effects have often been thought either as prematuration or as dyshomeostasis of age. However, maintaining these processes throughout life seems to result in extension. Instead, they may be adaptations which are important to longevity.

Building on previous ideas,[28] one theory of how CR acts can be termed the Adaptive-Longevity Related Process Theory of CR:

1) CR mimics a situation very common in the wild, *i.e.*, food scarcity at different times of year, or years on end;

2) A successful species preserves itself during these difficult times by either forming some vegetative stage (*e.g.*, a spore) or adapting the organism through some method so it will live long enough to reproduce when times become better again. Reproduction is often discontinued;

3) The mechanisms used to increase life span are the specific LRPs that the species normally is subject to, and emerge in long-lived members of the species.

The most easily conceptualized candidates for these mechanisms are those directly related to reproduction or are tied to the processes which directly regulate reproduction. However other, more distal phenomena, such as growth hormone pulsatility and physical activity, seem to be important. Delayed growth or sexual maturation may be an important LRP whose selection may result in delayed reproduction, increased brain size and increased longevity, a factor that may have operated in the relatively rapid extension of human life span in prehistory.

4) The sum total effect of CR using current methodologies is to extend life span differentially in different strains/diet combinations. However, there are a number of negative effects of the paradigm, such as elevated physical activity and stress hormones, which may result in increased DNA damage. This may lead to mutation, which may balance the positive effects of CR for the long-term survival of the species.

By understanding how CR induces its positive effects, we can perhaps trigger the LRPs which increase longevity, while minimizing the negative effects of CR. In this manner, we can suggest methods for how to trigger these mechanisms in man significantly improving human health.

REFERENCES

1. OLSON, C. B. 1987. A review of why and how we age: a defense of multifactorial aging. Mech. Age. Dev. **41:** 1–28.
2. HART, R. & A. TURTURRO. 1981. Evolution and longevity-assurance processes. Naturwissenschaften **68:** 552–557.
3. SACHER, G. 1975. Maturation and longevity in relation to cranial capacity in hominid evolution. *In* Primates: Functional Morphology and Evolution. R. H. Tuttle, Ed. 417–441. Mouton. The Hague.
4. SACHER, G. & P. H. DUFFY. 1979. Genetic relation of life span to metabolic rate for inbred mouse strains and their hybrids. Fed. Proc. **38:** 184–189.
5. TURTURRO, A. & R. HART. 1984. DNA repair mechanisms in aging. *In* Comparative Biology of Major Age-Related Diseases. D. Schiapelli & G. Migaki, Eds. 19–45. Liss. New York.
6. ALLABEN, W. T. Dietary restriction and toxicological end points: an historical perspective. *In* Biological Effects of Dietary Restriction. L. Fishbein, Ed. Springer-Verlag. New York. In press.
7. SACHER, G. 1977. Life table modification and life prolongation. *In* Handbook of the Biology of Aging. C. Finch & L. Hayflick, Eds. 582–638. Van Nostrand. New York.
8. MASORO, E. J., YU, B. P. & H. BERTRAND. 1982. Action of food restriction in delaying the aging process. Proc. Nat. Acad. Sci. USA **79:** 4239–4241.
9. WITT, W., D. BRAND, V. ATTWOOD & O. SOAVE. 1989. A nationally supported study on claoric restriction in rodents. Lab. Anim. **18:** 37–43.
10. DUFFY, P. H., R. J. FEUERS, J. A. LEAKEY, A. TURTURRO & R. HART. 1989. Effect of chronic caloric restriction on physiological variables related to energy metabolism in the male Fischer 344 rat. Mech. Age. Dev. **48:** 117–133.
11. DUFFY, P. H., R. J. FEUERS & R. HART. Effect of chronic caloric restriction on the circadian regulation of physiological and behavioral variables in the male B6C3F1 mouse. Chronobiology International. In press.
12. LEAKEY, J., J. BAZARE, JR., J. HARMON, R. FEUERS, P. DUFFY & R. HART. Effects of long-term caloric restriction on hepatic drug metabolizing enzyme activities in the Fischer 344 rat. *In* Biological Effects of Dietary Restriction. L. Fishbein, Ed. Springer-Verlag. New York.
13. LIPMAN, J. M., A. TURTURRO & R. HART. 1989. The influence of dietary restriction on DNA repair in rodents: a preliminary study. Mech. Ageing Dev. **48:** 135–143.
14. WILLIAMS, G. C. 1957. Pleiotropy, natural selection and the evolution of senescence. Evolution **11:** 398–411.

15. MERRY, B. The effect of dietary restriction on the endocrine control of reproduction. *In* Biological Effects of Dietary Restriction. L. Fishbein, Ed. Springer-Verlag. New York.

16. WEINDRUCH, R. & R. WALFORD. 1988. The Retardation of Aging and Disease by Dietary Restriction. C. C. Thomas, Springfield, Ill.

17. ROSS, M. 1972. Length of life and caloric intake. Am. J. Clin. Nutr. **25:** 834–838.

18. BIDDER, G. P. 1932. Senescence. Br. Med. J. **2:** 5831.

19. SACHER, G. & R. HART. 1978. Longevity, aging and comparative cellular and molecular biology of the house mouse, *Mus musculus,* and the white-footed mouse, *Peromyscus leucopus.* In Birth Defects Original Article Series. D. Bergsma & D. Harrison, Eds. Vol. 14(1): 71–96. Plenum. New York.

20. DUFFY, P. H., R. J. FEUERS & R. HART. 1987. Effect of age and torpor on the circadian rhythms of body temperature, activity and body weight in the mouse (*Peromyscus leucopus*). *In* Advances in Chronobiology. J. Pauly & L. Scheving, Eds. Part B: 111–120. Liss. New York.

21. REED, J. & E. SCHNEIDER. 1985. Modulations of aging processes. *In* Handbook of the Biology of Aging. C. Finch & E. Schneider, Eds. 45–78. Van Nostrand. New York.

22. KEYS, A., J. BROZEK, A. HENSCHEL, O. MICKELSON & H. TAYLOR. 1950. Cancer and other neoplasms. *In* The Biology of Human Starvation. Vol. 2. U. Minn. Press. Minneapolis.

23. RANDERRATH, E., R. HART, A. TURTURRO, T. F. DANNA, R. REDDY & K. RANDERRATH. Effects of aging and caloric restriction on I-compounds in liver, kidney, and white blood cell DNA of male Brown-Norway rats. Mech. Ageing Dev. In press.

24. WERAARCHAKULL, N., R. STRONG, W. G. WOOD & A. RICHARDSON. 1989. The effect of aging and dietary restriction on DNA repair. Exp. Cell Res. **181:** 197–204.

25. LICASTRO, F., R. WEINDRUCH, L. J. DAVIS & R. L. WALFORD. 1988. Effect of dietary restriction upon the age-associated decline of lymphocyte DNA-repair activity in mice. Age **11:** 48–52.

26. BRAUN, R. J., T. RATKO, J. PEZZUTO & C. BEATTIE. 1987. Estrous cycle modification of rat uterine DNA alkylation by N-methylnitrosourea. Cancer Lett. **37:** 345–352.

27. RATKO, T., R. J. BRAUN, J. PEZZUTO & C. BEATTIE. 1988. Estrous cycle modification or rat mammary gland DNA alkylation by N-methyl-N-nitrosourea. Cancer Res. **48:** 3090–3093.

28. TURTURRO, A. & R. HART. Effect of caloric restriction in maintenance of genetic fidelity. *In* DNA Damage and Repair in Human Tissue. Brookhaven Symposia in Biology Number 36. Brookhaven, NY. In press.

Effects of Factors Prolonging Life Span on Carcinogenesis

VLADIMIR N. ANISIMOV

Laboratory of Experimental Tumors
N. N. Petrov Research Institute of Oncology
68, Leningradskaya Str.
Pesochny-2
Leningrad 189646, USSR

INTRODUCTION

Cancer is well known to be a common cause of disability and death in the elderly with over 50 percent of all cancers occurring in those who are over 65.[1,2] It is generally accepted that age is the single greatest risk factor for cancer development. However, at present there is no common opinion on the nature of the relation between aging and carcinogenesis and on causes of this phenomenon. A number of data support the concept that an age-related accumulation of total dose of carcinogens account for cancer induction as a function of age in sensitive individuals.[3] Another concept is that natural changes in the internal milieu of the organism (immune, endocrine, metabolic) provide increasingly favorable conditions for malignant transformation of cell with increasing age.[4,5] Both approaches and numerous data and arguments *pro et contra* have been reviewed by us before.[6,7] The elucidation of the causes of the age-related increase in cancer incidence is essential to the elaboration of a strategy for primary cancer prevention. Comparative analysis of the effects of agents or factors which could influence both life span and incidence of spontaneous and exogenously induced tumors could help us to understand the mechanisms, both common and different, of aging and carcinogenesis, and to reveal the nature of the interrelation of these two fundamental biological processes.

Aging and Multistage Model of Carcinogenesis

Recently R. G. Cutler and I. Semsei[8] concluded that there is indeed much evidence for common causes of cancer and aging. The authors based this conclusion on the positive correlation between the aging rates of different species with their cancer rates and on the fact that both processes—aging and cancer development—may be initiated and promoted by impairments of gene regulation driven by destabilizing processes (affecting regulatory elements). In discussing processes of initiation and promotion of aging and carcinogenesis, it is necessary to define these events briefly.

The idea that carcinogenesis includes several (two or more) stages was proposed in early 1940s on the basis of studies of skin tumor induction by chemical carcinogens.[9,10] During the following 20 years, qualitative characteristics of initiation and promotion phenomena were described, using this model. During recent years, the multistage character of carcinogenesis has been demonstrated both *in vivo* and *in vitro*.[9] Carcinogenic agents (chemical, radiation, virus) are considered to interact with nucleic acids and proteins during the first stage of carcinogenesis (initiation), causing genetic damages that lead to irreversible changes in the genome of a normal cell, determining its predisposition to malignancy (latent, immortalized cell). During the second stage of carcinogenesis (promotion), the initiated cell, under the influence of a carcinogenetic agent (full carcinogen) or tumor promoters, acquires properties of a transformed cell, due to the changes in gene expression. Tumor promoters influence the cell in different ways, including activation of protein kinase C, intensification of hexose transport, increase in activity of ornithine-decarboxylase and polyamine production, influence on cell differentiation, and blocking cell-to-cell contacts.[9,11] Recently, the promoters, namely, 12-O-tetradecanoylphorbol-13-acetate (TPA), were found to cause damage of DNA, mediated by free radical formation, induction of sister chromatid exchange, and stimulation of DNA proviruses and some retroviruses expression.[11]

Different animal tumors induced by chemical carcinogenes *in vivo* and *in vitro* were found to contain active transforming genes. Not a single oncogene, but a cascade of oncogenes appeared to participate in neoplastic transformation, defining different stages of this process.[12–14]

An important role in the mechanism of neoplastic transformation may be played by the depressive influence of carcinogenetic agents on antioncogene activity and its expression.[13,14] Tumor promoters, especially TPA, were shown to increase activity of some activated cell oncogenes at different stages of carcinogenesis.[11] Protooncogene activation and its transformation to oncogenes as well as repression of antioncogenes may occur in different ways. Exact mechanisms of this process are still obscure.[12,14]

The mathematical formulation of a carcinogenesis multistage model facilitated the development of this concept. Despite some differences in the models described by several authors the main principles of them were the following.[10] Firstly, a normal cell was presumed to pass at least one intermediate stage on its way to complete malignant transformation. Secondly, the passages from one state to another may be considered stochastic events, the rate of which depends on the dose of a carcinogen which influences the cell. Finally, all cells at any stage of carcinogenesis may enter the next stage independently of each other.

According to this model, the tumor develops only if at least one cell passes through all the necessary stages, and due to clonal growth can be clinically identified. In this model, exact origin of stages is ignored and the changes in the cell function in the process of malignant transformation are not assessed. The grade of malignancy is considered to increase with every stage. Various carcinogenic agents are suggested to modify the rate of multistage malignant transformation in different ways. Besides, some agents act at early stages of carcinogenesis, while others act at late stages.[10] Epidemiological data, analyzed in frames of a multistage model of carcinogenesis, helped to estimate the value of such factors as the time after the beginning of carcinogenic action, the duration of exposure, the time after cessation of carcinogenic action, and the age at the onset of exposure. In cases when carcinogenic agents act at an early stage of carcinogenesis, the number of cells that ought to pass through all prior stages to become malignant, may increase. An elevated incidence of tumors induced by such an agent depends on time, and would not go down immediately upon withdrawal of this agent. If a carcinogenic agent affects late stages of carcinogenesis, the tumor incidence rate goes up without a prolonged latency. The increased rate of tumor incidence will be reversed immediately upon cessation of exposure.[10]

It should be noted that the subdivision of carcinogens to carcinogens of early and late stage is rather conventional. At the same time, epidemiologically defined terms "early" and "late" could not be regarded as analogues to specific experimental events. Among carcinogens affecting early stages, there are some agents that influence not only DNA directly, but also prevent the action of extracellular inhibitors, suppress DNA repair, and stimulate replication, thus leading to genome damage. Among late-stage carcinogens, there might be not only promoters, but also antagonists of some homeostatic mechanisms such as immune surveillance and nonspecific resistance, the agents stimulating tumor cell progression and some others. Some carcinogens, under special conditions, are considered to be able to affect early or late stages, or both of them. Moreover, the agent may act as an "early-stage agent" or a "late-stage agent" depending upon localization.

It should be taken into account that terms such as "initiation," "promotion," "early" and "late" stages describe only phenomena, but not the mechanisms of carcinogenesis. Each of these stages involves numerous mechanisms and different events, that include the process of induction, selection and others.[10-12]

The accumulation of knowledge of the mechanisms of carcinogenesis seems to diminish our arguments in favor of differences between initiators and promoters, "early" and "late" stages.[10] At the same time, the efforts of investigators aimed at deciphering events leading to transition of a cell from one state to another on its way to malignancy revealed the multistage nature of carcinogenesis, and established the role of separate events occurring at the molecular level, and a monoclonal origin of a malignant cell.[9-12,14]

The analysis of the problem of aging and carcinogenesis interrelations will be based on epidemiologically and experimentally confirmed statements revealing carcinogenesis as a process occurring in time, with a scale of chronological time or an account of events (stages) passed by the cell on its way to transformation from the norm to malignancy. FIGURE 1 shows an integrated scheme of multistage carcinogenesis. On the level of organism, carcinogenic agents not only influence a cell, causing genome damages that lead to neoplastic transformation, but also indirectly create in the cell microenvironment the conditions that facilitate proliferation and clonal selection.[6]

Thus multistage carcinogenesis is accompanied by different, sometimes profound disturbances in tissue homeostatic regulation and in the antitumor resistance system that, in turn, are under the influence of systemic nervous, hormonal and metabolic factors. The time of realization of these changes depends on the state of those systems at the moment of exposure to a carcinogen or tumor promoter (or on the contrary, the antipromoting factors) and intensity of the dose, and determines the probability of key changes in a target stem cell, probability of its delay at each intermediate stage for a certain period of time, or even reversion. All these factors determine the frequency of cell division (the rate of proliferation), the total period of carcinogenesis and accordingly the latency of tumor development.

It is worth noting that according to the multistage model, the carcinogen whose effect increases in proportion to age at exposure is supposed to affect the partially transformed cell. In this case the tumor latency would decrease and/or the incidence of tumor would increase, as compared to a population exposed to the same dose of carcinogen at a young age (FIG. 2). The data supporting this

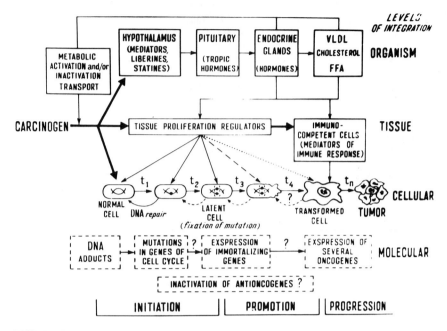

FIGURE 1. Integral scheme of multistage carcinogenesis. $t_1 \ldots t_{ii}$: time of passage of cell from stage k_1 to stage $k_2 \ldots k_n$.

conclusion, including the results of experiments with carcinogens and/or promoters administrated to animals at various age were presented previously.[6,7,15,16] These data suggest age-related accumulation of initiated cells in some tissues during natural aging.

Molecular Events in Senile DNA Are Sufficient for Carcinogenesis

According to some modern concepts both cancer and aging may arise from a common set of genetic alterations.[8] DNA damage is implicated in the etiology of cancer and there is good evidence that DNA damage is a major causative factor in aging.[17-19] One of the hypotheses explaining the interrelation between aging and carcinogenesis suggests an alteration of methylation in some genes as a clue to understanding reasons for the increase of cancer incidence in old individuals.[20-22] Recent data suggest that there is no common pattern of age-related alteration in methylation and protooncogene expression patterns in various tissues.[16,21-23] It is necessary to obtain more knowledge in this field. At the same time, it should be noted that age- and cancer-associated changes in DNA methylation did not occur in all tested genes.[14,16,26]

The formation of DNA adducts in target-tissues is one of the key events in the process of chemical carcinogenesis.[12,24] Of great interest are the data reporting that the DNA of various tissues in intact rats contain adduct-like compounds which accumulate with age.[25] Being identical to adducts of DNA biologically, these adduct-like substances (named as I-compounds) might play a critical role in the initiation of spontaneous carcinogenesis and aging. On the other hand, accumulation of I-compounds in the cells' DNA with age could control age-related changes in the cell differentiation.[25] The formation of I-compounds is not caused by the action of the specific DNA modifying enzymes such as cytozine-5-methyltransferase and might involve microsomal oxydases or other xenobiotic metabolizing enzymes.[26] The most important characteristic of I-compounds might be their capability to cause mutations (point or frame shift), DNA chain breaks and gene rearrangements.[25] However, it is too early to conclude that these I-compounds are involved in spontaneous tumor induction or are markers of aging in rodents.[27] Besides, the age-related accumulation of adduct 7-methylguanine in nuclear and mitochondrial DNA might play an important role in the process of aging and carcinogenesis.[28]

Thus, the data available indicate that fundamental changes in separate DNA structures and functions are developing in the process of normal aging. The character of these changes may vary in different tissues and might cause uneven tissue aging and thus different patterns of age-related increases in spontaneous incidence of tumors in various organs.

Geroprotectors as Anticarcinogenic Drugs

It is worthy of note that carcinogens could also accelerate the aging rate in target tissues as well as in the organism as a whole. The data on such effects of carcinogenic agents of various origin (chemical, hormonal and radiational) were reported elsewhere.[6,15] At the same time, the factors or drugs which increase life span in laboratory animals (geroprotectors) could influence spontaneous and induced carcinogenesis. Available data from other laboratories and the results of our studies on spontaneous tumor incidence in animals exposed to geroprotectors

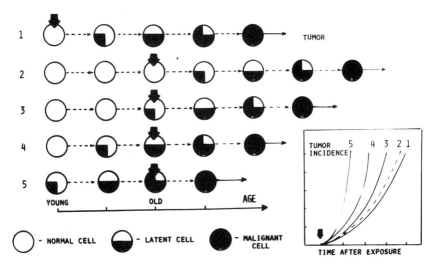

FIGURE 2. The multistage carcinogenesis induced by single exposure to carcinogenic agent at different ages. Groups 3–5 demonstrate carcinogenic effect produced on cell that has passed through one or more stages in accordance with multistage model of carcinogenesis.

demonstrated a good correlation between the type of induced aging delay and the pattern of tumor development (TABLE 1). In particular, some geroprotectors postpone the beginning of aging of the population. In this case the tumor latency increases without significant alterations in their incidence. On the contrary, drugs and factors that slow down the population aging rate (aging rate could be estimated as α in the Gompertz equation: $R = R_0e^{\alpha t}$, where R is mortality, $R_0 = R$ at $t = 0$; α is constant) decrease tumor incidence and increase tumor latency against the background. On the one hand, the geroprotectors which increase the aging rate thus give rectangularity to the Gompertz curve increasing tumor development (FIG. 3). It should be noted that the mean life span of animals increased equally in all three cases (FIG. 3) revealing no correlation between this parameter and tumor incidence in the population. On the other hand, the correlation between the aging rate and the constant that characterizes the rate of age-related cancer incidence increases (indicated as m in the equation $Q = Q_0e^{mt}$, where Q is the cumulative incidence of spontaneous malignant tumors, $Q_0 = Q$ at $t = 0$, and m is constant) appeared to be very high ($r = 0.82$).[6] From the standpoint of a multistage model, geroprotectors of one or another type may either inhibit or accelerate the passage of cells exposed to a carcinogen from one stage to another. In this case, the efficacy of geroprotectors as measures preventing tumor development would decrease in accord with the age of exposure onset. This suggestion is in accord with the results of a number of experiments.[6,42] But there is an increase of tumors in premature aging in humans, and also under the influence of drugs that increase the rate of aging.[6,15] It is important to stress that geroprotectors that slow down the aging rate (type II) do it by influencing the "main" regulatory systems of the organism (nervous, endocrine, immune). Therefore, they slow down age-related changes in the microenvironment of cells exposed to carcinogenic agents or stochastic hits.

According to their mechanism of action, all geroprotectors may also be classified into two main groups. The first group includes those drugs that mainly prevent stochastic lesions of macromolecules. The theoretical basis for using these preparations is provided for by variants of the "catastrophe errors" theory, which regards aging as a result of the accumulation of stochastic damage. The second group includes drugs and influences which are thought to slow down the program of aging and the development of age-related pathology.

Antioxidants are the most typical representatives of the first group. Their geroprotectors and antitumor effects depend upon the age at which their administration has begun and inversely upon the dose of the damaging agent. Antioxidants are sometimes thought not to slow down aging *per se* but to inhibit the action of the environmental factors which decrease the survival of control (intact) animals by, say, preventing the action of dietary components capable of producing free radicals.[49] The tumor-inhibiting effect of antioxidants is more pronounced in the case of carcinogenesis which is induced externally, by chemical carcinogens, for example.[50]

The second group of geroprotectors is represented by the antidiabetic biguanides, phenformin and buformin, pineal factors and caloric-restricted diet. These influences cause diverse effects on the hormonal, metabolic and immunological parameters of an organism, causing the the normalization of their age-dependent shifts and, thus, providing their antitumor effects.[6,15] Among life-span-prolonging mechanisms induced by caloric restriction are those that have the same effects as the above drugs, including antioxidants.[6,33] It should be noted that these influences were also capable of pronounced inhibition of chemical and radiation-induced carcinogenesis (TABLE 2). Of course, this classification is not absolutely

TABLE 1. Effects of Geroprotectors on Spontaneous Tumor Development in Rodents

Type of Aging Delay	Geroprotector	Effect on		Authors
		Tumor Latency	Tumor Incidence	
1	2-mercaptoethylamin	increases	no effect	Harman, 1972[29]
	2-ethyl-6-methyl-3--oxipyridine	increases	no effect	Emanuel, Obukhova, 1978[30]
2	Procaine/gerovital/	no effect	no effect	Aslan et al., 1965[31]
	Caloric restriction	increases	decreases	Tannenbaum, Silverstoun, 1953[32]
	Phenformin	increases	decreases	Dilman, Anisimov, 1980[34]; Anisimov, 1982[35]
	Buformin	increases	decreases	Anisimov, 1980[36]
	L-DOPA	no effect	decreases	Dilman, Anisimov, 1980[34]
	Phenytoin	no effect	decreases	Dilman, Anisimov, 1980[34]
	Tryptophan-deficient diet	no data	decreases	Segall, Timiras, 1976[37]
3	Dehydroepiandrosteron	increases	decreases	Schwartz et al., 1988[38]
	Succinic acid	no effect	decreases	Anisimov, Kondrashova, 1979[39]
	Epithalamin	increases	decreases	Dilman et al., 1979[40]; Anisimov et al., 1982, 1989[41,42]
	Thymalin	increases	decreases	Anisimov et al., 1982, 1989[41,42]
	Levamisole	increases	decreases	Bruley-Rosset et al., 1980[43]
	Selenium	no data	increases	Cherkas et al., 1962[44]; Schroeder, Mitchener, 1971[45]; Dubina, Razumovich, 1975[46]
	Ethylenediaminetetraacetate-Na2	no data	increases	
	Tritium oxide (low doses)	no data	increases	Muksinova et al., 1983[47]
	Tocopherol (vit.E): Benign tumor	increases	increases	Porta et al., 1980[48]
	Malignant tumor	increases	decreases	

rigid. It was shown, for instance, that some antioxidants were able to enhance an immune response in old mice.[6]

We believe that the data presented above enable us to understand possible causes of the increase in cancer incidence in the present century. The survival curves of human populations were noted to become more and more "rectangular".[59,60] This is caused by the decrease in child and early mortality, which is connected with infectious and noninfectious diseases. As a result, a significant increase in the mean life span in human populations occurred, while the maximum human life span has stayed the same for centuries.[59,61]

Thus, the changes in the shapes of the survival curves of human populations respond to the third type of aging delay presented in FIGURE 3. The changes of this type were shown experimentally and epidemiologically to be associated with an increase in tumor incidence. In other words, for the increase in mean life span achieved by the decrease in mortality at an early age, mankind pays at a later age by an increased risk of cancer or some other disease of civilization like atherosclerosis or diabetes mellitus.

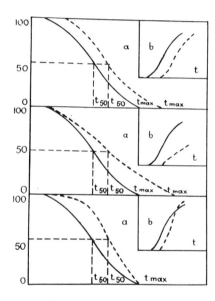

FIGURE 3. Types of aging delay (a) and incidence of spontaneous tumors (b) under influence of geroprotectors. Ordinate: (a) number of survival animals, %; (b) tumor rate, %. Abscissa: age; *solid line* = control, *broken line* = administration of geroprotector.

We believe that further progress in modern preventive medicine is impossible without radical changes in approaches to public health and to prolongation of the human life span. In the burst of industrialization, urbanization, and increasing environmental pollution, one may hope only for a partial alleviation of their unfavorable effects on human health. The achievement of more significant results in this field will require the solution of very complex scientific and technological problems as well as considerable economic expense.

It is probably true that, even at present, changes in life-style, *i.e.,* dietary and sexual habits, smoking and alcohol consumption, etc., may be the most promising approach to achieving a decrease in cancer incidence and, hence, and increase in life span.[62] It seems to become more and more clear that the measures which

TABLE 2. Effect of Some Geroprotectors on Induced Carcinogenesis in Rats

Carcinogen	Drug	Total Tumor Incidence %	Main Tumor Localization	Incidence Tumors of Main Site	Authors
DMBA, i.v.	control	97.3	mammary gland	81.1	Anisimov et al., 1980[51]
	buformin	54.4*		36.4*	
	phenytoin	71.0*		55.3*	
	epithalamin	80.0		25.7*	
	DOPA	50.0*		25.0*	
DMBA, i.v.	control	96.9	mammary gland	68.8	Anisimov et al., 1980[52]
	thymalin	72.8*		18.2*	
NMU, i.v.	control	100.0	mammary gland	71.4	Anisimov et al., 1980[53]
	phenformin	75.0*		37.5*	
NMU, trans-placentally	control	54.2	nervous system	33.3	Alexandrov et al., 1980[54]
	buformin	27.0*		9.5*	
NEU, trans-placentally	control	97.8	spinal cord	61.8	Bespalov et al., 1984[55]
	thymalin	90.4		28.8*	
	epithalamin	87.5*		33.9*	
	phenformin	82.6*		39.1*	
DMH, s.c.	control	94.7	colon	94.7	Anisimov et al., 1980[56]
	phenformin	90.8		90.8**	
Total body X-ray	control	74.1	malignant tumors at different sites	36.2	Anisimov et al., 1982[57]
	thymalin	69.4		18.9*	
	epithalamin	57.9		13.2*	
Total body X-ray	control	78.0	malignant tumors at different sites	42.0	Anisimov et al., 1982[58]
	phenformin	48.0*		30.0	

*Difference with control is significant, $p < 0.05$.
**Treatment with phenformin reduced the multiplicity of colon cancer and mean tumor size.

normalize the age-related changes in hormonal status, metabolism and immunity, and thus slow down the realization of the genetic program of aging (not postponing aging but decelerating its rate) are most effective in protection from aging and prevention of cancer development. The influences which protect against the initiating action of damaging agents (antioxidants, antimutagens) may be important additional means of prophylaxis of cancer and accelerated aging, especially under conditions of increased risk of exposure to damaging environmental factors (FIG. 4).

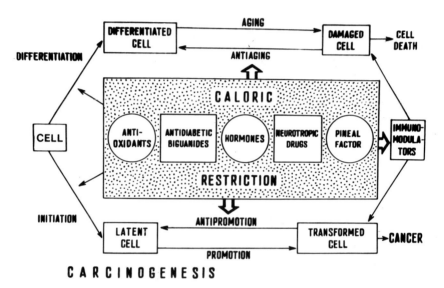

FIGURE 4. Targets in effects of geroprotectors on aging and carcinogenesis.

REFERENCES

1. NAPALKOV, N. P. 1985. *In* Age-Related Factors in Carcinogenesis. A. Likhachev, V. Anisimov & R. Montesano, Eds. IARC Sci. Publ. No. 58: 9–20. IARC. Lyon.
2. DIX, D. 1989. J. Gerontol. **44:** 10–18.
3. PETO, R., S. E. PARISH & R. G. GRAY. 1985. *In* Age-Related Factors in Carcinogenesis. A. Likhachev, V. Anisimov & R. Montesano, Eds. IARC Sci. Publ. No. 58: 43–53. IARC. Lyon.
4. BURNET, F. M. 1976. Immunology, Aging and Cancer. Medical Aspects of Mutation and Selection. Freeman and Co. San Francisco.
5. DILMAN, V. M. 1981. The Law of Deviation of Homeostatis and Diseases of Aging. Wright PSG. Boston.
6. ANISIMOV, V. N. 1987. Carcinogenesis and Aging. Vol. 1 & 2 CRC Press, Inc. Boca Raton, FL.
7. ANISIMOV, V. N. 1989. Semin. Oncol. **16:** 10–19.
8. CUTLER, R. G. & I. SEMSEI. 1989. J. Gerontol. **44:** 25–34.
9. SLAGA, T. J., ED. 1983/1984. Mechanisms of Tumor Promotion. Vols. 1–4. CRC Press, Inc. Boca Raton, FL.
10. KALDOR, J. M. & N. E. DAY. 1987. *In* Mechanisms of Environmental Carcinogenesis. J. C. Barret, Ed. Vol. 2: 21–57. CRC Press, Inc. Boca Raton, FL.

11. SLAGA, T. J. 1984. *In* Models, Mechanisms and Etiology of Tumor Promotion. M. Börzonyi, N. E. Day, K. Lapis & H. Yamasaki, Eds. IARC Sci. Publ. No. 56: 497–506. IARC. Lyon.
12. NAPALKOV, N. P., V. N. ANISIMOV, P. G. KNYAZEV & A. J. LIKHACHEV. 1989. *In* General Oncology. Handbook for Physicians. N. P. Napalkov, Ed. 28–52. Meditsina. Leningrad.
13. BALMAIN, A. & K. BROWN. 1988. Adv. Cancer Res. **51:** 147–182.
14. TANOOKA, H. 1988. Jpn. J. Cancer Res. **79:** 657–665.
15. ANISIMOV, V. N. 1987. *In* Concepts and Theories in Carcinogenesis. A. P. Maskens, P. Ebbesesn & A. Burny, Eds. 271–303. Exerpta Medica. Amsterdam.
16. ANISIMOV, V. N. 1990. Vopr. Onkol. **36**(7): 775–786.
17. KIRKWOOD, T. B. L. 1989. Mutat. Res. **219:** 1–7.
18. STREHLER, B. L. 1986. Exp. Gerontol. **21:** 283–319.
19. NAPALKOV, N. P., V. N. ANISIMOV, A. J. LIKHACHEV & L. TOMATIS. 1989. Cancer Res. **49:** 318–323.
20. NYCE, J., S. WEINHOUSE & P. MAGEE. 1985. Br. J. Cancer **48:** 463–475.
21. ONO, T., N. TAKAHASHI & S. OKADA. 1989. Mutat. Res. **219:** 39–50.
22. MAYS-HOOPES, L. L. 1989. Int. Rev. Cytol. **114:** 181–220.
23. SEMSEI, I., S. MA & R. G. CUTLER. 1989. Oncogene **4:** 465–470.
24. SINGER, B. & D. GRUNBERGER. 1983. Molecular Biology of Mutagens and Carcinogens. Plenum Press. New York and London.
25. RANDERATH, K., J. G. LIEHR, A. GLADEK & E. RANDERATH. 1989. Mutat. Res. **219:** 121–133.
26. RANDERATH, K., M. V. REDDY & R. M. DISHER. 1986. Carcinogenesis. **7:** 1615–1617.
27. WARNER, H. R. & A. R. PRICE. 1989. J. Gerontol. **44:** 45–54.
28. PARK, J.-W. & B. N. AMES. 1988. Proc. Natl. Acad. Sci. USA **85:** 7467–7470.
29. HARMAN, D. 1972. Am. J. Clin. Nutr. **25:** 839–843.
30. EMANUEL, N. M. & L. K. OBUKHOVA. 1978. Exp. Gerontol. **13:** 25–29.
31. ASLAN, A., A. VRABILESKU & C. DOMILESKU. 1965. J. Gerontol. **20:** 1–8.
32. TANNENBAUM, A. & H. SILVERSTONE. 1953. Adv. Cancer Res. **1:** 451–501.
33. WEINDRUCH, R. & R. L. WALFORD. 1988. The Retardation of Aging and Disease by Dietary Restriction. CC Thomas Publ. Springfield.
34. DILMAN, V. M. & V. N. ANISIMOV. 1980. Gerontology **26:** 241–246.
35. ANISIMOV, V. N. 1982. Farmakol. Toksikol. **45:** 127.
36. ANISIMOV V. N. 1980. Vopr. Onkol. **26**(6): 42–48.
37. SEGALL, P. E. & P. S. TIMIRAS. 1976. Mech. Ageing Dev. **5:** 109–124.
38. SCHWARTZ, A. G., J. M. WHITECOMB, J. W. NYCE, M. L. LEWBART & L. L. PASHKO. 1988. Adv. Cancer Res. **51:** 391–424.
39. ANISIMOV, V. N. & M. N. KONDRASHOVA. 1979. Dokl. Akad. Nauk SSSR **248:** 1242–1245.
40. DILMAN, V. M., V. N. ANISIMOV, M. N. OSTROUMOVA, V. G. MOROZOV, V. KH. KHAVINSON & M. A. AZAROVA. 1979. Exp. Pathol. **17:** 539–545.
41. ANISIMOV, V. N., V. KH. KHAVINSON & V. G. MOROZOV. 1982. Mech. Ageing Dev. **19:** 245–258.
42. ANISIMOV, V. N., A. S. LOKTIONOV, V. KH. KHAVINSON & V. G. MOROZOV. 1989. Mech. Ageing Dev. **49:** 245–257.
43. BRULEY-ROSSET, M., I. FLORENTIN, N. KIGER, J. I. SCULZ & G. MATHE. 1980. *In* Cancer Chemo- and Immunopharmacology. Vol. 2. Immunopharmacology, Relations, and General Problems. G. Mathe & F. M. Muggia, Eds. 139–146. Springer-Verlag. Berlin.
44. CHERKES, L. A., S. G. APTEKAR & M. N. VOLGAREV. 1962. Bull. Eksp. Biol. Med. **53**(3): 78–83.
45. SCHROEDER, H. A. & M. MITCHEMER. 1971. J. Nutr. **101:** 1531–1540.
46. DUBINA, T. L. & A. N. RAZUMOVICH. 1975. Introduction in Experimental Gerontology. Nauka & Tekhnika. Minsk.
47. MUKSINOVA, K. N., V. S. VORONINA & E. N. KIRILLOVA. 1983. *In* Biologic Effects of Low-level Radiation. Y. I. Moskalev, Ed. 70–74. Inst. Biophysics Publ. Moscow.
48. PORTA, E. A., N. S. JOUN & R. T. NITTA. 1980. Mech. Ageing Dev. **13:** 1–39.

49. KOHN, R. R. 1971. J. Gerontol. **26:** 378–380.
50. WATTENBERG, L. W. 1985. Cancer Res. **45:** 1–8.
51. ANISIMOV, V. N., M. N. OSTROUMOVA & V. M. DILMAN. 1980. Bull. Eksp. Biol. Med. **89:** 723–725.
52. ANISIMOV, V. N., E. V. DANETSKAYA, V. G. MOROZOV & V. KH. KHAVINSON. 1980. Dokl. Akad. Nauk SSSR **250:** 1485–1487.
53. ANISIMOV, V. N., E. V. DANETSKAYA, V. G. MOROZOV & V. M. DILMAN. 1980. Eksp. Onkol. **2**(3): 40–43.
54. ALEXANDROV, V. A., V. N. ANISIMOV, N. M. BELOUS, I. A. VASILYEVA & V. B. MAZON. 1980. Carcinogenesis **1:** 975–978.
55. BESPALOV, V. G., V. A. ALEXANDROV, V. N. ANISIMOV, V. G. MOROZOV & V. KH. KHAVINSON. 1984. Eksp. Onkol. **6**(5): 27–30.
56. ANISIMOV, V. N., V. M. DILMAN & K. M. POZHARISSKY. 1980. Vopr. Onkol. **26**(8): 54–58.
57. ANISIMOV, V. N., G. I. MIRETSKY, V. G. MOROZOV & V. KH. KHAVINSON. 1982. Bull. Eksp. Biol. Med. **94:** 80–82.
58. ANISIMOV, V. N., N. M. BELOUS & E. A. PROKUDINA. 1982. Eksp. Onkol. **4**(6): 26–29.
59. CUTLER, R. G. 1985. *In* Principles of Geriatric Medicine. R. Andres, E. L. Bierman & W. R. Hazzard, Eds. 22–79. McGraw-Hill. New York.
60. HIRSCH, H. R. 1982. J. Theor. Biol. **98:** 321–346.
61. GAVRILOV, L. A. & N. S. GAVRILOVA. 1986. The Biology of Life Span: Quantitative Aspects. Nauka. Moscow.
62. TOMATIS, L. 1985. Cancer Lett. **26:** 5–16.

Pathogenetic Approaches to Prevention of Age-Associated Increase of Cancer Incidence

V. M. DILMAN

Laboratory of Endocrinology
The N. N. Petrov Research Institute of Oncology
Pesochny-2, Leningradskaya, 68
Leningrad 189646, USSR

INTRODUCTION

At present, several controversial ideas concerning the cause of age-dependent increase in cancer incidence are discussed in the literature. For example, Peto *et al.*[1] distinguished two basic hypotheses. According the first, the age-dependent increase in cancer incidence is attributed to the increased exposure of the body to carcinogens with aging. The second hypothesis assumes that age-dependent increase in cancer incidence is the result of immune deficiency[2] and hormonal-metabolic shifts caused by age-associated hypothalamic dysfunction.[3] Peto *et al.*[1] completely rejected the second hypothesis and expressed their position in the rather extraordinary title of their article: "There is no such thing as aging, and cancer is not related to it."[4]

Meanwhile, there is no need to contrast the two hypotheses, but it is crucial to strictly distinguish two phenomena in carcinogenesis: (1) factors determining the initiation of carcinogenesis and (2) conditions promoting tumor development. Initiation is caused by certain damage to the cell genome. The probability of the occurrence of such lesions caused by chemical carcinogens, ionizing radiation, some viruses and endogenous damaging factors, such as free radicals, increase with aging.

The conditions promoting tumor process may be illustrated by events related to hormonal carcinogenesis. Hormones are not capable of causing damage to genetic apparatus. Therefore, hormones cannot act as initiators of carcinogenesis (except in cases when hormone metabolism leads to production of damaging agents such as free radicals). Meanwhile, certain hormones are known invariably to induce cancer. Analysis of data concerning hormonal carcinogenesis shows that a hormone is capable of promoting tumor development if (1) it causes the pool of dividing cells in target tissue to increase; or (2) it suppresses the immune system.

Taking into account these two statements the following well-known factors of cancer risk should be mentioned: obesity and overeating, and particularly, a diet high in saturated fat; essential hypertension; maturity-onset diabetes mellitus; extremely low or high blood cholesterol level; high blood cortisol level; decreased production of some androgen-like steroids, particularly, dehydroepiandrosterone and its metabolites;[5] disturbances of menstrual cycle including uterine bleeding, sterility and climacteric, and some other risk factors which will be discussed below.

It is easy to notice that the majority of these factors are inherent in normal aging. Naturally, a question arises as to the origin of cancer risk factors in the course of normal aging. The answer to this question is directly associated with general problems of etiology of pathologic processes.

Modern medicine suggests two models of pathologic process: genetic and ecological (TABLE 1).

Development of disease due to the influence of genetic and ecological pathogenic factors is a random event. Correspondingly, in modern medicine, formation of diseases is considered a random event which either may or may not take place in an individual. On the contrary, with time, the organism accumulates lesions induced by endogenous damaging agents, for example, free radicals. The accumulation of lesions is a regular event. This phenomenon is considered the key factor of aging.[6] Moreover, endogenous damaging agents greatly contribute to carcinogenesis and atherogenesis. In these cases the development of these diseases is a random (stochastic) event. To summarize, at present it is common to distinguish strictly between disease as a random event and normal aging as a regular event.

Meanwhile, I suggested that delimitation of mechanisms of aging and those underlying certain age-associated diseases is unjustified.[7] In this case we deal with another model of disease formation, namely, the ontogenetic model.

According to this model, disease is a by-product of the realization of developmental program of the organism (see in detail REF. 7). A few diseases follow the ontogenetic model of development. These are: climacteric, age-related obesity, prediabetes, hyperadaptosis,[7] age-related mental depression, essential hypertension, metabolic immunodepression, metabolic type of autoimmune disturbances, atherosclerosis and cancrophilia, *i.e.,* the sum of hormonal and metabolic conditions contributing to cancer development[7]. Theoretically, these diseases could sooner or later appear in every individual, even in the absence of pathogenic genetic and ecological factors. Therefore, the above diseases should be considered major noninfectious diseases. Moreover, the ontogenetic mechanisms underlying these diseases are the same as those involved in normal aging. Therefore, it is impossible to delimit the mechanism of normal aging from the ontogenetic mechanism of major diseases. This means that certain regular diseases including cancrophilia increase the risk of cancer development in the course of aging. This problem and, especially, the mechanism of age-associated disturbances inherit in three main homeostatic systems of the body, are worthy of separate discussion.

Age-Dependent Alterations in the Reproductive System

As we know, the mechanism of age-dependent switching-on of the female reproductive function seems to be realized through a decrease in hypothalamo-gonadotropic system sensitivity to inhibition by estrogens (see in detail REF. 7). Many years ago I suggested[8] that age-dependent switching-off of reproductive function is caused by the same hypothalamic mechanism which continues to operate after sexual maturation (see REF. 7).

This postulate was experimentally verified in rodents.[9] However, until now it has been a general belief that age-associated switching-off of the reproductive function in women is caused by a decrease in the hormonal activity of the ovaries. For example, Meites and associates[9] wrote: "The primary cause for termination of menstrual cycles in women appears to lie in the ovaries, whereas in female rats termination of estrous cycles lies in the hypothalamo-pituitary system." TABLE 2 shows that reproductive females are characterized by a gradual increase in blood

TABLE 1. Four Models of Major Diseases Formation (Some Examples)

Etiology	Ecological	Genetic	Accumulative	Ontogenetic
Atherosclerosis	external damaging factor	genetic defect	damages produced by side products of metabolic processes	by-product of realization of developmental program
	overfeeding	lack of LDL receptors	damages produced by free radicals	age-dependent glucose intolerance
Immunosuppression	overfeeding	some genetic syndromes	free radical damage to lymphocytes	metabolic immunodepression
Aging	carcinogenic stress-induced, x-ray-induced	progeria and other syndromes	accumulation of lipofuscin, glycosylation of proteins	by-product of developmental program
Cancer	chemicals, viruses, x-ray	genetic syndromes (xeroderma pigmentosa, etc.)	free radical damages to genome	cancrophilia

levels of gonadotropic hormones (FSH and LH) whereas blood estradiol concentration is elevated rather than decreased. Hence, female aging does not involve primary disturbance of the ovarian function. On the contrary, it may be supposed that a rise in blood gonadotropins concentration gradually leads to a decrease in ovarian sensitivity to the stimulating effect of these hormones and, therefore, to a decrease in estrogen synthesis in menopause.

TABLE 2. Age-Associated Changes of the Blood Gonadotropins (FSH and LH) and Estradiol Levels in Healthy Females

Age (Yrs)	FSH (mIU/ml)	LH (mIU/ml)	Estradiol (pg/ml)
20–29	6.7 ± 1.8	6.7 ± 1.9	95 ± 32
30–39	7.6 ± 2.8	11.0 ± 2.3	125 ± 23
40–49	10.0 ± 1.7	12.9 ± 2.0	134 ± 21
>50 years	42.0 ± 13.0	25.0 ± 11.0	82 ± 18

Several important conclusions may be drawn on the basis of the above data: (a) homeostatic disturbances involved in age-dependent switching-off of the reproductive function (defined as climacteric) causes concentrations of both gonadotropic hormones and estrogen in the blood to increase. These hormones stimulate proliferation of target tissue, thus increasing the probability of cancer development. Therefore, prolonged use of contraceptive steroid drugs is associated with a lower frequency of ovarian and endometrial cancer; (b) climacteric is part of normal aging as well as a disease. Indeed, any persisting disturbance in the homeostasis which increases death risk should be defined as disease. However, climacteric is an unusual disease because age-dependent switching-off of female reproductive function is a regular event, and (c) climacteric is a reversible phenomenon. For example, the prolonged use of contraceptive steroids postpones the onset of menopause. Climacteric reversibility, *i.e.*, the possibility for pharmacological regulation of the onset of climacteric must be studied to prevent age-dependent increase in tumor incidence (see below).

Age-Dependent Alterations in the Adaptive System

Rats and some other mammals reveal age-associated decrease in the sensitivity of hypothalamo-pituitary complex to the inhibiting effect of glucocorticoids.[7] As a result, the adaptive system capacity is increased providing the development of this system in ontogeny. Meanwhile, maintenance of this mechanism after the completion of the developmental part of ontogeny leads to the disturbance of homeostasis in the adaptive system, since the shift of the set-point of hypothalamic sensitivity decreases efficiency of negative feedback signals. For example, FIGURE 1 illustrates age-associated prolongation of surgery-associated stress reaction in breast cancer patients. Undoubtedly, excessive stress reaction is a disease since it assures higher probability of death.[10] This newly coined disease was defined as "hyperadaptosis."[7] Hyperadaptosis implies excessive activity of adaptive system in response to stressors caused by age-dependent decrease in the sensitivity of controlling centers to feedback signals.

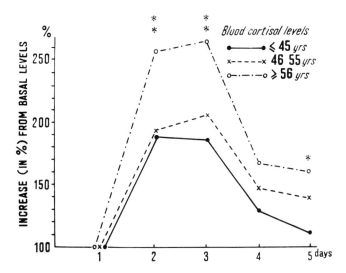

FIGURE 1. Influence of age of breast cancer patients on the blood cortisol level increment induced by operative stress. Difference is significant as compared with levels observed in patients younger than 45 yrs old: *$p < 0.05$; **$p < 0.01$.

Hyperadaptosis formed in the course of normal aging might be responsible for many age-associated pathologies.[11,12] TABLE 3 shows that in gastric and colonic cancer resistance to dexamethasone inhibition is prognostically less favorable than dexamethasone sensitivity.

The mechanisms underlying hyperadaptosis are partially explained by age-related decrease in levels of biogenic amines, especially catecholamines, in the hypothalamus. Therefore, hyperadoptosis is a reversible phenomenon. Drugs which improve sensitivity to dexamethasone inhibition in patients with affective disorders are listed in TABLE 4. Mechanisms underlying hypothalamic disturbances in these disorders may differ from those of the age-dependent alterations in the adaptive system. However, administration of polypeptide pineal gland extract to old rats is followed by improvement in hypothalamo-pituitary complex sensitivity to prednisolone.[13]

Certainly a rise in blood glucocorticoid levels induced by age-dependent regu-

TABLE 3. The 5-Year Cumulative Survival Rates of Cancer Patients and Dexamethasone (DM) Inhibition (%)

Tumor Site DM-Inhibition	Cumulative Survival Rates (Years)			
	0–1	2–3	4–5	P
Stomach cancer (stage III)				
>48%	0.833	0.581	0.492	<0.001
<34%	0.727	0.545	0.218	
Colon cancer (stage III)				
>50%	1.000	0.646	0.600	<0.05
<50%	0.806	0.607	0.494	

TABLE 4. The Effect of Pharmacological Drugs on the Sensitivity of the Hypothalamo-Pituitary Axis to Dexamethasone Inhibition (in Patients with Affective Psychoses)

Drugs	Blood 11-HOCS Level ($\mu g\%$)					
	Before Treatment		Inhibition (%)	After Treatment		Inhibition (%)
Diazepam	23.4 ± 2.1	20.1 ± 2.3	−14 ± 12	16.4 ± 1.8	6.7 ± 1.1	−59 ± 4
Phentolamine	13.3 ± 0.5	8.9 ± 10	−33 ± 1	12.4 ± 1.1	5.5 ± 0.3	−56 ± 0.3
L-Tryptophan	19.6 ± 2.0	16.1 ± 1.2	−18 ± 7	21.7 ± 2.3	10.5 ± 2.0	−52 ± 7
Levodopa	20.9 ± 2.8	15.8 ± 1.3	−24 ± 7	20.1 ± 3.0	5.9 ± 0.9	−71 ± 13
Bromocriptine	16.5 ± 2.0	13.8 ± 0.7	−16 ± 7	20.5 ± 5.5	8.0 ± 2.0	−61 ± 13
Phenformin	17.9 ± 4.9	11.6 ± 0.7	−35 ± 10	14.1 ± 1.2	4.4 ± 0.3	−69 ± 4

latory hypothalamic disorders exerts additional damage to regulatory, particularly hippocampal systems.[11,12] This mechanism is relevant to the interaction between ontogenetic and accumulative models of aging (see below).

Age-Dependent Alterations in the Energy System

The energy system of the body undergoes specific changes with age: low tolerance to glucose and, therefore, high postprandial blood insulin levels, increased utilization of free fatty acids as the energy substance, and high cholesterol and triglyceride concentrations in the blood which are typical for the aging pattern.

Hypothalamus-growth hormone-glucose system dysfunction might be one of the factors responsible for age-dependent metabolic shifts. TABLE 5 shows that in young persons (mean age 29 ± 1 yrs), distinct decrease in growth hormone levels are observed at 60 minutes following glucose loading whereas in the middle-aged subjects (mean age 53.4 ± 1.2 yrs) growth hormone secretion controlling systems are resistant to inhibition by glucose. The dysfunction is even more apparent in breast and endometrial cancer patients. In such patients, a pattern of delayed hyperinsulinemia after glucose loading is observed. It is common knowledge that age-dependent hyperinsulinemia plays an essential role in the pathogenesis of major diseases.

Let us consider some issues concerning two newly coined major diseases—metabolic immunodepression and cancrophilia, since hyperinsulinemia plays the key role in the pathogenesis of these diseases.

Metabolic Immunodepression

Metabolic immunodepression is defined as a decrease in cellular immunity and phagocytic function of monocyte-derived macrophages caused by certain disturbances of carbohydrate and lipid metabolism.[14] The following factors play key roles in the pathogenesis of metabolic immunodepression: high plasma membrane cholesterol concentration in T-lymphocytes; hyperinsulinemia resulting in reduction of insulin receptor concentration in T-lymphocytes and macrophages; increased utilization of free fatty acids, and, possibly, some other factors. In particular, the above-mentioned metabolic shifts inhibit growth hormone secretion and thyroid function.[7] However, growth and thyroid hormones are known to stimulate the immune system.[15,16] Metabolic shifts may exert an inhibitory effect on protein hormone production by activated T-lymphocytes which in turn, may lead to attenuation of hormonal signals activating the central neuroendocrine system. In addition, sensitivity of the controlling systems to hormonal signals may be lowered due to cholesterol accumulation in neurons[17] and age-dependent alterations in the adaptive system (see above). Metabolic factors obviously reduce natural killer cell activity as well.[18]

Metabolic immunodepression is a regular disease responsible for age-dependent increase in cancer incidence. Meanwhile, metabolic immunodepression developing in the course of aging is partially or completely reversible. Results obtained with the administration of an antidiabetic drug—phenformin—to ischemic heart disease patients support the role of age-dependent disturbances in carbohydrate and lipid metabolism in the pathogenesis of metabolic immunodepression.[7] Phenformin-induced improvement or normalization of metabolic indices was ac-

TABLE 5. Sensitivity to Glucose Loading of Hypotholamic Mechanisms Controlling Growth Hormone Secretion

	Blood Growth Hormone Level (ng/ml)		Blood Insulin Level 2 Hours After Glucose Load (μU/ml)
	Before Glucose Load	1 Hour After Glucose Load	
Healthy females (average age)			
29.1 ± 1 yrs	1.53 ± 026	0.99 ± 0.16	73.9 ± 20
53.4 ± 12 yrs	0.87 ± 0.26	0.83 ± 0.14	114 ± 12
Breast cancer patients			
(56 ± 2.8 yrs)	0.7 ± 0.2	1.7 ± 0.8	139 ± 76
Endometrial cancer patients			
(55.3 ± 1.3 yrs)	1.14 ± 0.4	1.5 ± 0.3	132 ± 5

companied by improvement or normalization of such parameters as blastogenic reaction of lymphocytes stimulated by mitogens, phagocytic activity of macrophages and skin tests to various antigens.[7,14]

Cancrophilia

The conditions promoting tumor development have been described above. One such condition is an increase in the pool of dividing cells. Regulation of cell division is known to be controlled by signals generated by hormones and growth factors. Such metabolic factors, as, for instance, elevated blood cholesterol concentration may also play an essential role in maintaining division of nonlymphoid cells.[7] Particularly, low density lipoproteins activate protein-kinase C,[19] the event playing an essential role in cancer promotion. In this respect, it is noteworthy that patients with familial polyposis and colon cancer show elevated cholesterol excretion.

Studies conducted in our laboratory showed enhanced blood somatomedin-like activity (as assessed biologically) in patients with obesity, diabetes mellitus, atherosclerosis and cancer (TABLE 6). Besides, our data showed a negative correlation between serum cholesterol level and the ability of lymphocytes to repair DNA damage caused by ultraviolet light.[19a]

Therefore, if metabolic factors which induce metabolic immunodepression and thus inhibit antitumor immunity, (and, possibly inhibit activity of DNA repair system) and those stimulating nonlymphoid cell division, *i.e.*, creating conditions promoting cancer development are the same, then a syndrome of cancrophilia may be coined.[7,14] Cancrophilia, as a disease, develops in the course of normal aging, whereas, as a pathological syndrome, it may be induced by certain ecological factors, for example, overeating. The above-mentioned data may explain why such diseases as diabetes mellitus type II, essential hypertension, *i.e.*, diseases which involve hyperinsulinemia as an essential factor of pathogenesis, are risk factors of cancer development. Some examples of coexistence of cancrophilia and cancer are worth discussion.

Cancrophilia and Cancer

Endometrial Carcinoma

Attention has long been paid to the triad of diseases often observed in endometrial carcinoma patients: obesity, diabetes mellitus and hypertension. Presence of this triad was first regarded as a sign of pituitary gland hyperfunction. Combination of these diseases was subsequently attributed to hypothalamic dysfunction.[20] Investigations performed in our laboratory identified a high frequency of metabolic and hormonal disturbances in endometrial cancer patients (TABLE 7). These disturbances may promote endometrial carcinoma development. It is noteworthy that high body weight at birth is a sign of latent diabetic-like metabolic disturbance which may occur 15–25 years prior to development of detectable tumor.[21]

Our study identified the hypothalamic type of endometrial carcinoma.[20] On the contrary, patients suffering type II endometrial carcinoma lack the above symptoms. Type I (hypothalamic) carcinoma is characterized by a relatively high level of tumor differentiation, increased blood estradiol concentration (316.3 ± 54.9 pmol/l and 188.3 ± 41.4 pmol/l in type I and II cancer, respectively) and high sensitivity of tumor to therapy with progestins. Furthermore, positive correlation between postprandial hyperinsulinemia, on the one hand, and concentration of estrogens ($r = 0.36$) and progesterone ($r = 0.56$) receptors in the tumor tissue, on the other, was observed.

Therefore, it should be kept in mind that hormonal factors play the essential role in promoting tumor development, and may determine some peculiarities of tumor biology. For example, it is quite possible that in patients with hypothalamic type of endometrial carcinoma, hyperestrogenemia provides the conditions for increased probability of lesions of certain loci of the genome assuring both malignant transformation of cells and a high degree of tumor differentiation.

TABLE 6. Blood Somatomedin-Like Activity in Patients with Obesity, Diabetes Mellitus, Atherosclerosis and Cancer

Group	Age	Percent Overweight	Somatomedin-Like Activity (Units)
Healthy subject			
Women	44.1 ± 0.7	+10.2 ± 2.3	0.55 ± 0.06
Men	51.0 ± 3.4	+9.8 ± 4.5	0.65 ± 0.18
Obesity	44.0 ± 1.96	+36.7 ± 1.9	1.49 ± 0.36
Diabetes mellitus	60.0 ± 2.5	+13.3 ± 6.2	1.62 ± 0.32
Atherosclerosis (women)	49.7 ± 3.1	+27.1 ± 4.9	2.59 ± 0.87
Cancer			
Breast	49.8 ± 1.36	+20.0 ± 2.5	1.49 ± 0.29
Prostate	68.0 ± 1.47	+15.4 ± 1.7	1.17 ± 0.02
Stomach	51.2 ± 3.4	+2.24 ± 4.4	1.03 ± 0.19
Breast cancer			
Before phenformin treatment	52.0 ± 1.5	+27.2 ± 3.68	1.22 ± 0.18
After phenformin treatment	52.0 ± 1.5	+22.6 ± 3.8	0.54 ± 0.04

TABLE 7. Hormonal-Metabolic Patterns in Healthy Women and Endometrial Cancer Patients

Test	Normal Subject	Endometrial Carcinoma
1. Percent overweight	+17.9 ± 2.0	+40.2 ± 4
2. Birth of large baby (≥4.0 kg)	14.2 ± 2.9	42.6 ± 5.7
3. Glucose intolerance (%)	12	72
Free fatty acids (μEq/L)	693 + 26	915 + 57
4. Hypercholesterolemia (%)	18	64.1
5. Blood 11-hydroxycorticosteroid level (mcg/%)		
Before DM-test	12.7 + 1.1	16.0 + 1.7
After DM-test	7.5 + 0.9	10.7 + 0.8
6. Blood growth hormone level (ng/ml)		
Before glucose load	2.4 + 0.5*	1.4 + 0.3
After glucose load	1.2 + 0.1*	1.4 + 0.3

* Data for the 20–35-year-old age bracket.

Colon Cancer

Endocrine-metabolic disorders are frequently observed in patients with colon cancer (TABLE 8). Particularly, we identified a considerable decrease in the sensitivity to insulin in these patients.[22] Changes in carbohydrate and lipid metabolism (hyperlipidemia or overweight) are accompanied by an increase in blood insulin, glucagon and gastrin levels. Colon cancer tissue revealed high levels of free cholesterol.[23] These data allow us to distinguish two types of colon cancer: (I) hormone-dependent and (II) hormone-independent. Relatively frequent coexistence of colon cancer and breast or endometrial cancer is characteristic for type I colon cancer. It should be especially emphasized that in hyperlipidemic colon cancer patients, metabolic rehabilitation measures (diet, and antidiabetic biguanides) taken after radical treatment were followed by a decrease in the frequency of tumor dissemination and recurrence within 5 years of follow-up.[24]

It must be stressed that longitudinal investigations to identify risk factors for

TABLE 8. Hormonal-Metabolic Patterns in Healthy Subjects and in Patients Suffering from Cancer of the Colon or Rectum

Test	Healthy Subject	Colon Cancer	Rectal Cancer
Birth of large baby (≥4.0 kg)	18.1 ± 1.8%	39.5 ± 7.5%	35.8 ± 5.3%
Blood 11-hydroxy-corticosteroid level (μg/%)			
Before DM-test	13.4 ± 0.19	16.7 ± 1.2	15.8 ± 0.6
After DM-test	4.9 ± 0.6	11.3 ± 0.8	9.8 ± 0.2
Blood triglyceride level (mg/%)	99 ± 3	128 ± 6	121 ± 5

ischemic heart disease usually showed a high frequency of colon cancer in males having considerably decreased blood cholesterol levels. It has been a point of concern that measures aimed at reduction of blood cholesterol level to normal in order to prevent ischemic heart disease might promote colon cancer. However, I feel that this apprehension is unjustified. Observation of abnormally low blood cholesterol levels at the age of 40–60 years is suggestive of a genetic defect because, at this time, age-associated hypercholesterolemia is usually seen.[7,25] Consequently, it may be supposed that such genetic defect is accompanied by other genetic defects (for instance, excessive cholesterol excretion by intestines or hereditary decrease in the immunity) which promote colon cancer. In the course of follow-up these subjects develop cancer more often than those with normal lipid metabolism. However, the frequency of colon cancer arising in this "defective" subpopulation is relatively low. TABLE 9 shows that in primary patients admitted to an oncological hospital (representing a general population), blood cholesterol levels are only slightly decreased. (However, this may be partially explained by increased cholesterol utilization by tumor.)

In the light of the existence of ontogenetic, genetic, accumulative and ecological pathogenic factors it is necessary to look at the interrelation between mechanisms of aging, major diseases and cancer.

TABLE 9. Blood-Cholesterol Level in Healthy Subjects and Patients Suffering from Colon Cancer

Group	Age (Years)	Blood-Cholesterol (mg%)
Healthy subject (n = 47)	58.1	241 ± 5
Cancer (total group) (n = 171)	57.1	234 ± 1
Subgroup with low blood cholesterol (n = 7)	64 + 2	156 ± 4

Four Models of Pathogenesis of Major Diseases and Aging

Let us go back to TABLE 1. Diseases which belong to the same class of major noninfectious diseases are formed by four different models of pathogenesis. However, only the ontogenetic model allows us to explain pathogenetic interrelationships between these diseases.[25] For example, a decrease in the concentration of biogenic amines in the hypothalamus, which is the major component of the mechanism of age-dependent switching-off of the reproductive function, simultaneously plays the key role in the mechanism of hyperadaptosis and age-dependent mental depression. Of great interest along with this, are the interrelations between different models, primarily, between accumulative and ontogenetic models of aging and disease. In this respect, it should be considered that regulatory shifts relevant to the ontogenetic model may be formed due to stochastic processes related to the accumulative model.[25a] In particular, the action of estrogens on the catecholaminergetic hypothalamic neurons of sex centers involves generation of potentially destructive free radicals. There are data showing that damage to these neurons plays a role in the mechanism of decreasing sensitivity of the hypothalamic sex center to feedback signals.[27,28] Similar data are available for glucocorticoids, which (as it was demonstrated in rodents) produce damage specifically to the hippocampal neurons of the brain.[11,12] Perhaps such damage creates a mechanism of age-associated increase in the adaptive system capacity in ontogeny and prolongation of stress reactions in the old organism (see above). Therefore, measures counteracting the accumulation of lesions, for example, antioxidants, should be used to prevent disorders developing within the framework of the ontogenetic model (see below).

Naturally, a question arises as to why systems hindering the accumulation of damage, the so-called antibiosenescence mechanisms according to Cutler,[27] such as antioxidant systems, have not become (in the course of evolution) effective enough to prevent the accumulation of lesions. I believe that such improvement (in the course of evolution) could not be the case, since maximum life span is restricted by events occurring in the ontogenetic model of aging and diseases. Thus, the presence of ontogenetic mechanisms of aging, disease and natural death would not give any advantages in natural selection to organisms possessing perfect defense systems. That is why measures intended to slow down the rate of aging and decrease the rate of age-dependent increase in cancer incidence must be directed to the ontogenetic and accumulative mechanisms of major disease formation.

Some Approaches to Aging Retardation and Cancer Prevention

As has been noticed above, traditional medicine considers aging and disease as different phenomena in terms of origin. However, mechanisms underlying both aging and regular diseases have been described within the framework of the ontogenetic model.[7,25] In the light of this model, pathogenesis of major diseases should be viewed as the by-product of realization of genetic developmental program. For this reason major diseases, while not genetically programmed, develop at varying speed in every individual if the developmental program is normally realized. The speed of disease formation, according to the ontogenetic model, depends consequently on the speed of aging of an individual. Therefore, the search for means for retarding the rate of aging is of crucial importance for the prevention of major diseases, cancrophilia included.[7,20,25] Several key elements in the mechanisms of the ontogenetic model of aging must be primarily influenced.

Hypothalamic (Neuroendocrine) Element of the Ontogenetic Model

Initially, the neuroendocrine theory of aging was presented as a hypothalamic theory.[3,20] At that time, my concept was described in physiological terms, namely, as elevation of the threshold of hypothalamic sensitivity to feedback signals without any specification of actual mechanisms responsible for the realization of this phenomenon. Later, from a biochemical viewpoint, this phenomenon was described as a neurotransmitter mechanism of aging,[28] as the receptor mechanism of aging,[29] as a neuroendocrine "clock" theory,[30] etc. Meanwhile, as the primary theory was developing, it was transformed into an ontogenetic theory, with the law of deviation from homeostasis as the main postulate.[7] This specifically implied that mechanisms of this phenomenon realization are present not only in the hypothalamus but in any other structures mediating hormonal-metabolic shifts required for the genetic program of development to operate. Correspondingly our choice in search of various ways and means for affecting aging and related diseases became wider.

Three important tasks are presented for future studies: 1. The role of increase in hypothalamo-pituitary complex sensitivity to feedback signals; 2. The effect of removal of compensatory hyperinsulinemia (in response to decrease in carbohydrate tolerance); and 3. The effect of a decrease in glucocorticoid production by adrenal glands.

Correspondingly, bearing in mind the first task, it has been proposed to use pineal gland hormones.[3] As has been shown further, the polypeptide extract of the pineal gland increases hypothalamo-pituitary system sensitivity to glucocorticoids[13] and estrogens[7] and, correspondingly, in rodents it increases life span and decreases the frequency of cancer development.[31,32]

At present, interesting data concerning various properties of melatonin are available. This hormone possesses geroprotective antitumor, antistressor and immunomodulating properties.[33,34]

It is therefore crucial to ascertain whether melatonin increases hypothalamo-pituitary complex sensitivity to feedback signals. The means influencing in such a way, must naturally possess a wide spectrum of therapeutic activity. For instance, polypeptide extract of the pineal gland, according to the data of our laboratory, improves glucose utilization, increases sensitivity to insulin, and decreases blood insulin and triglyceride concentration.[35] Thus, the search for some definite class of geroprotectors should be based on the evaluation of their influence upon the threshold of sensitivity of hypothalamo-pituitary system to regulatory signals. In particular, levodopa increases this system sensitivity to feedback signals[7] and increases rodents' life span.[36] It is the future's task to clarify whether dehydroepiandrosterone increases hypothalamus sensitivity to regulatory signals since many effects of this hormone and pineal gland hormones coincide.

Metabolic Component of the Ontogenetic Model

It is known nowadays that hyperinsulinemia is a pathogenetic factor of obesity, type II diabetes mellitus, metabolic immunodepression, atherosclerosis, cancrophilia, essential hypertension and ontogenetic mechanism of aging. More than 20 years ago I proposed to use phenformin, an antidiabetic drug increasing tissue sensitivity to insulin and therapy decreasing blood insulin and cholesterol concentration—to prevent atherosclerosis and cancer.[3,20] Indeed, phenformin administration decreases cancer incidence and increases mice's and rats' life span[25,37] (TABLE 10). Besides, phenformin eliminates age-associated metabolic immunodepression.[14] In this respect, it is necessary to stress that Fabris *et al.*[38] have shown that somatotropin and thyroxine treatment restore structure and function of murine thymus gland which has undergone age-dependent involution. Therefore, the question arises as to the possibility of reaching such an effect via elimination of metabolic disturbances. Probably, phenformin (or other drugs decreasing blood insulin level) may be effective for essential hypertension treatment. The spectrum of phenformin normalizing action may turn out to be even wider. In general, one may assume that any means improving glucose utilization and thereby decreasing fatty acids utilization as fuel can retard the rate of aging and counteract the age-dependent increase in cancer incidence. It should be emphasized that phenformin increases hypothalamo-pituitary complex sensitivity to the inhibiting action of glucocorticoids (TABLE 4) and estrogens.[7] For this reason, it cannot be excluded that the combination of the two properties of phenformin—"hypothalamic" and "metabolic"—determines the expressiveness of its geroprotecting and tumor-preventing influence. Rational restriction of food intake in many cases has the same influence as phenformin treatment, though the influence of calorie restriction on the hypothalamic system has not been sufficiently studied.

Adrenal Gland Component of the Ontogenetic Model

The effect of glucocorticoids on the body is increased in the course of aging (see above). In this respect, it is of interest that phenformin somehow improves the given situation as can be seen in the results of the dexamethasone suppression test (TABLE 11). One can see that phenformin treatment leads to a decrease in glucocorticoids' metabolites excretion and an increase in adrogen-like hormones' metabolites excretion. Taking into account these data one may suppose that an age-dependent decrease of dehydroepiandrosterone production by adrenal glands[39] may be counteracted by a decrease in insulin levels.

Taking into consideration the pathogenetic role of excessive glucocorticoids in the organism I have proposed to use in clinical oncology an antiepileptic drug diphenylhydantoin, which decreases glucocorticoids and insulin production.[40] As shown in TABLE 10 diphenylhydantoin (dilantin) decreases the frequency of tumor development and increases life span in mice.[37]

Summing up the above data it should be concluded that drugs such as phenformin, pineal gland hormones and dilantin may influence the conditions promoting age-dependent increase of cancer incidence, i.e., they may be used for prevention of cancer emergence, but it is doubtful whether they may act directly as antitumor drugs. This conclusion also relates to such influences as food restriction and drugs such as dehydroepiandrosterone which may, however, decrease the frequency of cancer incidence.[41] All these means may turn out to be useful for the prevention (via improvement of metabolic and hormonal parameters) of recurrence and metastases after radical treatment. At the same time, all these means may slow down the rate of aging and, correspondingly, the speed of development of major diseases. In this respect it is important to stress that ontogenetic and accumulative mechanisms determine the pattern of normal aging and, correspondingly, the value of species-specific life span, whereas ecological and genetic factors determine the speed of aging and the speed of the formation of major diseases, that is,

TABLE 10. The Effect of Phenformin and Dilantin Treatment on the Life Span and Tumor Incidence in Female C3H Mice[37]

	Control (N = 30)	Phenformin (N = 25)	Dilantin (N = 23)
Mean life span (days)	450 ± 19	555 ± 32*	558 ± 28*
No. of tumor-bearing mice	24(80%)	5(20%)*	8(34.8%)*
Mammary gland adenocarcinoma			
No. of mice	19(63%)	4(16%)*	7(30.4%)*
Total No. of tumors	30	4	7
Mammary tumors per animal	1.58	1.00	1.00
Leukemia			
No. of mice	4(13.3%)	1(4%)	2(8.7%)
Other tumors	5	1	0

* Difference is significant as compared with control group.

TABLE 11. The Influence of Phenformin Treatment on Excretion of 17-Hydroxycorticosteroids (17-HOCS) and 17-Ketosteroids in Patients with Atherosclerosis Before and After Dexamethasone Test (DM-Test)

Parameter	Before Treatment	3 Months After Treatment
17-HOCS (mg/g creatinine)		
Before DM-test	5.8 ± 1.1	4.6 ± 1.0
After DM-test	2.7 ± 0.5	1.7 ± 0.3
Inhibition (%)	−43 ± 21	−69 ± 5
17-ketosteroids (mg/g creatinine)		
Before DM-test	3.8 ± 0.3	5.9 ± 0.9
After DM-test	3.2 ± 0.4	2.8 ± 0.6
Inhibition (%)	−18 ± 12	−52 ± 8

the value of average life span. But, as it is known, modern medicine discusses only ecological and genetic mechanisms of major diseases development. Therefore, it is usually considered possible both to eliminate diseases (as random events) or to compress the period of time during which diseases may develop.[42] In this view it is expected that the termination of life of a long-lived individual will result in a majority of cases, either from physiological aging or from diseases appearing during a short period of time. However, my conception shows and warns that these fundamental positions of modern medicine are not correct, since there exist ontogenetic causes of major diseases. During longer life span due to the diminished pressure of unfavorable ecological and genetic pathogenic factors, the frequency of major diseases induced by ontogenetic and accumulative mechanisms will grow in the aged population. Therefore, I believe that prevention of major diseases, cancrophilia included, is impossible without intervention into the ontogenetic component of their mechanism. At the same time, interference with the ontogenetic and accumulative mechanisms of aging may result in the increase in the maximum life span since these characteristics are species-specific but not programmed, and are determined by the evolutionarily-developed speed of ontogenetic and accumulative processes realization in a given species.[43]

REFERENCES

1. PETO, R., F. J. C. ROE, P. N. LEE et al. 1975. Br. J. Cancer **32:** 418–426.
2. BURNET, F. M. 1970. Immunological Surveillance. Pergamon Press. Oxford.
3. DILMAN, V. M. 1971. Lancet. **1:** 1211–1219.
4. PETO, R., S. E. PARISH & R. G. GRAY. 1985. There is no such thing as ageing, and cancer is not related to it. In Age-Related Factors in Carcinogenesis. A. Likhachev, V. Anisimov & R. Montesano, Eds. **58:** 43–53. IARC Scientific Publ. No. 58. Lyon.
5. BULBROOK, R. D. 1972. J. Natl. Cancer Inst. **48:** 1039–1042.
6. STREHLER, B. L. 1981. In CRC Handbook of Immunology in Aging. M. Kay & T. Makinodan, Eds. CRC Press, Inc. Boca Raton, FL.
7. DILMAN, V. M. 1981. The Law of Deviation of Homeostasis and Diseases of Aging. H. T. Blumental, Ed. John Wright, PSG, Inc. Boston.
8. DILMAN, V. M. 1958. Trans. Inst. Physiol. Acad. Sci. USSR **7:**326–336.
9. MEITES, J., H. H. HUANG & E. W. SIMKINS. 1978. Recent studies on neuroendocrine

control of reproductive senescence in rats. *In* The Aging Reproductive System. E. L. Schneider, Ed. 213–235. Plenum Press. New York.

10. DILMAN, V. M. & M. N. OSTROUMOVA. 1984. Hypothalamic metabolic and immune mechanisms of the influence of stress on the tumor process. *In* Impact of Psychoendocrine System in Cancer and Immunity. B. Fox & B. Newberry, Eds. 58–87. C. J. Hogrefe, Inc. Lewinston.

11. LANDFIELD, P. W. 1987. Progr. Brain Res. **72:** 279–300.

12. SAPOLSKY, R. M., L. C. KREY & B. S. MCEWEN. 1986. Endocrine Rev. **7:** 284–301.

13. OSTROUMOVA, M. N. & V. M. DILMAN. 1972. Vopr. Onkol. **18:** 53–55.

14. DILMAN, V. M. 1978. Mech. Ageing Dev. **8:** 153–173.

15. PIERPAOLI, W., N. FABRIS & E. SORKIN. 1970. Ciba Found Symp. **36:** 126–143.

16. FABRIS, N., W. PIERPAOLI & E. SORKIN. 1972. Nature **240:** 557–559.

17. SHINITSKY, M. 1987. Gerontology **33:** 149–154.

18. PROVINCIALI, M., N. FABRIS & C. PIERI. Mech. Ageing Dev. In press.

19. BLOCK, L. H., M. KNORR & E. VOGT. 1988. Proc. Natl. Acad. Sci. USA **85:** 885–889.

19a. DILMAN, V. M. & YU . REVSKOY. 1981. Hum. Physiol. **7:**125–129.

20. DILMAN, V. M. 1968. Aging, Climacteric and Cancer. Meditsina. Leningrad.

21. BERSTEIN, L. M. 1988. Adv. Cancer Res. **50:** 231–273.

22. VASILJEVA, I. A. & V. M. DILMAN. 1973. Vopr. Onkol. **19:** 35–38.

23. BERSTEIN, L. M., YU. F. BOBROV, M. N. OSTROUMOVA, I. G. KOVALEVA, I. G. KOVALENKO, JE. V. TZYRLINA, JE. L. STRUKOV & V. M. DILMAN. 1988. Exp. Onkol. **10:** 38–41.

24. DILMAN, V. M., L. M. BERSTEIN & T. P. YEVTUSHENKO. 1988. Arch. Geschwulstforsch. **58:** 175–183.

25. DILMAN, V. M. 1987. Four Models of Medicine. Meditsina. Leningrad. Translated by Gordon and Breach Science Publishers, Inc. 1991. New York.

25a. DILMAN, V. U. 1984. Med. Hypotheses. **15:** 185–208.

26. FINCH, C. E., L. S. FELICIO, C. V. MOBBS & J. F. NELSON. 1984. Endocr. Rev. **5:** 467–497.

27. CUTLER, R. G. 1984. Evolutionary biology of aging and longevity in mammalian species. *In* Aging and Cell Function. J. E. Johnson, Ed. **2:** 371–428. Plenum Press. New York.

28. FINCH, C. E. 1973. Brain Res. **52:** 261–276.

29. ROTH, G. S. & G. D. HESS. 1982. Mech. Ageing Dev. **20:** 175–194.

30. EVERITT, A. V. 1973. Exp. Gerontol. **8:** 265–277.

31. DILMAN, V. M., V. N. ANISIMOV, M. N. OSTROUMOVA, V. KH. KHAVINSON & V. G. MOROZOV. 1979. Exp. Path. **17:** 539–545.

32. DILMAN, V. M., V. N. ANISIMOV, M. N. ANISIMOVA, V. G. MOROZOV, V. KH. KHAVINSON & M. A. ASAROVA. 1979. Oncology **36:** 274–280.

33. MAESTRONI, G. J. N., A. CONTI & W. PIERPAOLI. 1988. Ann. N.Y. Acad. Sci. **521:** 140–148.

34. PIERPAOLI, W. & G. J. M. MAESTRONI. 1987. Immunol. Lett. **16:** 355–362.

35. VASILJEVA, I. A. & M. N. OSTROUMOVA. 1976. Probl. Endokrinol. **3:** 66–69.

36. COTZIAS, G. C., S. T. MILLER, A. R. NICHOLSON *et al.* 1974. Proc. Natl. Acad. Sci. USA **71:** 2466–2469.

37. DILMAN, V. M. & V. N. ANISIMOV. 1980. Gerontology. **26:** 241–246.

38. FABRIS, N., E. MOCCHEGIANI, M. MUZZIOLI & M. PROVINCIALI. 1988. Ann. N.Y. Acad. Sci. **521:** 72–87.

39. NESTLER, J. E., K. S. USISKIN, C. O. BARLASCINI, D. F. WELTY, J. N. CLORE & W. G. BLACKARD. 1989. J. Clin. Endocrinol. **69:** 1040–1046.

40. DILMAN, V. M., G. O. ELUBAJEVA, A. S. VISHNEVSKY *et al.* 1971. Vopr. Onkol. **17:** 70–72.

41. REGELSON, W., R. LORIA & M. KALIMI. 1988. Ann. N.Y. Acad. Sci. **521:** 260–273.

42. FRIES, J. F. 1980. N. Engl. J. Med. **303:** 130–135.

43. DILMAN, V. M. 1986. J. Theor. Biol. **118:** 73–81.

Genetic and Environmental Modulations of Chromosomal Stability: Their Roles in Aging and Oncogenesis

GEORGE M. MARTIN

Departments of Pathology and Genetics
University of Washington
Seattle, Washington 98195

INTRODUCTION AND DEFINITIONS

We shall define aging (or senescing) in terms of the discernible phenotype that slowly and insidiously unfolds beginning around the time of sexual maturity in iteroparous species (*i.e.,* species that undergo repeated bouts of reproduction). Thus, for purposes of this paper, the types of rearrangements of the long arms of chromosomes 7 and 14 that are prevalent in the peripheral T cells of newborns[4] might best be regarded as a feature of the phenotype of development and not of aging.

What is this senescent phenotype? At the population level, there is an exponential increase in the age-specific death rate (the Gompertz relationship);[5] the ages at which such increments begin and their rates of progress are characteristic for the species. At the organismal level, one observes a decline in the efficiencies of various types of homeostatic mechanisms, including the responses to extreme fluctuations in ambient temperatures[6,7] and various types of enzyme induction— for example, those related to the response to severe dietary restriction.[8] At the organ system level, numerous decrements of function have been documented;[9] in cross-sectional studies, these decrements are typically linear, but in longitudinal studies, considerable variations are observed from subject to subject.[10] Cellular alterations have included declines in the proliferative potentials of various cell types, regional cell loss, loss of nucleolar volume, and accumulations of lipofuscin pigments in secondary lysosomes within certain cell types.[11] At the molecular level, various posttranslational alterations of proteins appear to be particularly well documented, including those related to oxidative attack[12] and those resulting from glycation.[13] There is evidence of a general decline in both rates of protein synthesis and turnover that might underlie, in part, the increasing prevalence of such altered proteins.[14,15] Transcription at certain loci appears to be diminished[16] and there is some evidence of epigenetic alterations in gene expression,[17] or "epimutation."[18] Certain classes of somatic mutations accumulate in some tissues of some species,[19] including chromosomal mutations, the primary subject of this review. Chromosomal mutations may be defined as alterations in the primary nucleotide sequences and/or alterations in gene dosage that involve multiple contiguous genetic loci, often to an extent such that they may be visible with the light microscope. They thus differ from point mutations, which can be defined as intragenic mutations that are either transitions (the substitution of one pyrimidine by the other, or of one purine by the other), or transversions (the replacement of a pyrimidine by a purine or vice versa). The term mutagen can be used generically to describe any agent capable of producing any type of alteration in the primary sequence of nucleotides or in gene dosage. I shall use the term clastogen to refer to agents that can result in chromosomal breakage, with the production of a variety of both stable and unstable chromosmal aberrations (see below). I shall differentiate such agents from aneugens, which can be defined as agents that increase the frequencies of aneuploid cells—*i.e.,* cells with chromosome numbers other than multiples of the haploid karyotype (1n, 2n, 3n, 4n, etc.). This leaves open a nomenclature for agents that produce increased frequencies of polyploidy or of endoreduplication.

The term "gerontogens" was introduced to describe hypothetical agents that could accelerate the times of onset and/or the rates of progression of particular aging processes.[11] Since there is as yet no proof of any single mechanism of aging, we can only think in terms of candidate gerontogens. Obviously, mutagens, including clastogens and aneugens might be such candidates.

The increasing probability of organismal death is accompanied by increasing prevalence of a wide variety of degenerative and proliferative disorders, including a number of neoplasms.[20] The oncogenetic process is believed to evolve via a series of discrete steps leading to increasing degrees of loss of the physiological controls of mitotic cell cycle function in both the primary and secondary (metastatic) microenvironments. This loss of "proliferative homeostasis"[21] may result in tissue atrophy as well as hyperplasia and neoplasia.

Evidence for a Tight Coupling of Abnormalities in Proliferative Homeostasis with Intrinsic Biological Aging

Before discussing evidence linking intrinsic aging with aberrations in proliferative homeostasis, it is useful to review some major arguments that have been raised against this proposition, in particular, the arguments of those who believe that the biology of cancer may be unrelated to intrinsic biological aging. A common theme in such arguments is that, while the prevalence of most cancers does indeed increase during the second half of an animal's life span, a systematic, continued rate of increase, paralleling that of the mortality rate, is observed for only occasional types of cancers.[2,3] This is a fallacious argument, in my opinion. There is no necessity that the kinetics of mortality, a *population* parameter, need necessarily parallel the kinetics of an intrinsic aging process occurring at the *organismal, organ system, tissue, cell and molecular* levels. A good example is the loss of visual accommodation, which is likely due primarily to posttranslational alterations in lens proteins.[22] For the case of human subjects, essentially all individuals will have lost the ability to accommodate by around age 60, with a rapid decline between the ages of 20 and 40.[23] Another example is the loss of reproductive fitness in the human female; a major contributor to this phenotype is a dramatic loss of ovarian primordial follicles, a process that is essentially complete by the early forties.[24]

A second argument is based upon the view that intrinsic aging must be genetically programmed: ("Cancer does not appear to be the inevitable consequence of aging, that is a preprogrammed genetic time bomb ticking away just waiting to go off.")[1] This argument is fallacious as there is no genetic or biochemical evidence that aging results from systematic, determinative switches in gene expression analogous to what happens during development. Moreover, there are persuasive evolutionary arguments against the notion that aging evolved adaptively.[25] Stochastic events clearly are part of the aging processes, as evidenced, for example, by the fact that genetically inbred strains of animals exhibit survival curves very similar to those of randomly bred genetically heterogeneous stocks.

A third commonly cited argument derives from the careful experiments of Peto et al.,[26] in which a course of local chemical carcinogen (benzpyrene) treatments was applied to the skin of mice of various ages (10–55 weeks). The cancer incidence rates increased as a power of the duration of exposure to the carcinogen and did not depend upon the age at which the treatments were commenced. It was thus concluded that age per se was irrelevant, carcinogenesis occurring merely as a result of calendar time. In the discussion of this same paper, however, reference was made to the intrinsic mutagenesis hypothesis of aging,[27] and it was noted that somatic mutation might be a common mechanism underlying both aging and carcinogenesis: "This postulated common cause for ageing rates and for cancer incidence rates might be the reason why most species suffer some cancer of old age, whether old age occurs at 80 weeks or 80 years, even though ageing itself does not affect oncogenesis." Thus, even Peto et al.[26] apparently agree that, given the striking species specificity of age of onset of neoplasia, that phenotype could be a biomarker of an underlying aging process or processes.

The species specificity referred to above is, of course, the most compelling evidence of the coupling of neoplasia with intrinsic biological aging. While we need much more detailed information from our colleagues in veterinary pathology (geriatric pathology has been comparatively neglected), a generalization is emerging that a number of different neoplasms begin to appear with high frequencies about halfway through the maximum life span of a variety of mammalian species: e.g., circa 2 years for *Mus musculus domesticus;*[28] circa 4 years for *Peromyscus leucopus* (REF. 29 and Sacher, personal communication); circa 7–12 years for canine species;[30–32] circa 55 years for man. (See also review in REF. 33.)

In addition to benign and malignant neoplasms, a variety of hyperplasias, typically multifocal, are prevalent during the latter half of the life span of mammals. A partial tabulation is given in TABLE 1 (modified from Martin).[21] It is of interest that these lesions often develop within a region of atrophic tissue (*e.g.,* leukoplakia and endometrial hyperplasia) or develop along with degenerative types of pathology (*e.g.,* atherosclerosis and osteoarthritis).

Classification of Chromosomal Mutations

TABLE 2 provides a brief functional classification of chromosomal mutations as they occur in somatic cells. There are essentially three types of consequences. The most frequent chromosomal lesions lead to one or more alterations in gene dosage. For the case of such lesions as unbalanced translocations, this can include both an increase in gene dosage for a subset of loci and a decrease of gene dosage for another subset of loci. Haploidy and nulliploidy are rare, although the latter occurs physiologically during the terminal differentiation of erythropoietic cells in mammals. Various types of aneuploidy are commonly observed in our species, as are a variety of chromosomal lesions leading to deletions, a number of which are lethal events at the cellular level. Spontaneous amplification of segments of DNA is commonly observed in cell cultures and also occurs *in vivo* in a variety of organisms, including man, where it can be one mechanism for resistance to chemotherapeutic agents.[34] Amplification of genomic units of infectious protozoa may also account for some forms of drug resistance.[35]

The second major functional effect of a chromosomal mutation may be the

TABLE 1. Examples of Multifocal Hyperplasias Which Accompany Senescence in Humans or Other Mammals

Cell Type Which Proliferates	Associated Age-Related Disorder
Adipocyte	regional obesity
Arterial myointimal cell	atherosclerosis
Cartilage osteocyte and synovial cells	osteoarthrosis (osteoarthritis)
Central nervous system astrocyte	gliosis
Epidermal basal cell	verruca senilis (seborrheic keratosis) (basal cell papilloma)
Epidermal melanocyte	senile lentigo ("liver spots")
Epidermal squamous cell	senile keratosis
Fibroblast	interstitital fibrosis (multiple tissues; ex., thyroid)
Fibromuscular stromal cell and glandular epithelium of prostate	nodular hyperplasia (benign prostatic hypertrophy)
Lymphocyte	ectopic lymphoid tissue
Lymphocyte (suppressor T cell)	immunologic deficiency
Oral mucosal squamous cell	leukoplakia
Ovarian cortical stromal cell	cortical stromal hyperplasia
Endometrial glandular epithelium	postmenopausal hyperplasia
Pancreatic ductal epithelial cell	ductal epithelial hyperplasia and metasplasia
Sebaceous glandular epithelium	senile sebaceous hyperplasia (skin) fordyce disease (oral mucosa)

[a]Adapted from Martin, 1979.[21]

expression of new genetic information. This can occur as a result of a reciprocal translocation, with the emergence of a new gene product, as has been documented for the case of the rearrangement involving the breakage cluster region of the long arm of chromosome 22 and the Abelson oncogene of the long arm of chromosome 9.[36] This rearrangement generates a novel fusion protein with a greatly increased tyrosine, kinase activity as compared to the normal Abelson gene product.[36,37] Mitotic recombinational events may also result in the appearance of new genetic information, as somatic crossing over can produce haplotypes not found in the constitutional genotype.

A third mechanism involves a position effect, whereby, as a result of a translocation or inversion or insertion, a gene or genes may be either downregulated (for example, because of their presence in a domain of constitutive heterochromatin) or upregulated (for example, because of a juxtaposition to a strong promoter).

Role of Chromosomal Mutations in Oncogenesis

A thorough review of this subject is, of course, beyond the scope of this paper. In recent years there has been an explosion of information vindicating the pioneering vision of Theodor Boveri regarding the seminal role of chromosomal mutations in the genesis of neoplasms.[38] It is now clear that many different types of nonrandom lesions are associated with specific neoplasms, both benign and malignant.[39] Typically, there is a sequence of lesions, each clonally selected, resulting in greater and greater degrees of escape from mitotic controls. An excellent example is the cytogenetic evolution of chronic myelogenous leukemia.[39] As indicated in the previous section, these phenotypic changes result from either alterations in gene dosage or the expression of new types of genetic information. For the case of recessive tumor suppressor genes, monosomy, deletion or recombination can lead to phenotypic expression.[40] For the case of dominant oncogenes, a position effect can result in activation, as noted above.[36]

Constitutional Genetic Determinants of Chromosomal Stability: Role in Oncogenesis and Gerotogenesis

Ongoing cytogenetic observations in our laboratory and in a number of other laboratories have expanded upon the pioneering work of the late Howard Curtis and his colleagues.[41–43] FIGURE 1 is a summary of much of that early work from the Curtis lab. Using squash preparations of regenerating livers of animals of varying ages and species of contrasting maximal life-span potentials, they showed, with a limited number of species, a correlation between the degree of chromosomal stability and life span. We have confirmed a remarkable degree of chromosomal instability in *Mus musculus domesticus* in first metaphases of cells from several tissues (Martin *et al.,* REF. 44 and unpublished). Using identical methods and homologous cell types, human and canine cells exhibit strikingly fewer lesions as they age. In contrast, we found little evidence for an increase in the frequencies of point mutations with age in *Mus musculus domesticus,* at least for the case of the HPRT locus.[45] Such point mutations do appear to increase in the cells of aging dogs (Martin *et al.,* unpublished observations) and man (REF. 46 and Martin *et al.,* unpublished observations), although it remains to be seen to

TABLE 2. Functional Classification of Somatic Chromosomal Mutations

I.	Alterations in gene dosage			
	A.	Changes in ploidy		
		1.	Nulliploidy	
		2.	Haploidy	
		3.	Polyploidy	
			a.	Triploidy
			b.	Tetraploidy
			c.	Octaploidy
	B.	Aneuploidy		
		1.	Nullisomy	
		2.	Monosomy	
		3.	Polysomy	
			a.	Trisomy
			b.	Tetrasomy
			c.	Pentasomy
	C.	Deletion (partial monosomy)		
	D.	Duplication (partial trisomy)		
	E.	DNA amplification		
II.	Expression of new genetic information			
	A.	Fusion gene products via translocation or inversion		
	B.	New haplotypes via mitotic recombination		
III.	Position effects			
	A.	Downregulation		
	B.	Upregulation		

what extent this is substantially related to chronological time as opposed to intrinsic biological aging.

At the intraspecific level of analysis, there are a number of constitutional mutations in man that result in chromosomal instability syndromes.[47,48] The phenotype includes a marked increase in the susceptibility to neoplasia, sometimes even in the heterozygotes, for the case of ataxia telangiectasia[49] and, possibly, Werner's syndrome.[50] Certain of these disorders can also be classified as "segmental progeroid syndromes," since the phenotype includes aspects that might be interpretable as evidence of the premature onset and/or the accelerated progress of aspects of aging.[51]

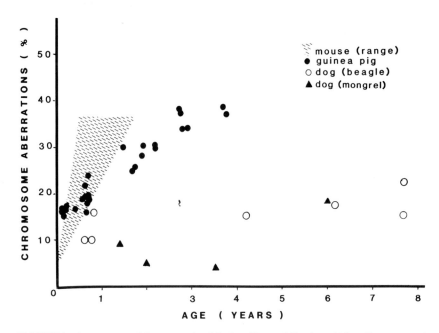

FIGURE 1. A summary of the research of the late Howard Curtis and his colleagues on the frequencies of chromosomal aberrations scored in squash preparations of the regenerating livers of mice, guinea pigs and dogs. For experimental details, consult References 41 and 42 and the references cited therein.

We have been investigating one such segmental progeroid syndrome in some detail. It is known variously as Werner's syndrome or as Progeria of the Adult. A major segment of the literature on this subject has been conveniently summarized in a monograph, which includes an English translation of the original doctoral thesis of Otto Werner and reprints of several seminal review articles.[52] A particularly useful review, not included in that monograph, is by Tollefsbol and Cohen.[53]

Patients with Werner's syndrome are normal at birth. The parents (who are typically consanguineous, as the disorder is a rare autosomal recessive) first seek the attention of a physician at around the time of adolescence, when it becomes evident that the patient is not enjoying the usual pubertal growth spurt. As a consequence, there is a very short adult stature. There then ensues premature greying and thinning of the hair, atrophic, hyperkeratotic and pigmentary changes in the skin, regional subcutaneous atrophy (stocky trunk with thin limbs), ocular cataracts, muscular weakness, a high-pitched squeaky or weak voice, diabetes mellitus, osteoporosis, various types of arteriosclerosis, including coronary atherosclerosis (the usual cause of death at a median age of 47 years) and a striking variety of neoplasms (the second most common cause of death), including many mesenchymal neoplasms and a number of benign as well as malignant tumors. Meningiomas and thyroid neoplasms may be particularly common.[54] Among Japanese, heterozygotic carriers, who are otherwise normal, may be subject to a higher prevalence of neoplasms.[50]

Cultured somatic cells from subjects with Werner's syndrome exhibit a striking limitation of their replicative life spans.[55] Cytogenetic analysis of these cells reveals a variety of translocations, deletions and inversions ("variegated translocation mosaicism").[56,57] There may be "hot spots" within the genome where chromosomal breaks are relatively common.[57]

This propensity to undergo chromosomal types of mutation is also evident at the single gene level. Even with the relatively crude methodology of Southern blotting, some 76% of all spontaneous forward mutations at the HPRT locus were found to have resulted from relatively large deletions, sometimes eliminating the entire gene and sometimes large segments within the gene.[58] That such aberrations may be occurring *in vivo* is supported by several lines of evidence, including cytogenetic studies[59] and autoradiographic studies of presumptive HPRT-deficient cells in fresh peripheral blood lymphocytes; the frequencies of such cells are some 8 times higher than those observed in lymphocytes from control subjects.[60]

Thus, in this experiment of nature, we see a striking correlation between chromosomal instability, oncogenesis and a number of aspects of gerontogenesis.

Environmental Chemical Clastogens and Aneugens

The indirect lines of evidence we have reviewed that are suggestive of a coupling between chromosomal instability, cancer and aging raise the question of the potential importance of environmental agents that break chromosomes (clastogens) or that result in a decrease in the fidelity of the transmission of chromosomes during mitosis (aneugens); such agents could be candidate "gerontogens."

In a comprehensive review of the literature on the cytogenetic effects of 851 chemical substances, covering the period between 1964–1985, Ishidate et al.[61] have noted that numerical aberrations can be induced with or without structural abnormalities. Many of the reviewed studies, however, did not rigorously investigate both phenotypes; our knowledge is thus quite incomplete for many classes of chemicals. It is clear, however, that some substances are predominately aneugens (e.g., vincristine and nocodazole) while others (e.g., ethylmethanesulfonate and cyclophosphamide) are predominately clastogens.[62]

The most potent clastogen so far detected is the alkylating agent, (2,3,5-Trisethyleniminobenzoquinone-1,4) (triaziquone) (Trenimon); for the case of Chinese hamster fibroblast cultures, significant clastogenicity appears at concentrations of about 10 picograms per ml.[63] An example of a relatively potent aneugen (at least for the case of a fungal assay) is chloracetaldehyde, thought to be the principal metabolite of the human and animal carcinogen, vinyl chloride; it is effective at concentrations as low as 16 μM.[64]

While there is a some correlation between potency in clastogenicity assays and in the Ames Salmonella reversion assay, the degree of correlation is poor when one discounts the data for weakly mutagenic agents that may have more global toxicity effects (FIG. 2).[61] Thus, it will be useful, for future work, to continue to pursue a variety of genotoxic assays for suspect compounds.

Other Environmental Clastogens

Ionizing radiation is, of course, a classical clastogenic agent. It is thought to break DNA strands via a free radical mechanism (see below), the hydroxyl ion being a major contributor. Deletions, inversions and translocations are the predominant types of resulting somatic mutations. Its role in the genesis of the Philadelphia chromosome of chronic myelogenous leukemia is exceedingly well established via epidemiologic studies; the seminal importance of that lesion in pathogenesis was recently underscored via the genesis of transgenic, leukemic mice bearing the rearranged Abelson oncogene.[65] A recent reevaluation of the atom bomb dosimetry at Hiroshima and Nagasaki revealed that the lifetime risk of cancer attributable to a given dose of gamma radiation is somewhat larger than

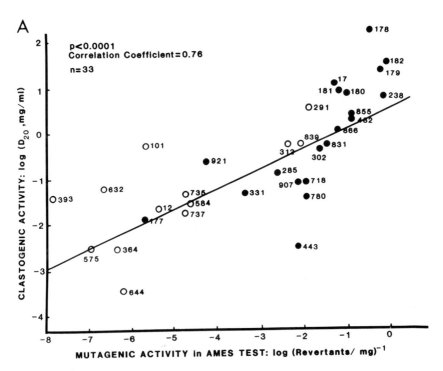

FIGURE 2. (A) Results of statistical regression analysis of the survey of Ishidate *et al.*[61] concerning the relationship between clastogenic and mutagenic activities of a range of chemical compounds. *Open circles* represent data derived by Ishidate and colleagues.

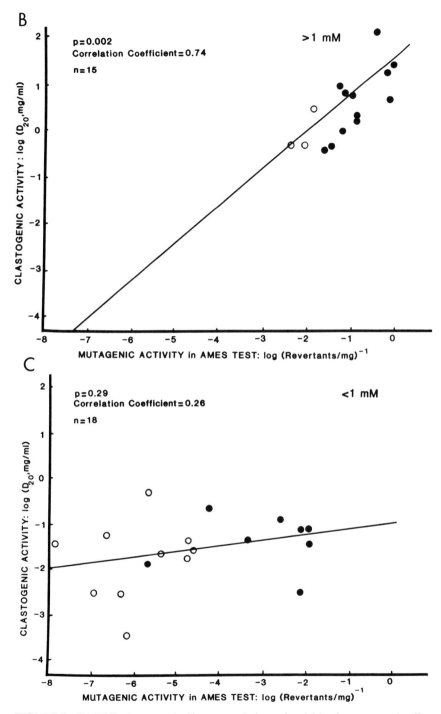

FIGURE 2. (B) While there are significant correlations of activities for compounds effective at comparatively high concentrations (>1 mM), **(C)** no correlation is evident for the subset of compounds for which activities were apparent at low concentrations (<1 mM).

formerly estimated;[66] consequently, we should be more concerned about the somatic effects of low level radiation.

Is ionizing radiation gerontogenic? There is a relatively large literature on this subject, with major reviewers concluding that it is not because the observations do not fit with the "Casarett rule."[67] This dictum states that, in order for an agent to be considered to accelerate aging, it must reproduce all of the phenotypic features associated with senescence and, moreover, in the same temporal sequence. Implicit in this view is the notion that aging is due to a single mechanism or process, something that is quite improbable on theoretical grounds.[68,69] Even dietary calories, the "agent" that comes closest to fulfilling the Casarett rule, does not modulate all aspects of the phenotype.[70]

The association of cytogenetic pathology with a variety of exogenous (as well as endogenous) viral agents is also well established.[71]

Pathogenetic Mechanisms

The cytogenetic pathology associated with aging and with cancer is diverse and presumably results from a variety of pathogenetic mechanisms. For example, one novel mechanism for the role of viral agents may be via a cell fusogen; resulting heterokaryons between cells in different stages of the mitotic cell cycle can result to the premature chromosome condensation or "pulverization."[72]

As already indicated, there are classes of chemical agents that act primarily as aneugens or that induce changes in ploidy. Some such agents act via alterations in the polymerization of microtubular proteins (*e.g.*, colchicine, vincritine, nocodazole). Similarly, there are genetic mutations that primarily affect the frequencies of aneuploidy via effects of microtubule stability.[73] It is conceivable that age-associated posttranslational modifications of spindle proteins and other centromere-associated proteins, together with an age-associated decline in protein turnover, may also be responsible, in part, for the age-associated increase in aneuploidy.

An area of current active research that may prove to be highly significant for our understanding of both age-associated aneuploidy and other types of chromosomal pathology has to do with the metabolism of telomeric DNA and other moieties of tandem, simple repeated DNA sequences (interstitial, pericentromeric; centromeric) that may be subject to recombinations, fusions and deletions.[74-77] An intriguing recent observation is the correlation between deletion of telomeric sequences and the decline in replicative potential of cultivated human somatic cells (widely regarded as an *in vitro* model for cellular aging).[78,79]

Derepression of one or more classes of mobile elements[80,81] could also play a role in the generation of age-related chromosomal abnormalities. There is considerable evidence of differential expression of such elements during development in some organisms.[80,82-84]

Segmental DNA amplification has been suggested as a mechanism for the generation of a great variety of chromosomal aberrations.[85] Its frequency may be on the order of one per thousand per DNA domain per cell generation in some cell lines.[86] It is conceivable that the interruptions and reinitiations of DNA synthesis demonstrated to be precursors of DNA amplification and chromosomal rearrangements[85] might be more common in older animals. DNA amplification appears to be far less common, however, in normal diploid human and rodent cell cultures.[87,88]

Most gerontologists would probably regard chemical free radicals (especially active oxygen species) as prime suspects for the alteration of both proteins[12] and DNA.[89,90] The free radical theory of aging[91] would invoke several classes of intrinsic, constitutional genetic differences among species as being primarily responsible for differing rates of aging and differing susceptibilities to age-related neoplasia. In TABLE 3, I have summarized the several subsets of relevant genetic loci, allelic variation at which might underlie such differences. These loci fall into seven groups: I) genes that modulate the degree to which free radicals are generated; II) genes that control the structure and, probably more significantly, the regulation of enzymes (such as catalase) that scavenge such free radicals; III) genes that regulate the flux of nonenzymatic scavengers of free radicals, such as glutathione; IV) genes that regulate the copy number of target macromolecules, such as mitochondrial DNA; V) genes that determine the structure of the macromolecular targets—for example, chromatin-associated proteins; VI) structural and regulatory genes for the repair of the damaged macromolecular targets, such as the excision repair system; and VII) genes that influence the orderly replacement of dead or damaged somatic cells, such as those that code for various growth factors.

The picture that emerges is that, even for the case of a single molecular mechanism of clastogenicity and gerontogenicity, there is a rich diversity of genetic and environmental variables that can interplay to result in striking interspecific and intraspecific differences in the rates at which oncogenesis and gerontogenesis progress.

SUMMARY

The primary objective of this review is to suggest a major role of cytogenetic pathology in the genesis of both the neoplastic phenotype and the senescent phenotype of aging mammalian organisms. It is hypothesized that allelic variation at a number of genetic loci that have the potential to modulate various types of chromosomal mutation could account, in part, for species-specific variations in maximum life-span potentials and the times of onset of characteristic age-related neoplasms. As a corollary to this proposition, attention is directed to the potential importance of environmental clastogens and aneugens as both oncogenic and "gerontogenic" agents.

By way of introduction, a series of definitions of our subject material is given (aging, oncogenesis, proliferative homeostasis, point mutation, chromosomal mutation, epimutation, mutagens, clastogens, aneugens, gerontogens). There follows a defense of the view that there is a tight coupling of abnormalities in proliferative homeostasis (including atrophies, hyperplasias, benign neoplasias and malignant neoplasias) with intrinsic biological aging. This view differs from those of other authors who either: 1) believe that, to qualify as a bona fide component of aging, the phenotype in question (in this case, neoplasia) must be "genetically programmed" (e.g., see REF. 1) or 2) insist that the rate of development of the neoplastic phenotype should parallel species-specific Gompertz kinetics for the survival of the *population* of organisms (e.g., see REFS. 2 and 3).

After briefly reviewing the classification of chromosomal lesions, we consider evidence for constitutional genetic determinants of chromosomal stability, oncogenesis, and some other aspects of the senescent phenotype, both with respect to interspecific and intraspecific differences. The discussion will include the recent evidence characterizing a human segmental progeroid syndrome (Werner's syndrome) as a deletor mutator strain.

TABLE 3. Free Radical Theory of Aging: Some Candidate Loci

I. Structural and regulatory genes modulating genesis of free radicals
    A. Cytochrome c oxidase
        1. Mitochondrial genes
            Subunit I. Binds heme a, a3, CuA, B. Performs basic processes of cataly-
            sis and proton pump
            Subunit II. Binds to cytochrome c
            Subunit III. Folding/assembly of catalytic subunits
        2. Nuclear genes
            Subunits IV, VI, VIIa, Va, Vb
            Subunits VII, VIII, IX, X, XI, XII, XIII. Regulatory?
    B. NADPH oxidase
    C. P450 family
    D. Peroxidsomal enzymes
    E. Metabolism of catechol amines

II. Structural and regulatory genes for scavenger enzymes
    A. SOD-1
    B. SOD-2
    C. Catalase
    D. Hydrogen peroxidase
    E. Glutathione peroxidase

III. Genes regulating flux on nonenzymatic scavengers
    A. Glutathione
    B. Uric acid
    C. Ascorbic acid
    D. Vitamin E
    E. Beta carotenes

IV. Genes regulating target copy number
    A. Regulation of mitochondrial DNA copy number
    B. Regulation of fidelity of chromosome transmission
        1. Microtubular proteins
        2. Microtubule-associated proteins

V. Genes regulating target structure
    A. Structural genes for membrane lipoproteins
    B. Structural genes for chromatin proteins

VI. Structural and regulatory genes for repair of targets
    A. Reversal of DNA damage
        1. Enzymatic photoreactivation
        2. Repair of 06-alkylguanine
        3. Purine insertion
        4. Ligation of DNA strand breaks
    B. Excision of damage
        1. DNA glycosylases
        2. AP endonucleases
        3. Nucleotide excision repair
        4. Mismatch excision repair
    C. Tolerance of DNA damage
        1. DNA polymerases performing replicative bypass
        2. DNA polymerases performing translesion synthesis

VII. Genes determining orderly replacement of effete cells
    A. Growth factor receptors
    B. Growth factors
    C. Tumor suppressor genes
    D. Oncogenes

A summary of research on environmental chemical clastogens and aneugens is given, showing both discordances and concordances of such assays with assays for point mutagens. An analysis of the literature indicates that there is no statistical evidence for the positive correlations when substances showing effects only at comparatively high concentrations (>1 mM) are excluded from the analysis. Brief mention is also made of the roles of viral agents and ionizing radiation in the genesis of chromosomal mutations.

Finally, some possible pathogenetic mechanisms common to chromosomal mutagenicity, oncogenicity and gerontogenicity are considered, including chemical free radicals (active oxygen species), DNA transposition, DNA amplification, DNA glycation, virally induced cell fusion, posttranslational modifications of centromeric and mitotic spindle proteins, and alterations in the metabolism of telomeric DNA.

REFERENCES

1. BENNINGTON, J. L. 1986. Cancer and aging—pathology. Front. Radiat. Ther. Onc. **20:** 45–51.
2. MACIEIRA-COELHO, A. 1986. Cancer and aging. Exp. Gerontol. **21:** 483–495.
3. ANISIMOV, V. N. 1989. Dependence of susceptibility to carcinogenesis on species life span. Arch. Geschwulstforsch. **59:** S205–213.
4. PRIEUR, M., W. A. ACHKAR, A. AURIAS, J. COUTURIER, A. M. DUTRILLAUX, B. DUTRILLAUX, A. FLÜRY-HERARD, M. GERBAULT-SEUREAU, F. HOFFSCHIR, E. LAMOLIATTE, D. LEFRANÇOIS, M. LOMBARD, M. MULERIS, M. RICOUL, I. SABATIER & E. VIEGAS-PÉQUIGNOT. 1988. Acquired chromosome rearrangements in human lymphocytes: effect of aging. Hum. Genet. **79:** 147–150.
5. GOMPERTZ, B. 1825. On the nature of the function expressive of the law of human mortality and on a new mode of determining life contingencies. Philos. Trans. R. Soc. Lond. **II:** 513–585.
6. TRUJILLO, T. T., J. F. SPALDING & W. H. LANGHAM. 1962. A study of radiation-induced aging: Response of irradiated and nonirradiated mice to cold stress. Radiat. Res. **16:** 144–150.
7. LYE, M. & A. KAMAL. 1977. Effects of heatwave on mortality-rates in elderly inpatients. Lancet **1:** 529–533.
8. FINCH, C. E. 1972. Enzyme activities, gene function and ageing in mammals. Exp. Gerontol. **7:** 53–67.
9. FINCH, C. E. & E. L. SCHNEIDER, EDS. 1985. Handbook of The Biology of Aging, 2nd ed. Van Nostrand Reinhold Company, New York.
10. SHOCK, N. W., R. C. GREULICH, P. T. COSTA, JR., R. ANDRES, E. G. LAKATTA, D. ARENBERG & J. D. TOBIN. 1984. Normal Human Aging: The Baltimore Longitudinal Study of Aging. U.S. Department of Health and Human Services, NIH Publication No. 84-2450, Washington, DC.
11. MARTIN, G. M. 1987. Interactions of aging and environmental agents: The gerontological perspective. *In* Environmental Toxicity and the Aging Processes. 25–80. Alan R. Liss, Inc. New York.
12. STADTMAN, E. R. 1988. Protein modification in aging. J. Gerontol. **43:**B112–B120.
13. HARDING, J. J., H. T. BESWICK, R. AJIBOYE, R. HUBY, R. BLAKYTNY & K. C. RIXON. 1989. Non-enzymic post-translational modification of proteins in aging. A review. Mech. Ageing Dev. **50:** 7–16.
14. BUTLER, J. A., A. R. HEYDARI & A. RICHARDSON. 1989. Analysis of effect of age on synthesis of specific proteins by hepatocytes. J. Cell. Physiol. **141:** 400–409.
15. GRACY, R. W., K. Ü. YÜKSEL, M. L. CHAPMAN, J. K. CINI, M. JAHANI, H. S. LU, B. ORAY & J. M. TALENT. 1985. Impaired protein degradation may account for the accumulation of "abnormal" proteins in aging cells. *In* Modification of Proteins during aging. R. C. Adelman & E. E. Dekker, Eds. Alan R. Liss. New York. Mod. Aging Res. **7:** 1–18.

16. RICHARDSON, A., J. A. BUTLER, M. S. RUTHERFORD, I. SEMSEI, M. Z. GU, G. FERNANDES & W. H. CHIANG. 1987. Effect of age and dietary restriction on the expression of alpha 2u-globulin. J. Biol. Chem. **262:** 12821–12825.
17. ONO, T., R. G. DEAN, S. K. CHATTOPADHYAY & R. G. CUTLER. 1985. Dysdifferentiative nature of aging: age-dependent expression of MuLV and globin genes in thymus, liver and brain in the AKR mouse strain. Gerontology **31:** 362–372.
18. HOLLIDAY, R. 1990. DNA methylation and epigenetic inheritance. Philos. Trans. R. Soc. Lond. Biol. Sci. **326:** 329–338.
19. MARTIN, G. M., M. FRY & L. A. LOEB. 1985. Somatic mutation and aging in mammalian cells. *In* Molecular Biology of Aging: Gene Stability and Gene Expression. R. S. Sohal, L. S. Birnbaum & R. G. Cutler, Eds. 7–21. Raven Press. New York.
20. KOHN, R. R. 1963. Human aging and disease. J. Chron. Dis. **16:** 5–21.
21. MARTIN, G. M. 1979. Proliferative homeostasis and its age-related aberrations. Mech. Ageing Dev. **9:** 385–391.
22. MOSES, R. A. 1981. Accommodation. *In* Adler's Physiology of the Eye: Clinical Application, 7th edit. R. A. Moses, Ed. 304–325. The C.V. Mosby Company. St. Louis.
23. FRIEDENWALD, J. S. 1952. The eye. *In* Cowdry's Problems of Ageing, Biological and Medical Aspects. A. Lansing, Ed. 239–259. Williams and Wilkins. Baltimore.
24. MARTIN, G. M. 1977. Cellular aging—postreplicative cells. Am. J. Pathol. **89:** 513–530.
25. ROSE, M. R. 1989. Genetics of increased lifespan in Drosopholia. Bioessays **11:** 132–135.
26. PETO, R., F. J. C. ROE, P. N. LEE, L. LEVY & J. CLACK. 1975. Cancer and ageing in mice and men. Br. J. Cancer **32:** 411–426.
27. BURNET, M. 1974. Intrinsic Mutagenesis: A Genetic Approach to Ageing. John Wiley and Sons. New York.
28. WOLF, N.S., W. E. GIDDENS & G. M. MARTIN. 1988. Life table analysis and pathologic observations in male mice of a long-lived hybrid strain ($A_f \times$ C57BL/6)F$_1$. J. Gerontol. **43:** B71–B78.
29. SACHER, G. A. & R. W. HART. 1978. Longevity, aging and comparative cellular and molecular biology of the house mouse, *Mus musculus,* and the white-footed mouse, *Peromyscus leucopus.* Birth Defects Orig. Artic. Ser. **14:** 71–96.
30. HOWARD, E. B. & S. W. NIELSEN. 1965. Neoplasia of the boxer dog. Am. J. Vet. Res. **26:** 1121–1131.
31. ZALDÏVAR, R. 1967. Incidence of spontaneous diseases in a Beagle colony. J. Am. Vet. Med. Assoc. **151:** 1186–1189.
32. PRIESTER, W. A. & F. W. MCKAY. 1980. The occurrence of tumors in domestic animals. Natl. Cancer Inst. Monogr. **54:** 1–210.
33. CUTLER, R. G. & I. SEMSEI. 1989. Development, cancer and aging: possible common mechanisms of action and regulation. J. Gerontol. **44:** 25–34.
34. MOSCOW, J. A. & K. H. COWAN. 1988. Multidrug resistance. J. Natl. Cancer Inst. **80:** 14–20.
35. ELLENBERGER, T. E. & S. M. BEVERLEY. 1989. Multiple drug resistance and conservative amplification of the H region in Leishmania major. J. Biol. Chem. **264:** 15094–15103.
36. KONOPKA, J. B., S. M. WATANABE, J. W. SINGER, S. J. COLLINS & O. N. WITTE. 1985. Cell lines and clinical isolates derived from Ph1-positive chronic myelogenous leukemia patients express c-abl proteins with a common structural alteration. Proc. Natl. Acad. Sci. USA **82:** 1810–1814.
37. LEIBOWITZ, D. & K. S. YOUNG. 1989. The molecular biology of CML: a review. Cancer Invest. **7:** 195–203.
38. WOLF, U. 1974. Theodor Boveri and his book "On the Problem of the Origin of Malignant Tumors." *In* Chromosomes and Cancer. J. German, Ed. 3–20. John Wiley & Sons. New York.
39. HEIM, S. & F. MITELMAN. 1987. Cancer Cytogenetics. Alan R. Liss. New York.
40. SKUSE, G. R. & P. T. ROWLEY. 1989. Tumor suppressor genes and inherited predisposition to malignancy. Semin. Oncol. **16:** 128–137.
41. CURTIS, H. J. 1971. Genetic factors in aging. Adv. Genet. **16:** 305–324.
42. CURTIS, H. J. & K. MILLER. 1971. Chromosome aberrations in liver cells of guinea pigs. J. Gerontol. **26:** 292–293.

43. CURTIS, H. J., J. LEITH & J. TILLEY. 1966. Chromosome aberrations in liver cells of dogs of different ages. J. Gerontol. **21:** 268–270.
44. MARTIN, G. M., A. C. SMITH, D. J. KETTERER, C. E. OGBURN & C. M. DISTECHE. 1985. Increased chromosomal aberrations in first metaphases of cells isolated from the kidneys of aged mice. Isr. J. Med. Sci. **21:** 296–301.
45. HORN, P. L., M. S. TURKER, C. E. OGBURN, C. M. DISTECHE & G. M. MARTIN. 1984. A cloning assay for 6-thioguanine resistance provides evidence against certain somatic mutational theories of aging. J. Cell. Physiol. **121:** 309–315.
46. TRAINOR, K. J., D. J. WIGMORE, A. CHRYSOSTOMOU, J. L. DEMPSEY, R. SESHADRI & A. A. MORLEY. 1984. Mutation frequency in human lymphocytes increases with age. Mech. Ageing Dev. **27:** 83–86.
47. HEIM, S., B. JOHANSSON & F. MERTENS. 1989. Constitutional chromosome instability and cancer risk. Mutat. Res. **221:** 39–51.
48. COHEN, M. M. & H. P. LEVY. 1989. Chromosome instability syndromes. *In* Advances in Human Genetics. Vol. 18. H. Harris & K. Kirschhorn, Eds. 43–149. Plenum Publishing Corporation. New York.
49. COHEN, M. M. &. H. P. LEVY. 1989. Chromosome instability syndromes. Adv. Hum. Genet. **18:** 43–149, 365–371.
50. GOTO, M., K. TANIMOTO, Y. HORIUCHI & T. SASAZUKI. 1981. Family analysis of Werner's syndrome: a survey of 42 Japanese families with a review of the literature. Clin. Genet. **19:** 8–15.
51. MARTIN, G. M. 1978. Genetic syndromes in man with potential relevance to the pathobiology of aging. Birth Defects Orig. Artic. Ser. **14:** 5–39.
52. SALK, D., Y. FUJIWARA & G. M. MARTIN, EDS. 1985. Werner's Syndrome and Human Aging. Adv. Exp. Med. Biol. Vol. 190. Plenum Press. New York.
53. TOLLEFSBOL, T. O. & H. J. COHEN. 1984. Werner's syndrome: an underdiagnosed disorder resembling premature aging. Age **7:** 75–88.
54. SATO, K., M. GOTO, K. NISHIOKA, K. ARIMA, N. HORI, N. YAMASHITA, Y. FUJIMOTO, H. NANKO, K. OHARA & K. OHARA. 1988. Werner's syndrome associated with malignancies: five case reports with a survey of case histories in Japan. Gerontology **34:** 212–218.
55. MARTIN, G. M., C. A. SPRAGUE & C. J. EPSTEIN. 1970. Replicative life-span of cultivated human cells. Effects of donor's age, tissue, and genotype. Lab. Invest. **23:** 86–92.
56. HOEHN, H., E. M. BRYANT, K. AU, T. H. NORWOOD, H. BOMAN & G. M. MARTIN. 1975. Variegated translocation mosaicism in human skin fibroblast cultures. Cytogenet. Cell Genet. **15:** 282–298.
57. SALK, D., K. AU, H. HOEHN & G. M. MARTIN. 1981. Cytogenetics of Werner's syndrome cultured skin fibroblasts: variegated translocation mosaicism. Cytogenet. Cell Genet. **30:** 92–107.
58. FUKUCHI, K., G. M. MARTIN & R. J. MONNAT, JR. 1989. Mutator phenotype of Werner syndrome is characterized by extensive deletions. Proc. Natl. Acad. Sci. USA **86:** 5893–5897.
59. SALK, D., K. AU, H. HOEHN & G. M. MARTIN. 1985. Cytogenetic aspects of Werner syndrome. Adv. Exp. Med. Biol. **190:** 541–546.
60. FUKUCHI, K., K. TANAKA, Y. KUMAHARA, K. MARUMO, M. B. PRIDE, G. M. MARTIN & R. J. MONNAT, JR. 1990. Increased frequency of 6-thioguanine-resistant peripheral blood lymphocytes in Werner syndrome patients. Hum. Genet. **84:** 249–252.
61. ISHIDATE, M., JR., M. C. HARNOIS & T. SOFUNI. 1988. A comparative analysis of data on the clastogenicity of 951 chemical substances tested in mammalian cell cultures. Mutat. Res. **195:** 151–213.
62. VANDERKERKEN, K., P. VANPARYS, L. VERSCHAEVE & M. KIRSCH-VOLDERS. 1989. The mouse bone marrow micronucleus assay can be used to distinguish aneugens from clastogens. Mutagenesis **4:** 6–11.
63. ARAKAKI, D. T. & W. SCHMID. 1971. Chemical mutagenesis: the Chinese hamster bone marrow as an *in vivo* test system. II. Correlation with *in vitro* results on Chinese hamster fibroblasts and human fibroblasts and lymphocytes. Humangenetik **11:** 119–131.
64. CREBELLI, R., G. CONTI, L. CONTI & A. CARERE. 1990. Chloroacetaldehyde is a

powerful inducer of mitotic aneuploidy in *Aspergillus nidulans*. Mutagenesis **5:** 165–168.

65. HEISTERKAMP, N., G. JENSTER, J. TEN HOEVE, D. ZOVICH, P. K. PATTENGALE & J. GROFFEN. 1990. Acute leukaemia in bcr/abl transgenic mice. Nature **344:** 251–253.
66. COMMITTEE ON THE BIOLOGICAL EFFECTS OF IONIZING RADIATION. 1990. Health Effects of Exposure to Low Levels of Ionizing Radiation: Beir V. National Academy Press. Washington, DC.
67. CASARETT, G. W. 1964. Similarities and contrasts between radiation and time pathology. Adv. Gerontol. Res. **1:** 109–163.
68. MARTIN, G. M. & M. S. TURKER. 1988. Model systems for the genetic analysis of mechanisms of aging. J. Gerontol. **43:** B33–B39.
69. ROSE, M. R. 1991. Evolutionary Biology of Senescence. Oxford University Press. Oxford.
70. WEINDRUCH, R. & R. L. WALFORD. 1988. The Retardation of Aging and Disease by Dietary Restriction. Charles C Thomas. Springfield, IL.
71. NICHOLS, W. W. 1972. Chromosomal changes due to viruses. Triangle **11:** 103–106.
72. RAO, P. N., R. T. JOHNSON & K. SPERLING. 1982. Premature Chromosome Condensation. Academic Press. New York.
73. HOYT, M. A., T. STEARNS & D. BOTSTEIN. 1990. Chromosome instability mutants of *Saccharomyces cerevisiae* that are defective in microtubule-mediated processes. Mol. Cell Biol. **10:** 223–234.
74. BELIAEV, I. IA. & A. P. AKIF'EV. 1988. [Genetic processes and the problem of the target in chromosomal mutagenesis.] Genetika **24:** 1384–1392.
75. HASTIE, N. D. & R. C. ALLSHIRE. 1989. Human telomeres: fusion and interstitial sites. Trends Genet. **5:** 326–331.
76. YU, G. L., J. D. BRADLEY, L. D. ATTARDI & E. H. BLACKBURN. 1990. *In vivo* alteration of telomere sequences and senescence caused by mutated tetrahymena telomerase RNAs. Nature **344:** 126–132.
77. VOGT, P. 1990. Potential genetic functions of tandem repeated DNA sequence blocks in the human genome are based on a highly conserved chromatin folding code. Hum. Genet. **84:** 301–336.
78. HARLEY, C. B., A. B. FUTCHER & C. W. GREIDER. 1990. Telomeres shorten during aging of human fibroblasts. Nature. In press.
79. BOEKE, J. D. 1990. Reverse transcriptase, the end of the chromosome, and the end of life. Cell **61:** 193–195.
80. COPELAND, N. G. & N. A. JENKINS. 1987. Eukaryotic transposable elements: probes for identifying and studying genes important in mammalian development. Birth Defects **23:** 123–135.
81. JENKINS, N. A. & N. G. COPELAND. 1987. Retroviral DNA content of the mouse genome. Birth Defects **23:** 109–122.
82. KAISER, D. 1986. Control of multicellular development: Dictyostelium and Myxococcus. Annu. Rev. Genet. **20:** 539–566.
83. WESSLER, S. R. 1988. Phenotypic diversity mediated by the maize transposable elements Ac and Spm. Science **242:** 399–405.
84. FEDOROFF, N., P. MASSON & J. A. BANKS. 1989. Mutations, epimutations, and the developmental programming of the maize suppressor-mutator transposable element. Bioessays **10:** 139–144.
85. SCHIMKE, R. T., S. W. SHERWOOD, A. B. HILL & R. N. JOHNSTON. 1986. Overreplication and recombination of DNA in higher eukaryotes: potential consequences and biological implications. Proc. Natl. Acad. Sci. USA **83:** 2157–2161.
86. STARK, G. R. & G. M. WAHL. 1984. Gene amplification. Annu. Rev. Biochem. **53:** 447–491.
87. WRIGHT, J. A., H. S. SMITH, F. M. WATT, M. C. HANCOCK, D. L. HUDSON & G. R. STARK. 1990. DNA amplification is rare in normal human cells. Proc. Natl. Acad. Sci. USA **87:** 1791–1795.
88. TLSTY, T. D. 1990. Normal diploid human and rodent cells lack a detectable frequency of gene amplification. Proc. Natl. Acad. Sci. USA **87:** 3132–3136.
89. BUCALA, R., P. MODEL, M. RUSSEL & A. CERAMI. 1985. Modification of DNA by

glucose 6-phosphate induces DNA rearrangements in an *Escherichia coli* plasmid. Proc. Natl. Acad. Sci. USA **82:** 8439–8442.

90. LEE, A. T. & A. CERAMI. 1987. Elevated glucose 6-phosphate levels are associated with plasmid mutations *in vivo*. Proc. Natl. Acad. Sci. USA **84:** 8311–8314.

91. HARMAN, D. 1986. Free radical theory of aging: role of free radicals in the origination and evolution of life, aging, and disease processes. *In* Free Radicals, Aging, and Degenerative Diseases. J. E. Johnson, Jr., R. Walford, D. Harman & J. Miquel, Eds. 3–49. Alan R. Liss, Inc. New York.

Monoclonal B-Cell Proliferative Disorders and Aging

JIRI RADL

TNO Institute for Experimental Gerontology
P.O. Box 5815
2280 HV Rijswijk, The Netherlands

A restriction of immunoglobulin (Ig) heterogeneity and the appearance of homogeneous immunoglobulin components (H-Ig) in serum belong to the most frequent phenomena of aging of the immune system (IS).[1,2] What kind of aging processes do these changes represent at the cellular level? The immunoglobulin spectrum reflects the antibody production of enormous numbers of B-cell clones which are continuously active in response to antigenic stimulation. Most of these responses are regulated by T cells. In normal young individuals, this results in a polyclonal, heterogeneous Ig spectrum. Only under certain experimental conditions, *i.e.*, (hyper)immunization with some T-cell independent antigens (polysaccharides or haptens) on a suitable genetic background, has an oligo- or monoclonal excess antibody production been observed.[3,4] It is highly unlikely that this mechanism is responsible for the frequent H-Ig found in aging individuals. Clinical studies have demonstrated that various conditions can be accompanied by an excess H-Ig production; they all have a common name: monoclonal gammapathies (MG). However, very little is known about the biology, pathogenesis and significance of the individual disorders. B-cell malignancies, such as multiple myeloma (MM) or Waldenström's macroglobulinaemia (WM) are known to increase in frequency with aging, but the vast majority of MG appearing during aging do not show any signs of malignant behavior. They are given different names, such as: benign monoclonal gammapathy (BMG), idiopathic paraproteinaemia (IP), monoclonal gammopathy of undetermined significance (MGUS), essential paraproteinaemia and the like. With the improvement of techniques for the detection of H-Ig in serum, the number of reports on these MG steadily increased and nowadays the literature on this subject is very voluminous. When using techniques with 100 μg/ml as a lower sensitivity limit for H-Ig detection, MG were found in frequencies increasing from ± 0% in the third decade up to 20% in the tenth decade of human life.[1,5] When increasing the sensitivity limit of the H-Ig detection techniques to 0.5 μg/ml, MG were detected in the sera of more than 80% of persons older than 95 years.[6] Some of those MG were persistent (malignant MG and BMG), others, mainly those of low concentration, were transient. These findings indicated that the involved B-cell clones expanded to various sizes and probably by different mechanisms. So much regarding the clinical observations. Our understanding of age-related MG has improved substantially only after recognition that aging C57BL/KaLwRij mice develop very similar disorders which could be studied in experimental model situations.

The C57BL Mouse Model

C57BL mice were shown to develop various B-cell proliferative disorders with aging. Up to 80% of mice of this strain develop BMG with all the features of human BMG.[7-10] Nearly 1% of mice older than two years develop WM or MM, again very similar to the corresponding human diseases.[11,12] In more than 30% of old mice at necropsy and histopathology examination, a lymphoma, mainly of the follicle center cell type (earlier known as reticulum cell sarcoma B) can be found. The greater part of this latter malignancy is most likely of B-cell origin, but is not accompanied by an excess of H-Ig production (REF. 8 and unpublished). Transient, low level and often multiple H-Ig components can also frequently be found, especially when more sensitive techniques for the detection of H-Ig are used and they complete the picture of age-related MG in C57BL mice. Since all these age-related mouse MG have been shown to be very similar to, if not identical with those in humans, results of studies on the biology and the pathogenesis of these disorders in both species have been considered to be complementary. Of all these disorders, BMG has been the subject of most of the studies.

BMG

Just as in man, BMG in mice represents an excessive but nonprogressive proliferation of an Ig (most often IgG) producing clone. This clone resides mainly in the bone marrow in a diffuse pattern and its cells keep morphological features of a normal plasma cell. The corresponding H-Ig component in the serum is usually detected at a concentration below 0.5 mg/ml and it persists for months, usually till the death of the animal. The concentration of the other Ig remains usually within normal values. Excess production of a Bence-Jones protein has not yet been detected in mice with BMG.

Transplantation experiments demonstrated that the cells of the BMG clone are "autonomous" but not immortal.[13] BMG can be transplanted and propagated in syngeneic young mice, but with decreasing 'take' frequency and for a limited number (maximum 3 to 4) of generations. This is in sharp contrast with the results of transplantation experiments using MM and MW cells of the 5T series.[11,12] Those can be transplanted indefinitely and with a 'take' frequency approaching 100%. Even the very slowly growing and relatively 'benign' 5T7 MM, comparable to the so-called smoldering MM (SMM) as described in man,[14] exhibits an immortal nature. These results were very important in showing that, in its final form, BMG represents an intrinsic defect within the given B-cell clone and not an extrinsic one due to some aging factors; this defect, however, is fundamentally different from that in B-cell malignancies.

Further studies showed that factors extrinsic to the BMG clone play an important role in the early stages of its development. A deficiency in the T immune system can have an important influence here. Experiments performed in neonatally and adult thymectomized mice[15] and in nude athymic mice[16] demonstrated a close correlation between the increase of the frequencies of age-related MG and the grade of the T-cell defect. Vice versa, supplementation of nude mice with T cells leads to the decrease of the incidence of these MG.[17] A defect in the regulatory function of the T cells was postulated to be responsible for this effect.[18] An impairment in the T-suppressor cell activity was shown to contribute to the increased frequencies of MG in the aging C57BL mice.[19] A role for the contribution of a defective T-helper cell function to the development of B-cell proliferative disorders is indicated by increased frequencies of these disorders in humans with AIDS, but this mechanism has not been tested experimentally. In the above mentioned studies performed in the C57BL mice, a T-cell defect clearly increased the frequency of low level transient MG and persistent BMG. When similar experiments were performed in a strain with low incidence of BMG, the results were different. Transient MG were found in high frequencies, but the development of BMG was less frequent than in the C57BL mice.[15,20] This indicates that genetic factors may be of basic importance in the pathogenesis of BMG.

The role of genetic factors in the development of BMG was indicated already by differences in the frequency and the onset of MG among mice of different strains.[8] This was confirmed in subsequent experiments. In radiation chimeras of the C57BL (high frequency BMG) and the CBA (low frequency of BMG) mice, BMG of the IgG2a isotype developed only in mice with B cells of C57BL and not of CBA origin.[21] The F1 hybrid mice of these two strains showed high frequency of BMG (of the IgG2a and IgD isotypes tested) carrying the C57BL Igh[b] allotype and only a few BMG of the CBA Igh[a] allotype.[22] Further studies in H2 and Igh congenic C57BL and BALB strains indicated that the genetic influences in the pathogenesis of BMG are complex and cannot simply be ascribed to a certain H2 or Igh locus.[23,24] It seems that the H2 complex does not clearly influence the development of BMG. The Igh locus may contribute to BMG development but only to a limited extent. Other subcellular C57BL-related genetic factors which regulate B-cell proliferation, such as activated oncogenes, are postulated to play a more important role in this respect.[25]

Finally, the potential role which an antigenic stimulation may play in the development of age-related MG should be considered. An indication for such an effect has repeatedly been suggested in reports on MG where the H-Ig had antibody activity to an antigen encountered in the patient's history.[26,27] In mice, the role of antigenic stimulation on the development of MG was indicated by clear-cut differences in the frequency of MG between barrier-maintained and conventionally kept nude mice.[16] However, it was difficult to evaluate in that experiment in how many cases only transient MG or BMG had developed. Later, a contributory role of an (intensive) antigenic stimulation on the development of BMG was demonstrated in follow-up studies using various antigens which were applied at a young age of the C57BL mice.[27–29] When aging, some of the mice developed BMG with antibody activity to the corresponding antigens. These results indicate that memory cells of the B-cell clones involved in the original specific responses to some proteins and haptens (but not to a polysaccharide) may become targets for events leading to the development of BMG. Data of an analysis on clonal properties and the relationship of BMG in one aging female C57BL mouse suggest that selection by antigen might have occurred in that B-cell clone before the intrinsic B-cell defect appeared and that antigen selection no longer plays a role afterwards.[30]

Multiple Myeloma and Waldenström's Macroglobulinemia

The mouse B-cell malignancies of spontaneous origin, the 5TMM and 5TMW series, occur with about 200 times lower frequency than BMG. 5TMM are readily transplantable in syngeneic recipients, maintaining their original properties, and most of them are kept *in vivo* as stable lines. In contrast to mineral oil induced plasmacytomas in BALB/c mice having consistent translocations of the c-*myc* oncogene, a rearrangement of c-*myc* oncogene in human MM as well as in mouse 5TMM and MW is a very rare finding.[31,32] Analysis of the development of the 5T malignancies from the beginning was possible in 5 cases. They all developed in aging mice within three months (*i.e.*, the time period between blood sampling), with a progressive increase of the H-Ig concentration up to levels surpassing 10 mg/ml. In each case they developed *de novo* and not from a preexisting MG with features of BMG. More details on the clinical and laboratory findings in the 5TMM and 5TMW and their use in preclinical studies can be found in recent reviews.[11,12]

Transient MG

Single or multiple MG of low concentration (usually <2.5 mg/ml) which can be detected in the serum temporarily (for a couple of months but in some cases even for a couple of years) are frequent findings in aging humans.[6,33] However, they can also be found in young persons and even in children.[34,35] The most consistent appearances of these MG have been described in some primary immunodeficiencies (*e.g.*, Wiskott-Aldrich, Nezelof and DiGeorge syndromes and combined immunodeficiency), and in secondary immunodeficiencies (after treatment with immunosuppressiva or cytostatics, in malignancies of the components of the immune system other than B cells, and in acquired, viral or idiopathic immunodeficiencies); they typically appear during the reconstitution period after bone marrow transplantation for whatever disease it was applied.[36] Sometimes they were reported in newborns from mothers with an intrauterine infection. Mechanisms of the development of these MG have been studied in animal models (reviewed in REF. 37). Results of these studies can briefly be summarized as suggesting that in all the above-mentioned conditions mono- or oligoclonal B-cell proliferation was the result of an insufficient T-cell regulation of the more or less properly functioning B cells. Diminished help from T_H cells may result in fewer activated B-cell clones; those clones, however, will expand in excess if suppression fails. A direct and clear-cut influence of the antigenic load on their incidence has been shown in both clinical and experimental studies.[16,38] All the data indicated that transient MG are very sensitive indicators of this kind of immunodeficiency with T- and B-cell imbalance. It is very likely that the transient MG which frequently appear in old individuals reflect similar changes and mechanisms within their gradually aging immune system.[33]

An additional immunosuppression (*e.g.*, iatrogenic in graft recipients, late effects of irradiation or due to viral infections) can accelerate the aging process within the immune system and increase the frequencies not only of transient MG but also of BMG and possibly of B-cell malignancies.[39,40] All the above-mentioned studies improved our understanding of MG to such an extent that a new classification of MG on the basis of their biology and possible pathogenesis became possible for the first time.[41–43]

Four Major Categories of MG

On the basis of biological features and possible pathogenetic factors (see TABLE 1), four major categories of MG can be distinguished:[42,43]

B-Cell Malignancies

MG reflects a progressive proliferation of a malignant B-cell clone at a maturation stage of Ig production; the serum H-Ig concentration more or less reflects the size of the clone. This is not the case in nonsecretory MM, in Bence Jones MM, J-chain MM and lymphomas of a less differentiated nature.[42] Experiments in animal models have shown that the involved B-cell clone is immortal and indefinitely transplantable in syngeneic recipients. It often contains chromosomal derangement, its subcellular control is largely lost, but some extrinsic control within the immune system (*e.g.*, via the T cells) may remain preserved with a wide variation among individual cases. This is possibly one of the reasons for the so pronounced differences in the clinical course of individual cases.

Benign B-Cell Neoplasia (BMG)

BMG is a nonmalignant excessive proliferation of a B-cell clone at a maturation stage of the plasma cell. H-Ig concentration reflects the size of the clone, which may be relatively large, but does not show any clear-cut progression. In animal experiments, the BMG clone shows an 'autonomous' proliferation but is not immortal, *i.e.*, it is transplantable but it dies out after three to four transplantation generations. Subcellular control of the cell proliferation seems to be lost, but other properties and functions of the cell probably remain unaffected. A transition from BMG into MM has not been documented yet in large follow-up studies.

TABLE 1. Possible Pathogenetic Factors in Age-Related Monoclonal Gammapathies[a]

Category	1. MMG	2. BMG	3. ARID	Remark
Aging	+	+	+	
Regulatory				
T cell defect	?	+	+	
Genetic influences	+	+	+	strong*
(Onco)gene dysfunction	multiple?	single?	−	
Failure of				
immunosurveillance	+	+?	−	
Additive effect of				
immunosuppression	+	+	+	
(Hyper)immunization				
at young-adult age	?	+	−	

[a] MMG: malignant monoclonal gammapathies (specifically multiple myeloma); BMG: benign monoclonal gammapathy; ARID: age-related immunodeficiency. *: acting possibly at different sites and stages.

Immunodeficiency with T<B Cell Imbalance

MG in these immunodeficiencies represent an excess proliferation of a normal B-cell clone due to an insufficient regulation by T (helper and/or suppressor) cells. H-Ig reflects the size of the clone. The duration of the MG depends on the antigenic stimulation; it is transient, but it can last for months and even for a couple of years. This MG is considered to be a very sensitive indicator of immunodeficiency with preserved B-cell functions but impaired regulatory T-cell functions. Studies in animal models showed that the clone proliferating in excess is not transplantable, thus without signs indicating intrinsic abnormalities in its control of cell proliferation. On susceptible genetic background, however, a transition into BMG may be possible. A similar possibility of transformation of such a clone into malignancy is suspected but not yet proved.

Antigen Driven MG

An antibody response towards some polysaccharides, haptens and autoantigens may on a genetic basis be excessive and restricted even to a single clone. The H-Ig component reflects its size.

Clearly age-related are MG of the categories 1, 2 and a part of category 3. Together, they represent more than 90% of all MG. How do they develop?

Hypothesis on the Three-Stage Development of BMG

An explanation of the development of MG of the second and the third (age-related) categories was offered by the so called "Three-stage hypothesis" in 1979.[18] It postulates that BMG, a benign B-cell neoplasia, develops as a consequence of an age-related immunodeficiency within the T-immune system. Involution of the thymus is followed by selective decline in some T-cell subpopulations, which is genetically determined. The function of the mainly regulatory T cells becomes impaired; the onset, progress and extent of this process can be influenced by some extrinsic factors, such as chronic antigenic stimulation, viral infections and iatrogenic immunosuppression (Stage 1). The control of the B-cell responses to antigenic stimulation becomes insufficient; fewer B-cell clones respond, but those which do, expand in excess (MG of the third category). This Stage 2 is still reversible. On a susceptible genetic background, the repeated mono- or oligoclonal expansions lead to a bigger chance for mutation. If it happens within the regulatory gene sequences controlling the cell proliferation, the clone will continue to proliferate even in the absence of the original antigenic stimulus (Stage 3). This stage is irreversible.

The genetic susceptibility for a B-cell malignancy may have the same background and its development may go along a similar pathway; however, it certainly is much more complex and the intrinsic cellular defect in the B-cell malignancy is different from that in BMG. It consists most likely of more than a single (onco)gene dysfunction,[44] as may be the case in BMG. The validity of the three-stage hypothesis has been tested in several experiments in the last 10 years; so far all the results support it.

CONCLUSIONS

What is the significance and what are the practical consequences of the results of all these studies? First of all, they elucidate some phenomena of the aging process and indicate how the B and T cells participate in the gradually developing age-related deficiency of the immune system. Secondly, they give a realistic background for a new classification of MG, for the first time on the basis of their biology and possible pathogenesis. Further, they attack the old dogma saying that BMG represents a premalignant condition, a premyeloma. BMG and MM are clearly two different conditions and a transition of BMG into MM is very rare, if it occurs at all.[45] The fundamental differences between the two conditions, especially that of the clonal cell mortality, indicate that a reliable test for an early detection of (smoldering) MM and WM and for their differential diagnosis from BMG may be possible and could be developed in the clinical laboratory. Finally, the recognition of MG of the immunodeficiency category opened a new research field which should receive more attention. Not only because they seem to be very sensitive indicators of an immunodeficiency with T<B cell imbalance but also because these proliferative disorders may be in a causative relationship with at least some of the B-cell neoplasias.

It seems worthwhile to study whether individuals (on the basis of their genetic susceptibility) at an increased risk for the development of B-cell proliferative disorders can be revealed already at a younger age. An indication for such a possibility can be derived from observations in mice. In contrast to mice of the CBA strain with low frequency of B-cell proliferative disorders, many mice of the C57BL strain seem to respond to T-cell dependent antigenic stimulation with a clear-cut mono- or oligoclonal dominancy (REFS. 27, 29, 46 and unpublished) and this already at a young age. This pattern, detected only by very sensitive techniques of antigen-specific immunoblotting,[29,47] may reflect the very first stage of the T<B cell imbalance. If this is true and could be confirmed in humans, tests on the heterogeneity of the antibody response to a vaccination may be useful in members of families with a high incidence of B-cell proliferative disorders or in persons undergoing an immunosuppressive treatment or where such a treatment is being considered.

REFERENCES

1. RADL, J. 1982. Effects of aging on immunoglobulins. *In* Pathology of Immunoglobulins: Diagnostic and Clinical Aspects, Protein Abnormalities. S. E. Ritzmann, Ed. Vol. 2: 55–69. Alan R. Liss, Inc. New York.
2. RADL, J. 1971. Immunoglobulin levels and abnormalities in aging humans and mice. *In* Immunological techniques applied to aging research. W. A. Adler & A. A. Nordin, Eds. 121–139. CRC Press. Boca Raton, FL.
3. KRAUSE, R. M. 1970. Factors controlling the occurrence of antibodies with uniform properties. Fed. Proc. **29:** 59–65.
4. BRAUN, D. G. & J.-C. JATON. 1974. Homogeneous antibodies: induction and value as probe for the antibody problem. Curr. Top. Microbiol. Immunol. **66:** 29–76.
5. RADL, J., J. M. SEPERS, F. SKVARIL, A. MORELL & W. HIJMANS. 1975. Immunoglobulin patterns in humans over 95 years of age. Clin. Exp. Immunol. **22:** 84–90.
6. RADL, J., J. WELS & C. M. HOOGEVEEN. 1988. Immunoblotting with (sub)class-specific antibodies reveals a high frequency of monoclonal gammopathies in persons thought to be immunodeficient. Clin. Chem. **34:** 1839–1842.
7. RADL, J. & C. F. HOLLANDER. 1974. Homogeneous immunoglobulins in sera of mice during aging. J. Immunol. **112:** 2271–2273.
8. RADL, J., C. F. HOLLANDER, P. VAN DEN BERG & E. DE GLOPPER. 1978. Idiopathic paraproteinaemia. I. Studies in an animal model—the ageing C57BL/KaLwRij mouse. Clin. Exp. Immunol. **33:** 395–402.
9. RADL, J. 1981. Benign monoclonal gammopathy (Idiopathic paraproteinemia). Am. J. Pathol. **105:** 91–93.
10. RADL, J. 1989. Benign monoclonal gammopathy, model no. 234. supplemental update. *In* Handbook: Animal Models of Human Disease. Fasc. 17. C. C. Capen, T. C. Jones & G. Migaki, Eds. Registry of Comparative Pathology, Armed Forces Institute of Pathology. Washington, DC.
11. RADL, J., J. W. CROESE, C. ZURCHER, M. H. M. V.D. ENDEN-VIEVEEN & A. M. DE LEEUW. 1988. Animal model of human disease: multiple myeloma. Am. J. Pathol. **132:** 177–181.

12. RADL, J., M. H. M. VAN DEN ENDEN-VIEVEEN, C. ZURCHER, P. J. M. ROHOLL & E. BLAUW. 1989. Morbus Waldenström-like B-cell lymphoma in the aging C57BL/KaLwRij mouse. In Monoclonal Gammapathies. II. Clinical Significance and Basic mechanisms. J. Radl & B. van Camp, Eds. Topics in Aging Research in Europe. Vol. 12: 233–238. EURAGE. Rijswijk.

13. RADL, J., E. DE GLOPPER, H. R. E. SCHUIT & C. ZURCHER. 1979. Idiopathic paraproteinemia. II. Transplantation of the paraprotein producing clone from old to young C57BL/KaLwRij mice. J. Immunol. 122: 609–613.

14. KYLE, R. A. & P. R. GREIPP. 1980. Smoldering multiple myeloma. N. Engl. J. Med. 302: 1347–1349.

15. RADL, J., E. DE GLOPPER, P. VAN DEN BERG & M. J. VAN ZWIETEN. 1980. Idiopathic paraproteinemia. III. Increased frequency of paraproteinemia in thymectomized aging C57BL/KaLwRij and CBA/BrARij mice. J. Immunol. 125: 31–35.

16. RADL, J., J. G. MINK, P. VAN DEN BERG, M. J. VAN ZWIETEN & R. BENNER. 1980. Increased frequency of homogeneous immunoglobulins in the sera of nude athymic mice with age. Clin. Immunol. Immunopathol. 17: 469–476.

17. VAN DEN AKKER, T. W., A. P. TIO-GILLEN, H. A. SOLLEVELD, R. BENNER & J. RADL. 1988. The influence of T cells on homogeneous immunoglobulins in sera of athymic nude mice during aging. Scand. J. Immunol. 28: 359–365.

18. RADL, J. 1979. Idiopathic paraproteinemia. A consequence of an age-related deficiency in the T immune system. Clin. Immunol. Immunopathol. 14: 251–255.

19. VAN DEN AKKER, TH. W., A. P. GILLEN, W. BRIL, R. BENNER & J. RADL. 1983. Increased incidence of transient homogeneous immunoglobulins in irradiated and reconstituted C57BL/KaLwRij mice treated with 2'-deoxyguanosine. Clin. Exp. Immunol. 54: 411–417.

20. RADL, J. 1986. Aging of the immune system and B cell monoclonal proliferative disorders. In Immunoregulation in Aging. A. Facchini, J. J. Haaijman & G. Labo', Eds. Topics in Aging Research in Europe. Vol. 9: 295–298. EURAGE. Rijswijk.

21. RADL, J., P. J. HEIDT, S. KNAAN-SHANZER & M. J. VAN ZWIETEN. 1984. Idiopathic paraproteinaemia. IV. The role of genetic factors in the development of monoclonal B cell proliferative disorders—a study in the ageing C57BL/KaLwRij and CBA/BrARij mouse radiation chimeras. Clin. Exp. Immunol. 57: 213–216.

22. RADL, J., M. H. M. VAN DEN ENDEN-VIEVEN, T. W. VAN DE AKKER, R. BENNER, J. J. HAAIJMAN & C. ZURCHER. 1985. Idiopathic paraproteinaemia. V. Expression of Igh1 and Igh5 allotypes within the homogeneous immunoglobulins of ageing (C57BL/LiARij × CBA/BrARij) F1 mouse. Clin. Exp. Immunol. 62: 405–411.

23. VAN DEN AKKER, T. W., A. P. TIO-GILLEN, R. BENNER, C. ZURCHER & J. RADL. 1987. The influence of H-2 genetic factors on the development of benign monoclonal gammopathy in ageing H-2 congenic C57BL and BALB mice. Immunology 61: 403–408.

24. VAN DEN AKKER, TH. W., E. DE GLOPPER-V.D. VEER, J. RADL & R. BENNER. 1988. The influence of genetic factors associated with the immunoglobulin heavy chain locus on the development of benign monoclonal gammapathy in aging Igh congenic mice. Immunology 65: 31–35.

25. RADL, J. 1986. Benign monoclonal gammapathy (BMG). Curr. Top. Microbiol. Immunol. 132: 221–224.

26. MERLINI, G., M. FARHANGI & E. F. OSSERMAN. 1986. Monoclonal immunoglobulins with antibody activity in myeloma, macroglobulinemia and related plasma cell dyscrasias. Semin. Oncol. 13: 350–365.

27. NOOIJ, F. J. M., A. J. VAN DER SLUIJS-GELLING, R. J. MINKMAN-BRONDIJK & J. RADL. 1989. The role of antigenic stimulation in the development of monoclonal gammapathies in aging mice. In Monoclonal Gammapathies. II. Clinical Significance and Basic Mechanisms. J. Radl & B. van Camp, Eds. Topics in Aging Research in Europe. Vol. 12: 91–96. EURAGE. Rijswijk.

28. VAN DEN AKKER, TH. W., R. BRONDIJK & J. RADL. 1988. Influence of long-term antigenic stimulation started in young C57BL mice on the development of age-related monoclonal gammapathies. Int. Arch. Allergy Appl. Immunol. 87: 165–170.

29. RADL, J., A. J. VAN DER SLUIJS-GELLING, C. M. HOOGEVEEN, R. J. MINKMAN-

BRONDIJK & F. J. M. NOOIJ. 1989. Influence of antigenic stimulation at young age on the development of monoclonal gammapathies in the aging C57BL mice. *In* Monoclonal Gammapathies. II. Clinical Significance and Basic Mechanisms. J. Radl & B. van Camp, Eds. Topics in Aging Research in Europe. Vol. 12: 229–232. EURAGE. Rijswijk.

30. BOS, N. A., C. G. MEEUWSEN, E. DE GLOPPER-V.D. VEER, TH.W. VAN DEN AKKER, J. RADL, K. A. ZWAAGSTRA & R. BENNER. Isolation and molecular characterization of the B cells producing the paraprotein in a case of benign monoclonal gammopathy in C57BL mice. Submitted.

31. RADL, J., Y. A. PUNT, M. H. M. VAN DEN ENDEN-VIEVEEN, P. A. J. BENTVELZEN, M. H. C. BAKKUS, TH. W. VAN DEN AKKER & R. BENNER. 1990. The 5T mouse multiple myeloma model: absence of c-*myc* oncogene rearrangement in early transplant generations. Br. J. Cancer **61**: 276–278.

32. VAN DEN ENDEN-VIEVEEN, M. H. M., Y. A. PUNT, M. BAKKUS, R. BENNER & J. RADL. 1989. Rearrangement of the c-*myc* oncogene in mouse multiple myeloma, morbus Waldenström and plasmacytoma. *In* Monoclonal Gammapathies. II. Clinical Significance and Basic Mechanisms. J. Radl & B. van Camp, Eds. Topics in Aging Research in Europe. Vol. 12: 245–248. EURAGE. Rijswijk.

33. RADL, J. 1989. Monoclonal gammapathies in immunodeficient adults. *In* Monoclonal Gammapathies. II. Clinical Significance and Basic Mechanisms. J. Radl & B. van Camp, Eds. Topics in Aging Research in Europe. Vol. 12: 45–50. EURAGE. Rijswijk.

34. RADL, J. 1979. The influence of the T immune system on the appearance of homogeneous immunoglobulins in man and experimental animals (a minireview). *In* Humoral Immunity in Neurological Diseases. D. Karcher, A. Lowenthal & A. D. Strosberg, Eds. NATO Advanced Study Institutes Series (A-Life Sciences). Vol. 24: 517–522. Plenum Press. New York.

35. GERRITSEN, E., J. VOSSEN, M. VAN TOL, C. JOL-VAN DER ZIJDE, R. VAN DER WEIJDEN-RAGAS & J. RADL. 1989. Monoclonal Gammopathies in Children. J. Clin. Immunol. **9**: 296–305.

36. VOSSEN, J. M., R. A. HOLL, G. E. M. ASMA, R. LANGLOIS-VAN DEN BERGH, C. P. M. VAN DER WEIJDEN-RAGAS & J. RADL. 1986. Reconstitution of the B cell system following allogeneic BMT: an accelerated recapitulation of ontogenic development. *In* Primary Immunodeficiency Diseases. M. M. Eibl & F. S. Rosen, Eds. 309–314. Elsevier Sci. Publ. Amsterdam.

37. BENNER, R., TH. W. VAN DEN AKKER & J. RADL. 1985. Monoclonal gammapathies in immunodeficient animals—a review. *In* Monoclonal Gammapathies. II. Clinical Significance and Basic Mechanisms. J. Radl, W. Hijmans & B. van Camp, Eds. Topics in Aging Research in Europe. Vol. 5: 97–102. EURAGE. Rijswijk.

38. LIGTHART, G. J., J. RADL, J. X. CORBERAND, J. A. VAN NIEUWKOOP, G. J. VAN STAALDUINEN, D. J. WESSELMAN VAN HELMOND & W. HIJMANS. 1990. Monoclonal gammopathies in human aging: increased occurrence with age and correlation with health status. Mech. Ageing Dev. **52**: 235–243.

39. RADL, J., R. M. VALENTIJN, J. J. HAAIJMAN & L. C. PAUL. 1985. Monoclonal gammapathies in patients undergoing immunosuppressive treatment after renal transplantation. Clin. Immunol. Immunopathol. **37**: 98–102.

40. PEEST, D., B. SCHAPER, B. NASHAN, K. WONIGEIT, E. RAUDE, R. PICHLMAYR, A. HAVERICH & H. DEICHER. 1988. High incidence of monoclonal immunoglobulins in patients after liver or heart transplantation. Transplantation **46**: 389–393.

41. RADL, J. 1984. Differences among the three major categories of paraproteinaemias in aging man and the mouse. A minireview. Mech. Ageing Dev. **28**: 167–170.

42. RADL, J. 1985. Monoclonal gammapathies—an attempt at a new classification. Neth. J. Med. **28**: 134–137.

43. RADL, J. 1985. Four major categories of monoclonal gammapathies—introductory remarks. *In* Monoclonal Gammapathies. II. Clinical Significance and Basic mechanisms. J. Radl, W. Hijmans & B. van Camp, Eds. Topics in Aging Research in Europe. Vol. 5: 3–8. EURAGE. Rijswijk.

44. MELCHERS, F. 1984. Multiple steps in the transformation of normal B cells towards neoplasia. Curr. Top. Microbiol. Immunol. **113:** 56–61.
45. WALDENSTROM, J. G. 1990. Concluding remarks. *In* Monoclonal Gammapathies. II. Clinical Significance and Basic Mechanisms. J. Radl & B. van Camp, Eds. Topics in Aging Research in Europe. Vol. 12: 97–102. EURAGE. Rijswijk.
46. TAKIGUCHI, T., W. H. ADLER & R. T. SMITH. 1979. Strain specificity of monodisperse gamma-globulin appearance after immunization of inbred mice. Proc. Soc. Exp. Biol. Med. **145:** 868–873.
47. NOOIJ, F. J. M., A. J. VAN DER SLUIJS-GELLING, C. M. JOL-VAN DER ZIJDE, M. J. D. VAN TOL, H. HAAS & J. RADL. 1990. Immunoblotting techniques for the detection of low level homogeneous immunoglobulin components in serum. J. Immunol. Methods **134:** 273–281.

Aging, Longevity, and Cancer: Studies in Down's Syndrome and Centenarians[a]

CLAUDIO FRANCESCHI, DANIELA MONTI,
ANDREA COSSARIZZA, FRANCESCO FAGNONI,[b]
GIOVANNI PASSERI,[b] AND PAOLO SANSONI[b]

Department of Immunology
Institute of General Pathology
University of Modena School of Medicine
Via Campi, 287
41100 Modena, Italy

[b]Clinica Medica Generale e Terapia Medica
University of Parma School of Medicine
Via Gramsci, 14
43100 Parma, Italy

Despite the enormous amount of data available in the literature, physiological aging is still a poorly understood phenomenon. However, very little is known about environmental factors and genes which control aging. The problem is even more complicated if we consider longevity. Usually, hypotheses of aging do not account for longevity differences between species and between individuals within a species.[1]

Aging, Longevity and the Network of the Cellular Defense System

The theories proposed to explain the aging process may be schematically grouped in two main categories. The first suggests that aging is indirectly controlled by genes which have been selected for reproductive fitness before maturity. Such genes could exert pleiotropic undesirable effects later in life. Evidence favoring this hypothesis comes from studies in *Drosophila,* where selection for late fecundity increases life span.[2,3] Moreover, a gene responsible for high fecundity and reducing life span has been found in *Caenorhabditis elegans.*[4–6]

The second type of theory proposes that aging is the consequence of a stocastic process of deterioration caused by the accumulation of unavoidable errors in the synthesis and processing of macromolecules, *i.e.,* DNA, RNA and proteins.[7,8] Probably the most elaborate theories of this kind are the somatic mutation theory of aging and the error hypothesis of aging.[9,10]

At the DNA level, the aging process appears to be the result of a balance between mechanisms that tend to destabilize DNA information, and mechanisms that tend to maintain and preserve DNA integrity.[11]

[a] The authors gratefully acknowledge EURAGE, the Italian National Research Council, the Ministry of Education and Scientific Research, Sigma Tau, Sandoz Foundation for Gerontological Research, and Associazione Italiana per la Ricerca sul Cancro, which supported the research whose results are reported in this review.

Cells continuously exposed to exogenous and endogenous stressors such as heat, radiations, reducing sugars and oxygen free radicals, have developed a variety of defense and repair mechanisms, such as DNA repair mechanisms, antioxidant defense systems and production of stress proteins. These mechanisms are interconnected and constitute a network of integrated cellular defense systems that must be considered all together, and not one by one.[12]

In fact, when cells are exposed to a potential genotoxic agent such as oxygen free radicals (OFR), all the above-mentioned defense mechanisms are triggered.[12] The final result, *i.e.*, cell survival with or without heavy DNA damage or cell death, will depend on the coordinated capability of the network to cope with the attrition caused by the damaging agent.

Our hypothesis is that longevity determinant genes proposed by Cutler[1] are in fact the genes responsible for the above-mentioned network of defense mechanisms, and that the global level of efficiency of this network is genetically controlled. We assume that the efficiency of such genes has been evolutionarily set at different levels in different species, thus accounting for the different life span among them.[12–15] We also assume that interindividual differences in life span within a species depend on the different efficiency of the network.[13–15]

These considerations are particularly important to understand the role of the immune and the neuroendocrine systems in maintaining the homeostasis and the integrity of the body. These systems, which are profoundly interconnected and probably share a common evolutionary origin,[16] are composed of a variety of cells continuously exposed to damaging agents, and could be severely impaired if a derangement occurs in their repair and defense mechanisms.[12] In fact, immune alterations are present in classical syndromes characterized by DNA repair defects, such as *xeroderma pigmentosum*.[17]

We assume that the correct function of the network of defense mechanisms is essential for the performance of the immunoneuroendocrine system.

Age-related attrition of the network of defense mechanisms could alter the balance between DNA stability and instability, favoring the accumulation of mutations and rearrangements with time.[11] Disastrous consequences can be predicted if different cells of the same organ or lineage accumulate different types of DNA lesions, thus increasing cell heterogeneity and altering cell-cell interactions, which are particularly important in the immune and in the nervous systems.[8,11,15]

We also assume that the network of cellular defense mechanisms which counteract the aging process and favor longevity is fundamentally the same as that which offsets the development of cancer, as its main purpose is to maintain the integrity of genetic information in somatic cells and eliminate damaged or mutated cells.[12–15,17]

Down's Syndrome and Centenarians as Models for the Study of Aging, Longevity and Cancer in Humans

Several animal models and strategies are available to test these hypotheses, such as short and long living species and strains, caloric restriction and transgenic animals. However, the situation in humans is much more complicated, due to the extreme genetic heterogeneity and variability of our species and to confounding variables related to cultural attitudes and life style habits. Also, the effect of the strategies used to retard the aging process are very difficult to ascertain, because of human longevity.

Two conditions have been chosen by our laboratory as possible suitable candidates to analyze the aging process and longevity assuring determinants in humans, *i.e.,* Down's syndrome (DS) and centenarians.

Down's Syndrome

Down's syndrome is the most frequent chromosomal aberration in humans, characterized, in most cases, by an extra chromosome 21 (trisomy 21). In addition to mental retardation, DS patients have an increased cancer incidence,[17] and show signs of precocious aging of various organs and tissues.[18] According to some investigators, DS ranks first among human "segmental progeroid syndromes," defined as those genetic disorders in which multiple major aspects of the senescent phenotype appear.[19] The derangement of the immune system is thought to be responsible, at least in part, for the increased susceptibility to infectious diseases and the increased frequency of cancer; indeed, infections are still among the major causes of death in DS patients.[20]

In the last decade, our studies have focused on the precocious aging of the immune system in DS.[18,20–31] Recently obtained data on this topic which may be relevant for the understanding of the biochemical and molecular mechanisms involved in the precocious aging of DS will be reviewed.

It is likely that this data will help in understanding the processes involved in physiological aging.

TABLES 1 and 2 show that immune cells and their activity are profoundly deranged in DS subjects. Apart from a reduced number of $CD4^+$ T lymphocytes in DS children (743 ± 72 cells/mm³ vs 1,256 ± 141 in karyotypically normal controls, $p <0.02$), most of the immune parameters deteriorate with age. In particular, a marked increase of $CD8^+$, $CD16^+$ and $CD57^+$ cells is observed in older DS patients. In our laboratory, the normal values (mean ± s.e.) of these cells in 20 young healthy controls are 595 ± 33, 179 ± 31 and 327 ± 41, respectively. These subsets include most of the cytotoxic T lymphocytes ($CD8^+$) and NK cells ($CD16^+$ and $CD57^+$ cells). However, the non-MHC restricted cytotoxic capacity of DS lymphocytes is markedly reduced despite the high proportion of cells with NK markers. A similar phenomenon was observed by several groups, including our own, in physiological aging, even if the increase in cells bearing NK markers and the reduction of their activity with advancing age were less marked than in DS.

TABLE 1. Phenotypical Analysis of Peripheral Blood Lymphocytes (PBL) from Children and Adults Affected by Down's Syndrome[a]

mAb Anti-	Children	Adults
CD3	2,183 ± 149	2,502 ± 232
CD4	743 ± 72	705 ± 68
CD8	797 ± 64	1,126 ± 134
CD19	163 ± 24	142 ± 24
CD57	417 ± 46	1,139 ± 225
CD16	151 ± 24	286 ± 161

[a] Data are expressed as number of PBL/mm³ (mean ± s.e.) expressing the marker recognized by the indicated monoclonal antibody (mAb). Data refer to 28 children (mean age: 9.2 ± 0.3 years) and 9 adults (mean age: 44.2 ± 3.0 years). (Data are from Cossarizza *et al.*[27] and Cossarizza *et al.*[28])

TABLE 2. NK Activity in PBL from Children and Adults Affected by Down's Syndrome[a]

E/T Ratio[b]	Children	Adults
50:1	32 ± 4	28 ± 3
25:1	24 ± 3	18 ± 2

[a] Data are expressed as percentage of specific lysis of the human erythromyeloid target cell line K562 in a classical 4 hr ⁵¹Cr release test. Similar results were obtained with other E/T ratios. Data refer to 10 children (mean age: 9.2 ± 1.2 years) and 7 adults (mean age 43.9 ± 3.5 years). (Data are from Cossarizza et al.[28])

[b] E/T ratio: effector/target cell ratio.

Lymphocytes from DS subjects show a reduced capability to proliferate after mitogenic stimuli. This defect is very mild in children and quite evident in older subjects (TABLES 3 and 4). The same defect, present in lymphocytes from normal old subjects[23,32] could play a role in explaining the reduced efficiency of the immune system in aged people by limiting the clonal expansion of lymphocytes after antigenic challenge.

Recently, we demonstrated that exposure to low frequency pulsed electromagnetic fields (PEMFs) was able to increase the mitogen-induced proliferation of PBL from young and old subjects, but was much more evident in the latter.[33] Critical steps of cell proliferation such as the expression of interleukin-2 (IL-2) receptor and IL-2 utilization, were altered in cells from aged donors and appear to be modulated by PEMF-exposure.[34] The same pattern of responsiveness to PEMF-exposure was observed in DS subjects. Cells from relatively old patients (46–55 years old), whose responsiveness to PHA is dramatically decreased, responded to PEMF-exposure much more than cells from young patients (TABLE 3). Quantitatively, the response was similar to that of cells from karyotypically normal donors of much more advanced age.[33,34]

On the whole, these data suggest that the defect of cell proliferation in DS as well as in physiological aging is not irreversible, and can be modulated at least in part by physical and chemical interventions.[23,29] Moreover, the sensitivity to PEMFs can be considered a reliable biomarker of aging, being increased both in physiological aging and in syndromes of precocious aging.

DNA changes and accumulation of point mutations and rearrangements are most likely involved in the aging process.[8,11] OFR appear to play a crucial role as they are continuously produced during normal metabolism. An inverse relationship between OFR-induced DNA damage and life span has been observed in mammals.[35] Moreover, antioxidant systems have been proposed as one of the most important longevity determinant mechanisms.[1]

Besides the classical enzymatic and nonenzymatic antioxidant systems, it has been suggested that a nuclear enzyme, i.e., poly(ADP-ribosyl)polymerase (ADPRP), plays a crucial role in cells exposed to OFR and other genotoxic agents. The physiological role of ADPRP is poorly understood, even if several data indicate that it is perhaps involved in cell proliferation and differentiation, and in DNA repair.[12] ADPRP, once activated by single DNA strand breaks, utilizes NAD⁺ as substrate to add chains of poly(ADP-ribose) to several nuclear proteins. A great number of breaks may lead to a marked depletion in intracellular NAD⁺ pool and eventually to cell suicide.[12] The activity of ADPRP can be inhibited by several compounds such as benzamides and nicotinamide.[36,37] We have proposed that programmed cell death or apoptosis should be considered a sort of defense mechanism devoted to the elimination of heavily damaged and/or mutated cells, which can have an important role in the aging process.[12]

Accordingly, a decreased efficiency in the antioxidant defense mechanisms can be predicted in subjects with a shorter life span. These considerations are particularly pertinent for DS subjects, who show a shorter life span and several alterations in OFR production and processing, probably related to the presence of an extra copy of the Cu/Zn SOD gene in most cases.[18]

We tested this hypothesis by using an *in vitro* system which allows the exposure of human cells to graded doses of OFR produced by an enzymatic system which mimics pathophysiological situations.[36,37]

TABLE 3. Lymphocyte Proliferation and Sensitivity to Low Frequency Pulsed Electromagnetic Fields (PEMFs) in Children and Adults Affected by Down's Syndrome[a]

PHA Dose (µl/ml)	Children		Adults	
	− PEMFs	+ PEMFs	− PEMFs	+ PEMFs
0	100 (446 ± 87)	138 ± 19	100 (254 ± 53)	140 ± 24
0.1	100 (16,672 ± 1,658)	93 ± 6	100 (3,750 ± 1,025)	91 ± 3
1	100 (73,096 ± 6,225)	110 ± 5	100 (10,574 ± 2,864)	176 ± 34
5	100 (56,916 ± 4,938)	126 ± 9	100 (8,772 ± 1,672)	170 ± 10
10	100 (37,358 ± 4,226)	122 ± 9	100 (5,362 ± 1,139)	185 ± 22

[a] PBL were separated following standard methods, stimulated with different doses of phytohemagglutinin (PHA) and cultured for 72 hr. Data are expressed as percentage of ^{3}H-thymidine incorporation in PEMF-exposed cultures in comparison with control unexposed ones, taken as 100% at each PHA dose. Data in brackets represent the values of ^{3}H-thymidine incorporation in the control cultures (mean c.p.m. ± s.e.). Data refer to 21 children (mean age: 9.9 ± 1.2 years) and 4 adults (mean age: 50.3 ± 2.3 years). (Data are from Cossarizza *et al.*[29])

In this experimental system cells are exposed for one hour to OFR produced extracellularly by a classic enzymatic system (xanthine oxidase plus hypoxanthine), and then washed and stimulated with phytohemagglutinin. Under these conditions, the susceptibility of PBL from older patients with DS is consistently higher than that of cells from DS children[38] (TABLE 4). A similar age-related increase in sensitivity of OFR was observed in physiological aging.[39,40] In this case the phenomenon spans over 80–90 years, while in DS it is evident within 30–40 years, suggesting, once again, that DS cells behave like normal cells that are several decades older.

OFR-damaged cells can be rescued if an ADPRP inhibitor, such as 3-aminobenzamide (3-ABA), is present during the damaging period.[36,37] The protective effect of 3-ABA is less evident in cells from older DS patients, suggesting that the damage induced by OFR is partially different in cells from young and old DS patients. In both cases, ADPRP activation appears to play a role in mediating OFR damage, but its importance varies according to the donor's age.

TABLE 4. Sensitivity to Oxygen Free Radicals (OFR) of Lymphocytes from Children and Adults Affected by Down's Syndrome[a]

Treatment	Children	Adults
PHA	100	100
	(72,315 ± 7,484)	(24,280 ± 5,064)
PHA + HYP 25 μM	94.9 ± 11.5	41.8 ± 12.6
PHA + HYP 25 μM + 3 ABA	98.5 ± 6.4	75.6 ± 11.9
PHA + HYP 50 μM	50.4 ± 10.2	11.8 ± 2.4
PHA + HYP 50 μM + 3 ABA	107.1 ± 8.8	51.9 ± 11.0

[a] Data are expressed as percentage of ^{3}H-thymidine incorporation in cultures exposed to an OFR-producing system in comparison with control unexposed ones, taken as 100%. The OFR-producing system was composed by xanthine-oxidase (fixed dose, 0.5 I.U./ml) plus hypoxanthine (HYP, graded doses), in the presence or in the absence of the poly(ADP-ribosyl)polymerase inhibitor 3-aminobenzamide (3-ABA, 5 mM). Data in brackets represent the values of ^{3}H-thymidine incorporation in the control cultures (mean c.p.m. ± s.e.). Data refer to 15 children (mean age: 9.5 ± 1.0 years) and 4 adults (mean age: 51.7 ± 1.7 years). (Data are from Monti et al.[38])

We have evidence that in physiological aging as well, the protective effect of 3-ABA against OFR-induced damage is age-related.[39,40]

OFR are genotoxic, and a reduced ability to cope with their effects suggests that cells from DS patients may be more sensitive to other genotoxic substances, in an age-related manner. In order to test this prediction, lymphocytes from young and adult DS subjects were exposed to mitomycin-C (MMC), and its genotoxic effect was assessed by using a very sensitive cytogenetic technique, i.e., the induction of micronuclei (MN) by the cytokinesis block method.[31] A significant increase of MMC-induced MN frequency was observed in older DS patients, even if the spontaneous frequency of MN was similar in young and adult DS subjects (TABLE 5). We predict that this phenomenon, although not present in normal age-matched control subjects, will be evident in older subjects. An increased formation of MN in old subjects has been described using a less sensitive method.[41]

As far as the signs of precocious aging are concerned, we would like to stress that they appear at different ages and with varying intensity. In any case, most are absent in DS children, but appear in young adults and become dramatically evident in patients older than 40 years, as shown in TABLE 6.

TABLE 5. Spontaneous and Mitomycin-C-Induced Frequency of Micronuclei (MN) in Lymphocytes from Children and Adults Affected by Down's Syndrome[a]

% MN	Children	Adults
Spontaneous	0.64 ± 0.06	0.86 ± 0.10
MMC-Induced	2.45 ± 0.22	4.94 ± 0.55

[a] PHA-stimulated PBL were cultured for 44 hr in the absence or in the presence of mitomycin-C (MMC), then cytochalasin-B was added in order to block cytokinesis. After 28 hr cells were harvested and scored for the presence of micronuclei (MN). Data are expressed as percentage of binucleated cells showing the presence of at least one micronucleus (mean ± s.e.). Data refers to 3 children (mean age: 13 ± 1.7 years) and 4 adults (mean age: 44.7 ± 3.8 years). (Data are from Scarfí et al.[31])

TABLE 6. Age-Related Alterations of Immune Responses and Sensitivity to Genotoxic Agents in Patients Affected by Down's Syndrome

	Children	Adults	Ref.
Lymphocyte subsets:			
CD4 T lymphocytes	−	− −	27
CD8 T lymphocytes	+	+ + +	27
B lymphocytes	−	− −	27
NK cells	+	+ + +	28
NK activity	− −	− −	28
Lymphocyte proliferation	=/−	− −	21, 23
Sensitivity to PEMFs	=	+ + +	29
Sensitivity to OFR	=	+ + +	30
MMC-induced micronuclei	=	+ + +	31

This is also true for other phenotypic signs of precocious aging not studied by our group, such as cataract and the number of plaques and tangles in the brain, accompanied in most cases by the clinical signs of Alzheimer's type dementia.[42] The great majority of DS subjects over 35–40 years have the above-mentioned anatomopathological signs of brain dementia.

Centenarians

People older than 100 years represent a highly selected group, considering that 1 individual out of 7,000–10,000 will reach this extreme limit of human life. Centenarians apparently escaped from the major age-related diseases, including cancer, thus suggesting that their defense mechanisms against most of the threatening agents in the internal or in the external environment and uncontrolled cell proliferation are particularly efficient.

Surprisingly, the literature on centenarians is scanty, episodic and primarily devoted to clinical aspects. We think that much more attention should be paid instead to this selected group of human beings, who certainly have "something special" as far as their genetic makeup or their life-style is concerned.

As stated above, the prediction is that centenarians, considered as a group,

TABLE 7. Phenotypical Analysis of PBL from Centenarians and Healthy Adults[a]

mAB Anti-	Centenarians	Adults
Lymph./mm³	1,667 ± 301	2,182 ± 148
CD3	1,108 ± 204	1,570 ± 35
CD4	669 ± 180	1,008 ± 39
CD8	422 ± 26	595 ± 33
CD19	29 ± 5	215 ± 16
CD57	370 ± 91	327 ± 41
CD16	301 ± 51	179 ± 31
CD56	402 ± 115	316 ± 28

[a] Data are expressed as number of PBL/mm³ (mean ± s.e.) expressing the marker recognized by the indicated monoclonal antibody (mAb). Data refers to 6 centenarians and 20 healthy adults (mean age: 45 ± 3 years). (Data are from Cossarizza et al.[43])

TABLE 8. NK Activity in PBL from Centenarians and Young Adults[a]

E/T Ratio	Centenarians	Adults
50 : 1	43 ± 6	50 ± 6
25 : 1	32 ± 5	41 ± 5

[a] Data are expressed as percentage of specific lysis of the human target cell line K562 in a classical 4 hr ^{51}Cr release test. Similar results were obtained with other E/T ratios. Data refer to 12 centenarians and 9 young healthy adults (mean age: 25 ± 4 years). (Data are from Sansoni *et al.*[44])

should have a more efficient network of cellular defense mechanisms. Owing to the great importance of OFR in the aging process, we further hypothesized that the antioxidant defense mechanisms of centenarians should be set at a higher level or should decay more slowly than those of subjects not so far advanced in age.

Assuming that a well preserved immune system should help in reaching the limit of human life we studied several immune parameters in these subjects.

Accordingly, our group has started a research program with the aim of characterizing several biochemical and immune parameters of centenarians. Preliminary evidence suggests that some of the previously illustrated hypotheses may be correct, and that in any case centenarians differ from "normal aged people" in several responses and parameters.

Some relevant results are reported in TABLES 7–9. Centenarians and their controls were studied with the same methods used in the study of DS patients and their age-matched controls.

As far as the phenotypical analysis of PBL is concerned, centenarians show a decreased absolute number of lymphocytes, with a proportional reduction in CD3$^+$, CD4$^+$ and CD8$^+$ subsets, in contrast with DS, where a marked subversion of CD4/CD8 ratio is present, as a consequence of a dramatic increase of CD8$^+$ cells[43] (TABLE 7).

TABLE 9. Sensitivity to Oxygen Free Radicals (OFR) of PBL from Centenarians and Young Subjects[a]

Treatment	Days of Culture	Centenarians	Young Donors
PHA	4	78,651 ± 6,422	105,570 ± 15,313
PHA	6	38,884 ± 6,061	20,782 ± 4,054
PHA	7	28,450 ± 3,357	7,848 ± 1,632
PHA + HYP 25 μM	4	55,564 ± 7,228	76,529 ± 14,389
PHA + HYP 25 μM	6	48,371 ± 10,659	22,987 ± 6,833
PHA + HYP 25 μM	7	34,571 ± 7,606	8,954 ± 2,447
PHA + HYP 50 μM	4	35,328 ± 7,239	38,081 ± 8,855
PHA + HYP 50 μM	6	52,115 ± 8,910	39,345 ± 11,160
PHA + HYP 50 μM	7	36,425 ± 8,011	15,216 ± 4,442

[a] Values of ^{3}H-thymidine (^{3}H-TdR) incorporation are expressed in c.p.m., mean ± s.e. Lymphocytes were damaged for 1 hr by the OFR-producing system as described in note to TABLE 4, washed and stimulated with an optimal dose of PHA (1 μl/ml) and cultured for different days. Six hrs before the end of the culture, cells were pulsed with ^{3}H-TdR. Data refer to 17 centenarians and 12 young subjects (mean age: 26 ± 4 years). (Data are from Monti *et al.*[46])

B lymphocytes, *i.e.,* CD19$^+$ cells, are markedly decreased in centenarians. This result is difficult to interpret, considering that preliminary data suggest that several Ig classes and subclasses are augmented in the serum. Further investigations are needed to clarify possible alterations in B cell differentiation and compartmentalization in far advanced age.

Markers present on NK cells, such as CD16, CD56 and CD57 suggest that this peripheral blood mononuclear cell subset is highly expanded in centenarians, particularly the CD16$^+$ cells, which in humans have the strongest natural cytotoxic activity. A trend towards an age-related increase in NK cells has been observed by several groups, including our own, although controversial data have been reported.[28] The functional activity of NK cells appears to be well preserved in centenarians[44] (TABLE 8). However, alterations in NK activity at a single cell level cannot be excluded.

The ability of lymphocytes from old people to repair DNA damage is markedly reduced.[45] However, an increased resistance to DNA damage could be predicted in centenarians. Accordingly, it was interesting to test the sensitivity of lymphocytes from centenarians to genotoxic agents.

The sensitivity of PBL from centenarians to OFR in comparison with young donors is reported in TABLE 9.[46] The ability to proliferate after PHA-stimulation is well preserved in centenarians, and the kinetics of the phenomenon are quite different from those observed in young control; the thymidine uptake on the sixth and seventh days of culture remained quite consistent in comparison to the marked drop observed in young subjects. Centenarian PBL appear quite resistant to the oxidative stress that apparently retards entrance into the cell cycle rather than causing irreversible cell damage. The reverse seems to be true for cells from young donors, where the oxidative stress apparently caused an unrescued damage rather than a delay in cell cycling.

Possible Strategies to Retard the Aging Process

Preliminary evidence suggests that it is possible to protect cells from oxidative stress by using natural substances such as carnitine. The rationale to use carnitine as an antiaging substance is that cells from old donors as well as cells from persons with syndromes of precocious aging, such as DS, have decreased levels of ATP. Moreover, one of the most crucial factors deterring the survival of cells exposed to genotoxic agents is the energy crisis due to the marked decrease in the endogenous pools of NAD$^+$ and ATP.[12] Carnitine could increase the energy charge of the cells thus rendering them less prone to cell death. Moreover, we demonstrated that carnitines were able to increase mitogen-induced proliferation of human lymphocytes, and this effect was more evident in cells from old donors.[47] To test this hypothesis, lymphocytes were preincubated with L-carnitine for 48 hr and then exposed to the above described OFR-producing system. The results shown in TABLE 10 indicate that a consistent degree of protection is evident, particularly when lymphocytes from old subjects are exposed to oxidative stress of medium intensity.[48]

CONCLUSIONS

The results obtained in the two models we have proposed to study aging and longevity suggest that:

a) Down's syndrome appears to be a reliable model to study several aspects of the aging process, and to test the role and importance of some pathogenetic mechanisms. In particular, it is evident that most DS patients show phenotypical signs of aging several decades in advance.

The appearance of age-related immune derangements follows accelerated kinetics even if these derangements may differ quantitatively from those found in physiological aging. The alterations in cells bearing NK markers and the decreased proliferative capability of T lymphocytes may be taken as examples;

TABLE 10. Effect of L-Carnitine (LC) Preloading (48 Hrs) on the Proliferation of PBL from Old and Young Subjects Damaged with OFR

Subject (Age, Sex)[a]	L-Carnitine Pretreatment (5 mM)	Xanthine Oxidase (0.5 U/ml)	Hypoxanthine (μM)				
			5	10	25	50	100
n. 1 (81, F)	−	+	−	95[b]	3	−	0.2
	+	+	−	101	98	−	0.8
n. 2 (70, M)	−	+	−	4	6	2	0.2
	+	+	−	57	2	0.1	0.1
n. 3 (81, M)	−	+	51	56	7	2	1
	+	+	95	65	21	3	0.4
n. 4 (22, M)	−	+	102	105	96	76	7
	+	+	111	114	102	26	3
n. 5 (23, F)	−	+	104	105	91	6	0.1
	+	+	113	113	42	5	0.3
n. 6 (22, M)	−	+	111	113	0.5	0.2	0.2
	+	+	122	70	0.6	0.3	0.2

[a] Age in years; M = male, F = female.
[b] Data refer to ³H-TdR incorporation and are expressed as percentage of control cultures:

subject 1: without LC = 74,443 ± 7,240; with LC = 65,244 ± 2,135
"   2   "   = 50,904 ± 2,601;   "   = 59,043 ± 3,348
"   3   "   = 68,979 ± 3,170;   "   = 67,639 ± 2,920
"   4   "   = 45,646 ± 1,416;   "   = 42,532 ± 1,974
"   5   "   = 130,149 ± 4,458;   "   = 137,881 ± 7,400
"   6   "   = 85,912 ± 2,573;   "   = 87,766 ± 1,730

(Data are from Franceschi *et al.*[48])

b) precocious aging and longevity are both characterized by modifications in the immune status. The most important changes seem to be the decrease in CD4$^+$ T lymphocytes, the decrease in circulating B lymphocytes (CD19$^+$) and the increase in cells with NK markers. However, NK activity follows opposite patterns, being dramatically decreased in DS but well preserved in centenarians. Thus, a good NK activity appears to be correlated with a long life span, and inversely correlated with a short life span, thus suggesting that it is a relevant biological function. We advance that such activity is a possible biomarker of longevity;

c) similar considerations apply to the capacity of cells to cope with oxidative stress. In this case as well, DS patients and centenarians behave in an opposite way. DS cells show an increased sensitivity to OFR that increases with age, and is similar to that of normal subjects 30–40 years older. Cells from centenarians appear to have a great capacity to survive and proliferate after OFR-exposure.

We do not know the reasons for this increased resistance to oxidants, and it will be interesting to investigate this problem thoroughly in order to identify the responsible mechanisms and biochemical pathways.

The preliminary data illustrated above suggest that the PBL sensitivity to oxidative stress is a biomarker of aging and longevity. Further studies in a larger number of cases and in a broader spectrum of physiological and pathological conditions are needed to verify this hypothesis;

d) an increased sensitivity to genotoxic agents such as mitomycin-C and OFR appears to be a characteristic of cells from old donors or from patients affected by syndromes of precocious aging, such as DS. This fact would fit the hypothesis that an age-related deterioration in the antiaging network of cellular defense mechanisms occurs during life;

e) one of the main age-related defects, *i.e.*, a loss of proliferative vigor, is not irreversible, since a variety of agents can modulate and restore this function, at least in part. We presented evidence that exposure to nonionizing radiations can be used to improve the proliferative performance of cells from both DS patients and normal aged donors;

f) natural substances such as carnitine and nicotinamide are possible candidates as antiaging compounds, owing to their ability to rescue cells from the damage caused by oxidative stress.

REFERENCES

1. CUTLER, R. G. 1984. Evolutionary biology of aging and longevity in mammalian species. *In* Aging and Cell Function. J. E. Johnson, Jr., Ed. 1–147. Plenum Press. New York.
2. ROSE, M. & B. CHARLESWORTH. 1980. A test of evolutionary theories of senescence. Nature **287:** 141–142.
3. ROSE, M. R. & J. L. GRAVES, JR. 1989. What evolutionary biology can do for gerontology. J. Gerontol. **44:** B27–B29.
4. FRIEDMAN, D. B. & T. E. JOHNSON. 1988. A mutation in the *age-1* gene in *Caenorhabditis elegans* lengthens life and reduces hermaphrodite fertility. Genetics **118:** 75–86.
5. FRIEDMAN, D. B. & T. E. JOHNSON. 1988. Three mutants that extend both mean and maximum life span of the nematode *Caenorhabditis elegans* define the *age-1* gene. J. Gerontol. **43:** B102–109.
6. JOHNSON, T. E. 1988. Genetic specification of life span: processes, problems and potentials. J. Gerontol. **43:** B87–92.
7. KIRKWOOD, T. B. L. 1989. DNA, mutations and aging. Mutat. Res. **219:** 1–7.
8. VIJG, J. 1990. DNA sequence changes in aging: how frequent, how important? Aging **2:** 105–123.
9. BURNET, F. M. 1974. Intrinsic Mutagenesis: a Genetic Approach to Aging. J. Wiley and Sons. New York.
10. ORGEL, L. 1973. Ageing of clones of mammalian cells. Nature **243:** 441–445.
11. FRANCESCHI, C. 1990. Genomic instability: a challenge for aging research. Aging **2:** 101–104.
12. FRANCESCHI, C. 1989. Cell proliferation, cell death and aging. Aging **1:** 3–15.
13. FRANCESCHI, C., D. MONTI & A. COSSARIZZA. 1989. Biologia molecolare dell'invecchiamento e neoplasie. Nuovi argomenti di Medicina **5:** 522–529.
14. FRANCESCHI, C., D. MONTI, L. TROIANO, F. TROPEA & A. COSSARIZZA. 1990. Aging and cellular defense mechanisms. *In* Stress and the Aging Brain. G. Nappi *et al.,* Eds. 185–192. Raven Press. New York.
15. FRANCESCHI, C. & D. MONTI. 1990. Il controllo genetico dell'invecchiamento e della longevità: peculiarità e paradossi. Giorn. Geront. **38:** 127–134.

16. OTTAVIANI, E., F. PETRAGLIA, G. MONTAGNANI, A. COSSARIZZA, D. MONTI & C. FRANCESCHI. 1990. Presence of ACTH and beta-endorphin immunoreactive molecules in the freshwater snail *Planorbarius corneus* (L.) (Gastropoda, Pulmonata) and their possible role in phagocytosis. Regul. Pept. **27:** 1–9.

17. FRANCESCHI, C. & M. CHIRICOLO. 1987. DNA repair, aging and cancer in immunodeficient subjects. Giorn. Ital. Chirurgia Dermatol. Oncol. **2:** 325–331.

18. FRANCESCHI, C., F. LICASTRO, M. CHIRICOLO, M. ZANNOTTI & M. MASI. 1986. Premature senility in Down's syndrome: a model for and an approach to the molecular genetics of the ageing process. *In* Immunoregulation in Aging. A. Facchini, J. J. Haaijman & G. Labò, Eds. 77–83. EURAGE. Rijswijk, The Netherlands.

19. MARTIN, G. M. 1978. Genetic syndromes in man with potential relevance to the pathobiology of aging. *In* Genetic Effects on Aging. D. Bergsma & D. E. Harrison, Eds. The National Foundation March of Dimes, Birth Defects. Vol. 14: 5–39. Alan R. Liss, Inc. London.

20. FRANCESCHI, C., M. CHIRICOLO, F. LICASTRO, M. ZANNOTTI, M. MASI, E. MOCCHEGIANI & N. FABRIS. 1988. Oral zinc supplementation in Down's syndrome. Restoration of thymic endocrine activity and of some immune defects. J. Ment. Defic. Res. **32:** 169–181.

21. FRANCESCHI, C., F. LICASTRO, P. PAOLUCCI, M. MASI, S. CAVICCHI & M. ZANNOTTI. T and B lymphocyte subpopulations in Down's syndrome. Study on not-institutionalized subjects. J. Ment. Defic. Res. **22:** 179–181.

22. FRANCESCHI, C., F. LICASTRO, M. CHIRICOLO, F. BONETTI, M. ZANNOTTI, N. FABRIS, E. MOCCHEGIANI, M. P. FANTINI, P. PAOLUCCI & M. MASI. 1981. Deficiency of autologous mixed lymphocyte reactions and serum thymic factor level in Down's syndrome. J. Immunol. **126:** 2161–2164.

23. LICASTRO, F., M. CHIRICOLO, P. L. TABACCHI, F. BARBONI, M. ZANNOTTI & C. FRANCESCHI. 1983. Enhancing effect of lithium and potassium ions on lectin-induced lymphocyte proliferation in aging and Down's syndrome subjects. Cell. Immunol. **75:** 111–121.

24. CHIRICOLO, M., L. MINELLI, F. LICASTRO, P. L. TABACCHI, M. ZANNOTTI & C. FRANCESCHI. 1984. Alteration of the capping phenomenon on lymphocytes from aged and Down's syndrome subjects. Gerontology **30:** 145–152.

25. FABRIS, N., E. MOCCHEGIANI, L. AMADIO, M. ZANNOTTI, F. LICASTRO & C. FRANCESCHI. 1984. Thymic hormone deficiency in normal ageing and Down's syndrome: is there a primary failure of the thymus? Lancet. **i:** 983–986.

26. COSSARIZZA, A., D. MONTI, G. MONTAGNANI, F. DAGNA-BRICARELLI, A. FORABOSCO & C. FRANCESCHI. 1989. Fetal thymic differentiation in Down's syndrome. Thymus **14:** 163–170.

27. COSSARIZZA, A., D. MONTI, G. MONTAGNANI, C. ORTOLANI, M. MASI, M. ZANNOTTI & C. FRANCESCHI. 1990. Precocious aging of the immune system in Down's syndrome: alterations of B-lymphocytes, T-lymphocyte subsets and of cells with NK markers in DS children. Am. J. Med. Genet. 7(Suppl.): 213–218.

28. COSSARIZZA, A., C. ORTOLANI, E. FORTI, G. MONTAGNANI, R. PAGANELLI, M. ZANNOTTI, M. MARINI, D. MONTI & C. FRANCESCHI. 1991. Age-related expansion of functionally inefficient cells with markers of NK activity in Down's syndrome. Blood **77:** 1263–1270.

29. COSSARIZZA, A., D. MONTI, F. BERSANI, M. R. SCARFÍ, M. ZANNOTTI, R. CADOSSI & C. FRANCESCHI. 1991. Lymphocyte sensitivity to low frequency pulsed electromagnetic field as a biomarker of precocious aging in Down's syndrome. Aging. In press.

30. FRANCESCHI, C., D. MONTI, A. COSSARIZZA, A. TOMASI, P. SOLA & M. ZANNOTTI. 1990. Oxidative stress, poly(ADP-ribosyl)ation and aging: *in vitro* studies on lymphocytes from normal and Down's syndrome subjects of different age and from patients with Alzheimer's dementia. *In* Antioxidants in Therapy and Preventive Medicine. I. Emerit, L. Packer & C. Auclair, Eds. 499–502. Plenum Press. New York.

31. SCARFÍ, M. R., A. COSSARIZZA, D. MONTI, F. BERSANI, M. ZANNOTTI, M. B. LIOI & C. FRANCESCHI. 1990. Age-related increase of mitomycin-C-induced micronuclei in lymphocytes from Down's syndrome subjects. Mutat. Res. **237:** 217–222.

32. LICASTRO, F., M. CHIRICOLO, P. L. TABACCHI, R. PARENTE, M. CENCI, F. BARBONI

& C. FRANCESCHI. 1983. Defective self-recognition in subjects of far advanced age. Gerontology **29:** 64–72.

33. COSSARIZZA, A., D. MONTI, F. BERSANI, M. CANTINI, R. CADOSSI, A. SACCHI & C. FRANCESCHI. 1989. Extremely low frequency pulsed electromagnetic fields increase cell proliferation in lymphocytes from young and aged subjects. Biochem. Biophys. Res. Commun. **160:** 692–699.

34. COSSARIZZA, A., D. MONTI, M. CANTINI, R. PAGANELLI, G. MONTAGNANI, R. CADOSSI, F. BERSANI & C. FRANCESCHI. 1989. Extremely low frequency pulsed electromagnetic fields increase interleukin-2 (IL-2) utilization and IL-2 receptor expression in lymphocytes from aged subjects. FEBS Lett. **248:** 141–144.

35. ADELMAN, R., R. L. SAUL & B. N. AMES. 1988. Oxidative damage to DNA: relation to species metabolic rate and life span. Proc. Natl. Acad. Sci. USA **85:** 2706–2708.

36. FRANCESCHI, C., M. MARINI, G. ZUNICA, D. MONTI, A. COSSARIZZA, A. BOLOGNI, C. GATTI & M. A. BRUNELLI. 1988. Effect of ADP-ribosyl transferase inhibitors on the survival of human lymphocytes after exposure to different DNA-damaging agents. Ann. N.Y. Acad. Sci. **551:** 446–447.

37. MARINI, M., G. ZUNICA, M. TAMBA, A. COSSARIZZA, D. MONTI & C. FRANCESCHI. 1990. Recovery of human lymphocytes damaged with gamma radiation or enzymatically-produced oxygen radicals: different effects of poly(ADP-ribosyl) transferase inhibitors. Int. J. Radiat. Biol. **58:** 279–291.

38. MONTI, D., P. SOLA, A. COSSARIZZA, M. ZANNOTTI, M. MARINI, P. FAGLIONI, F. TROPEA, D. TROIANO & C. FRANCESCHI. 1990. Age-related increased sensitivity to oxygen free radicals in Down's syndrome. Submitted for publication.

39. MONTI, D., A. COSSARIZZA, L. TROIANO, A. TOMASI, G. SARTOR, V. COMASCHI, G. FARRUGGIA, L. MASOTTI & C. FRANCESCHI. 1990. Oxygen free radicals and cellular ageing. I. DNA damage in lymphocytes from young and old subjects. *In* Protein Metabolism in Aging. 381–386. Alan R. Liss, Inc. New York.

40. MONTI, D., A. COSSARIZZA, M. MARINI, P. FAGLIONI, P. SOLA, F. TROPEA, D. TROIANO, D. BAROZZI & C. FRANCESCHI. 1990. Age-related increased sensitivity to oxygen free radicals in human healthy subjects. Submitted for publication.

41. FENECH, M. & A. A. MORLEY. 1985. Effect of donor age on spontaneous and induced micronuclei. Mutat. Res. **148:** 99–105.

42. WISNIEWSKI, K. E., H. M. WISNIEWSKI & G. Y. WEN. 1985. Occurrence of neuropathological changes and dementia of Alzheimer's disease in Down's syndrome. Ann. Neurol. **17:** 278–282.

43. COSSARIZZA, A., C. ORTOLANI, D. MONTI, G. PASSERI, P. SANSONI, M. PASSERI, S. MARCATO & C. FRANCESCHI. 1990. Peryphel blood lymphocyte subsets in centenarians. In preparation.

44. SANSONI, P., G. PASSERI, F. FAGNONI, S. MARCATO, D. MONTI, A. COSSARIZZA, C. FRANCESCHI & M. PASSERI. 1990. NK subsets and activity in centenarians. Submitted for publication.

45. LICASTRO, F., C. FRANCESCHI, M. CHIRICOLO, M. G. BATTELLI, P. TABACCHI, M. CENCI, F. BARBONI & D. PALLENZONA. 1982. DNA repair after gamma radiation and superoxide dismutase activity in lymphocytes from subjects with far advanced age. Carcinogenesis **3:** 45–48.

46. MONTI, D., D. BAROZZI, P. BUTTAFOCO, M. C. PELLONI, F. TROPEA, L. TROIANO, A. COSSARIZZA, P. SANSONI, G. PASSERI, F. FAGNONI, M. PASSERI & C. FRANCESCHI. 1990. Highly preserved ability to cope with oxidative stress in cells from centenarians. In preparation.

47. MONTI, D., A. COSSARIZZA, L. TROIANO, E. ARRIGONI-MARTELLI & C. FRANCESCHI. 1989. Immunomodulatory properties of L-acetylcarnitine on lymphocytes from young and old humans. *In* Stress, Immunity and Aging. A Role for L-Acetylcarnitine. C. De Simone & E. Arrigoni-Martelli, Eds. 83–96. Elsevier. Amsterdam, The Netherlands.

48. FRANCESCHI, C., A. COSSARIZZA, L. TROIANO & D. MONTI. 1990. Immunological parameters in aging. Studies on natural immunomodulatory and immunoprotective substances. Int. J. Clin. Pharmacol. Res. **10:** 53–57.

Concluding Remarks

Two Dozen Current Problems in Neuroimmunomodulation, Aging, and Cancer Research; the Second Stromboli Cocktail; Further Rambunctious Remarks

NOVERA HERBERT SPECTOR

Division of Fundamental Neurosciences
National Institutes of Health
Federal Building, Room 916
Bethesda, Maryland 20892

Under the ever-watchful eye of Mother Stromboli* was gathered a small band of intrepid scientists, scratching at the Gates of Immortality. Many silver bullets (the Second Stromboli Cocktail!) were fired at the locks. But the Gates remained firmly closed, while the ever-rumbling volcano seemed to be paraphrasing the words of the ancient Persian poet:

> What, without knowing, hither hurried
> hence?
> and, without adequate controls, quickly hurried
> whence?
> Another and another cup to drown
> the memory of this
> impertinence!

Almost unbelievably, thanks to the combined genius of Walter Pierpaoli and Nicola Fabris, this Second Stromboli Conference has exceeded the First Stromboli Conference on Aging and Cancer in depth and quality of science and in good fellowship. Dr. Bianca Marchetti described this assemblage of scientists as "challenging." This is an apt description. We could add as well that this group was merciless in discussion, but always friendly.

To open not the gates of immortality but, more modestly, a continuing discussion, I pose two dozen questions, which I hope contributors and readers alike will try to answer, using ever-better experimental tools, freshly inspired from having drunk from the fountains of knowledge and, especially, having in hand the formula for the Second Stromboli Cocktail.

Some of these problems were posed at this conference, while others were implied. Despite this volcanic assemblage of some of the best minds in modern science, most of the key questions that were addressed still are not answered. Three years hence, at the Third Stromboli Conference, after we have tackled these dilemmas in our laboratories, some answers will be newly evident . . . and, of course, still newer problems will need to be solved.

Meanwhile, with the exponential explosion of new experimental data confirming and detailing the continuous interactions among the nervous, endocrine and

---

* Stromboli is one of the most active volcanoes in the world.

immune systems (neuroimmunomodulation, NIM), we shall witness a revolution in the practice of the healing arts. Not only will there be a reduction in the use of harmful drugs now used to treat cancer and old age but, even more importantly, the practice of *preventive* medicine will be greatly enhanced and broadened.

Stromboli Cocktails

In summarizing the proceedings of the First Stromboli Conference,[1] I remarked:

> As at any good scientific gathering we come away with at least a half a dozen new cures for cancer, but what is even more amazing is at least a half a dozen new elixirs of youth. Most of us will rush home and immediately make a cocktail consisting of all of the ingredients shown in TABLE 1, and then we'll all live long enough to have at least ten more—maybe thirty more reunions on this wonderful volcano. [See TABLE 1.]

At the 1990 conference, many new ingredients were proposed, either to reverse cancer, or to postpone old age, or even in a few cases, to do both. Thus we must revise the cocktail, and try to incorporate all these wonderful substances into a complex miracle molecule (FIG. 1).

TABLE 1. R_x: [The First] Stromboli (i.v.) Cocktail[a] (1987)

Volcanic Ash
Thymus (whole)
Thymus (dessicated, from calf)
Thymus (all fractions)
Haloperidol
Superoxide Dismutase
Selected Catalases
Activated Charcoal
Epsom Salts
Butterfly Wings
Milk of Magnesia
Beta-Carotene
Vitamin A
Melatonin
Arginine
Thioproline
PCPA
Vitamin E
Enkephalins
Zinc
Selenium
DHEA
Estrogens
Prolactin
Growth Hormone
3,4-Dimethyl Pyridine
Levamysol

[a] To be taken with social support, exercise, sex, and electrical stimulation of the hypothalamus.

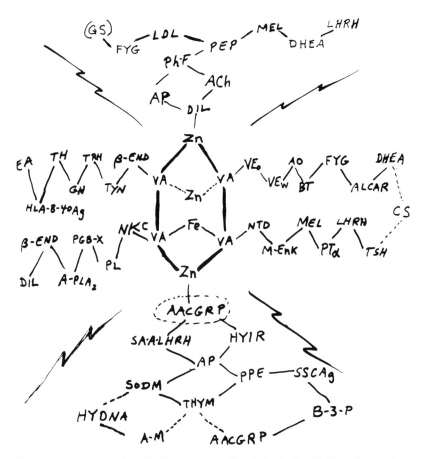

FIGURE 1. R_x: Stromboli Cocktail #2 (1990). 10% solution in fine Sicilian wine (or Stromboli rain water) p.o.—10 cc/kg wet body wt., as needed for relief of signs or symptoms of aging and/or cancer. Key to the molecular structure: AACGRP = anti-calcitonin-gene-related-peptide (hypothetical); ACH = acetylcholine; ALCAR = acetyl-l-carnitine; AO = all other antoxidants; AP = assorted other peptides; A-PLA$_2$ = anti-PLA$_2$; β-End = beta-endorphin; BT = bretylium tosylate; CS = chronic starvation; DHEA = dihydroepiandrosterone; DIL = Dilantin; Dil'man; EA = ethanolamine; Fe = iron; FYG = fresh young genes; GH = growth hormone; (GS) = gene stabilizers (hypothetical-?); HLA-B40-Ag = HLA-B-40-Ag; HYDNA = healthy young DNA; HYIR = healthy young insulin receptors; LDL = low density lipids and lipoproteins; LHRH = luteinizing hormone-releasing factor; Mel = melatonin; M-Enk = metenkephalin; NKC = natural killer cells; NTD = nootropic drugs; PEP = polypeptide extract of pineal; PGB-X = PGB-X; PhF = phenformin; PL = assorted phospholipids; PPE = polypeptide pineal extract; PT = pro-thymosin alpha; SA-A-LHRH = superactive analogs of LHRH; TH = T$_3$, T$_4$; TRH = thyrotropin-releasing hormone; TSH = thyroid-stimulating hormone; TYN = thymulin; VA = volcanic ash; VA = more volcanic ash; VE$_o$ = vit. E, lipid-soluble; VE$_w$ = vit. E, aqueous; Zn = zinc; Zn = more zinc. *Note:* 42 ingredients: at least a dozen more than in Stromboli Cocktail #1 (1987) (see TABLE 1).

Two Dozen Problems

Two dozen problems raised or implied by this conference are:

1. Is there an evolutionary survival value to individual death?
2. Why do different species have different "maximum" life spans?
3. How immutable are these maxima?
4. Why do some cells in multicellular animals seem to be immortal, while others age?
5. How many viable stem cells remain in the aging brain?
6. Under what conditions can neurons proliferate?
7. Is there a master aging clock, and if so does it reside in the hypothalamus, the *epiphysis* (the pineal), the *hypophysis* (the pituitary), the heart, the bone marrow, or the genes?
8. By tinkering with this clock, can we get the gears to move more smoothly, and can we reset the clock to make it last longer?
9. Can we improve immune functions in the aging individual without increasing the risk of autoimmune diseases?
10. Is there a link between cancers and other diseases of old age?
11. What common mechanisms do different types of cancer share?
12. What common features are shared by lymphocytes, macrophage, glial cells, neurons, hepatocytes, and cardiac cells?
13. In the feedback loops between the nervous and immune systems, how many are open, and which ones are closed? Are there any positive feedback loops which are not fatal?
14. (a) What afferent messages are transmitted to the central nervous system (CNS) by means of hard-wired (neuronal) fibers?
    (b) Are these of equal importance with chemical messengers in the circulation? Such messages, by means of nerve fibers, would have the advantage of much greater speed of transmission, and would not be subject to impedance by the blood-brain barrier.
    (c) How are various forms of energy transduced into nerve membrane depolarization, and how are these messages decoded in the CNS?
15. What do the afferent terminals look like?
16. How do ultradian, circadian, menstrual, lunar, and other chronobiological factors coalesce into the lifetime rhythm? How do their alterations affect life span?
17. What are the links among the pineal, superchiasmatic nucleus and immune functions?
18. What common features are shared in the transduction of signals across all cellular and intercellular membranes?
19. See FIGURE 2.
20. Would it be reasonable to simplify our nomenclature, to make our thinking about biological problems easier? For example, could we stop using the horrible word "stress?" This word means all things to all people, and is used to mean "distress," "eustress," "stimulus," and often even "*strain*," in which case the *stimulus is totally confused with the response*. Also, could we clarify such terms as lymphokine, monokine, neuromodulator, immunomodulator, and so on? Does the word cytokine encompass all of these? What about aging *versus* senescence?
21. Does senescence begin with conception? When does aging begin?

22. To what degree and by what mechanisms does the macroenvironment influence the microenvironment, and *vice versa*?
23. Will we ever have a single equation which quantitatively describes all of the factors and their interactions, in the twin cascades of anabolism and catabolism, from conception to death (a sort of biological "unified field theory")?
24. If, by pharmacologic, genetic, or other manipulation, we can get a lab mouse to live 4 years, have we raised the pre-set life-span maximum? How does this affect the potential life span of a mouse in the wild? How does this affect the practical or potential maximum life span of a human in today's quasi-civilized society?
25. Two of our conferees have spoken of a "death hormone." Is there a death gene or a set of death genes? If we were to eliminate or to alter this gene (or genes) how would this alter the biological balance of the individual? Of society?
26. Can the biological problems of aging and cancer be solved while we live in an increasingly maddened society, threatened with overpopulation, biologic and "nuclear" warfare, and thus the imminent extinction of our species? In other words, is there a link between molecular biology and sociobiology?

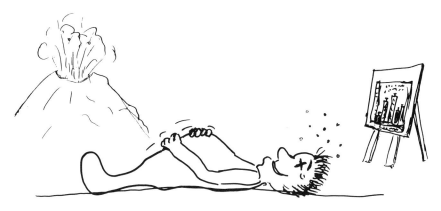

FIGURE 2. Are the organizers of this conference trying to shorten our life spans by caloric overload?

NOTES OF APPRECIATION

I have already expressed our gratitude to the generals, Pierpaoli and Fabris, for the organization of this remarkable conference. Too often, however, the colonels, the captains and the foot soldiers, without whom such conferences are impossible, are ignored. Thus I want to relate the appreciation of all conferees to Anna Fabris and Massimo Bazzano who worked tirelessly before, during, and after the meeting to make it a complete success.

I take this opportunity also to express the profound appreciation of all the editors of and contributors to this and previous volumes of these *Annals* to the wonderful, highly competent, very professional, and personally delightful editors and staff of the New York Academy of Sciences.

REFERENCE

1. SPECTOR, N. H. 1988. Rambunctious remarks and a look to the future. *In* Neuroimmunomodulation: Interventions in Aging and Cancer. W. Pierpaoli & N. H. Spector, Eds. Annals of the New York Academy of Sciences. Vol. 521: 323–335. New York Academy of Sciences. New York.

Subject Index

447

Index of Contributors